**This book is to be returned on or before
the last date stamped below.**

27 OCT 1982

18 NOV 1991

Huvos

BONE TUMORS
Diagnosis, Treatment and Prognosis

ANDREW G. HUVOS, M.D.

Attending Pathologist,
Memorial Sloan-Kettering Cancer Center;
Associate Professor of Pathology,
Cornell University Medical College, New York, N.Y.

W. B. SAUNDERS COMPANY
Philadelphia / London / Toronto

W. B. Saunders Company: West Washington Square
Philadelphia, PA   19105

1 St. Anne's Road
Eastbourne, East Sussex BN21 3UN, England

1 Goldthorne Avenue
Toronto, Ontario M8Z 5T9, Canada

Bone Tumors   ISBN   0-7216-4862-2

Last digit is the print number: 9   8   7   6   5   4   3

PREFACE

"Few books today are forgivable," says R. D. Laing, and this one may not be an exception. It is written about a relatively obscure but important subject in which a few are interested and even fewer care to master.

This book is intended to be authoritative but not authoritarian, balanced and lucid, reflecting my inherently conservative philosophy influenced by the teachings and long-term association with Dr. Henry L. Jaffe, who stimulated my interest in the diseases of bone. This interest was fostered by many former and present colleagues at Memorial Hospital for Cancer and Allied Diseases who pioneered the diagnosis and treatment of bone tumors not only as a science but also as an art. Among these, Dr. Ralph C. Marcove should be especially mentioned for his infectious enthusiasm and many original ideas.

I should like to acknowledge the cooperation of several people in the writing of this book. Dr. Norman L. Higinbotham gave me ready access to his files, a treasure-trove of clinical and pathological information, which were of great help to me. Particular appreciation is due to the many members of the Medical Illustration Department at Memorial Hospital for Cancer and Allied Diseases for the preparation of illustrative material and reproduction of the many radiographs. Miss Lynn B. McDowell, M.A., deserves special thanks for designing the innovative skeletons and age and sex distribution prototypes and for making me aware of the importance of good visuals. Mr. George C. Vilk, Associate Medical Editor, and the staff at W. B. Saunders Company were most helpful during the production of this book.

My wife, Phyllis, patiently typed and meticulously prepared the entire manuscript from the very beginning to the end, in addition to offering innumerable helpful suggestions for improving it. Without her help and untiring efforts this book would never have been completed. My gratitude to her cannot be totally expressed.

ANDREW G. HUVOS

CONTENTS

CARTILAGE-FORMING TUMORS – BENIGN
Chapters 10, 11 and 12

CARTILAGE-FORMING TUMORS – MALIGNANT
Chapters 13 and 14

TUMORS OF FIBROUS CONNECTIVE TISSUE ORIGIN
Chapters 15 and 16

TUMORS OF HISTIOCYTIC OR FIBROHISTIOCYTIC ORIGIN
Chapters 17 through 20

TUMORS AND TUMOR-LIKE LESIONS OF BLOOD VESSELS ARISING IN THE SKELETAL SYSTEM
Chapters 22 and 23

Bone-forming Tumors — Benign
Chapters 1 through 4

1

OSTEOMA AND GARDNER'S SYNDROME

OSTEOMA

DEFINITION

Osteomas are benign bone lesions characterized by bony excrescences usually arising in membranous bones.

They are benign lesions in which a major component is mature, lamellar, or woven bone. They are well-circumscribed and localized and appear to be sessile or pedunculated with expansile, not infiltrative, borders. Smooth or lobulated surfaces and peripheral resorption of normal bone are demonstrated by these lesions.

SYNONYMS

The extensive literature on this subject loosely employs the term "osteoma" to cover a wide variety of osseous lesions, some of which are clearly nonneoplastic but are of traumatic origin. Included in these categories are old osteochondromas with eburnated cartilaginous caps, traumatic and inflammatory bony protuberances, examples of hyperostosis frontalis interna, and monostotic fibrous dysplasia involving the skull, as well as hyperostotic lesions of the calvarium.

HISTORICAL ASPECTS

There are clear-cut examples of osteomas from ancient times. A fine example of an ivory osteoma has been demonstrated on the right side of an Egyptian skull of Roman vintage. Seventeen skull osteomas found in Neolithic Anglo-Saxon graves have been described by Brothwell.[4] Thirteen examples of skull "button osteomas" have been encountered in Indians of the Pecos Pueblo.[13] A pre-Columbian skull found in Ancon, Peru, shows an osteoma occurring in the left orbit. The often discussed "exostosis" of the femur of the *Pithecanthropus erectus* most likely represents a post-traumatic periosteal myositis ossificans.[9]

INCIDENCE

Since many osteomas are asymptomatic, their true prevalence is not known. In 1941, Teed collected 321 cases from the pertinent literature between 1886 and 1939 involving the frontal sinuses.[35] Childrey noted 15 cases among 3510 (0.42 per cent) largely asymptomatic patients with paranasal sinus roentgenograms. Data from Finland[34] and West Germany[31] vary from 0.1 to 1 per cent of the patients examined in larger otolaryngology clinics.

The most frequent involvement of the frontal sinus among the paranasal sinuses has been confirmed by other, larger studies as well.

SIGNS AND SYMPTOMS

Most osteomas present as a painless, slowly enlarging, hard lump noticed by the patient for at least two years. The lesion's bulk and pressure produce headaches, facial asymmetry, and difficulty in nasal breathing. Patients with large osteomas of the orbit may present with ophthalmic complaints, such as exophthalmos, blindness, or even pneumoencephalos in association with a frontoethmoidal localization. In a review of 21 patients treated in Oxford, England, the cranial vault lesions were asymptomatic and were removed for cosmesis only. Among the 14 nasal sinus tumors, the left frontal sinus presentation (10 instances) was most common, with symptoms of frontal headaches, bulging of the eyes, recurrent sinusitis, and visual alterations.[6]

Some of these lesions cause severe debilitating symptoms, as in the patient reported by Hudolin et al. who had a large frontal sinus osteoma that extended into the cranial fossa and caused mental deterioration, headaches, incontinence, epileptic seizures, and habitual alcoholism.[14] Large osteomas of the mandible may cause bizarre defects in vision and balance by their close proximity to the carotid sinus and internal carotid artery.[19]

LOCATION, AGE, AND SEX DISTRIBUTION

Lautenbach from the University Dental Clinic in Bonn, Germany, reports 36 cases equally distributed in the maxilla and the mandible. A 3:1 female to male ratio was noted. Ages varied from 16 to 74 years, with the sixth decade of life having the most lesions. Histologic examination of the 36 lesions revealed 22 compact, 8 mixed spongy and compact, and 6 spongy types.[16]

The presence of multiple osteomas should arouse the suspicion of an associated Gardner's syndrome, although cases have been reported in which multiple osteomas occurred in the absence of this syndrome complex.[19]

HISTOGENESIS

There is considerable doubt and controversy about the exact derivation of this lesion. Lichtenstein regards osteomas, like osteoid osteomas, as a special type of benign osteoblastoma, i.e., related benign tumor entities of osteoblastic derivation.[18] Aegerter and Kirkpatrick describe these lesions as hamartomas of the periosteum; they believe that the lesion is always formed by intramembranous ossification

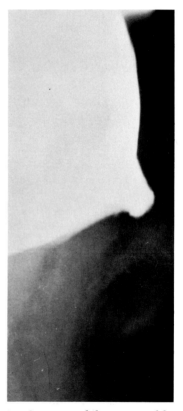

Figure 1–1. Osteoma of the occipital bone in a 34-year-old man. No history of trauma.

that represents only a simple exaggeration of a normal physiologic process.[1] Similarly, Vinogradova considers osteomas to be developmental anomalies of bone but not true tumors.[37] According to Jaffe, this lesion may represent the terminal, ossified stage of a fibrous dysplasia.[15] Smith and Zavaleta[33] and Reed and Hagy[28] believe that ossifying fibromas may differentiate into more mature osteomas.

Some of the skull lesions classified as osteomas may in fact be a reaction to a low grade inflammatory process with subsequent progressive osseous reparative reaction (Fig. 1–1). Based on study of three sequential biopsies, a case of Garré's sclerosing osteomyelitis was diagnosed in its final form clinically, radiographically, and microscopically as an osteoma.[28]

Animal Studies

Long-term multigeneration studies in CF-1 mice regularly found the incidence of spontaneous osteomas to be approximately 10 per cent, the skull being involved in about 90 per cent of this minimally inbred strain, over a period of six consecutive generations.[7a]

Osteomas in mice may also be induced by injection of the RFB osteoma virus of CF-1 mice. These periosteally located exostoses occur two to three months following the injection of the murine virus into the newborn. A rapid growth spurt can be observed in these osteomas for a few weeks, as many as 36 have been seen in a single rodent, after which the lesions increase only slowly in size.[10] This osteoma-producing virus (RFB) is distinct from the osteosarcoma virus (FBJ).

HISTOLOGIC STUDIES

Compact or Ivory Osteoma

Compact or ivory osteoma (ivory exostosis) consists of dense, compact, mature lamellar bone (Fig. 1–2). The periphery of these lesions shows interanastomosing trabeculae of mature cancellous bone. The periosteal surface of the compact osteoma exhibits layers of lamellar bone without attempt at remodeling. In the deeper portions of this lesion, a coarse mosaic pattern of the lamellar bone is present. No attempt at haversian system formation is made, and only occasionally can one encounter marrow spaces (Fig. 1–3). It seems that the original haversian systems of the central portion of the lesions became obliterated and the osteocytes degenerated.

Trabecular or Spongy Osteoma

The trabecular or spongy osteoma may be central (endosteal) or peripheral (subperiosteal) in its location. Histologically, they reveal a chiefly cancellous, trabecular

Figure 1–2. Compact, or ivory, osteoma (also known as ivory exostosis) represents a protuberance on the surface of a membrane type of bone without evidence of a cartilage cap. (Hematoxylin-eosin stain. Magnification ×4.)

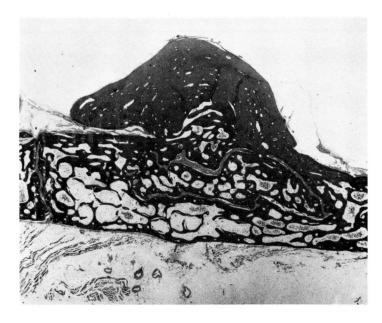

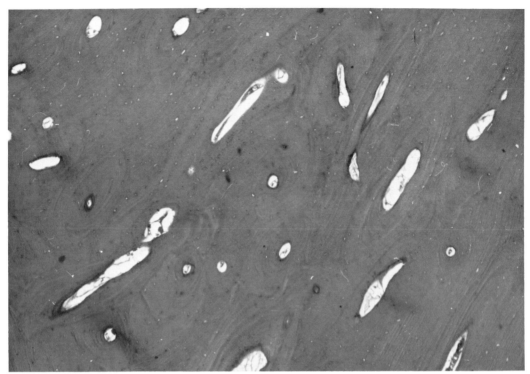

Figure 1–3. Ivory osteoma showing densely compact mature lamellar bone without marrow spaces. (Hematoxylin-eosin stain. Magnification × 50.)

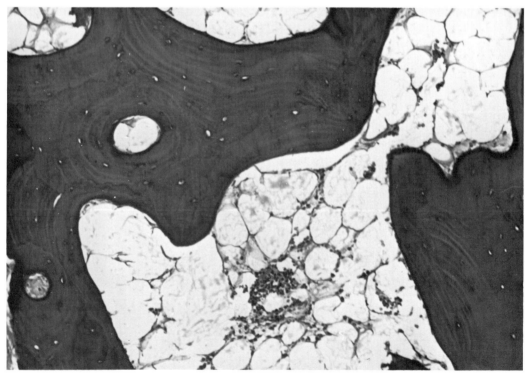

Figure 1–4. Trabecular osteoma with cancellous bony architecture and fatty marrow. (Hematoxylin-eosin stain. Magnification × 50.)

architecture with peripheral cortical bony margin (Fig. 1–4). The trabeculae are thin with fatty marrow present in the intertrabecular spaces. Radiographically, the subperiosteal, or peripheral, osteoma presents as a dense radiopaque lesion protruding from the surface of the bone. The central, or endosteal, type appears as a well-delineated sclerotic mass with clear outlines and smooth borders. No destruction of adjacent bone is noted.

The so-called cancellous osteoma of the long bones referred to in earlier literature is now considered to be an osteochondroma (osteocartilaginous exostosis) in which the cartilaginous cap is eburnated and replaced by fibrous tissue following the cessation of skeletal maturation. Occasionally, osteoma diagnosed as such may represent the final complete ossification of an osteochondroma.

TREATMENT

Treatment consists of surgical excision if the lesion is symptomatic and painful. Large lesions should also be removed for diagnostic purposes, and complete removal yields curative recurrence-free results. Otherwise, no treatment is necessary.

REFERENCES

1. Aegerter, E. E., and Kirkpatrick, J. A., Jr.: Orthopedic Diseases. 4th ed. Philadelphia, W. B. Saunders Company, 1975.
2. Appalanarasayya, K., Murthy, A. S. R., Viswanath, C. K., et al.: Osteoma involving the orbit. Case report and review of the literature. Int. Surg., 54:449–453, 1970.
3. Béraud, C., Morel, P., and Boyer, R.: Ostéome géant fronto-ethmoidal découvert sur un crâne médiéval du Var. J. Radiol. Electrol. Med. Nucl., 42:45–47, 1961.
4. Brothwell, D. R.: The palaeopathology of early British man: an essay on the problems of diagnosis and analysis. J. R. Anthrop. Inst., 91:318–344, 1961.
5. Brunner, H., and Spiesman, I. G.: Osteoma of the frontal and ethmoid sinuses. Ann. Otol. Rhinol. Laryngol., 57:714–737, 1948.
6. Bullough, P. G.: Ivory exostosis of the skull. Postgrad. Med. J., 41:277–281, 1965.
7. Calhoun, N. R., Jackson, S., and Wright, M. C.: Multiple osteomas of the mandible. Report of a case. J. Oral Surg., 15:325–328, 1957.
7a. Charles, R. T., and Turusov, V. S.: Bone tumors in CF-1 mice. Lab. Anim., 8:137–144, 1974.

8. Childrey, J. H.: Osteomas of the sinuses, of the frontal and sphenoid bone. Arch. Otolaryngol., 30:63–72, 1939.
9. Dubois, E.: Über die Hauptmerkmale des Femur von Pithecanthropus erectus. Anthropol. Anz., 4:131–146, 1927.
10. Finkel, M. P., Reilly, C. A., Jr., and Biskis, B. O.: Pathogenesis of radiation and virus-induced bone tumors. In: Grundmann, E. (ed.): Malignant Bone Tumors. New York, Springer-Verlag, 1976, pp. 97–98.
11. Green, A. E., and Bowerman, J. E.: An osteoma of the mandible. Br. J. Oral Surg., 12:225–228, 1974.
12. Hallberg, O. E., and Begley, J. W., Jr.: Origin and treatment of osteomas of the paranasal sinuses. Arch. Otolaryngol., 51:750–760, 1950.
13. Hooton, E. A.: The Indians of Pecos Pueblo. A Study of Their Skeletal Remains. New Haven, Yale University Press, 1930.
14. Hudolin, V., Riessner, D., Kadrnka, S., et al.: A huge osteoma in the anterior cranial fossa. J. Neurol. Neurosurg. Psychiatry, 24:80–83, 1961.
15. Jaffe, H. L.: Tumors and Tumorous Conditions of the Bones and Joints. Philadelphia, Lea & Febiger, 1958.
16. Lautenbach, E.: Klinische und Histologische Studien an Osteomen. Dtsch. Zahn. Mund. Kieferheilkd., 43:434–456, 1964.
17. Lewars, P. H. D.: Osteoma of the mandible. Br. J. Plast. Surg., 12:277–283, 1959–1960.
18. Lichtenstein, L.: Bone Tumors. 4th ed. St. Louis, C. V. Mosby Co., 1972, p. 112.
19. MacLennan, W. D., and Brown, R. D.: Osteoma of the mandible. Br. J. Oral Surg., 12:219–224, 1974.
20. Malan, E.: Chirurgia degli osteomi delle cavita pneumatiche perifacciali. Arch. Ital. Chir., 48:1–124, 1938.
21. Mehta, B. S., and Grewal, G. S.: Osteoma of the paranasal sinuses along with a case report of an orbito-ethmoidal osteoma. J. Laryngol., 77:601–610, 1963.
22. Mikaelian, D. O., Lewis, W. J., and Behringer, W. H.: Primary osteoma of the sphenoid sinus. Laryngoscope, 86:728–733, 1976.
23. Montgomery, W. W.: Osteoma of the frontal sinus. Ann. Otol. Rhinol. Laryngol., 69:245–255, 1960.
24. Moodie, R. L.: Studies in paleopathology. XVIII. Tumors of the head among pre-Columbia Peruvians. Ann. Med. Hist., 8:394–412, 1926.
25. Nelson, D. F., Miller, F. E., and Gross, B. D.: Osteoma of the mandibular condyle: report of a case. J. Oral Surg., 30:761–763, 1972.
26. Olumide, A. A., Fajemisin, A. A., and Adeloye, A.: Osteoma of the ethmofrontal sinus. Case report. J. Neurosurg., 42:343–345, 1975.
27. Pell, L. H., and Carroll, D.: Peumocephalus in association with fronto-ethmoidal osteoma. Clin. Radiol., 14:110–112, 1963.
28. Reed, R. J., and Hagy, D. M.: Benign nonodontogenic fibro-osseous lesions of the skull. Report of two cases. Oral Surg., 19:214–227, 1965.
29. Rowbotham, G. F.: Neoplasms that grow from the bone-forming elements of the skull. A survey of 20 cases. Br. J. Surg., 45:123–134, 1957.
30. Samy, L. L., and Mostafa, H.: Osteomata of the

nose and paranasal sinuses with a report of twenty-one cases. J. Laryngol. Otol., *85*:449–469, 1971.

31. Schertel, L.: Die Höhlenosteome. Radiologe, *15*:62–68, 1975.
32. Schwenzer, N.: Zur Klinik und Therapie Knochenbildender Geschwülste im Kiefergelenkbereich. Dtsch. Zahnaerztl. Z., *27*:848–852, 1972.
33. Smith, A. G., and Zavaleta, A.: Osteoma, ossifying fibroma and fibrous dysplasia of facial and cranial bones. Arch. Pathol., *54*:507–527, 1952.

34. Tarkkanen, J., Paljakka, P., and Holopainen, E.: Die Osteome der Nasennebenhöhlen. Mschr. Ohrenheilk., *102*:320–325, 1968.
35. Teed, R. W.: Primary osteoma of the frontal sinus. Arch. Otolaryngol., *33*:255–292, 1941.
36. Van Dellen, J. R.: A mastoid osteoma causing intracranial complications. A case report. S. Afr. Med. J., *51*:597–598, 1977.
37. Vinogradova, T.: Bone Neoplasms. Moscow, Izdatelstvo Meditsina, 1973.

GARDNER'S SYNDROME

Gardner's syndrome consists of the tetrad of abnormal growths: intestinal polyposis involving the small and large bowel, osteomas, fibromas of the soft tissues, and sebaceous cysts of the skin. This was described in a single Utah family group during the period 1950 to 1953.[14, 15, 27] Although it was Gardner and his coworkers who, in the 1950's, first postulated a mendelian dominant role of predictable inheritance of a single defective gene for the tetrad of physical characteristics of this syndrome, there were several cases with similar attributes reported as early as 1912.[3, 10] These studies firmly established the various associated traits as a definite genetic entity and demonstrated that this syndrome is inherited as an autosomal mendelian dominant disorder with the pleiotropic effects of a single mutant gene, as well as additional heterogeneity in hereditary polyposis.[26] Several separate, but

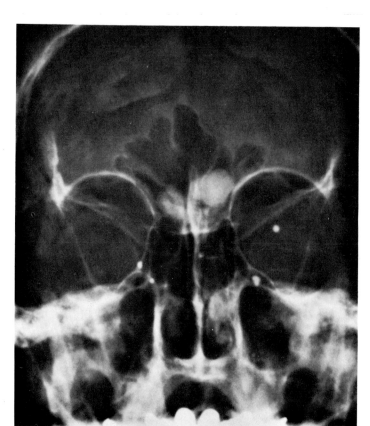

Figure 1–5. Bilateral frontal sinus osteomas in a 62-year-old woman with Gardner's syndrome.

closely linked, defective genes may also account for this syndrome. Fibrosarcoma, dental abnormalities characterized by supernumerary and unerupted teeth, and carcinoma of the ampulla of Vater, as well as thyroid carcinoma, have since been described in association with this syndrome.[2, 12, 13, 16]

Less than 10 per cent of all patients exhibit the complete tetrad of skin and soft tissue lesions with bone tumors and intestinal polyps. About 45 per cent of the patients at risk display some or all aspects of the symptoms. In a survey of 280 patients with this syndrome, 40 (14 per cent) showed bone abnormalities.[5, 35] The multiple and solitary osteomas so characteristic of this disease appear most frequently in the frontal bone (Fig. 1–5). The mandible, maxilla, sphenoid, ethmoid, zygoma, and temporal bones, in descending order of frequency, are involved. Other bones of the appendicular skeleton, usually femur or fibula, can also be affected. It is important to remember that the bony tumors usually precede the other manifestations and continue to develop regardless of any other lesion. In addition to the osteomas, localized cortical thickening of long and short tubular bones, reminiscent of Leri's melorheostosis, are also present with abnormal tubulation.[28, 29] In none of the cases reported in the literature could a malignant transformation in the benign bony lesions be established. A case of osteogenic sarcoma occurring in a 15-year-old girl, a member of a family with Gardner's syndrome,[5, 35] and an instance of chondrosarcoma of the hyoid bone also associated with this syndrome have been reported.[17] A familial sarcoma of bone arising in the tibia of the mother and in the femur of her 13-year-old son has been described in a polyposis coli family.[19] The clinical significance of the progressive (size and number) intestinal polyps lies in the fact that practically all patients with untreated colonic polyposis will indeed develop carcinoma. Since some of the cancers are multiple in the colon or rectum and are detected only in advanced stages, the crude survival rate is about 27 per cent.

Danes has done extensive genetic studies on Gardner's syndrome and found that when only the classic clinical methods of study are employed, this syndrome is rarely diagnosed before the age of 30 years, which is generally too late for useful genetic counselling.[6, 7, 8] Using skin fibroblast markers in tissue cultures of affected individuals and certain family members, 11 to 31 per cent heteroploidy was noted; in contradistinction, fibroblasts obtained from skin biopsies of those with familial polyposis showed only up to 1 per cent heteroploidy. Since this marker is present in individuals at risk before the syndrome is clinically diagnosable, an earlier detection of the affliction is feasible, making effective genetic counselling a stronger reality. The lack of fibroblast markers in patients with familial polyposis strengthens the thesis that Gardner's syndrome is a truly separate and distinct entity.[6, 7, 8]

Bone Abnormalities in Gardner's Syndrome

There are various bony proliferations (osteomatosis) varying from slight, localized, occasionally wavy thickening to large protuberant masses. In their analysis of the roentgenologic features of the bony abnormalities, Chang and his associates found that the character of these lesions depended on the location and the type of bone.[5]

Osteomas of the skull are of two major types: (1) Those that arise from the inner or outer tables are protuberant, frequently have a broad base, and present as a lump. These lesions are best detected in somewhat underexposed tangential roentgenograms. (2) Those that appear next to the paranasal sinuses are without corresponding lumps on the facial surface. Special tomographic views are often necessary to appreciate these lesions.

The most characteristic bone lesion appears to be a protuberant, dense, lobulated osteoma involving the cortex of the mandibular angle. Central enostoses, irregularly eburnated lesions next to teeth also showing other dental abnormalities, were often noted.

Whenever an examining physician or dentist discovers any bony or soft tissue stigmata of a presumed Gardner's syndrome, he is obligated to refer the patient for proctosigmoidoscopy and roentgenographic barium enema to exclude the asymptomatic presence of familial intestinal polyposis. It is also suggested that other members of the family be examined.

REFERENCES

1. Amato, A. E., and Small, E. W.: Oral manifestations of Gardner's syndrome: report of a case. J. Oral Surg., 28:458–460, 1970.
2. Camiel, M. R., Mulé, J. E., Alexander, L. L., et al.: Association of thyroid carcinoma with Gardner's syndrome in siblings. N. Engl. J. Med., 278:1056–1058, 1968.
3. Case records of the Massachusetts General Hospital. Case 21061. N. Engl. J. Med., 212:263–267, 1935.
4. Case records of the Massachusetts General Hospital. Case 53–1976. N. Engl. J. Med., 295:1526–1532, 1976.
5. Chang, C. H., Piatt, E. D., Thomas, K. E., et al.: Bone abnormalities in Gardner's syndrome. Am. J. Roentgenol. Radium Ther. Nucl. Med., 103:645–652, 1968.
6. Danes, B. S.: The Gardner syndrome. A study in cell culture. Cancer, 36:2327–2333, 1975.
7. Danes, B. S.: Increased tetraploidy: cell-specific for the Gardner gene in the cultured cell. Cancer, 38:1983–1988, 1976.
8. Danes, B. S., and Krush, A. J.: The Gardner syndrome: a family study in cell culture. J. Natl. Cancer Inst., 58:771–775, 1977.
9. Delaney, T. J., Findlay, J. M., and Haggart, B. G.: A case of Gardner's syndrome. Br. J. Surg., 53:826–827, 1966.
10. Devic and Bussy: Un cas de polypose adénomateuse généralisée à tout de l'intestin. Arch. Mal. App. Dig., 6:278–289, 1912.
11. Dolan, K. D., Seibert, J., and Seibert, R. W.: Gardner's syndrome. A model for correlative radiology. Am. J. Roentgenol. Radium Ther. Nucl. Med., 119:359–364, 1973.
12. Fader, M., Kline, S. N., Spatz, S. S., et al.: Gardner's syndrome (intestinal polyposis, osteomas, sebaceous cysts), a new dental discovery. Oral Surg., 15:153–156, 1962.
13. Fitzgerald, G. M.: Multiple composite odontomes coincidental with other tumorous conditions: report of a case. J. Am. Dent. Assoc., 30:1408–1417, 1943.
14. Gardner, E. J.: Discovery of the Gardner syndrome. Birth Defects, 13:48–51, 1972.
15. Gardner, E. J., and Richards, R. C.: Multiple cutaneous and subcutaneous lesions occurring simultaneously with hereditary polyposis and osteomatosis. Am. J. Hum. Genet., 5:139–147, 1953.
16. Gorlin, R. J., and Chaudhry, A. P.: Multiple osteomatosis, fibromas, lipomas and fibrosarcomas of the skin and mesentery, epidermoid inclusion cysts of the skin, leiomyomas and multiple intestinal polyposis. N. Engl. J. Med., 263:1151–1158, 1960.
17. Greer, J. A., Jr., Devine, K. D., and Dahlin, D. C.: Gardner's syndrome and chondrosarcoma of the hyoid bone. Arch. Otolaryngol., 103:425–427, 1977.
18. Halse, A., Roed-Petersen, B., and Lund, K.: Gardner's syndrome. J. Oral. Surg., 33:673–675, 1975.
19. Hoffmann, D. C., and Brooke, B. N.: Familial sarcoma of bone in polyposis coli family. Dis. Colon Rectum, 13:119–120, 1970.
20. Jones, E. L., and Cornell, W. P.: Gardner's syndrome. Review of the literature and report on a family. Arch. Surg., 92:287–300, 1966.
21. Kaczurba, M., Biedrzycki, T., Buraczewska-Lipinska, H., et al.: A case of Gardner's syndrome with malignant transformation in one of osseous lesions (osteoblastoma malignum). Pol. Przegl. Radiol., 40:213–217, 1976.
22. Lazar, H. P., Crow, N. S., and Brogdon, B. G.: External manifestations of multiple polyposis. Report of a case with negative family history. Arch. Intern. Med., 100:290–295, 1957.
23. Leppard, B., and Bussey, H. J. R.: Epidermoid cysts, polyposis coli and Gardner's syndrome. Br. J. Surg., 62:387–393, 1975.
24. Martel, A. J., and Bonanno, C. A.: Multiple polyposis of the gastrointestinal tract with osteoma and soft tissue tumors. Am. J. Dig. Dis., 13:588–591, 1968.
25. Neale, H. W., Pickrell, K. L., and Quinn, G. W.: Extra-abdominal manifestations of Gardner's syndrome. Case report. Plast. Reconstr. Surg., 56:92–96, 1975.
26. Pierce, E. R.: Pleiotropism and heterogeneity in hereditary intestinal polyposis. Birth Defects, 13:52–62, 1972.
27. Plenk, H. P., and Gardner, E. J.: Osteomatosis (Leontiasis ossea). Hereditary disease of membranous bone formation associated in one family with polyposis of the colon. Radiology, 62:830–840, 1954.
28. Rayne, J.: Gardner's syndrome. Br. J. Oral Surg., 6:11–17, 1968–1969.
29. Rayne, J., and Bullough, P.: A case of Gardner's syndrome. Br. J. Surg., 53:824–826, 1966.
30. Shiffman, M. A.: Familial multiple polyposis associated with soft-tissue and hard-tissue tumors. J.A.M.A., 179:138–146, 1962.
31. Singer, R.: Ein Beitrag zum Gardner-Syndrom. Dtsch. Zahn. Mund. Kieferheilkd., 62:18–31, 1974.
32. Teramoto, T., Motegi, M., Murayama, N., et al.: Three cases of Gardner's syndrome. Jpn. J. Clin. Oncol., 6:69–76, 1974.
33. Terao, H., Sato, S., and Kim, S.: Gardner's syndrome involving the skull, dura, and brain. J. Neurosurg., 44:638–641, 1976.
34. Utsunomiya, J., and Nakamura, T.: The occult osteomatous changes in the mandible in patients with familial polyposis coli. Br. J. Surg., 62:45–51, 1975.
35. Watne, A. L., Core, S. K., and Carrier, J. M.: Gardner's syndrome. Surg. Gynecol. Obstet., 141:53–56, 1975.
36. Watne, A. L., Lai, H.-Y., Carrier, J., et al.: The diagnosis and surgical treatment of patients with Gardner's syndrome. Surgery, 82:327–333, 1977.
37. Wiener, R. S., and Cooper, P.: Multiple polyposis of the colon, osteomatosis and soft-tissue tumors. Report of a familial syndrome. N. Engl. J. Med., 253:795–799, 1955.

2

OSSIFYING FIBROMA

DEFINITION

Ossifying fibroma is a gradually expansile, well-marginated, often asymptomatic, central fibro-osseous lesion most commonly found in jawbones that may, owing to its large size, cause pain, swelling, or paresthesia. If left untreated, the tumor may reach enormous proportions and have a grotesque appearance (Fig. 2–1).

SYNONYMS

1. Cemento-ossifying fibroma.[23, 49]
2. Benign fibro-osseous lesion of periodontal ligament origin.[24, 59]
3. Fibro-osseous lesion of bone.
4. Osteofibroma.[33]
5. Fibro-osteoma.[14]
6. Ossifying fibroma (fibrous dysplasia).[17]
7. Fibrous osteoma.[37]
8. Benign nonodontogenic tumor of jaw.[60]

Fibro-osseous lesions of the mandible and maxilla are one of the more confusing and controversial groups of lesions faced by a diagnostician. There are endless numbers of synonyms, and, in the absence of clear-cut distinctions between the various entities, the terminology is hopelessly confusing and nebulous. It is difficult to establish whether the lesions in question are truly neoplastic or simply developmental anomalies or reactive processes.

HISTORICAL ASPECTS

Ossifying fibrous tumors of the jaw and the maxilla were reported as early as 1865 in British literature. Menzel[33] from Vienna seems to have been the first in 1872 to describe the first case of ossifying fibroma as osteofibroma (Fig. 2–1). Montgomery[34] popularized the term "ossifying fibroma," Figi[14] designated the lesion "fibrous osteoma," and Furedi[16] named it "fibro-osteoma."

INCIDENCE

Since several authorities accept various divergent lesions as fibro-osteoma, ossifying fibroma, and fibrous dysplasia, the incidence and predominant location data are widely variable and not very useful. For instance, about 90 per cent of the ossifying fibromas reported by Waldron occurred in the mandible and almost exclusively in women.[57] Others, however, maintain that this lesion is most common in the maxil-

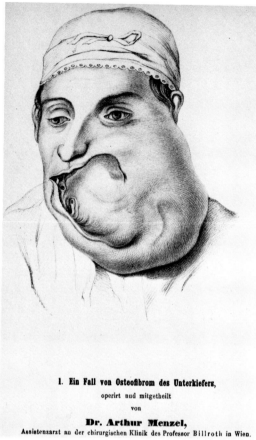

1. Ein Fall von Osteofibrom des Unterkiefers,

operirt und mitgetheilt

von

Dr. Arthur Menzel,

Assistenzarzt an der chirurgischen Klinik des Professor Billroth in Wien.

Figure 2–1. Ossifying fibroma of the jaw with a 25 year history of slowly increasing size in a 35-year-old Hungarian woman.

la,[17] with no significant sexual predilection.[23, 24]

LOCATION, AGE AND SEX DISTRIBUTION

Except for the juvenile variety, the lesion seems to occur after the second decade of life, mostly in the third and fourth decades. It predominantly affects women and arises close to the roots of the teeth or the periapical aspects of the jaws. The antrum and the molar area of the mandible are the favored sites, although occurrences in other locations in the craniofacial bones have also been reported.[7, 29]

Ossifying fibromas have been reported in extragnathic long bones.[20, 26, 31a] In the 14 cases encountered, all but two occurred in the tibia. One lesion involved the hu-

merus and another arose in the femur (Fig. 2–2). The clinical differential diagnosis may include bone cyst, fibrous dysplasia, nonossifying fibroma, fibromyxoma, or even adamantinoma. Although it is more common to see solitary lesions, multiple ossifying fibromas may occur, especially in Negroes.[25, 41] According to Markel, ossifying fibroma and adamantinoma of long bones are somehow related.[31a]

VARIOUS TYPES

In contrast to ossifying fibroma, *fibro-osteoma* is defined as a more solid, well-circumscribed tumor most commonly involving the maxilla and the paranasal sinuses.[41] Many authors interchange the terms "ossifying fibroma" and "fibro-osteoma," depending on whether the fibrous or the bony tissue component predominates in the lesion. Others believe fibro-osteoma to be larger in size, often producing clinical swelling.[24] On radiographic examination, these lesions appear to be radiopaque with a ground-glass appearance. They frequently involve several teeth but are not closely associated with the periodontal membrane. Hamner et al. feel that fibro-osteoma is microscopically separable from ossifying fibroma, the former lesion showing larger trabeculae of lamellar bone with artifactual space surrounding them. The fibroblastic stroma is more myxoid, less collagenized, with adequate blood supply.[23] Some believe that fibrous osteomas can mature into osteomas on the one hand or into ossifying fibromas on the other.[15, 40, 50] Those in favor of this histologic separation cite the clinical features of fibrous osteomas that occur in older patients and have a lower recurrence rate than ossifying fibromas.

In 1946, Billing and Ringertz[2] distinguished four distinct developmental stages in the maturation process of fibro-osteoma: (1) Least differentiated, "osteoid fibroma," a soft fibroma-like tumor, (2) moderately mature; (3) mature, so-called osteomas; and (4) the most differentiated, "eburnifying fibromas," which most commonly occur in the ethmoid bone or the adjacent portion of the frontal bones.

Lesions originally diagnosed as ossifying fibroma may become quiescent, and micro-

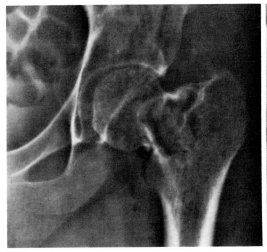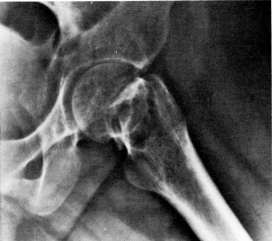

Figure 2-2. Ossifying fibroma of left femur in a 19-year-old girl showing a lytic femoral neck lesion and angulated pathologic fracture. Varus deformity.

scopic examination of a later biopsy may show the histologic features of an osteoma.[42]

Is it feasible or practical to separate *fibrous dysplasia* from ossifying fibroma? Schlumberger,[44] Dahlin,[6] Pindborg,[38] and Waldron,[57] among others, believe that both entities have a similar histologic appearance, although ossifying fibroma demonstrates the presence of a capsule. Others, such as Thoma,[56] Reed,[40] Reed and Hagy,[41] and Kempson,[26] put forward rather convincing data to prove the two lesions to be clinically and pathologically separate. The author shares this latter view. Lichtenstein[30] considers fibrous osteomas or ossifying fibromas as variants of benign osteoblastoma.

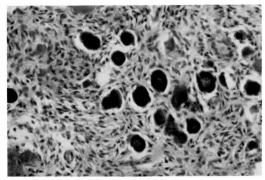

Figure 2-3. Cementifying fibroma showing cellular fibroblastic tissue surrounding rounded, calcified, strongly basophilic, cementum-like material. (Hematoxylin-eosin stain. Magnification × 40.)

Cementifying fibromas, ossifying fibromas, and periapical cementomas are considered by some oral pathologists to be variants of the same disease arising in the periodontal ligament.[24, 59] The lesion is labelled "ossifying" or "cementifying," depending on the predominant tissue (Fig. 2–3). The difficulties in separating these lesions result in the all-encompassing term "cemento-ossifying fibroma."[23, 49]

RADIOGRAPHIC FEATURES

Radiographically, in the early stages, the lesions are osteolytic and radiolucent and appear to be solitary and cystlike, without periosteal reaction (Fig. 2–4). The initial radiolucent stage progresses from a predominantly fibrous lesion to an increasingly calcified osseous structure. This process of maturation is represented on the roentgenograms by the appearance and then coalescence of radiopaque calcified spicules within a well-described radiolucency. At later stages of evolution, a well-circumscribed radiopaque lesion can be seen surrounded by a uniformly radiolucent periphery. Irrespective of its stage of maturation, the radiolucent borders are well-defined and smoothly contoured. Occasionally, peripheral sclerosis will be induced, represented on the radiograph by a hyperostotic, sclerotic margin. Sherman and Sternbergh made the first attempt to

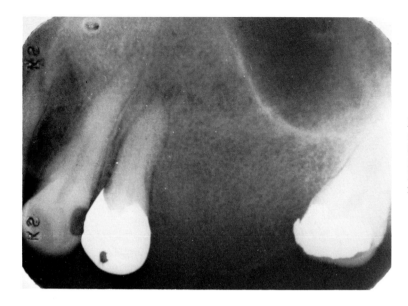

Figure 2-4. Typical ossifying fibroma of the maxilla in a 50-year-old woman presenting with a slowly growing localized lesion of the alveolar ridge of 10 years' duration.

distinguish between the neoplastic and the developmental, tumor-like osseous lesions. They described 11 cases of ossifying fibroma, five in the mandible and six in the maxilla, all of which appeared to be unilocular and rounded or oval with a surrounding thin rim of bone. They claim that, radiologically, fibrous dysplasia and ossifying fibroma may be distinguished by their appearance, namely that ossifying fibroma shows expansile, clearly defined margins while monostotic fibrous dysplasia appears to have a diffuse merging border.[48] (Table 2-1.)

DIFFERENTIAL DIAGNOSIS

Condensing or sclerosing osteitis is an osteosclerosis occurring as a sequel to an inflammatory process. Occasionally, it may be confused with an ossifying fibroma or fibrous dysplasia. It occurs most frequently as a periapical radiopacity, especially in the premolar and molar regions, and only rarely in edentulous jaws; it is limited to areas around decayed teeth, retained roots, or root tips.

Idiopathic osteosclerosis of the jaw is a periapical radiopaque lesion *not* usually found in association with roots of teeth. It occurs most often in the alveolus, between roots of teeth in the body, or in the crest of the ridge of the mandible.

HISTOLOGIC FEATURES

Histologically, this is a uniformly cellular fibrous spindle cell growth arranged in a whorled or matted pattern. Reflected by the radiographic appearance is the stage of lesional maturation, and varying amounts of smooth lamellar bone formation with

TABLE 2-1. Distinction Between Fibrous Dysplasia and Ossifying Fibroma

	Location	Sexual Predilection	Age Distribution	Radiographic Appearance	Jaw Expansion
Fibrous dysplasia	More common in maxilla	Equal sexual distribution	Most common during first and second decades of life	Poorly defined merging borders	Elongated fusiform
Ossifying fibroma	90 per cent in mandible	High predilection for women	Past second decade of life	Well-defined borders	Nodular, dome-shaped

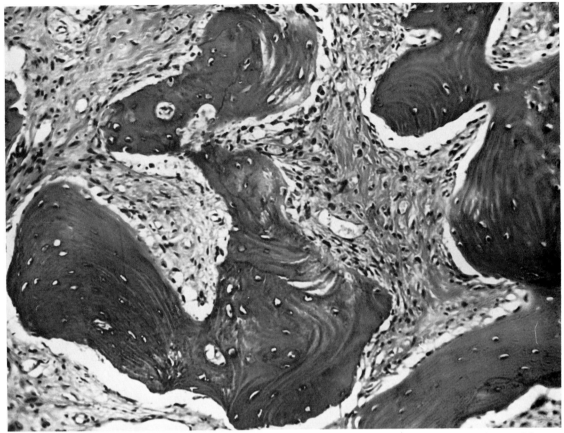

Figure 2–5. Ossifying fibroma with mature lamellar-type bone surrounded by a cellular fibroblastic tissue. Note brisk osteoblastic activity. (Hematoxylin-eosin stain. Magnification × 80.)

brisk osteoblastic activity are demonstrated (Fig. 2–5). Capsule formation is often clearly evident. The ossification process usually begins at the periphery and extends inward. The trabeculae of lamellar bone in ossifying fibroma polarize, with dark and light, widely spaced, parallel lines of birefringence (Table 2–2). Some believe that, histologically, fibrous dysplasia represents an arrest of maturation at the woven or fiber bone stage with high alkaline phosphatase activity of the stromal fibroblastic cells.[40] Accordingly, lamellar bone formation with osteoblastic cells rimming the bony trabeculae is inconsistent with a diagnosis of fibrous dysplasia. Others, however, maintain that lamellar bone formation with osteoblastic activity may be seen in fibrous dysplasia.[9, 13, 58]

Fibrous dysplasia is a specific pathologic process in which the woven (fiber) immature bone persists owing to an arrest of osseous maturation. Polarized light reveals random birefringence. Silver reticulin stain displays a twisted and tangled peripheral pattern of the individual bone trabeculae. The fibrous stromal pattern becomes more collagenized in older lesions, but the trabeculae never mature into lamellar types of bone. Since the lesion gradually and imperceptibly merges into surrounding normal bone, no encapsulation is evidenced and enucleation is not feasible. *Woven or fiber bone* is characterized by irregular bony trabeculae with large osteocytic lacunar spaces showing feathery margins. Special histologic stains demonstrate the various aspects of this type of osseous tissue. Masson's trichrome–stained histologic sections delineate central calcification with a peripheral osteoid rim blending imperceptibly into adjacent fibrous cellular stromal tissue. Silver impregnation techniques un-

TABLE 2–2.   Histologic Differential Diagnosis in Fibrous Dysplasia, Ossifying Fibroma, and Reactive Bone Formation

	Fibrous Dysplasia	Ossifying Fibroma	Reactive Bone Formation
Type of Bone	Strictly woven	Woven with peripheral lamellar maturation	Woven with complete lamellar maturation
Bony spicule distribution	Evenly placed random	Evenly placed random	Evenly placed regular
Osteoblastic and osteoclastic activity	Absent°	Present	Present
Fibrous stroma	Loose to dense according to age	Uniformly loose or dense with whorling	Loose or dense
Stromal hemorrhage Stromal inflammation Stromal giant cells	Present	Absent	Present
Endochondral ossification	Absent	Absent	Present
Capsule formation	Absent	Present	Absent
Silver reticulin stain	Tangled, twisted disoriented fibers; irregular borders	Regular, parallel lamellation with regular borders	Not useful
Polarized light	Randomly birefringent lines	Mostly birefringent parallel lines	Not useful

°After fracture or trauma, there may be osteoblastic or osteoclastic rimming of the bony spicules.

derline the feathery margins, and, under the polarizing light microscope, a parallel-oriented woven fiber pattern entirely devoid of lamellation is demonstrated. *Lamellar compact bone* is characterized by single or interanastomosing osseous tissue surrounded by a fibrous cellular stroma. Under the polarizing light, a broad lamellar, parallel-oriented fiber pattern is evident. In *reactive bone formation,* evenly placed, regularly distributed, bony spicules appear along the lines of trauma. Endochondral ossification is present, and the woven (fiber) bone matures completely into lamellar bone.

JUVENILE OSSIFYING FIBROMA

Juvenile ossifying fibroma is a fast-growing destructive lesion of the maxilla occurring in children and adolescents usually under the age of 15 years (Fig. 2–6). The rapidly increasing swelling of the cheek and intraorbital areas results in marked deformity of the face with symptoms of nasal blockage or orbital proptosis. It may cause death by aggressive local extension into adjacent structure with metastases.

In typical lesions, the radiographic examination reveals a radiolucent, homogeneously dense destruction of the maxilla with often ill-defined, thin, eggshell-like bony margins.

Histologically, the lesion is identical with ossifying fibroma occurring in adults. The stroma exhibits numerous osteoblasts often arranged in a trabecular growth pattern. Mature bone trabeculae may be present with brisk osteoblastic rimming. The clinical significance of this tumor's recognition lies in the fact that since it is fast-growing, a preliminary diagnosis of osteogenic sarcoma is suggested.[38]

TREATMENT

Appropriate therapy by necessity depends on the following important distinctions: duration and nature of symptomatology, duration and rate of tumor growth, roentgenologic appearance, and histologic presentation.

The preferred treatment is complete surgical removal by curettage, enucleation, or excision. Small maxillary lesions may be excised through an incision in the buccoalveolar sulcus, although larger tumors may

A

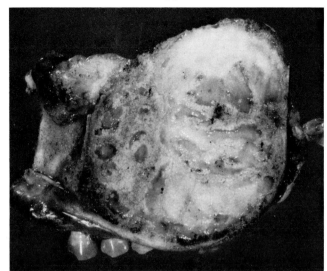

Figure 2–6. Rapidly enlarging destructive juvenile ossifying fibroma of maxilla in a 16-year-old boy. *A,* Maxillectomy specimen and *B,* radiograph. (Courtesy of Dr. R. H. Spiro.)

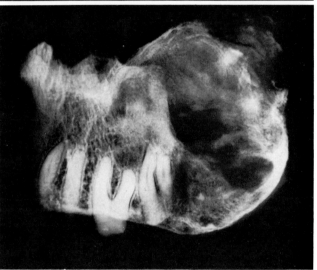

B

require a Weber-Fergusson lip-splitting procedure to facilitate adequate surgical exposure for complete extirpation.[39] Although radiation therapy has been reported in the treatment of these tumors, the risk of malignant transformation in such instances is too real for it to be of serious consideration.[31, 37] In some instances, the lesion may be so large that only subtotal removal can be accomplished for cosmesis and to improve function.[61] Curative attempts in long bones should include, in addition to removal of the periosteum at the time of initial treatment, a complete resection of the involved area of bone with placing of bone chips.

REFERENCES

1. Abrams, A. M., and Melrose, R. J.: Fibro-osseous lesion. J. Oral Pathol., *4*:158–165, 1975.
2. Billing, L., and Ringertz, N.: Fibro-osteoma. A pathologico-anatomical and roentgenological study. Acta Radiol., *27*:129–152, 1946.
3. Champion, A. H. R., Moule, A. W., and Wilkinson, F. C.: Case report of an endosteal fibroma of the mandible. Br. Dent. J., *86*:3–6, 1949.
4. Cooke, B. E. D.: Benign fibro-osseous enlargements of the jaws. Parts I and II. Br. Dent. J., *102*:1–14, 49–59, 1957.
5. Cornet, L., Vilasco, J., and Dadie, A.: Total extirpation of the mandible in a case of giant osteogenic fibroma. Rev. Stomatol. Chir. Maxillofac., *66*:693–699, 1965.
6. Dahlin, D. C.: Bone Tumors. 2nd ed. Springfield, Illinois, Charles C Thomas, 1967, pp. 238–241.

7. Darsie, J. L., and Kenan, P. D.: Ossifying fibromas of the frontal-ethmoid sinuses. South. Med. J., 64:1033–1038, 1971.

8. Dehner, L. P.: Tumors of the mandible and maxilla in children. I. Clinicopathologic study of 46 histologically benign lesions. Cancer, 31:364–384, 1973.

9. Dehner, L. P.: Fibro-osseous lesions of bone. In Ackerman, L. V., Spjut, H. J., and Abell, M. R. (eds.): Bones and Joints. Baltimore, Williams & Wilkins, 1976, pp. 209–235.

10. Dodge, O. G.: Tumors of the jaw, odontogenic tissues and maxillary antrum (excluding Burkitt lymphoma) in Uganda Africans. Cancer, 18:205–215, 1965.

11. Dolamore, W. H.: The importance of clinical observation in dental surgery. Proc. R. Soc. Med., 14:1–22, 1920–1921.

12. Eden, K. C.: The benign fibro-osseous tumours of the skull and facial bones. Br. J. Surg., 27:323–350, 1939.

13. Eversole, L. R., Sabes, W. R., and Rovin, S.: Fibrous dysplasia; a nosologic problem in the diagnosis of fibro-osseous lesions of the jaws. J. Oral Pathol., 1:189–220, 1972.

14. Figi, F. A.: Fibro-osteoma of the mandible. Surg. Clin. North Am., 10:101–113, 1930.

15. Fu, Y.-S., and Perzin, K. H.: Non-epithelial tumors of the nasal cavity, paranasal sinuses, and nasopharynx: a clinicopathologic study. II. Osseous and fibro-osseous lesions, including osteoma, fibrous dysplasia, ossifying fibroma, osteoblastoma, giant cell tumor, and osteosarcoma. Cancer, 33:1289–1305, 1974.

16. Furedi, A.: Study of so-called osteofibroma of the maxilla. Dent. Cosmos., 77:999–1010, 1935.

17. Georgiade, N., Masters, F., Horton, C., et al.: Ossifying fibromas (fibrous dysplasia) of the facial bones in children and adolescents. J. Pediatr., 46:36–43, 1955.

18. Gerughty, R. M.: Clinicopathologic characteristics of controversial lesions of bone. In Irby, W. B. (ed.): Current Advances in Oral Surgery. St. Louis, C. V. Mosby Co., 1974, Chapter 9.

19. Geschickter, C. F., and Copeland, M. M.: Tumors of Bone. 3rd ed. Philadelphia, J. B. Lippincott Co., 1949.

20. Goergen, T. G., Dickman, P. S., Resnick, D., et al.: Long bone ossifying fibromas. Cancer, 39:2067–2072, 1977.

21. Gögl, H.: Das Psammo-Osteoid-Fibrom der Nase und ihrer Nebenhöhlen. Monatsschr. Ohrenheilk. Laryngorhinol., 83:1–10, 1949.

22. Gullotta, F., and Lorenz, F.: Ossifying fibroma — an ultrastructural study. Riv. Patol. Clin. Sper., 13:37–42, 1972–1973.

23. Hamner, J. E., III, Lightbody, P. M., Ketcham, A. S., et al.: Cemento-ossifying fibroma of the maxilla. Oral Surg., 26:579–587, 1968.

24. Hamner, J. E., III, Scofield, H. H., and Cornyn, J.: Benign fibro-osseous jaw lesions of periodontal membrane origin. An analysis of 249 cases. Cancer, 22:861–878, 1968.

25. Jaffe, H. L.: Tumors and Tumorous Conditions of the Bones and Joints. Philadelphia, Lea & Febiger, 1958, pp. 136–138.

26. Kempson, R. L.: Ossifying fibroma of the long bones. Arch. Pathol., 82:218–233, 1966.

27. Langdon, J. D., Rapidis, A. D., and Patel, M. F.: Ossifying fibroma — one disease or six? An analysis of 39 fibro-osseous lesions of the jaws. Br. J. Oral Surg., 14:1–11, 1976.

28. Lazarov, G., and Peeva, I.: Ossifying fibroma, aneurysmal cyst and epidermoid cyst — three rare localizations in the short tubular bones of the hand treated with homo-osseous grafts. Onkologiia, 10:176–179, 1973.

29. Lehrer, H. Z.: Ossifying fibroma of the orbital roof. Its distinction from "blistering" or "intraosseous" meningioma. Arch. Neurol., 20:536–541, 1969.

30. Lichtenstein, L.: Bone Tumors. 4th ed. St. Louis, C. V. Mosby Co., 1972.

31. Maris, A. M.: Effect of roentgenotherapy on osteofibroma of the maxilla. J. Oral Surg., 5:223–226, 1947.

31a. Markel, S. F.: Ossifying fibroma of long bone. Its distinction from fibrous dysplasia and its association with adamantinoma of long bone. Am. J. Clin. Pathol., 69:91–97, 1978.

32. Meister, H. P.,Lufft, W., and Schlegel, D.: Differential diagnosis of fibro-osseous jaw lesions (fibrous dysplasia vs. ossifying fibroma). Beitr. Pathol., 148:221–229, 1973.

33. Menzel, A.: Ein Fall von Osteofibrom des Unterkiefers. Arch. Klin. Chir., 13:212–219, 1872.

34. Montgomery, A. H.: Ossifying fibromas of jaw. Arch. Surg., 15:30–44, 1927.

35. Paul, M., Thompson, L. W., and Morton, D., Jr.: An ossifying fibroma of the coronoid process. Case report. Plast. Reconstr. Surg., 60:118–120, 1977.

36. Pepler, W. J.: Ossifying fibromas and their relation to fibrous dysplasia, and other tumours. J. Pathol., 79:408–412, 1966.

37. Phemister, D. B., and Grimson, K. S.: Fibrous osteoma of the jaws. Ann. Surg., 105:564–583, 1937.

38. Pindborg, J. J.: Fibrous dysplasia or fibroosteoma. Report of a case. Acta. Radiol., 36:196–204, 1951.

39. Pound, E., Pickrell, K., Huger, W., et al.: Fibrous dysplasia (ossifying fibroma) of the maxilla. Analysis of 14 cases. Ann. Surg., 161:406–410, 1965.

40. Reed, R. J.: Fibrous dysplasia of bone. Arch. Pathol., 75:480–495, 1963.

41. Reed, R. J., and Hagy, D. M.: Benign nonodontogenic fibro-osseous lesions of the skull. Report of two cases. Oral Surg., 19:214–227, 1965.

42. Ringertz, N.: Fibro-osteoma, a pathological anatomical and roentgenographic study. Acta. Radiol., 27:129–152, 1946.

43. Scarff, R. W., and Walker, D. G.: Unilateral bony swelling of maxilla. Proc. R. Soc. Med., 41:485–489, 1948.

44. Schlumberger, H. G.: Fibrous dysplasia (ossifying fibroma) of the maxilla and mandible. Am. J. Orthod., 32:579–581, 1946.

45. Schlumberger, H. G.: Fibrous dysplasia of single bones (monostotic fibrous dysplasia). Milit. Surg., 99:504–527, 1946.

46. Schmaman, A., Smith, I., and Ackerman, L. V.: Benign fibro-osseous lesions of the mandible and maxilla. A review of 35 cases. Cancer, 26:303–312, 1970.

47. Schwarz, E.: Ossifying fibroma of the face and skull. Am. J. Roentgenol. Radium Ther. Nucl. Med., 91:1012–1015, 1964.
48. Sherman, R. S., and Sternbergh, W. C. A.: The roentgen appearance of ossifying fibroma of bone. Radiology, 50:595–609, 1948.
49. Small, I. A., and Goodman, P. A.: Giant cemento-ossifying fibroma of the maxilla; report of case and discussion. J. Oral Surg., 31:113–119, 1973.
50. Smith, A. G., and Zavaleta, A.: Osteoma, ossifying fibroma, and fibrous dysplasia of facial and cranial bones. Arch. Pathol., 54:507–527, 1952.
51. Smith, I., and Schmaman, A.: Benign fibro-osseous lesions of the mandible and maxilla: clinical features. S. Afr. Med. J., 44:1423–1428, 1970.
52. Solley, S.: Surgical Experiences, Lecture 41. London, Hardwicke, 1865.
53. Sonesson, A.: Fibro-osteoma in the mandible of a child. Acta Radiol., 34:17–24, 1950.
54. Stock, H. J.: Two unusual bone tumours of the hand. Zentralbl. Chir., 102:420–425, 1977.
55. Test, D., Schow, C., Cohen, D., et al.: Juvenile ossifying fibroma. J. Oral Surg., 34:907–910, 1976.
56. Thoma, K. H.: Differential diagnosis of fibrous dysplasia and fibro-osseous neoplastic lesions of the jaws and their treatment. J. Oral Surg., 14:185–194, 1956.
57. Waldron, C. A.: Fibro-osseous lesions of the jaws. J. Oral Surg., 28:58–64, 1970.
58. Waldron, C. A., and Giansanti, J. S.: Benign fibro-osseous lesions of the jaws: a clinical-radiologic-histologic review of sixty-five cases. Part I. Fibrous dysplasia of jaws. Oral Surg., 35:190–201, 1973.
59. Waldron, C. A., and Giansanti, J. S.: Benign fibro-osseous lesions of the jaws: a clinical-radiologic-histologic review of sixty-five cases. Part II. Benign fibro-osseous lesions of periodontal ligament origin. Oral Surg., 35:340–350, 1973.
60. Walker, D. G.: Benign nonodontogenic tumors of the jaws. J. Oral Surg., 28:39–57, 1970.
61. Young, F. W., and Putney, F. J.: Ossifying fibroma of the sinuses. Ann. Otol. Rhinol. Laryngol., 77:425–434, 1968.

3

OSTEOID OSTEOMA

DEFINITION

Osteoid osteoma is a benign osteoblastic lesion characterized by a well-demarcated core (nidus) of usually less than 1 cm and by a distinctive surrounding zone of reactive bone formation.

HISTORICAL ASPECTS

Individual cases of this lesion were noted before 1935, when Jaffe recognized and described five cases as definite clinicopathologic entities.[46, 47, 48] Heine, in 1927, described a case in the basal phalanx of the ring finger but interpreted it as a healing osteomyelitic sequestrum.[41] Hitzrot[43] referred to a case in 1930 as a "sclerosing osteomyelitis," and Bergstrand[3] reported two examples in that same year under the heading of "osteoblastic disease." Originally, it was thought that the lesions occurred only in the spongy bones, but later it became clear that osteoid osteoma may also develop in the cortices of long bones. These findings established Jaffe's concept of osteoid osteoma as a lesion *sui generis*.[48, 50] A paleopathologic and radiologic study revealed an example of an intracortical osteoid os-

teoma in the right tibia of a middle-aged man found in a 7th to 11th century Slavic grave in Abraham, Czechoslovakia.[121] Another such case was identified in a 7th century Anglo-Saxon femur.[122]

SIGNS AND SYMPTOMS

Pain is very characteristic of this lesion and is accompanied by vasomotor disturbances, namely increased skin temperatures in the affected region, and profuse perspiration. These features are more commonly noted with the smaller lesions and may persist for some time, even after complete removal of the lesion. Exquisite local tenderness can also be a striking feature.

Intermittent vague pain gradually increasing in severity and usually occurring nocturnally characterizes the early symptoms; boring or nagging constant pain becomes prevalent later (Fig. 3–1). In many cases, salicylates completely relieve the symptoms. Many of the studies record only the effective relief of pain and no negative results, and therefore these data are notoriously inaccurate.[7] It must be stated, however, that many otherwise typical lesions are pain-free, showing, in turn, the characteristic reactive bone formation.

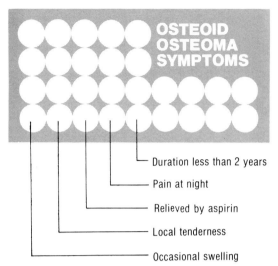

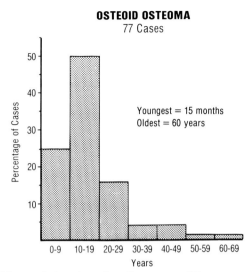

Figure 3-1. Symptomatology in osteoid osteoma.

Figure 3-2. Age distribution in 77 patients at Memorial Hospital with osteoid osteoma.

Such painless lesions have been noted by many.[23, 59, 67, 87, 99, 109]

Pain is not always localized at the exact site of the lesion but is often referred to a nearby joint. Muscle wasting, painful limping, and diminished stretch reflexes in the involved extremity, especially in children, may lead to misdiagnosis of a neurologic disorder.[95] Considerable interest concerning the true nature of the pain has evolved, and an interesting case was reported by Mauer in 1958. A small painful osteoid osteoma in the 12th rib of an adult was excised under thorough local anesthesia without any relief until the rib itself was actually cut through.[72] In 1965, Sherman and McFarland[102] described unmyelinated nerve fibers in the reactive fibrous zone surrounding the nidus accompanying blood vessels and postulated a possible mechanism for the pathognomonic pain in this lesion. Applying the Bielschowsky silver impregnation technique, Catto and Cairns (cited by Byers) and later, using other methods, Byers[7] demonstrated axonal fibers singly and in groups irregularly coursing and ramifying through several lesions. Such silver-impregnable nerve fibers were found in a similar way by Schulman and Dorfman, who, in addition, postulated that the pain was generated and transmitted by vascular pressure–sensitive autonomic nerves.[98]

AGE AND SEX DISTRIBUTION

This lesion occurs predominantly in children, adolescents, and young adults between the ages of 10 and 25 years. It is distinctly rare above the age of 30 years. The youngest patient reported was eight months old;[38] the oldest was 70 years. Overall, the lesion occurred twice as often in males as in females. In the cases that came to us . at Memorial Sloan-Kettering Cancer Center, the average age was 14 years, the youngest patient was 15 months and the oldest was 60 years (Fig. 3–2). About 75 per cent of our cases are under the age of 25 years, with the lesion occurring, in this group, four times as often in males as in females.

LOCATION

Osteoid osteoma may be found in the cortex (most frequent, classic) or the medulla (spongiosa) of bone. In cortical presentation, it may occupy the midcortex or its subperiosteal or endosteal surface (Fig. 3–3). The subperiosteal or exostotic form is the rarest.[10, 97, 116] Occasionally, the lesion abuts the joint cartilage and, at times, may erode through it.[87, 103]

Osteoid osteoma has been known to occur in practically every bone of the ap-

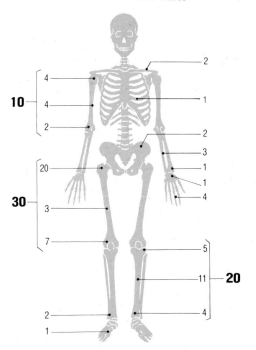

OSTEOID OSTEOMA
Distribution of 77 Cases

Figure 3-3. Skeletal distribution in 77 patients at Memorial Hospital with osteoid osteoma.

pendicular and axial skeleton, with special predilection for the bones of the legs (Fig. 3–4). In about half of the cases, the lesion was located in the femur or the tibia (Fig. 3–5). Involvement of the bones of the feet was also common, with lesser frequency in

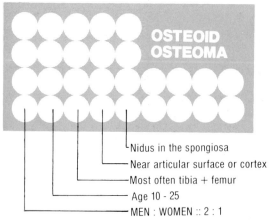

OSTEOID OSTEOMA

Nidus in the spongiosa
Near articular surface or cortex
Most often tibia + femur
Age 10 - 25
MEN : WOMEN :: 2 : 1

Figure 3-4. The most important clinical parameters in osteoid osteoma.

the upper limbs. Carroll[11] reported six cases found in the bones of the hand, and others have also encountered single cases. The toes may also be affected.[118] Spinal location occurred in about 10 per cent of the cases, most commonly in the posterior elements, the lamina, pedicle, facet, and spinous process being involved in descending order of frequency as listed here.[96] The ribs, the mandible, and the calvarium are the rarest sites of involvement (Fig. 3–6).[23, 24, 93] Distal phalangeal presentation in children may result in premature closure of the epiphysis[5] or other more severe bony growth disturbances.[29] Localized overgrowth or deformity of bone may be seen in approximately 10 per cent of children under the age of five.[82] Spinal location has been known to cause unexplained backache and painful scoliosis in children and adults.[26, 55, 68]

The rare localization of lesions close to articular surfaces may result in the presenting clinical symptoms of synovitis and concomitant pathologic changes in the joint surfaces and synovial tissues (hypertrophic degenerative arthritis), as demonstrated by Sherman.[100] Intracapsular, para-articular lesions, especially in the elbow joint area, may be mistaken for a tuberculous synovitis,[61] with regional osteoporosis or rheumatoid arthritis[70] The inflammatory and degenerative changes may resolve after the removal of the osteoid osteoma, depending on whether the removal of the nidus has been considerably delayed.[44] Marked hyperostotic reaction in adjacent bones may be seen.[77, 79]

In the approximately 50 to 60 cases reported in the literature to occur in the vertebral column,[8, 26, 68] the fact that plain films of routine roentgenograms usually do not demonstrate the lesion stands out. Laminagrams, or even angiograms, may be required to accurately pinpoint the nidus or to better delineate the extent of sclerosis. This is especially important when the posterior elements of the vertebrae are affected in order to avoid removal of normal bone.[123]

The true incidence in the skull is difficult to ascertain. If one accepts the Jaffe and Lichtenstein concept that osteoma is a developmental end stage of osteoid osteoma,[50] the number of lesions in that location increases considerably. Notwithstand-

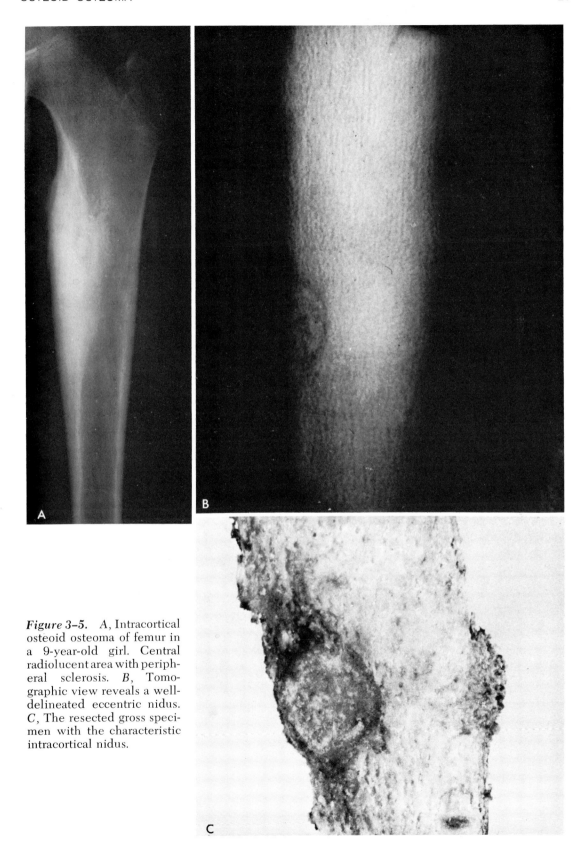

Figure 3–5. A, Intracortical osteoid osteoma of femur in a 9-year-old girl. Central radiolucent area with peripheral sclerosis. B, Tomographic view reveals a well-delineated eccentric nidus. C, The resected gross specimen with the characteristic intracortical nidus.

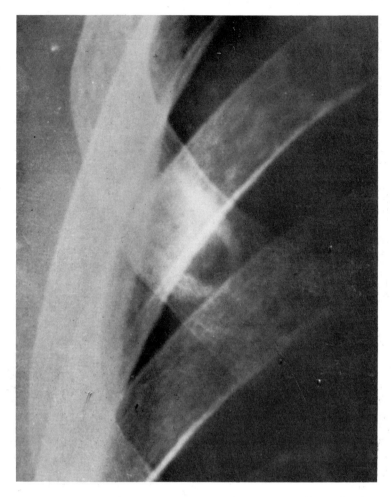

Figure 3–6. An unusual osteoid osteoma in the left third rib in a 43-year-old man. An oval, well-circumscribed, radiolucent lesion is seen with peripheral zone of dense sclerosis.

ing this, several well-documented examples of osteoid osteoma appear in the literature.[15, 81, 91] Multifocal but monostotic osteoid osteoma has been reported on several occasions.[30, 35, 119] The lesion may occur in adjacent bones (the ulna and radius).[83]

RADIOGRAPHIC FEATURES

The roentgenographic presentation provides the single most reliable diagnostic guide. When the osteoid osteoma arises in the spongiosa, the surrounding rim of spongy bone, which is of variable thickness, becomes densely sclerotic (Fig. 3–7). If the lesion develops in the cortex, the adjacent cortical bone becomes strikingly thickened by periosteal new bone formation (Fig. 3–5A).

The radiologic interpretation should account not only for the nestlike central lesion but also for the surrounding perifocal sclerotic area. The nidus proper is indicated by a radiolucent rarefied area that on subsequent maturation, i.e., deposition of well-calcified bone, becomes relatively radiopaque (Fig. 3–5B). In cases in which the cortical bone reaction becomes exuberant, the radiologic search for the nidus becomes difficult, since the cortical thickening overshadows and obscures the underlying lesion. It should be remembered that even the smallest nidus can incite excessive perilesional osseous changes. Experience has shown that by overpenetration with increased kilovoltage, the use of the Bucky diaphragm and radiographs in various oblique and tangential planes with a cone may be of help in recognizing the lesion.

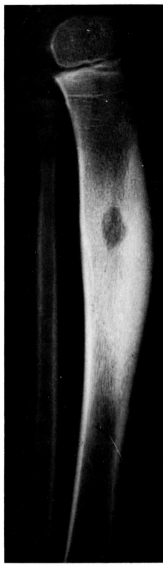

Figure 3–7. Typical osteoid osteoma located in the spongiosa of the left tibia in a 2½-year-old boy.

On radiographic examination, the nidus is most often homogeneously radiolucent, but cortical location occasionally produces a radiopaque center with a ringlike band of radiolucent zone ("ring sequestrum").

The great practical value of scintigraphic detection of osteoid osteoma has been well demonstrated in several case reports.[124] The use of angiography in the detection of osteoid osteoma may also result in improved recognition of the nidus. With this process, it is possible to demonstrate the appearance of a small blood vessel with an irregular lumen at the site of the actual lesion. The area of bone is highly vascularized with an intensely hypervascular, homogeneous circumscribed blush appearing in the arterial phase and persisting late into the venous phase.[65, 84, 113] This should aid in distinguishing it from an abscess. The osteolytic area in an abscess represents necrotic, nonviable tissue, hence no increased vascularity is expected. In small lesions or in lesions with excessive reaction perifocal bone formation, photographic subtraction may be of use.[60]

Intra-articular osteoid osteomas are often difficult to detect, since they do not have the classic clinical and radiographic features seen in extra-articular locations. In such locations, these lesions may present scanty bone sclerosis and the nidus may remain unrecognized radiographically. In this specific instance, an arteriogram would be of ideal use.[39]

The radiographic appearance of the nidus closely corresponds to histologic findings. If, in the center of the nidus, the irregularly calcified osseous tissue predominates, the lesion appears to be denser than normal bone and is more radiopaque. If the central portion of the nidus contains more nonmineralized osteoid tissue, a radiolucent nidus will result. The radiographic appearance of the so-called "annular sequestrum" is depicted by a centrally located nonmineralized osteoid material concentrically alternating with a densely calcified osseous tissue rim followed by a peripheral zone of an osteoid-containing tissue.

The radiographic differential diagnosis of an osteoid osteoma arising in the spongy areas of bone should include chronic osteomyelitis with a bone abscess or an annular, ring sequestrum formation, depending on the degree to which the osteoid osteoma has been ossified (Fig. 3–8). The rarefied and distinct area of cortical shadow with only slight cortical thickening, a common picture in a shaft location, usually elicits a diagnosis of a nonsuppurative osteomyelitis of Garré's type or a chronic intracortical bone abscess (Brodie's abscess).[6] It has been emphasized that distinguishing a stress fracture in the tibia from an osteoid osteoma may present a most difficult diagnostic problem.[84]

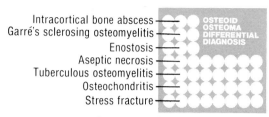

Intracortical bone abscess
Garré's sclerosing osteomyelitis
Enostosis
Aseptic necrosis
Tuberculous osteomyelitis
Osteochondritis
Stress fracture

Figure 3–8. Radiographic differential diagnosis in osteoid osteoma.

On roentgenographic examination, sclerosing osteogenic sarcoma may have at least a superficial resemblance to osteoid osteoma,[13] and accordingly, several cases have been referred to our hospital with that diagnosis. The reparative healing phase of so-called subperiosteal greenstick fracture, not discovered at the time of occurrence, may simulate osteoid osteoma fairly closely, but the perinidal focal radiolucent area, which is characteristic for osteoid osteoma, is conspicuously absent in osteogenic sarcomas and fractures. Occasionally, on a routine skeletal survey in entirely asymptomatic patients, one may find a solitary nidus-like core representing an enostosis (bone spot, bone island) originating in the spongiosa, probably due to a developmental anomaly.[107] Histologically, these enostoses are merely compressed trabeculae of normal spongy bone. Similar histologic characteristics are seen in the multiple compact islands of bone in osteopoikilosis.

The diagnostic difficulties include the following: (1) A nidus beneath articular cartilage, especially at the distal end of the femur or the proximal end of the tibia when the lesion is usually misinterpreted as an osteochondritis dissecans. (2) A nidus within transverse process or lamina of vertebral body (spot films, laminagrams, and tomograms may be required).

PATHOLOGIC FEATURES

Grossly, the osteoid osteoma nidus may appear entirely within the cortex, it may straddle the inner surface of the cortex, or it may be located completely in the spongiosa (Fig. 3–9). Most often, its configuration varies from oval to globular, with clear and distinct delimitation from the adjacent osseous tissue. The color and consistency vary considerably and do not always mirror the maturity of the lesion. Usually, the lesion is brownish-red and mottled, with granular, gritty consistency.

Histologically, the nidus is surrounded by thickened cortical bone (Fig. 3–10). The lesional tissue is characterized by varying intermixtures of osteoid, newly formed bone and highly vascular support-

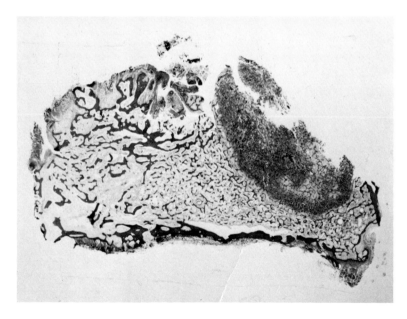

Figure 3–9. Photomicrograph showing an osteoid osteoma nidus in its cortical setting. (Hematoxylin-eosin stain. Magnification × 10.)

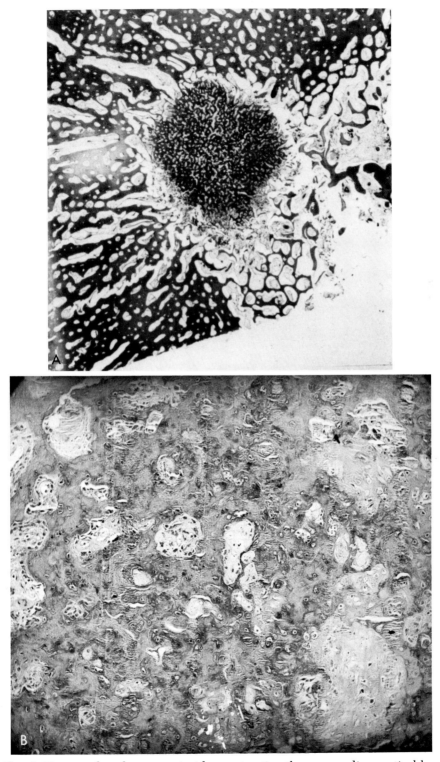

Figure 3–10. A, Topography of a compact nidus contrasting the surrounding cortical bone. (Hematoxylin-eosin stain. Magnification ×10.) B, Typical microscopic picture of an osteoid osteoma nidus. (Hematoxylin-eosin stain. Magnification ×100.)

ing osseous tissue. The osteoid may appear in broad sheets in some areas or may present bony trabeculae in the process of calcification or ossification. In some lesions, on the other hand, thin, newly formed bone dominates the histologic picture, with only a minor component of osteoid being present. Osteoclastic activity is readily apparent.

Three evolutionary stages of nidification can be ascertained, and the developmental phase of the lesion can thereby be approximated.[46, 56] It must be emphasized that the clinical symptomatology in no way corresponds to the various histologic phases. The *initial stage* is characterized by actively proliferating, densely packed, prominent osteoblasts in a background of highly vascularized stroma. This picture changes imperceptibly into an *intermediate phase* in which intercellular substance (osteoid) is deposited between the osteoblasts. The patches of intercellular osteoid and osteoid trabeculae show various degrees of calcification. This is the most characteristic phase of the evolution. In the *mature or osteoma stage*, the osteoid becomes well-calcified, compact trabeculae of atypical bone, which is histologically atypical since it is neither typically woven nor lamellar.

Electron-microscopic Appearance

Only a few reports deal with the ultrastructural aspects of osteoid osteoma.[16, 42, 112] These studies reveal the osteoblasts present to be basically similar to those in normal osteogenesis, with only minor variations. The osteoclasts and osteocytes in the nidus also resemble their normal counterparts. No morphologic differences were found in cells or cellular components of osteoid osteoma or osteoblastoma.[112] Two authors recognized virus-like particles in one case.[16] Ultrastructural and histologic studies show evidence of rapidly progressing bone formation on one side and forceful bone destruction on the other side focused in a relatively small volume of nidus. The osteoclastic resorption of bone is elicited by cells that have a marked aversion to osteoid.[52, 112]

In about 10 to 15 per cent of the cases, even in the best of circumstances, microscopic confirmation of a nidus cannot be secured. The reasons may be multifold. One reason may be that, at the time of operation, the lesion lacks the characteristic reddish-brown to cherry red color. It should be emphasized that every piece of tissue removed in the operating room should be examined microscopically. A better evaluation and orientation of the removed bone chips can be obtained if they are examined radiographically, and the nidus can then be readily identified.

Giant osteoid osteoma is an ill-chosen term in that it is applied to what is really a benign osteoblastoma and not an osteoid osteoma.[14] Since several osteoid osteomas larger than 1 cm (up to 6 cm in dimension) have now been diagnosed and described, the epithet "giant" blurs the differences between these two entities, especially as benign osteoblastomas may, in fact, be small (1 to 2 cm size range). As will be stated later, osteoid osteoma differs from benign osteoblastoma in that it has broader, longer, and more widely separated osteoid trabeculae; is generally less cellular and less vascular; and contains less abundant osteoblasts.[46, 47, 48, 50, 51]

PATHOGENESIS

The pathogenesis of this lesion still remains controversial, and some believe it to be a neoplasm or to arise on an inflammatory basis or to represent an unusual healing and reparative process. Whether it is a true neoplasm is also questioned, since it has a self-limiting growth potential (usually small size). The histologic appearance is usually independent of its duration, and there is a puzzling perifocal marginal bone sclerosis at a considerable distance from the center of the lesion. Contrary to typical neoplasms, the nidus contains a relatively immature central area with more mature calcified bone at the periphery. All of these aspects make the evolution very unlike a true neoplasm.

The author is in basic agreement with the opinion of James Ewing concerning pathogenesis, which the latter stated in a letter dated April 12, 1940, to Jaffe.

I find it somewhat difficult to interpret the process which you designate as osteoid-osteoma. The lesion is specific and peculiar.

There are several features which favor the interpretation as a neoplasm. The process is circumscribed and independent of the surrounding tissue hypertrophy. It has its own blood supply in the form of numerous dilated venous sinuses. The new growth of osteoid tissue is excessive and somewhat atypical. The cells from which the new bone is developed are hyperchromatic and atypical, and they are overnumerous. There are no definite traces of any strictly inflammatory process, no old blood pigment, no leukocytes, no remnants of old pus, and no old necrotic debris. On the basis of these features one is justified in regarding the process as a form of neoplasia. I cannot understand how such a process can result from infectious osteomyelitis.

Recently, vascular origin has been theorized.[33, 84]

The majority of the cases can be categorized by clinical, radiologic, and pathologic features, but some cases present difficulties at classification. These lesions are larger than 1 cm, growing in long bones associated with abundant reactive bone formation. Some, like Flaherty and his associates,[23] believe that osteoblastomas represent overgrown osteoid osteomas, while others, such as Lichtenstein,[64] regard these as special forms of osteoid osteomas.

In 1963, Marcove and Alpert[69] studied fifteen benign osteoblastomas and found definite histologic characteristics to differentiate an osteoblastoma from an osteoid osteoma nidus. Accordingly, type A osseous tissue in an osteoblastoma is char-

acterized by thin, small irregular spicules of cellular woven bone with an abundant fibrous stroma widely separating the spicules. Type B tumor tissue, in contrast, displays wide, smoothly contoured trabeculae of bone with a tendency toward maturation. Only a sparse fibrous stroma is present, with adjacent large bony masses. In their opinion, an osteoid osteoma nidus contains one type of osseous tissue (either type A or type B) and only very rarely (about 10 per cent) has both tumor tissue types. (See the description of type A and type B osseous tissues in Chapter 4, p. 42.) The nidus will also reveal less mature bone, increased numbers of osteocytes, and decreased numbers of cement lines, in contradistinction to the type B tissue of osteoblastoma. Osteoid osteoma, in addition, shows no tendency for progressive deposition of compact tumor bone, even after long periods of observation.

Based primarily on clinical and radiologic differences, and also on some histologic distinctions, it is well worth keeping osteoid osteomas and osteoblastomas as separate entities. Since 1970, because there are occasional borderline or overlapping cases in which definite, dogmatic differentiation is well nigh impossible, attempts have been made to amalgamate these lesions (Table 3–1).[80, 97, 111] These efforts at new classification, however laudable, seem to suffer from cumbersome and confusing terminology, which makes acceptance by all concerned rather doubtful.

TABLE 3–1. Attempts at Reclassification of Benign Osteoblastic Tumors of Bones

Schajowicz and Lemos – 1970	Morton, Vassar, and Knickerbocker – 1975	DeSouza Dias and Frost – 1974
Circumscribed osteoblastoma (formerly osteoid osteoma; nidus less than 2 cm) 1. Cortical, sclerosing 2. Medullary, cancellous 3. Periosteal	Circumscribed osteoblastoma 1. Cortical 2. Medullary 3. Periosteal	Cortical osteoblastoma
Genuine osteoblastoma (formerly benign osteoblastoma; nidus larger than 2 cm) 1. Cortical, sclerosing 2. Medullary, cancellous 3. Periosteal	Genuine osteoblastoma 1. Cortical 2. Medullary 3. Periosteal	Spongious osteoblastoma
Multifocal osteoblastoma 1. Medullary 2. Peripheral	Multifocal osteoblastoma 1. Medullary 2. Peripheral	Multifocal osteoblastoma
		Periosteal osteoblastoma

TREATMENT AND PROGNOSIS

Mayer's Method of Localizing Osteoid Osteoma

The center of the surgical incision, carefully measured before operation, should correspond with the radiographically demonstrated area of focal bone thickening.[73] To be absolutely certain of the exact location, a drill hole, or holes, can also be made and an intraoperative roentgen verification can be obtained. The deepest portion of the osseous incision should correspond to the nidus. Surgical excision of the thickened overlying cortical bone usually reveals the nidus, the removal of which should be accompanied by curettage of the immediately adjacent sclerotic bone to avoid recurrence of symptoms.

In the quest for the elusive nidus, if the lesion is located superficially in the cortex, the surgeon is helped by a surface cortical roughening that signals the presence of an underlying lesion. X-ray control during the operative procedure is mandatory, especially in those instances in which the nidus cannot be recognized preoperatively.

In most instances, removal of the inner nest of osteoid osteoma with thorough curettage of the perilesional bone will yield a cure. In other cases intact excision of the nidus *en bloc* with adjacent bone, especially in lesions located in the cortical shaft, is strongly indicated.[88] Wide *en bloc* resection with removal of surrounding sclerotic bone permits thorough pathologic and radiologic study of the specimen, facilitating the identification of the nidus. Even if the surgeon misses the nidus and removes only adjacent segments of sclerotic bone, symptoms may be ameliorated or even completely alleviated if the overlying bony cortex is unroofed and the nidus is exposed.[78] Closing of the wound in layers without drainage is emphasized for good results.[13, 73] For those rare lesions that occur in a vertebral body, irradiation may be indicated.

Recurrence of an adequately treated osteoid osteoma is seldom reported but was noted by Jaffe[48] 13 years after radical removal and by Dunlop and his coworkers,[21] whose case recurred twice after *en bloc* excision. Other instances of recurrent le-

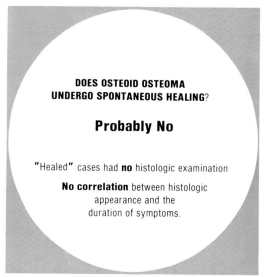

Figure 3–11. Is there spontaneous regression of osteoid osteoma?

sions, especially following curettage, have also been encountered.[27, 33, 88, 106]

Spontaneous regression of untreated osteoid osteomas has been reported, although no histologic confirmation was obtained in many of the cases (Fig. 3–11).[3, 65, 76, 77, 92, 120] Such spontaneous re-

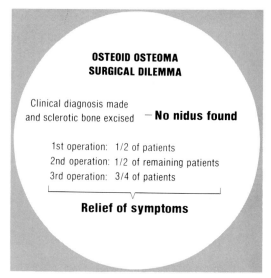

Figure 3–12. Surgical dilemma when no nidus is identified at exploration. (From Sim, F. H., Dahlin, D. C., and Beabout, J. W.: Osteoid-osteoma: diagnostic problems. J. Bone Joint Surg. [Am.], 57:154–159, 1975.)

gression has also been postulated based on the observation that osteoid osteoma is extremely rare after the age of 30 years.[101]

What happens to patients who have characteristic clinical signs and symptoms and distinctive roentgenographic features of an osteoid osteoma but in whom the subsequent surgical exploration and the pathologic identification of the nidus are not accomplished?[106] This dilemma and the ultimate fate of patients are described in Figure 3–12.

Osteoid osteoma may present a baffling diagnostic problem because the clinical symptoms, especially pain, may appear long before the characteristic roentgenographic findings become evident, and many months may pass before a definite diagnosis is made. It behooves the primary care physician to further investigate any unexplained persistent pain in a child or young adult in order to rule out the diagnosis of an osteoid osteoma.[115] Unfortunately, several patients have been labeled as malingerers or psychoneurotic and unnecessarily referred for psychiatric consultations in search of the etiological agents of their pain.[104]

REFERENCES

1. Belding, R. H., Thompson, J. D., Jr., and Hay, E. L.: Osteoid osteoma: a cause of monoarticular joint pain. Three case reports. J. S. C. Med. Assoc., 72:343–345, 1976.
2. Benjamins, C. E.: Das Osteoid-Fibrom mit atypischer Verkalkung in Sinus frontalis. Acta Otolaryngol., 26:26, 1938.
3. Bergstrand, H.: Über eine eigenartige, wahrscheinlich bisher nicht beschriebene osteoblastische Krankheit in den langen Knochen der Hand und des Fusses. Acta Radiol., 11:596–612, 1930.
4. Blair, W. F., and Kube, W. J.: Osteoid osteoma in a distal radial epiphysis. Case report. Clin. Orthop., 126:160–161, 1977.
5. Bordelon, R. L., Cracco, A., and Book, M. K.: Osteoid-osteoma producing premature fusion of the epiphysis of the distal phalanx of the big toe. J. Bone Joint Surg. [Am.], 57:120–121, 1975.
6. Brailsford, J. F.: Chronic sub-periosteal abscess. Br. J. Radiol., 15:313–317, 1942.
7. Byers, P. D.: Solitary benign osteoblastic lesions of bone. Osteoid osteoma and benign osteoblastoma. Cancer, 22:43–57, 1968.
8. Caldicott, W. J. H.: Diagnosis of spinal osteoid osteoma. Radiology, 92:1192–1195, 1969.
9. Campos, O. P.: Osteoid-osteoma of cervical spinous process. Report of a case. J. Internat. Coll. Surgeons, 9:112–115, 129, 1946.
10. Candiani, A.: Contributo anatomo-clinico alla conoscenza dell'osteoma-osteoide (Riassunto). Acta Chir. Patavina, 9:110–111, 1953.
11. Carroll, R. E.: Osteoid osteoma in the hand. J. Bone Joint Surg. [Am.], 35:888–893, 1953.
12. Ciccone, W. J.: Osteoid osteoma. A rare occurrence in the carpal navicular. Rocky Mt. Med. J., 73:325–327, 1976.
13. Coley, B. L., and Lenson, N.: Osteoid osteoma. Am. J. Surg., 77:3–9, 1949.
14. Dahlin, D. C., and Johnson, E. W.: Giant osteoid osteoma. J. Bone Joint Surg. [Am.] 36:559–572, 1954.
15. Daly, J. G.: Osteoid osteoma of the skull. Br. J. Radiol., 46:392–393, 1973.
16. De Giuli, C., and Frontino, G.: Rilievo al microscopio elettronico di particolari strutture endocellulari in un caso di osteoma osteoide. Arch. Ital. Patol. Clin. Tumori, 11:35–51, 1968.
17. De Santis, E., and Luppino, D.: Contributo allo studio dell'osteoma osteoide. Riv. Anat. Patol. Oncol., 36:52–76, 1970.
18. De Wet, I. S.: Osteoid osteomata. Review of the literature with a report of five cases. S. Afr. J. Surg., 5:13–24, 1967.
19. Döge, H., Schadeberg, A., and Widera, A.: Das Osteoidosteom und seiner Differentialdiagnose. Zentralbl. Chir., 97:1728–1733, 1972.
20. Dumler, B., and Haussmann, P.: Osteoid osteoma involving bones of the hand. Single observation on the middle finger basal phalanx. Handchirurgie, 9:41–42, 1977.
21. Dunlop, J. A. Y., Morton, K. S., and Elliott, G. B.: Recurrent osteoid osteoma. Report of a case with a review of the literature. J. Bone Joint Surg. [Br.], 52:128–133, 1970.
22. Edeiken, J., DePalma, A. F., and Hodes, P. J.: Osteoid osteoma (roentgenographic emphasis). Clin. Orthop., 49:201–206, 1966.
23. Flaherty, R. A., Pugh, D. G., and Dockerty, M. B.: Osteoid osteoma. Am. J. Roentgenol. Radium Ther. Nucl. Med., 76: 1041–1051, 1956.
24. Foss, E. L., Dockerty, M. B., and Good, C. A.: Osteoid osteoma of the mandible. Report of a case. Cancer, 8:592–594, 1955.
25. Fowles, S. J.: Osteoid osteoma. Br. J. Radiol., 37:245–252, 1964.
26. Freiberger, R. H.: Osteoid osteoma of the spine. A cause of backache and scoliosis in children and young adults. Radiology, 75:232–236, 1960.
27. Freiberger, R. H., Loitman, B. S., Helpern, M., et al.: Osteoid osteoma: a report on 80 cases. Am. J. Roentgenol. Radium Ther. Nucl. Med., 82:194–205, 1959.
28. Galway, R., Bobechko, W. P., and Heslin, J.: Osteoid osteoma in childhood. Abstract. J. Bone Joint Surg. [Br.], 51:196, 1969.
29. Giustra, P. E., and Freiberger, R. H.: Severe growth disturbance with osteoid osteoma. Radiology, 96:285–288, 1970.
30. Glynn, J. J. and Lichtenstein, L.: Osteoid osteoma with multicentric nidus. A report of 2 cases. J. Bone Joint Surg. [Am.], 55:855–858, 1973.

31. Goidanich, I. F., and Zanasi, R.: Osteoma osteoide ed osteomielite sclerosante: due entita cliniche definite e distinte. Chir. Organi Mov., 43:427–460, 1956.

32. Goldenberg, R. R.: Osteoid-osteoma. J. Med. Soc. N. J., 45:104–107, 1948.

33. Golding, J. S. R.: The natural history of osteoid osteoma: with a report of 20 cases. J. Bone Joint Surg. [Br.], 36:218–229, 1954.

34. Greene, G. W., Jr., Natiella, J. R., and Spring, P. N., Jr.: Osteoid osteoma of the jaws. Report of a case. Oral Surg., 26:342–351, 1968.

35. Greenspan, A., Elguezabel, A., and Bryk, D.: Multifocal osteoid osteoma. A case report and review of the literature. Am. J. Roentgenol. Radium Ther. Nucl. Med., 121:103–106, 1974.

36. Grundberg, A. B.: Osteoid osteoma of the thumb: report of a case. J. Hand Surg., 2:266, 1977.

37. Gschnitzer, F., and de Gennaro, P. F.: Das Osteoid-Osteom. Z. Orthop., 86:1–14, 1955.

38. Habermann, E. T., and Stern, R. E.: Osteoid-osteoma of the tibia in an eight-month-old boy. A case report. J. Bone Joint Surg. [Am.], 56:633–636, 1974.

39. Halpern, M., and Freiberger, R. H.: Arteriography as a diagnostic procedure in bone disease. Radiol. Clin. North Am., 8:277–288, 1970.

40. Heiman, M. L., Cooley, C. J., and Bradford, D. S.: Osteoid osteoma of a vertebral body. Report of a case with extension across the intervertebral disk. Clin. Orthop., 118:159–163, 1976.

41. Heine, J.: Einheilender Knochensequester an der Grundphalanx des rechten Ringfingers. Arch Klin. Chir., 146:737–753, 1927.

42. Hirohata, K., and Morimoto, K.: Ultrastructure of Bone and Joint Diseases. New York, Grune & Stratton, Inc. (Igaku Shoin Ltd.), 1971.

43. Hitzrot, J. M.: Sclerosing osteomyelitis of carpal scaphoid. Ann. Surg., 91:450–452, 1930.

44. Jackson, I. J.: Osteoid osteoma of the lamina and its treatment. Am. Surg., 19:17–23, 1953.

45. Jacobs, B., and Goldberg, V.: Osteoid osteoma about the hip in children. Abstract. J. Bone Joint Surg. [Am.],53:1029, 1971.

46. Jaffe, H. L.: "Osteoid-osteoma." A benign osteoblastic tumor composed of osteoid and atypical bone. Arch. Surg., 31:709–728, 1935.

47. Jaffe, H. L.: Osteoid-osteoma of bone. Radiology, 45:319–334, 1945.

48. Jaffe, H. L.: Osteoid-osteoma. Proc. R. Soc. Med., 46:1007–1012, 1953.

49. Jaffe, H. L.: Benign osteoblastoma. Bull. Hosp. Joint Dis., 17:141–151, 1956.

50. Jaffe, H. L., and Lichtenstein, L.: Osteoid osteoma: further experience with this benign tumor of bone. With special reference to cases showing the lesion in relation to shaft cortices and commonly misclassified as instances of sclerosing nonsuppurative osteomyelitis or cortical bone abscess. J. Bone Joint Surg., 22:645–682, 1940.

51. Jaffe, H. L., and Mayer, L.: An osteoblastic osteoid tissue-forming tumor of a metacarpal bone. Arch. Surg., 24:550–564, 1932.

52. Johnston, A. D.: Clinical problems in osteoid-osteoma. Evidence of osteoclastic aversion to osteoid. Bull. Hosp. Joint Dis., 23:80–94, 1962.

53. Jurgens, P. E.: Osteoid osteoma of the mandible: report of a case. J. Oral Surg., 26:129–132, 1968.

54. Kaye, J. J., and Arnold, W. D.: Osteoid osteomas in siblings. Case reports. Clin. Orthop., 126:273–275, 1977.

55. Keim, H. A., and Reina, E. G.: Osteoid-osteoma as a cause of scoliosis. J. Bone Joint Surg. [Am.], 57:159–163, 1975.

56. Kleinsasser, O., and Nigrisoli, P.: Das sog. Osteoid-Osteom und seine Entwicklungsstadien. Frankf. Z. Pathol., 68:1–10, 1957.

57. Kovalenko, K. N., Bekzadyan, G. R., and Talantov, V. A.: Osteoid osteoma in children. Vopr. Onkol., 20:37–44, 1974.

58. Lapidus, P. W., and Salem, E. P.: Osteoid osteoma. Report of a case with probably double lesion. Arch. Surg., 58:318–327, 1949.

59. Lawrie, T. R., and Sinclair, A. M.: Painless osteoid osteoma. J. Bone Joint Surg. [Am.], 52:1357–1363, 1970.

60. Lechner, G., Riedl, P., Knahr, K., et al.: Das angiographische Bild des Osteoid-Osteoms. Fortschr. Geb. Roentgenstr. Nuklearmed., 122:323—326, 1975.

61. Leonessa, C., and Savoini, E.: Osteoma osteoide paraarticolare del gomito. Chir. Organi Mov., 59:487–492, 1971.

62. Lester, P. D.: Osteoid osteoma. Letter to the editor. J. A. M. A., 218:741, 1971.

63. Levi-Valensin, G., Bernageau, J., Guérin, Cl., et al.: Ostéome ostéoïde. Problèms actuels. J. Radiol. Electrol. Med. Nucl., 57:640–642, 1976.

64. Lichtenstein, L.: Bone Tumors. 4th ed. St. Louis, C. V. Mosby Co., 1972.

65. Lindbom, A., Lindvall, N., Soderberg, G., et al.: Angiography in osteoid osteoma. Acta Radiol., 15:327–333, 1960.

66. Lloyd-Roberts, G. C.: Regional osteoporosis in osteoid osteoma. J. Bone Joint Surg. [Br.], 43:501–507, 1961.

67. Lofgren, L.: Osteoid-osteoma. Acta Chir. Scand., 104:383–404, 1953.

68. MacLellan, D. I., and Wilson, F. C., Jr.: Osteoid osteoma of the spine. J. Bone Joint Surg. [Am.], 49:111–121, 1967.

69. Marcove, R. C., and Alpert, M.: A pathologic study of benign osteoblastoma. Clin. Orthop., 30:175–181, 1963.

70. Marcove, R. C., and Freiberger, R. H.: Osteoid osteoma of the elbow—a diagnostic problem. Report of four cases. J. Bone Joint Surg. [Am.], 48:1185–1190, 1966.

71. Marzagalli, G.: Osteoma osteoide della 2ª vertebra lombare. Arch. Med. Chir., 7:505–511, 1938.

72. Mauer, I.: Osteoid osteoma of the 12th rib. Resection under local anesthesia. A case report. Milit. Med., 122:194, 1958.

73. Mayer, L.: The surgery of osteoid osteoma. Bull. Hosp. Joint Dis., 12:174–210, 1951.

74. Mazabraud, A.: Remarque à propos de l'ostéome ostéoïde et de l'ostéoblastome. Ann. Anat. Pathol. (Paris), 17:177–186, 1972.

75. McKeever, F. M.: Osteoid-osteoma. West. J. Surg., 58:213–218, 1950.

76. Moberg, E.: The natural course of osteoid osteoma. J. Bone Joint Surg. [Am.], 33:166–170, 1951.

77. Moberg, E.: Further observations on "corticalis-osteoide" or "osteoid osteoma." Acta Radiol., 38:279–293, 1952.

78. Morrison, G. M., Hawes, L. E., and Sacco, J. J.: Incomplete removal of osteoid-osteoma. Am. J. Surg., 80:476–481, 1950.

79. Morton, K. S., and Bartlett, L. H.: Benign osteoblastic change resembling osteoid osteoma. J. Bone Joint Surg. [Br.], 48:478–484, 1966.

80. Morton, K. S., Vassar, P. S., and Knickerbocker, W. J.: Osteoid osteoma and osteoblastoma: Reclassification of 43 cases using Schajowicz's classification. Can. J. Surg., 18:148–152, 1975.

81. Munk, J. E., Peyser, E., and Gellei, B.: Osteoid osteoma of frontal bone. Br. J. Radiol., 33:328–330, 1960.

82. Norman, A., and Dorfman, H. D.: Osteoid-osteoma inducing pronounced overgrowth and deformity of bone. Clin. Orthop., 110:233–238, 1975.

83. O'Dell, C. W., Jr., Resnick, D., Niwayama, G., et al.: Osteoid osteomas arising in adjacent bones: report of a case. J. Can. Assoc. Radiol., 27:298–300, 1976.

84. O'Hara, J. P., Tegtmeyer, C., Sweet, D. E., et al.: Angiography in the diagnosis of osteoid-osteoma of the hand. J. Bone Joint Surg. [Am.], 57:163–166, 1975.

85. Osteoid osteoma. Editorial. Br. Med. J., 3:395–396, 1975.

86. Paus, B. C., and Kim, T. K.: Osteoid osteoma of the spine. Acta Orthop. Scand., 33:24–29, 1963.

87. Pines, B., Lavine, L., and Grayzel, D. M.: Osteoid osteoma: etiology and pathogensis. Report of twelve new cases. J. Internat. Coll. Surgeons, 13:249–277, 1950.

88. Ponseti, I., and Barta, C. K.: Osteoid osteoma. J. Bone Joint Surg., 29:767–776, 1947.

89. Poulsen, J. O.: Osteoid osteoma. Acta Orthop. Scand., 40:198–204, 1969.

90. Powers, R. C.: Osteoid osteoma of the ulna in a Negro child. Clin. Orthop., 118:157–158, 1976.

91. Prabhakar, B., Reddy, D. R., Dayananda, B., et al.: Osteoid osteoma of the skull. J. Bone Joint Surg. [Br.], 54:146–148, 1972.

92. Pritchard, J. E., and McKay, J. W.: Osteoid osteoma. Can. Med. Assoc. J., 58:567–575, 1948.

93. Reinhardt, K.: Osteoid-Osteom im Os parietale. Fortschr. Geb. Roentgenstr. Nuklearmed., 116:563–565, 1972.

94. Rosborough, D.: Osteoid osteoma. Report of a lesion in the terminal phalanx of a finger. J. Bone Joint Surg. [Br.], 48:485–487, 1966.

95. Rushton, J. G., Mulder, D. W., and Lipscomb, P. R.: Neurologic symptoms with osteoid osteoma. Neurology, 5:794–797, 1955.

96. Sabanas, A. O., Bickel, W. H., and Moe, J. H.: Natural history of osteoid osteoma of the spine. Am. J. Surg., 91:880–889, 1956.

97. Schajowicz, F., and Lemos, C.: Osteoid osteoma and osteoblastoma. Closely related entities of osteoblastic derivation. Acta Orthop. Scand., 41:272–291, 1970.

98. Schulman, L., and Dorfman, H. D.: Nerve fibers in osteoid osteoma. J. Bone Joint Surg. [Am.], 52:1351–1356, 1970.

99. Sevitt, S., and Horn, J. S.: A painless and calcified osteoid osteoma of the little finger. J. Pathol., 67:571–574, 1954.

100. Sherman, M. S.: Osteoid osteoma associated with changes in adjacent joint. J. Bone Joint Surg., 29:483–490, 1947.

101. Sherman, M. S.: Osteoid osteoma. Review of the literature and report of thirty cases. J. Bone Joint Surg., 29:918–930, 1947.

102. Sherman, M. S., and McFarland, G., Jr.: Mechanism of pain in osteoid osteomas. South. Med. J., 58:163–166, 1965.

103. Shifrin, L. Z., and Reynolds, W. A.: Intra-articular osteoid osteoma of the elbow. A case report. Clin. Orthop., 81:126–129, 1971.

104. Silberman, W. W.: Osteoid osteoma. J. Internat. Coll. Surgeons, 38:53–66, 1962.

105. Sim, F. H., Dahlin, D. C., and Beabout, J. W.: Lesions which simulate osteoid-osteoma. Abstract. J. Bone Joint Surg. [Am.], 56:1541, 1974.

106. Sim, F. H., Dahlin, D. C., and Beabout, J. W.: Osteoid-osteoma: diagnostic problems. J. Bone Joint Surg. [Am.], 57:154–159, 1975.

107. Smith, J.: Giant bone islands. Radiology, 107:35–36, 1973.

108. Snarr, J. W., Abell, M. R., and Martel, W.: Lymphofollicular synovitis with osteoid osteoma. Radiology, 106:557–560, 1973.

109. Sobel, R.: Osteoid-osteoma: report of 2 cases and review of pertinent literature. Bull. Hosp. Joint Dis., 7:94–98, 1946.

110. Soukup, P. and Näkel, G.: Osteoid-Osteom des Os naviculare der Hand—eine Kasuistik. Beitr. Orthop. Traumatol., 24:131–133, 1977.

111. de Souza Dias, L., and Frost, H. M.: Osteoid osteoma—osteoblastoma. Cancer, 33:1075–1081, 1974.

112. Steiner, G. C.: Ultrastructure of osteoid osteoma. Hum. Pathol., 7:309–325, 1976.

113. Sullivan, M.: Osteoid osteoma of the fingers. Hand, 3:175–178, 1971.

114. Symeonides, P. P.: Osteoid osteoma of the lumbar spine. South. Med. J., 63:975–976, 1970.

115. Szepesi, K., Vizkelety, T. and Csato, Z.: Differential-diagnostische Probleme des osteoiden Osteoms im Kindesalter. Arch. Orthop. Unfallchir., 73:308–315, 1972.

116. Tavernier, L., Guilleminet, M., and Faysse, R.: Sur une forme speciale d'ostéome ostéoide à point de départ cortical et à évolution paraosseuse: l'ostéome ostéoide à forme exostosante. Lyon Chir., 45:133–144, 1950.

117. Toman, J.: To the occurrence of the osteoid osteoma in the jaws. Czas. Stomatol., 65.98–108, 1965.

118. Toth, S. P.: Bone cyst, osteoid-osteoma. A case report. J. Am. Podiatry Assoc., 60:404–406, 1970.

119. Uehlinger, E.: Multizentrisches Osteoid-Osteom des Tibiaschaftes mit atypischem Röntgenbild. Arch. Orthop. Unfallchir., 89:101–107, 1977.

120. Vickers, C. W., Pugh, D. C., and Ivins, J. C.: Osteoid osteoma. A 15 year follow-up of an

untreated patient. J. Bone Joint Surg. [Am.], *41*:357–358, 1959.

121. Vyhnanek, L.: Osteoma osteoideum. Eine Kasuistik aus dem frühmittelalterlichen Skelettmaterial. Z. Orthop., *109*:922–923, 1971.

122. Wells, C.: A pathological Anglo-Saxon femur. Br. J. Radiol., *38*:393–394, 1965.

123. Wilkinson, R. H.: Osteoid osteoma. Postgrad. Med., *49*:61–62, 1971.

124. Winter, P. F., Johnson, P. M., Hilal, S. K., et al.: Scintigraphic detection of osteoid osteoma. Radiology, *122:177*–178, 1977.

125. Worland, R. L., and Dick, H. M.: Osteoid-osteoma of the radius. Report of a case. Clin. Orthop., *106*:190–191, 1975.

4

OSTEOBLASTOMA

DEFINITION

Osteoblastoma, although histologically related to osteoid osteoma, is a progressively growing lesion of a larger size, is sometimes painful, and is characterized by the absence of any reactive perifocal bone formation.

Some consider progressively enlarging osteoblastic lesions in long bones, when associated with perifocal sclerosis, to be overgrown osteoid osteomas.[28] Others emphasize the close relationship between these two lesions and recommend reclassification to account for the sometimes overlapping radiologic and microscopic features (See Chapter 3, p. 27). Accordingly, in 1970, Schajowicz and Lemos proposed the designation of "osteoblastoma" for both osteoblastoma and osteoid osteoma.[79] The more significant distinguishing features of these two entities are summarized in Table 4-1.

SYNONYMS

1. Osteoblastic osteoid tissue-forming tumor.[45]
2. Spindle-cell variant of giant cell tumor.[33]

TABLE 4-1. Variation in Clinical Presentation, Radiographic Appearance and Microscopic Characteristics in Osteoblastoma and Osteoid Osteoma

	Osteoblastoma	Osteoid Osteoma
Clinical Presentation	Pain inconsistent Lesion >2 cm Rapid increase in size	Pain persistent, nocturnal Lesion 1–2 cm or less Limited growth potential
Radiography	Perifocal osseous reaction is missing or only slight Dense soft tissue mass	Perifocal osseous reaction is constant and marked No soft tissue mass
Histology	Osteoid trabeculae with discontinuous and irregular bone formation Abundant fibrous stromal reaction with many multinucleated osteoblastic giant cells	Osteoid trabeculae with continuous and regular bone formation Scanty stromal reaction Multinucleated osteoblastic giant cells rare

3. Osteogenic fibroma.[54]
4. Giant osteoid osteoma.[19]
5. Benign osteoblastoma.[44, 54]

INCIDENCE, AGE, AND SEX DISTRIBUTION

Benign osteoblastoma is a very uncommon lesion that constitutes about 1 per cent of all primary bone tumors, with approximately 360 cases reported in world literature (Fig. 4–1). In a tally of such reports, the incidence was 2:1 male to female ratio. The average age was 17 years, with the men averaging slightly older (19 years) than the women (15 years). The ages ranged from 3 to 78 years. Nearly 90 per cent of the patients were less than 30 years, and almost 75 per cent of the lesions appeared in the second and third decades of life.[64]

LOCATION

Osteoblastoma most commonly involves the vertebral column (34 per cent), the long bones of the appendicular skeleton (30 per cent), the small bones of the hands and feet (13.5 per cent), as well as the skull,[92] maxilla,[9, 10, 47] and mandible[3, 10, 11, 49] (totaling 14.6 per cent) (Fig. 4–1). Ribs are affected in 4 per cent of the reported cases [64, 76] (Fig. 4–2). The metaphysis and the diaphysis are preferentially, but about equally, implicated.[59] Epiphyseal involvement is rare and usually occurs in the small tubular bones of the hands and feet.[59, 95] Among the small flat bones of the feet, the tumor occurs chiefly on the dorsal aspects of the anterior portion of the talus. Preferential spinal sites are the spinous and transverse processes as well as the neural arches. The vertebral body is only rarely involved primarily but may be the secondary target in anterior tumor extension. The lesions may be intracortical or intramedullary, and their occurrence in these locations in the long tubular bones is equally frequent. As in cases of osteoid osteoma, osteoblastoma can occur in periosteal locations.[38, 47, 55, 79] Multifocal (or multicentric) osteoblastoma has been reported.[36, 65, 79] Since there is considerable overlapping in the diagnosis of osteoid os-

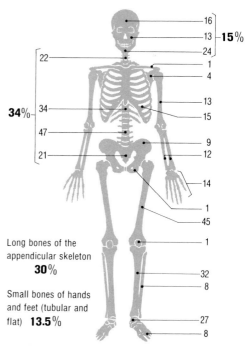

BENIGN OSTEOBLASTOMA
Location in 364 Cases

Long bones of the appendicular skeleton **30%**

Small bones of hands and feet (tubular and flat) **13.5%**

Figure 4–1. Osteoblastoma: Location in 364 cases. (Data culled from the literature.)

teoma and osteoblastoma in the pertinent literature, a number of these cases may be designated by some authors as osteoid osteoma with a multifocal nidus. Although the multifocal involvement is usually monostotic, a few cases have been reported involving two entirely separate bones (e.g., the ethmoid and pubis, as reported by Schajowicz and Lemos[79]). In these multifocal but monostotic cases, the surgical problem of curing the patient becomes quite difficult, since a minute tumor may be overlooked.

SIGNS AND SYMPTOMS

Dull, aching, usually localized pain, often insidiously occurring, is the main complaint. The pain pattern is not that pattern commonly experienced with osteoid osteoma; i.e., it is not nocturnal and is not particularly relieved by salicylates. The duration of pain varies from a few months to as long as two years. Slight local tenderness and palpable swelling of increasing

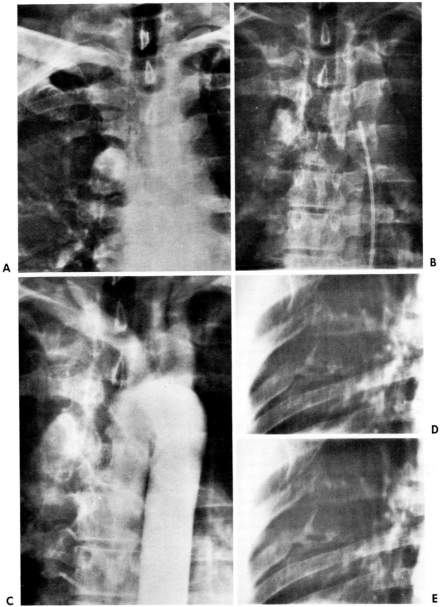

Figure 4–2. Osteoblastoma of fifth rib in a 47-year-old man who had pain of 2½ years duration. *A* and *B*, Radiographs reveal coarsening of the trabeculae of T₅ with poor definition of the transverse process accompanied by slight sclerosis. *C*, Thoracic aortogram shows no tumor staining or abnormal vascularity. *D* and *E*, Tomograms show partially resected fifth and sixth ribs following first attempt at excision.

size may also be noted. Lesions involving the neural arch of the vertebrae produce progressive symptoms of spinal cord and nerve root compression, with paresthesia and muscle weakness culminating in paraplegia. Location of the tumor in the lumbar vertebrae results in pains radiating down the legs associated with muscle spasms and iliolumbar extensor stiffness.[41] Extreme tenderness and swelling are an outstanding feature in mandibular and maxillary presentation but may also be present in other locations.

Scoliosis and muscle spasms appear in patients with spinal tumors. Lesions in the extremities predispose to tissue atrophy and limping. Occasionally, symptomatic cervical vertebrae lesions may be quite small and radiographically undetectable.[53]

RADIOGRAPHIC FEATURES

The radiographic features are not necessarily distinctive; they vary widely, depending on the location of the lesion. In general, the lesions, irrespective of their site or size, are well-circumscribed, radiolucent, and usually quite expansile and may occasionally contain a thin shell of peripheral new bone (Fig. 4–3). On occasion, irregularly mottled radiopacities appear. According to Lichtenstein and Sawyer,[55] if the peripheral sclerosis (pronounced cortical new bone formation) is marked, the lesion should be classified as osteoid osteoma, even if it is quite large. Even in cases in which the expanding lesion stretches the overlying cortex until it is delicately thin, a fine peripheral shell of periosteal new bone is still retained. The

slow rate of tumor expansion elicits a densely sclerotic bone reaction along the inner aspect that may, in turn, obscure the definite delimitation of the lesion. The presence and the extent of intralesional radiopaque granular mottling depends on the degree of focal or diffuse calcification of the osteoid and the conversion of primitive bone (osteoid) into mature bone. The radiologic picture of the lesion in the vertebrae demonstrates a definitely expansile radiolucent growth containing irregularly patchy or granular radiopacities. More often than not, it is well-defined and has a thin shell of bone. In larger tumors, the granular mottled areas coalesce into ill-defined radiopaque fields.

The differential diagnosis of the periosteal type of osteoblastoma includes periosteal osteoma, myositis ossificans, juxtacortical osteogenic sarcoma, and a sessile type of osteochondroma (Fig. 4–4). In those cases, the perifocal bony sclerotic margin is missing and only a thin shell of new periosteal bone is evident. Occasion-

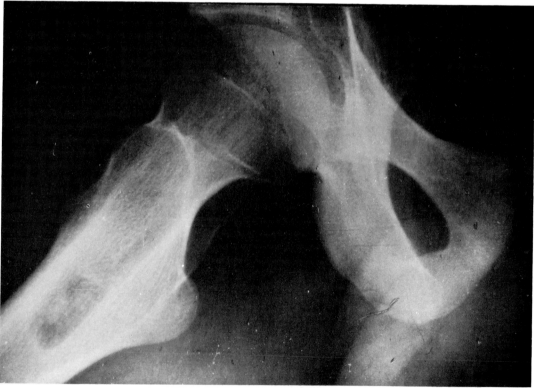

Figure 4–3. Eccentric diaphyseal intramedullary osteoblastoma of femur in a 20-year-old man. The oval lesion is well-delineated, showing intralesional sclerosis.

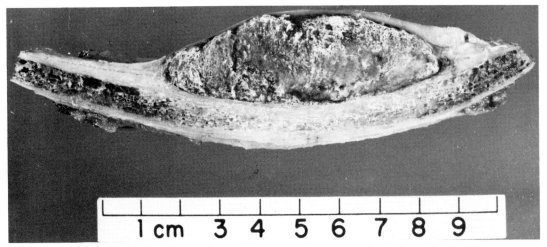

Figure 4–4.   Typical periosteal osteoblastoma of the seventh rib in a 32-year-old man.

ally, the cortex may be breached by an extension into soft tissues.

In the jaw, the interpretation of the radiographic presentation is complicated by the presence of teeth.[10] The typical osteolytic lesion is usually seen with a sprinkling of calcifications and ossification surrounded by an expanded and focally eroded cortex. In occasional instances, a "sun-ray" pattern of radiographic presentation may be evident, suggesting a diagnosis of an osteogenic sarcoma[10] (Table 4–2).

One of the first demonstrations of the usefulness of angiography in diagnosing osteoblastoma was in 1967 when Jeanmart and his coworkers decribed increased vascularity of the tumor in C_4 and C_5 vertebrae.[46] This additional method of diagnosis enables the surgeon to pinpoint the exact extent of involvement and may guide in the surgical approach to be taken (Fig. 4–5). The bone scan is of great practical value for properly localizing the exact site of the lesion (Fig. 4–6).

PATHOLOGIC FEATURES

On *gross examination,* the tumor is hemorrhagic, purplish red or reddish brown, gritty, and friable, although these features are not always evident, especially in those removed by fragmentary curettage from the vertebral column. Large lesions may show central softening and cystic degeneration. The size of the lesions varies from about 2 to 10 cm.

HISTOLOGIC FEATURES

On first impression, one is easily misled to a diagnosis of a highly malignant osteogenic sarcoma. On further examination, one notices the absence of cellular pleomorphism and the presence of abundant osteoid tissue. Adjacent to areas of necrosis and vascular channels, spindly fibroblastic tissue appears with focal calcification and woven bone. Due to the occasional focally dominant fibroblastic pattern, the

TABLE 4–2.   Radiologic Differential Diagnosis in Osteoblastoma

Osteogenic sarcoma: Irregular sclerosing type of bone formation, haphazard calcification, periosteal bone formation. Most often at the end of long bones. Poorly defined. Soft tissue extension not limited by a calcific shell.

Chondrosarcoma: Heavily and irregularly calcified. Indistinct borders.

Chondroblastoma: Epiphyseal location. May cross epiphyseal line. Soft tissue mass is denser.

Osteoid osteoma: Perifocal bone sclerosis around the nidus. No dense soft tissue mass.

Aneurysmal Bone Cyst: Balloon, soap bubble effect. Fine, incomplete septa-forming loculations. In vertebral column, indistinguishable from osteoblastoma.

(Modified from Pochaczevsky et al., 1960.)[72]

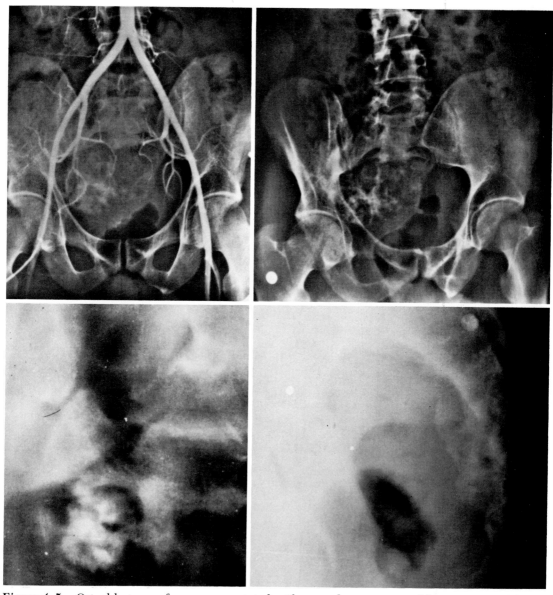

Figure 4–5. Osteoblastoma of sacrum associated with secondary aneurysmal bone cyst in a 27-year-old man. A partly calcified, large, destructive lesion is shown involving almost the entire sacrum and accompanied by dense new bone formation.

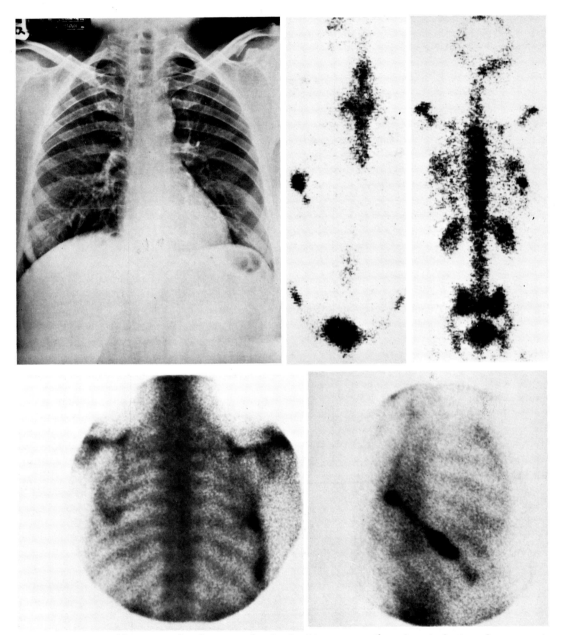

Figure 4–6. Osteoblastoma of right seventh rib showing expansile sclerotic lesion along anterior axillary line in a 55-year-old man. Minified bone scans reveal markedly increased uptake in a rib.

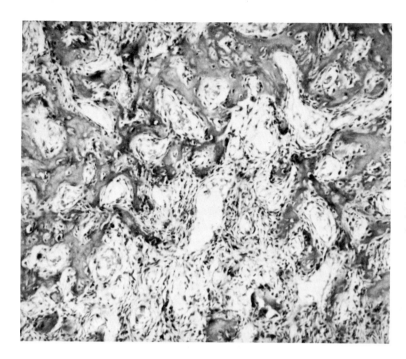

Figure 4–7. Osteoblastoma with partially calcified osteoid and immature bone formation associated with heavy osteoblastic activity. Note vascular fibroblastic stroma. (Hematoxylin-eosin stain. Magnification ×40.)

lesion was originally designated as an osteogenic fibroma by Lichtenstein.[54] This woven bone is directly produced by highly vascular connective tissue ossification and not by endochondral bone formation. The newly formed bony trabeculae are lined by osteoblasts. A loose, richly vascularized, areolar type of connective tissue can be observed between the osseous trabecular network. Areas of transformation from coarse woven bone to finely structured lamellar bone can also be seen. Unless a pathologic fracture has intervened, there is no evidence of cartilage cells in any stage of maturation. The complete lack of these cells is a very helpful feature in distinguishing this lesion from an osteogenic sarcoma. The histologic hallmark of an osteoblastoma is that of a cellular osteoblastic lesional tissue with ample intercellular osteoid material (Figs. 4–7, 4–8, and 4–9 and Table 4–3).

By means of painstaking, quantitative analysis in comparing 10 cases each of osteoblastoma and osteoid osteoma, Aszódi concluded that the former lesion has an increased amount of stroma, including capillaries and giant cells, as compared to the latter. Osteoid osteoma, however, possesses about 10 per cent more osteoid than osteoblastoma. The number of osteoblasts is essentially the same in both lesions.[5]

The relative number of osteoblasts, osteoclasts, and fibroblasts varies from lesion to lesion, as does the stroma, osteoid, and mature bone. In many instances, maturation, i.e., mineralization of the osteoid matrix, is seen progressing toward lamellar bone formation with heavily calcified central areas presenting a Paget disease–like mosaic pattern. The organizational interrelationship of osteoid and mature bone in osteoblastoma is, more often than not, quite haphazard. The lesion usually appears to be histologically in its entirety at the same stage of maturation. The prominent vascularization in association with osteoblastic hypertrophy is accompanied by active new bone formation. In many cases, large aneurysmally dilated vascular spaces appear within the lesion; accordingly, an aneurysmal bone cyst secondarily engrafted on an osteoblastoma can be diagnosed.[7]

An abundance of multinucleated giant cells usually appears around vascular channels and extravasated blood and adjacent to osteoid or newly formed bone (Fig. 4–10). The prominence of these cells in an osteolytic well-circumscribed lesion, especially in the vertebrae, may lead to a mistaken diagnosis of a giant cell tumor of bone, particularly if one deals with a needle aspiration biopsy. The presence of calcification, prominent osteoid, and bone

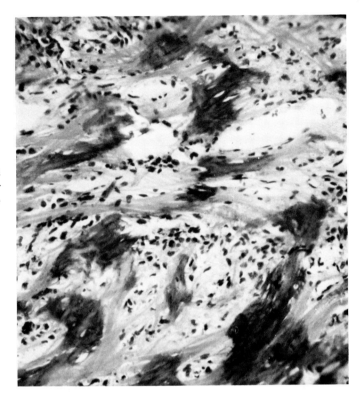

Figure 4-8. Osteoblastoma with heavy mottled calcific bone production and loose fibrous stroma. Hematoxylin-eosin stain. Magnification ×80.)

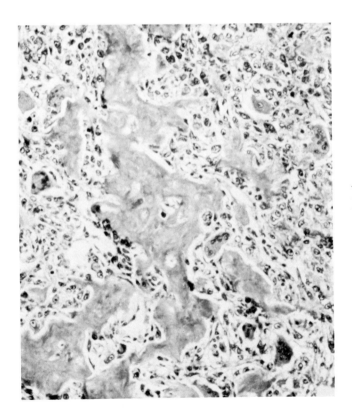

Figure 4-9. Osteoblastoma with heavy osteoid deposition in a filigree pattern with cellular stroma exhibiting numerous giant cells. (Hematoxylin-eosin stain. Magnification ×80.)

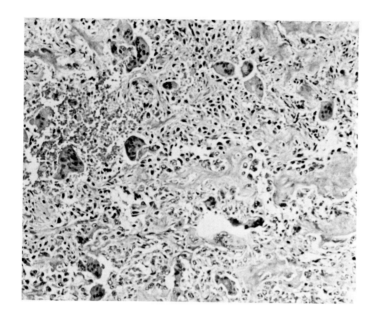

Figure 4–10. Osteoblastoma with large numbers of giant cells associated with hemorrhages and areas of osteoid deposition. (Hematoxylin-eosin stain. Magnification ×40.)

formation, however, is not conspicuously displayed in giant cell tumors and helps one to steer away from such a diagnosis.

The key to the differentiation between osteoblastoma and osteoblastic osteogenic sarcoma should be in the insistence of the diagnostician to obtain an adequate, well-oriented biopsy, with proper roentgenograms and clinical information as to size, location, symptoms, and so on. Careful microscopic examination will reveal stromal cells that are small and slender and do not resemble sarcomatous spindle cells; mitoses are rare; anaplastic giant tumor cells

are not present; tumor cartilage is not formed; and the tumor cells present in the osteoid matrix are small and inconspicuous (Table 4–4). The more important histologic distinctions are summarized in Table 4–1 (p. 33). It must be mentioned that, following several local recurrences, histologic examination may indeed reveal microscopic areas of metaplastic hyaline cartilage.[25, 36] According to Marcove and Alpert, the occasionally present peripheral sclerosis in osteoblastoma that is seen in the roentgenogram is largely due to type B tumor bone rather than to the distinctive reactive bone formation present in osteoid osteoma.[58] This type B tumor bone is char-

TABLE 4–3. Histologic Features of Osteoblastoma

Type A tissue: 1. Small, thin, irregular spicules of highly cellular woven bone
2. Stroma—fibrous connective tissue widely separating bony spicules

Type B tissue: 1. Wide, smooth-edged interconnecting trabeculae of bone
Tumor bone has tendency toward maturation (decreased number of osteocytes, increased number of cement lines)
2. Sparse fibrous connective tissue; large bony masses
3. Benign giant cells especially around hemorrhage of eroding bone
Presence of osteoblasts is not helpful!

(Slightly modified from Marcove and Alpert[58])

TABLE 4–4. Histologic Differential Diagnosis of Osteogenic Sarcoma and Osteoblastoma

	Cartilage Production	Bone and Osteoid Production
Osteogenic sarcoma	Yes	Fine compact strands of osteoid Poorly calcified woven bone Little stroma with sparse blood vessels
Osteoblastoma	None unless pathologic fracture	Thick osteoid and woven bone Irregular serrated margins Osteoclasts present Vascularized stroma

(Modified from Mirra et al., 1976[66])

acterized by wide sheets of interconnecting trabeculae of dense bone with sparse surrounding fibrous tissue, in contrast to a nonspecific reactive bone associated with the osteoid osteoma nidus.

The differential diagnosis of osteoblastoma of the jaw includes *cementoblastoma* (true cementoma). Since both lesions may be attached to or arise around the root of a premolar or molar tooth and occur in young adult males, in addition to having similar although not strictly identical histologic features, some consider them to be the same tumor.[64] On radiographic examination, both lesions show a mottled or densely opaque central mass, usually in the lower jaw with radiolucent periphery. The involved roots appear to be resorbed. Examined microscopically, cementoblastoma is characterized by a dense mass of sparsely cellular, cementum-like material with basophilic "reversal lines" resembling the Paget disease–like mosaic pattern adjacent to a vascular, loosely arranged, fibrous tissue with osteoclastic and osteoblastic giant cells. The peripheral portion of the lesional tissue lacks any attempt at mineralization, as well as remodeling, and large areas of uncalcified "cementoid" are present here. Some feel, however, that although these two lesions are separate entities distinguishable histologically by the lack of cementum-like material in true osteoblastomas, an occasional case may indeed overlap.[1, 26]

TREATMENT AND PROGNOSIS

When the lesion is of small to moderate size, conservative surgical treatment, consisting of thorough curettage with or without packing by bone chips, is the procedure of choice. Since a perilesional reactive zone of sclerosis is practically absent, no wide margin of intact bone resection is indicated. Local resection for lesions in the vertebral spinous processes is advised. Extreme care should be employed in resection for tumors arising in the neural arch of the vertebrae; decompression of the extradural component of the lesion should be attempted even if complete removal may not be achieved. For lesions in the small bones of feet, fibula, and rib, resection of the entire bone is performed and yields a cure.

It is noteworthy that, in spite of less than complete removal of the tumor by curettage, many years of a symptom-free existence can be achieved for the patients, with the residual tumor remaining quiescent and inactive for long periods of time.[59] Data suggest that postoperative radiation therapy is not usually indicated, and only aggressively expanding lesions or recurrent growths should receive this additional mode of therapy.[37, 62, 65, 72] Tumors in the spine require special consideration, since in approximately half of the cases reported, curettage was followed by irradiation because the complete removal of the tumor was technically difficult.

The recurrence rate varies with the reported series. Canepa and Defabiani, in 1965, reported that 11 of their 54 cases showed recurrence.[13] There are several reports of rare recurrences of up to four times in the spine when the tumor was extensive, and complete *en bloc* resection was not feasible.[25, 54, 65] Extreme vascularity of the lesion, most often due to an aneurysmal bone cyst component, hampers thorough curettage. In such cases, radiation therapy is recommended.[22] An entrance dose of approximately 6000 rads with 3500 rads minimal tumor dose in about 40 days, through a single posterior field using a Cobalt-60 unit, seems to be curative. Follow-up roentgenograms show marked increase in density, representing prominent sclerosis of bone in the irradiated area. A total tumor dose of at least 3000 rads in three weeks is advised by another investigator.[42]

In 1976, Schajowicz and Lemos[80] described under the heading of "malignant osteoblastoma" eight patients with locally aggressive growths microscopically characterized by increased mitotic rate as well as cellularity, plump hyperchromatic nuclei, nuclear atypia, and numerous osteoclastic giant cells. Since seven of the eight patients were alive, without evidence of disease, from 1½ to 11 years after the original surgical treatment, which in only two instances involved amputation, one wonders whether the epithet "malignant" is apt or fair.

Several cases discussed in detail, or

mentioned only in passing, in the literature deal with examples of malignant transformation in osteoblastoma, the coexistence of osteogenic sarcoma with microscopic areas of clear-cut osteoblastoma, and finally, osteoblastoma showing worrisome areas of marked cellular atypia.[61, 66] The problem is aptly stated by McLeod and his associates: "Does malignancy develop in osteoblastoma or can malignant tumors simulate osteoblastoma?"[64] The evaluation of the possible occurrence of malignant transformation in reported cases of osteoblastomas is obscured by the great likelihood that some of these examples were indeed sarcomas from the very onset.[20, 83]

Malignant transformation in the absence of, but also following, radiation therapy has been noted.[61, 79, 84, 88]

REFERENCES

1. Abrams, A. M., and Melrose, R. J.: Cementoblastoma. Oral Surg., 83:394–403, 1974.
2. Acquaviva, R., Bru, P. M., Tamic, J., et al.: L'ostéoblastome vertébral. J. Med. Maroc., 4:265–270, 1968.
3. Anand, S. V., Davey, W. W., and Cohen, B.: Tumours of the jaw in West Africa. Br. J. Surg., 54:901–917, 1967.
4. Anneroth, G., Isacsson, G., and Sigurdsson, A.: Benign cementoblastoma (true cementoma). Oral Surg., 40:141–146, 1975.
5. Aszódi, K.: Benign osteoblastoma: quantitative histological distinction from osteoid osteoma. Arch. Orthop. Unfallchir., 88:359–368, 1977.
6. Bethge, J. F. J.: Benignes Osteoblastom. Chirurg., 34:121–123, 1963.
7. Biesecker, J. L., Marcove, R. C., Huvos, A. G., et al: Aneurysmal bone cysts. A clinicopathologic study of 66 cases. Cancer, 26:615–625, 1970.
8. Bloom, M. H., and Bryan, R. S.: Benign osteoblastoma of the spine. Clin. Orthop., 65:157–162, 1969.
9. Borello, E. D., and Sedano, H. O.: Giant osteoid osteoma of the maxilla. Report of a case. Oral Surg., 23:563–566, 1967.
10. Brady, C. L., and Browne, R. M.: Benign osteoblastoma of the mandible. Cancer, 30:329–333, 1972.
11. Byers, P. D.: Solitary benign osteoblastic lesions of bone. Osteoid osteoma and benign osteoblastoma. Cancer, 22:43–57, 1968.
12. Calcagni, V., and Tos, L.: L'osteoblastoma del tarso. Chir. Organi Mov., 52:228–234, 1963.
13. Canepa, G., and Defabiani, F.: Osteoblastoma del radio. Minerva Ortop., 16:645–648, 1965.
14. Case records of the Massachusetts General Hospital. N. Engl. J. Med., 265:700–704, 1961.
15. Corio, R. L., Crawford, B. E., and Schaberg, S. J.:

16. Crabbe, W. A., and Wardill, J. C.: Benign osteoblastoma of the spine. Br. J. Surg., 50:571–575, 1962–1963.
17. Curran, J. B., and Collins, A. P.: Benign (true) cementoblastoma of the mandible. Oral Surg., 35:168–172, 1973.
18. Curtis, B. H.: Osteoblastoma of the spine. Abstract, J. Bone Joint Surg. [Am.], 54:201, 1972.
19. Dahlin, D. C., and Johnson, E. W.: Giant osteoid osteoma. J. Bone Joint Surg. [Am.], 36:559–572, 1954.
20. Dalinka, M. K., and Chunn, S. P.: Osteoblastoma — benign or malignant precursor? Report of a case. J. Can Assoc. Radiol., 23:214–216, 1972.
21. Davis, N. A., Dooley, B. J., and Bardsley, A.: Benign osteoblastoma. Aust. N. Z. J. Surg., 46:37–43, 1976.
22. Deffebach, R. R., and Phillips, T. L.: Benign osteoblastoma of the vertebra. Radiol. Clin. Biol. (Basel), 37:45–52, 1968.
23. DiGiglia, J. W., Bradford, J. K., Leonard, G. L., et al.: Benign osteoblastoma of the rib: Report of a case. South. Med. J., 64:624–626, 1971.
24. Doron, Y., Gruszkiewicz, J., Gelli, B., et al.: Benign osteoblastoma of vertebral column and skull. Surg. Neurol., 7:86–90, 1977.
25. Eisenbrey, A. B., Huber, P. J., and Rachmaninoff, N.: Benign osteoblastoma of the spine with multiple recurrences. Case report. J. Neurosurg., 31:468–473, 1969.
26. Eversole, L. R., Sabes, W. R., and Dauchess, V. G.: Benign cementoblastoma. Oral Surg., 36:824–830, 1973.
27. Farman, A. G., Nortjé, C. J., and Grotepass, F.: Periosteal benign osteoblastoma of the mandible. Report of a case and review of the literature pertaining to benign osteoblastic neoplasms of the jaws. Br. J. Oral Surg., 14:12–22, 1976.
28. Flaherty, R. A., Pugh, D. G., and Dockerty, M. B.: Osteoid osteoma. Am. J. Roentgenol. Radium Ther. Nucl. Med., 76:1041–1051, 1956.
29. Freedman, S. R.: Benign osteoblastoma of the ethmoid bone. Report of a case. Am. J. Clin. Pathol., 63:391–396, 1975.
30. Freedman, S., Taber, P., and Alter, A.: Benign osteoblastic lesion in the scapula of a child. Am. J. Dis. Child., 123:236–237, 1972.
31. Gallinaro, P.: Evoluzione del concetto di osteoblastoma benigno. Revisione della letteratura e presentazione di due casi. Arch. Ital. Chir., 93:634–660, 1967.
32. Gertzbein, S. D., Cruickshank, B., Hoffman, H., et al: Recurrent benign osteoblastoma of the second thoracic vertebra. J. Bone Joint Surg. [Br.], 55:841–847, 1973.
33. Geschickter, C. F., and Copeland, M. M.: Tumors of Bone. 3rd ed. Philadelphia, J. B. Lippincott Co., 1949.
34. Giannestras, N. J., and Diamond, J. R.: Benign osteoblastoma of the talus. J. Bone Joint Surg., [Am.], 40:469–478, 1958.
35. Gibbons, J. M., Jr., and Hammond, G.: Benign osteoblastoma. Lahey Clin. Bull. 13:97–103, 1963.

16. Benign cementoblastoma. Oral Surg., 41:524–530, 1976.

36. Goidanich, I. F., and Battaglia, L.: Osteoblastoma (fibroma osteogenetico). Neoplasia benigna di tessuto osteoblastico. Studio clinico, radiografico ed anatomo-patologico di 14 casi. Chir. Organi Mov., 46:353–388, 1958.

37. Golding, J. S. R., and Sissons, H. A.: Osteogenic fibroma of bone. J. Bone Joint Surg. [Br.], 36:428–435, 1954.

38. Goldman, R. L.: The periosteal counterpart of benign osteoblastoma. Am. J. Clin. Pathol., 56:73–78, 1971.

39. Greenspan, A., Elguezabal, A., and Bryk, D.: Benign osteoblastoma of a rib. J. Can. Assoc. Radiol., 26:208–209, 1975.

40. Guy, R., Lafond, G., Gagnon, P.-A., et al.: L'ostéoblastome bénin. Union Med. Can., 88:666–678, 1959.

41. Immenkamp, M.: Ein benignes Osteoblastom des 4. Lendenwirbels als Ursache einer Hüftlendenstrecksteife. Z. Orthop., 109:616–625, 1971.

42. Irwin, G. A. L.: Benign osteoblastoma of spine. N.Y. State J. Med., 70:687–689, 1970.

43. Jackson, J. R., and Bell, M. E. A.: Spurious "benign osteoblastoma." A case report. J. Bone Joint Surg. [Am.], 59:397–401, 1977.

44. Jaffe, H. L.: Benign osteoblastoma. Bull. Hosp. Joint Dis., 17:141–151, 1956.

45. Jaffe, H.L., and Mayer, L.: An osteoblastic osteoid tissue-forming tumor of a metacarpal bone. Arch. Surg., 24:550–564, 1932.

46. Jeanmart, L., Brihaye, J., and Gompel, C.: Tumeurs rares du rachis. J. Belge. Rhumatol. Med. Phys., 22:317–332, 1967.

47. Kent, J. N., Castro, H. F., and Girotti, W. R.: Benign osteoblastoma of the maxilla. Case report and review of the literature. Oral Surg., 27:209–219, 1969.

48. Kirkpatrick, H. J. R., and Murray, R. C.: Osteogenic fibroma of bone. Report of a case. J. Bone Joint Surg. [Br.], 37:606–611, 1955.

49. Kramer, H. S.: Benign osteoblastoma of the mandible. Oral Surg., 24:842–851, 1967.

50. Kwart, L., and Sikora-Gierowska, I.: Osteoblastoma benignum ossis mandibularis. Czas. Stomatol., 20:1073–1077, 1967.

51. Labayle, J., Bacular, J., and Chelloul, D.: Benign osteoblastoma. Apropos of a case localized in the upper maxilla. Ann. Otolaryngol. Chir. Cervicofac., 93:661–668, 1976.

52. Laskowski, A., Maj, T., and Koziol-Honorynski, E.: Nonmalignant embryonic osteoma of the maxilla. Patol. Pol., 22:391–395, 1971.

53. Leipold, D.: Ein Beitrag über das benigne Osteoblastom. Beitr. Orthop. Traumatol., 16:428–432, 1968.

54. Lichtenstein, L.: Benign osteoblastoma. A category of osteoid- and bone-forming tumors other than classical osteoma, which may be mistaken for giant-cell tumor or osteogenic sarcoma. Cancer, 9:1044–1052, 1956.

55. Lichtenstein, L., and Sawyer, W. R.: Benign osteoblastoma. Further observations and report of twenty additional cases. J. Bone Joint Surg. [Am.], 46:755–765, 1964.

56. Lievre, J. A. and Lievre, J. A.: Ostéoblastome bénin. Rev. Rhum., 28:95–100, 1961.

57. Maar, D., and Dornetzhuber, V.: Benign osteoblastoma ossis tali resembling ostitis tuberculosa. Acta Chir. Orthop. Traumatol. Cech., 41:362–366, 1974.

58. Marcove, R. C., and Alpert, M.: A pathologic study of benign osteoblastoma. Clin. Orthop., 30:175–181, 1963.

59. Marsh, B. W., Bonfiglio, M., Brady, L. P., et al.: Benign osteoblastoma: Range of manifestations. J. Bone Joint Surg. [Am.], 57:1–9, 1975.

60. Marsh, H. O., and Choi, C.-B.: Primary osteogenic sarcoma of the cervical spine originally mistaken for benign osteoblastoma. A case report. J. Bone Joint Surg. [Am.], 52:1467–1471, 1970.

61. Mayer, L.: Malignant degeneration of so-called benign oteoblastoma. Bull. Hosp. Joint Dis., 28:4–13, 1967.

62. Mayer, L.: Benign (?) osteoblastoma. Letter to the Editor. Bull. Hosp. Joint Dis., 29:236–240, 1968.

63. Mazabraud, A.: Remarques à propos de l'ostéome-osteoide et de l'ostéoblastome. Ann. Anat. Pathol., 17:177–186, 1972.

64. McLeod, R. A., Dahlin, D. C., and Beabout J. W.: The spectrum of osteoblastoma. Am. J. Roentgenol. Radium Ther. Nucl. Med., 126:321–335, 1976.

65. Meary, R., Merle d'Aubigné, R., and Mazabraud, A.: Ostéoblastomes bénins. Mém. Acad. Chir., 91:911–925, 1965.

66. Mirra, J. M., Kendrick, R. A., and Kendrick, R. E.: Pseudomalignant osteoblastoma versus arrested osteosarcoma. A case report. Cancer, 37:2005–2014, 1976.

67. Morton, K. S., Vassar, P. S., and Knickerbocker, W. J.: Osteoid osteoma and osteoblastoma: reclassification of 41 cases using Schajowicz's classification. Abstract. J. Bone Joint Surg. [Br.], 56:585, 1974.

68. Morton, K. S., Vassar, P. S., and Knickerbocker, W. J.: Osteoid osteoma and osteoblastoma: reclassification of 43 cases using Schajowicz's classification. Can. J. Surg., 18:148–152, 1975.

69. Navarra, S., Pedulla, G., and Romeo, G.: L'osteoblastoma benigno. Gazz. Int. Med. Chir., 65:2079–2112, 1960.

70. Netherlands Committee on Bone Tumours: Radiological Atlas of Bone Tumours. Vol. 2. Baltimore, Williams & Wilkins Co., 1973.

71. Otis, R. D., and Scoville, W. B.: Benign osteoblastoma of the vertebra. J. Neurosurg., 18:700–702, 1961

72. Pochaczevsky, R., Yen, Y. M., and Sherman, R. S.: The roentgen appearance of benign osteoblastoma. Radiology, 75:429—437, 1960.

73. Rajcev, R., Vasilev, H., and Komitovski, D.: On the question of benign osteoblastoma. Khirurgiia (Sofia), 14:883–887, 1961.

74. Remagen, W., and Prein, J.: Benign osteoblastoma. Oral Surg., 39:279—283, 1975.

75. Ronis, M.L., Obando, M., Bucko, M.I., et al.: Benign osteoblastoma of the temporal bone. Laryngoscope, 84:857–862, 1974.

76. Rosensweig, J., Mikail, M., and Mayman, A.: Benign osteoblastoma (giant osteoid osteoma): Report of an unusual rib tumour and review of the literature. Can. Med. Assoc. J., 89:1189–1192, 1963.

77. Salzer, M., and Salzer-Kuntschik, M.: Das benigne Osteoblastom. Langenbecks Arch. Chir., *302*:755–778, 1963.

78. Saylam, A., Boke, E., E., Bozer, A. Y., et al.: Benign osteoblastoma and aneurysmal bone cyst. Hacettepe Bull. Med. Surg., 5:172–177, 1972.

79. Schajowicz, F., and Lemos, C.: Osteoid osteoma and osteoblastoma. Closely related entities of osteoblastic derivation. Acta Orthop. Scand., *41*:272–291, 1970.

80. Schajowicz, F., and Lemos, C.: Malignant osteoblastoma. J. Bone Joint Surg. [Br.], *58*:202–211, 1976.

81. Schein, A. J.: Osteoblastoma of the scapula. A case report. J. Bone Joint Surg. [Am.], *41*:359–362, 1959.

82. Schreyvogel, R.: Benignes Osteoblastom. Schweiz. Med. Wochenschr., *98*:1009–1015, 1968.

83. Schulze, K. J.: Maligne Entartung eines benignen Osteoblastoms (Jaffe-Lichtenstein). Beitr. Orthop. Traumatol., *15*:136–137, 1968.

84. Seki, T., Fukuda, H., Ishii, Y., et al.: Malignant transformation of benign osteoblastoma. A case report. J. Bone Joint Surg. [Am.], 57:424–426, 1975.

85. de Souza Dias, L., and Frost, H. M.: Osteoblastoma of the spine. Clin. Orthop., *91*:141–151, 1973.

86. de Souza Dias, L., and Frost, H. M.: Osteoid osteoma — osteoblastoma. Cancer, *33*:1075–1081, 1974.

87. Steiner, G. C.: Ultrastructure of osteoblastoma. Cancer, *39*:2127–2136, 1977.

88. Stutch, R.: Osteoblastoma — a benign entity? Orthop. Rev., *4*:27–33, 1975.

89. Tate, R. C., Kim, S.-S., and Ogden, L.: Osteoblastoma of the sacrum with intra-abdominal manifestation. Am. J. Surg. *123*:735–738, 1972.

90. Trifaud, A., Payan, H., Bureau, H., et al.: Les ostéoblastomes bénins. A propos de cinq observations. Mém. Acad. Chir., *91*:890–895, 1965.

91. Tulloh, H. P., and Harry, D.: Osteoblastoma in a rib in childhood. Clin. Radiol., *20*:337–338, 1969.

92. Viallet, J. I., Degouilloux, B., Vanneuville, G., et al.: Ostéoblastome occipital. J. Radiol. Electrol. Med. Nucl., *49*:425–426, 1968.

93. Weickert, H., and Dominok, G. W.: Benignes Osteoblastom als Ursache einer Skoliose. Dtsch. Gesundh., *26*:102–105, 1971.

94. Wickenhauser, J., Strassl, H., and Hollmann, K.: Das benigne Osteoblastom. Seltene Lokalisation in der Maxilla? Fortschr. Geb. Roentgenstr. Nuklearmed., *119*:618–623, 1973.

95. Yllanes, H., and Compere, E. L.: Benign osteoblastoma. A rare tumor involving the humerus of a 5 year old boy. Clin. Orthop., *42*:147–150, 1965.

Bone-forming Tumors — Malignant
Chapters 5 through 8

5

OSTEOGENIC SARCOMA

DEFINITION

Osteogenic sarcoma is a malignant tumor of bone in which the malignant proliferating spindle-cell stroma directly produces osteoid or immature bone.

This definition of osteogenic sarcoma circumvents the disagreement regarding the exact histogenesis of these tumors and is based on the usually readily recognizable product of this neoplasm. "Osteogenic" carries a double meaning, namely "derived from bone" and "producing bone." A good discussion of the etymologic considerations that dates back to the times of Plato and Aristotle, in addition to more modern definitions and terminology, can be found in the exhaustive article by Acchiappati and his coworkers.[2]

The term "osteogenic sarcoma" is sometimes used to indicate a sarcoma that has arisen in skeletal connective tissue. This usage may lead to confusion, since chondrosarcomas and fibrosarcomas, for example, may also be called "osteogenic." In this chapter, the designation "osteogenic sarcoma" refers to a sarcoma of bone in which the sarcomatous stromal tumor cells directly form osteoid and immature bone. Some refer to this as "malignant" osteoid.

Uncalcified osteoid is difficult to differentiate from collagen formed by fibroblastic spindle cells.[102] Previously, one had to resort to a rather elementary method of identifying the cells with which the osteoid or collagen is in direct contact. Osteoblastic cells are cuboid or spheric, in contradistinction to fibroblasts, which are elongated or spindly.[428] Newly developed histochemical methods are helpful in establishing alkaline phosphatase activity in tissue sections of osteogenic sarcoma. The richly positive staining one sees with this enzyme is missing entirely in fibroblastic lesions producing collagen.[30, 177, 178, 264]

INCIDENCE, GEOGRAPHIC PATTERNS OF DISTRIBUTION, AND EPIDEMIOLOGIC CONSIDERATIONS

Excluding plasma cell myeloma, osteogenic sarcoma is the most frequent primary malignant bone tumor. It is approximately twice as common as chondrosarcoma and three times more frequent than Ewing's sarcoma.

The true incidence of bone cancer in general, or osteogenic sarcoma in particular, is difficult to estimate, since the population-based tumor registries record too few bone cancer cases to permit separation into the various types. Mortality figures are notoriously inaccurate because they only state which bone was involved and not the histologic type of the tumor. Osteogenic sarcoma is not listed separately from Ewing's sarcoma or other tumors. In the United States, 1934 deaths were attributed to osteogenic sarcoma or Ewing's sarcoma in patients under 15 years of age during an eight year period.[259] Bone sarcoma is estimated to occur in one out of every 100,000 inhabitants in the United States. In Great Britain, the estimation is between two and three tumors per one million persons. There are about 130 to 150 new primary osteogenic sarcoma cases annually in that country.[306] Osteogenic sarcoma is the most common primary malignant bone tumor save for multiple myeloma. It is calculated that approximately 1500 cases of osteogenic sarcoma exist at any one time in this country. Memorial Hospital in New York City, primarily a referral institution, annually diagnoses and treats 24 new patients with osteogenic sarcoma. This does not include cases referred for consultation only.

In 1971, the Swedish National Cancer Registry reported an annual incidence of 0.28 cases per 100,000 people. They found no significant variation between urban and rural environments in the geographic distribution of osteogenic sarcoma.[46] More recently, the same Cancer Registry data were analyzed employing different criteria, and a significantly increased incidence was noted in urban areas.[204] In a study based on data from East and West Malaysia, with known, clear-cut, geographic and racial distinctions, the annual incidence was 0.11 cases per 100,000 people in the Malays and 0.23 cases in the Chinese and Indian populations respectively. The urban incidence in contrast to the rural incidence was 0.22 cases to 0.09 in the Malays and 0.31 cases to 0.18 in the Chinese.[22]

A study of the geographic patterns of bone cancer mortality in individuals under the age of 20 in the United States between the years 1950 and 1969 showed a prominent pattern of very high mortality in *females* in the area from Oklahoma eastward through the South and into Appalachia. Among *males*, the pattern was less pronounced. Scattered high death rates occurred in Pennsylvania, West Virginia, Louisiana, Mississippi, and Kentucky.[243]

The epidemiology of osteogenic sarcoma should encompass a search for genetic and environmental factors in order to yield possible clues to the etiological causes of oteogenic sarcoma[121] (Table 5–1).

AGE AND SEX DISTRIBUTION

Osteogenic sarcoma can occur at any age, although it is chiefly an affliction of the young.[420] Adolescents in the second decade of life are most commonly involved (45.7 per cent) (Fig. 5–1). This age distribution essentially does not vary in any part of the world.[263] In our series at Memorial Hospital, the age of 27 years is the average for both sexes. The median age is 18 and 17 years in males and females respectively. The modal age is 18 years in males and 14 and 15 years in females. The youngest patients in our series were a two-year-old boy and a three-year-old girl. The oldest male was 82 years old, and the oldest female was 79 years old. The Mayo Clinic has reported occurrence in a 35-month-old girl.[352]

The diagnosis of primary osteogenic sarcoma in older patients should be accepted only after careful examination excludes association with other pre-existent bone diseases, such as Paget's disease, fibrous dysplasia, and so forth.

Males are affected slightly more frequently than females are. In the series at Memorial Hospital, the proportion is 1.3:1, and at the Mayo Clinic, it is 1.6:1. The higher number of tumors in men may be related to the longer period of skeletal growth and the additional volume of bone produced in the male. It is also notable that osteogenic sarcoma tends to start at an earlier age in females than in males. The sex distribution of patients does not vary essentially in any decade of life (Fig. 5–1).

The most frequent occurrences of osteogenic sarcoma correspond to the periods of peak skeletal growth in childhood (Fig. 5–1).[362] The growth potential of each individual long bone generally determines the frequency of tumor occurrence. Accordingly, the femur (41.5 per cent), the tibia (16 per cent), and the humerus (15 per cent) are the most common sites for osteogenic sarcoma.[124] Patients affected by osteogenic sarcoma have been found to be taller than

TABLE 5-1. Familial Aggregation of Osteogenic Sarcoma*

Age (in years) and sex at diagnosis	Site of lesions	Relation	Remarks	Reference
23 male	tibia	brother		Roberts and
13 female	humerus	sister		Roberts, 1935
17 female	femur	sister		
3 female	femur	sister		Pohle et al., 1936
11 female	ulna	sister		
15 female	humerus	sister	mother: soft tissue	Lee and
15 male	femur	brother	sarcoma of thigh	MacKenzie, 1964
14 male	femur	brother		Lee and
23 male	tibia	brother		MacKenzie, 1964
15 male	femur	brother		Harmon and
20 male	tibia	brother		Morton, 1966
11 female	tibia	sister		
22 male	tibia	brother		
22 male	cranium	first		Robbins, 1967
18 male	ulna	cousins		
15 and	tibia and	father	6 out of 15 members	Epstein et al., 1970
40 male	maxilla		of family have 7	
13 female	femur	daughter	cancers	
27 female	tibia (dedifferentiated chondrosarcoma)	mother	polyposis coli family	Hoffman and Brooke, 1970
13 male	femur	son		
25 male	humerus	father		Swaney, 1973
6 female	femur	daughter		
11 male	femur	brother		Swaney, 1973
4 male	tibia	brother		
15 female	femur	sister	mother and her sister:	Miller and
17 female	femur	sister	breast cancer maternal grandmother: colon cancer	McLaughlin, 1977
13 female	ilium	sister		Matejovsky, 1977
13 female	tibia	sister		
14 female	tibia	sister	American Indian	Mulvihill et al., 1977
7 female	femur	sister	family	
18 male	tibia	brother		

*Only primary cases are included.

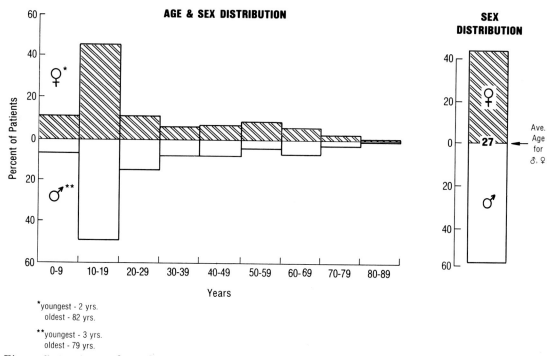

OSTEOGENIC SARCOMA (1949 - 1974)
605 Pts. (♂ = 338, ♀ = 267)

AGE & SEX DISTRIBUTION

SEX DISTRIBUTION

*youngest - 2 yrs.
oldest - 82 yrs.

**youngest - 3 yrs.
oldest - 79 yrs.

Figure 5–1.   Age and sex distribution of 605 patients with osteogenic sarcoma at Memorial Hospital.

their peers in the corresponding age group. Such children are found to have high plasma somatomedin levels.[253, 254] Fraumeni[105] was the first to point out that the recorded height of these patients is at or above the median, a finding that was subsequently corroborated at the University of Pittsburgh Health Center Hospitals.[347] Osteogenic sarcomas of the humerus form before those in the lower extremity, and Price ascribes this to the relatively advanced length of bone growth of the humerus in the young.[303] Until the cessation of the growth period, the long bones are the bones most frequently involved in osteogenic sarcoma.[123] After this growth period, the long and the flat bones are about equally affected.[416]

Incidence in Canines

Several studies have shown that osteogenic sarcoma of long bones has an increased incidence in canines of the giant breeds: Great Danes, St. Bernards, Great Pyrenees, and wolfhounds.[363] Tjalma estimates the risk of osteogenic sarcoma developing in giant dogs (over 80 lbs) varies anywhere from 61 to 185 times the risk of it developing in small breeds (20 lbs).[390] In dogs, more weight is borne by the front legs than by the hind legs. This fact may explain the greater frequency of osteogenic sarcoma in the front legs.[425]

CLINICAL FEATURES

The rate of tumor growth, the degree of bone destruction, and the severity of the symptoms vary widely. A sudden onset of severe symptoms is the general rule, although protracted, slowly developing, slight to moderate pain and tenderness are often observed. Since many of the lesions occur in the knee region, a blow or some other minor injury is usually related by the patient as an inciting or even causative factor. It is, however, much more likely that the occurrence of injury drew the patient's attention to an already existing neoplasm. Ewing referred to this occurrence as "traumatic determinism." Trauma *reveals* more malignant growths than it *produces.*[89]

The earliest symptom is pain in the involved bone. Initially, this is insidious and transitory, gradually but inexorably becoming persistent and severe. This pain finally develops into a throbbing, excruciating, and unremitting experience.

Swelling is minimal at first but becomes more prominent as times passes. It usually has a fusiform eccentric configuration based on the underlying bone. The larger the swelling, the easier it becomes to delineate its contours. There is a wide variation in the hardness of the tumor. The sclerosing type of osteogenic sarcoma is rock hard; the osteolytic type is rubbery firm. A pulsatile quality, even in the telangiectatic variety, is rarely if ever observed. The skin overlying the tumor is often shiny and stretched, with the superficial veins showing prominence and dilatation. Minor restriction in motion at the adjacent joint is often present with minimal limp and disability. Lung metastases, even if massive, are usually entirely symptomless.

PROGNOSTIC CONSIDERATIONS

The prognosis of osteogenic sarcoma is purported to depend on the histologic characteristics (type of tumor), grade of malignancy, site of tumor, radiologic features, presence or absence of pathologic fractures, size of tumor, rapidity of growth, age and sex of the patient, and finally, the mode of therapy.[220, 405] Several authors have suggested an improved survival rate among females.[69, 252, 416] The most recent study of 54 patients by McMaster and his associates showed that while 45.8 per cent of the females survived five years or more, only 16.6 per cent of the males were alive after the same time interval.

In a study of 85 patients with osteogenic sarcoma treated at the University of Michigan Medical Center in Ann Arbor, Nosanchuk and his coworkers found significantly more women than men surviving. When

survival results were analyzed with respect to epiphyseal closure of the involved bone, no male patients survived with lesions adjacent to an open epiphysis, in contrast to four female long-term survivors with similarly open epiphyses.[281] In three of the four pregnant patients reported, the presence of osteogenic sarcoma did not affect labor or the delivery of normal infants and did not exert a demonstrably deleterious effect on the maternal clinical course.[298]

PATHOLOGIC FRACTURE

The rare occurrence of a pathologic fracture in an osteogenic sarcoma was considered a sinister prognostic sign until McKenna and his associates questioned this in 1966.[252] Five of the 30 patients surviving for more than 10 years after treatment at Memorial Hospital for osteogenic sarcoma had this complication.[282] The survival results reported by Coley and Pool similarly suggest that a pathologic fracture is not an indicator of a poor prognosis.[55] Those patients with pathologic fractures who died of their disease, however, lived only half as long as the average period of survival for the entire group.

SECONDARY OSTEOGENIC SARCOMA

Children with bilateral *retinoblastoma,* a genetically transmissible tumor, have an increased incidence of femoral osteogenic sarcoma.[180, 193, 196] Only the familial, and not the sporadic, cases of retinoblastoma are at high risk. This occurrence may be due to the retinoblastoma gene predisposing the patient to other neoplasms, including bone tumors. Two siblings with bilateral retinoblastoma have been described, both of whom subsequently developed osteogenic sarcoma of the femur.[340]

Exuberant callus formation following fracture in patients with or without *osteogenesis imperfecta* may clinically simulate, especially roentgenographically, an osteogenic sarcoma.[12, 186, 401] True malignant transformation, e.g., osteogenic sarcoma in the pelvis of a 49-year-old man[181] and in the tibia of a 29-year-old woman,[145] has been reported in patients with osteogenesis imperfecta tarda. Other well-documented cases have also been published.[194, 418] Klenerman and his coworkers suggested that the osteogenic sarcomas arose spontaneously and were not related to the underlying osteogenesis imperfecta.

On rare occasions, osteogenic sarcoma may develop in a bone that is the site of an *infarct*. The patients are of varying types, including caisson workers, as discussed in the literature.[183, 260]

Osteogenic sarcoma may occasionally arise in a *solitary osteochondroma*,[9, 69, 344, 359] *solitary enchondroma*,[319] or in *enchondromatosis* (Ollier's disease).[24] A single example of an osteogenic sarcoma in an adult woman with *chronic osteomyelitis* of the tibia has been encountered. Three years following an above-the-knee amputation, the patient was without evidence of disease.[370] Another case of sarcoma developed following chronic osteomyelitis of the femur.[13] Osteogenic sarcoma may also arise in association with *nonossifying fibroma*.[144, 199]

LOCATION

The long bones of the extremities are the most common sites of osteogenic sarcoma, the femur being involved in 41.5 per cent of all cases, the tibia in 16 per cent, and the humerus in 15 per cent. The femoral involvement occurs most frequently in the distal part of the bone, especially in the metaphysis or diaphysis; when the humerus or the tibia are affected, the proximal portions are preferred. About 48 per cent of all lesions occur in the knee region. In 7 per cent of instances, bones of the cranium are predilected. Exceptionally, osteogenic sarcoma may be situated along the mid-shaft, thereby causing diagnostic difficulties. Osteogenic sarcoma developing in other than long tubular bones of the appendicular skeleton is a rare occurrence, especially in children. One such case involving the scapula in a 12-year-old girl has been reported by Salmon and his coworkers.[336]

The number of well-documented primary osteogenic sarcomas arising in the hand is extremely small.[48] Although the rarity of occurrence should make one wary of such

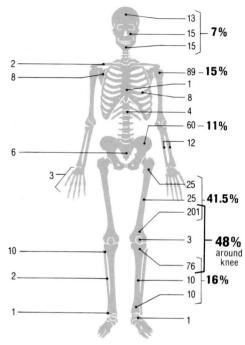

OSTEOGENIC SARCOMA
Skeletal Location
in 605 Cases

Multifocal cases - 5

Figure 5–2. Skeletal location in 605 cases of osteogenic sarcoma at Memorial Hospital (1949 through 1974).

a diagnosis unless histologically proved, the differential diagnostic considerations should also include this tumor of the hand. Primary osteogenic sarcoma of the spine, in the absence of previous irradiation or Paget's disease, is extremely rare and only a handful of cases have been reported.[96, 239]

SYNCHRONOUS AND METACHRONOUS MULTICENTRIC OSTEOGENIC SARCOMA

Although it is rare, osteogenic sarcoma may involve multiple skeletal sites in a patient at the same time (synchronous involvement). This involvement tends to be symmetric. In order to rule out the possibility of metastases, the acceptable cases should have no pulmonary or other visceral involvement at the time the multifocal skeletal affection is demonstrated. It is, of course, not inconceivable that one of these sarcomas has metastasized rapidly to other bone or bones without demonstrable visceral involvement.

In 1922, White reported the first case of a multifocal telangiectatic osteogenic sarcoma involving one extremity of a 27-year-old man.[419] Subsequent to this study, several patients with or without postmortem examinations were noted where multifocal skeletal osteogenic sarcoma could be demonstrated.[3, 8, 35, 57, 70, 136, 140, 187, 208, 221, 307, 341, 353, 407] These cases exclude those in which Paget's osteitis deformans or other preexisting skeletal conditions were present. This apparently simultaneous osteogenic sarcoma has been designated as "sclerosing osteogenic sarcomatosis."[66, 94, 247, 265, 267, 355, 426] The prominent feature of this condition is a densely sclerotic radiopaque lesion involving multiple bones. It is usually present at the metaphyseal ends of long bones but may also be seen in other flat or round bones or in the vertebrae.[66] Most of the patients reported in the literature are children in the first decade of life.

In a study of 600 patients with osteogenic sarcoma at the Mayo Clinic, 16 cases occurred in multiple primary sites.[69]

Patients with synchronously occurring polyostotic osteogenic sarcoma have a uniformly poor prognosis. In contrast to this rapidly fatal outcome the prognosis seemed to be markedly improved if curative surgery was attempted for those patients in whom another osteogenic sarcoma developed metachronously, either as a late metastasis or as a new primary tumor. In a study of 12 such patients with multiple metachronous osteogenic sarcomas, two long-term survivors were seen.[100]

SERUM AND TISSUE ALKALINE PHOSPHATASE IN NORMAL AND NEOPLASTIC CONDITIONS, ESPECIALLY OSTEOGENIC SARCOMA

The determination of serum alkaline phosphatase values can be studied by different assay methods. Since assayed serum levels may be expressed in various units, using different substrates at varying temperatures, it is important to establish which method is employed if comparisons are planned (Tables 5–2 and 5–3).

TABLE 5–2. The More Important Serum Alkaline Phosphatase Methods and the Normal Range in Adults

Method		Normal range
Bowers-McComb	I.U./L at 30°	6–110
Babson-Greeley-Coleman-Phillips	I.U./L at 37°	9–35
Klein-Read-Babson	Units/dl at 37°	1–3.5
Bessey-Lowry-Brock	Units/L at 37°	0.8–2.5
Bodansky	Units/dl at 37°	1.5–4
Shinowara-Jones-Reinhart	Units/dl at 37°	2–8.5
King-Armstrong	Units/dl at 37°	4–10

NOTE: Infants and children normally have a two- to fourfold increase in activity as compared to adults. (From Bowers, G. N., Jr., and McComb, R. B.: Measurement of total alkaline phosphatase activity in human serum. Clin. Chem., 21:1988–1995, 1975.)

McKenna and associates pointed out the possible prognostic value of the serum alkaline phosphatase.[252] This and other studies firmly established that these values are helpful in determining prognosis. Postoperative, postamputation, or postchemotherapy follow-up examinations should include alkaline phosphatase determination, since elevated or increasing values herald the presence of residual, reactivated, and spreading osteogenic sarcoma. Virus-induced murine osteogenic sarcomas reportedly elaborate alkaline phosphatase released in the culture medium.[6] Olson and Capen found significantly elevated serum

TABLE 5–3. Normal Serum Alkaline Phosphatase Values in Adults and Children (units/dl at 37°C).

Method	Adults		Children	
	Range	Average	Range	Average
Bodansky	1.5–4	2.6	5–14	7.7
King-Armstrong	4–10	8.0	10–25	20.0
International Unit (IUB)°	31–82°°	56.5	72–247°°	159.5

°The IUB unit of enzyme activity is micromoles per minute, and the corresponding activity concentration is in units per liter.
°°The substrate and the IUB values are expressed at Memorial Hospital in mmol/P-Nitrophenyl phosphate/min of ml serum at 37°C.

alkaline phosphatase values in Moloney virus–induced osteogenic sarcoma of New Zealand black rats.[284]

Serum phosphatase determinations have definite value in establishing a prognosis. Patients in whom the serum phosphatase levels remain high after amputation should be strongly suspected of harboring metastases. The same applies to patients whose previously elevated serum alkaline phosphatase falls to normal levels following amputation but rises again with the development of metastases or recurrence. The amount of phosphatase present also gives valuable clinical information as to the degree of tumor destruction produced by irradiation therapy. Changes in the tumor activity may frequently be detected by this means before other clear-cut physical signs are manifested.

The reduction of elevated serum alkaline phosphatase values following chemotherapy is a valuable guide to administration of therapy (Fig. 5–3). The return of abnormal levels signals the recrudescence of active disease, and administration of chemotherapy, if toxicity permits, should be undertaken forthwith.[325]

The elevated serum alkaline phosphatase readings correspond roughly to the degree and extent of bone involvement by Paget's disease; the lowest figures are usually those for the monostotic involvement (5 to 25 Bodansky units). In Paget's disease, the serum calcium and inorganic phosphorus show no abnormalities.[135] In widespread skeletal involvement, the phosphatase values range between 50 and 150 units (BU). The more active the process, the higher the value is. In cases of polyostotic involvement coupled with the presence of an osteogenic sarcoma, values over 230 units are not unexpected.

Serum alkaline phosphatase findings in children are difficult to interpret since values range from 72 to 247 international

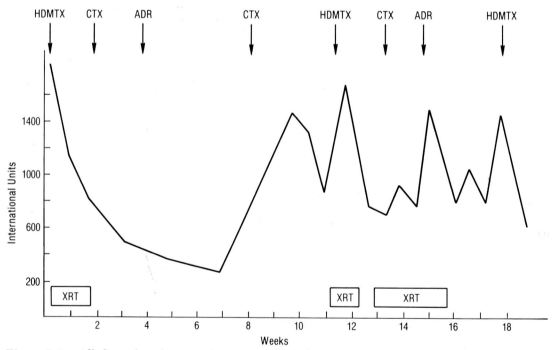

Figure 5–3. Alkaline phosphatase values in a patient during treatment for disseminated osteogenic sarcoma. (Courtesy of Dr. G. Rosen.)

units (5 to 14 Bodansky units), depending on the rate of the child's growth, and reaching their highest point in adolescence.

In general, there is a fairly good correspondence between the elevated phosphatase figures and the degree of osteoblastic activity within the osteogenic sarcoma.[427] Most osteolytic types of osteogenic sarcoma in which bone destruction is a prominent feature produce alkaline phosphatase, but not in amounts sufficient to elevate the serum levels considerably above normal limits. Rapidly growing anaplastic bone sarcomas have the microscopically demonstrable capacity to form osteoid but grow too fast to form calcified osseous tissue. In such instances, serum alkaline phosphatase values are either normal or only slightly elevated.

Jeffree and Price presented histochemical and microchemical analyses of osteogenic sarcoma tissue in 10 patients.[178] The sarcoma tissue showed high levels of alkaline phosphatase with richly positive staining for this enzyme in the tumor cells. In heavily collagenized fibrosarcomas of bone, the possibility of a fibroblastic osteogenic sarcoma should be entertained. In cases in which fresh, unfixed tumor tissue is available for histochemical studies, alkaline phosphatase reactions are negative in fibrosarcomas while increased tissue phosphatase values are registered in the fibroblastic osteogenic sarcomas.[30, 177, 264, 361]

In the report of multifocal but metachronously appearing osteogenic sarcoma, Amstutz noted that an alkaline phosphatase activity of 59 Bodansky units decreased to 26 units after removal of the tumor by hip disarticulation. With the appearance of new sites of osteogenic sarcoma, the enzyme levels rose again, this time to a value of 430 units one month prior to death.[8]

HISTOLOGIC FEATURES

Osteogenic sarcomas can be divided into histologic subtypes of fibroblastic (fibrosarcomatous), chondroblastic (chondrosarcomatous), osteoblastic, or telangiectatic, on the basis of the predominant cell forming the lesion or the pattern of growth, as in the case of the telangiectatic type (Figs. 5–4 through 5–8). This classification probably dates back to Simmons[354] and MacDonald and Budd.[222] Others, however, find the histologic appearance of osteogenic sarcoma too variable, complex, and pleomorphic to neatly categorize it.[125]

The different histologic types of osteogenic sarcoma vary according to their predominant stromal differentiation. The Bristol Bone Tumour Registry material reported by Ross enumerates five subtypes: osteoblastic (44.5 per cent), chondroblastic (26.6 per cent), fibroblastic (8.6 per cent), mixed (3.1 per cent), and anaplastic variants (17.2 per cent).[329]

Others, like Gravanis and Whitesides[132] or Dahlin and Coventry,[69] attempted to subdivide these sarcomas into osteoblastic, chondroblastic, and fibroblastic variants. No statistically significant differences could be established beyond some vague trends pointing to the osteoblastic type as having a worse prognosis than the fibroblastic variety. Price found the mitotic index useful in assessing prognosis. In his study, the chondroblastic variety of osteogenic sarcoma progressed more rapidly in comparison with the osteoblastic and fibroblastic types.[308] Others, like O'Hara and his coworkers at Memorial Hospital,[282] found absolutely no evidence that any such histologic parameters are of use in predicting the clinical behavior of a given tumor.

The five year survival rate of osteogenic sarcoma varies with the histologic subtypes, i.e., depending on whether the tumor is predominantly osteoblastic, chondroblastic (chondrosarcomatous), or fibroblastic (fibrosarcomatous) (Table 5–4).

A group of 27 patients with intramedullary well-differentiated osteogenic sarcoma has been reported, the tumors histologically showing a pattern of low-grade juxtacortical osteogenic sarcoma appearing in an intraosseous location.[403] A more recently recognized histologic variant is the small cell type, in which clear-cut osteoid is being produced directly by Ewing sarcoma–like tumor cells.

GRADING

The histologic grading of osteogenic sarcoma is a controversial and contested subject (Table 5–5). Several serious difficulties limit its usefulness for assessing

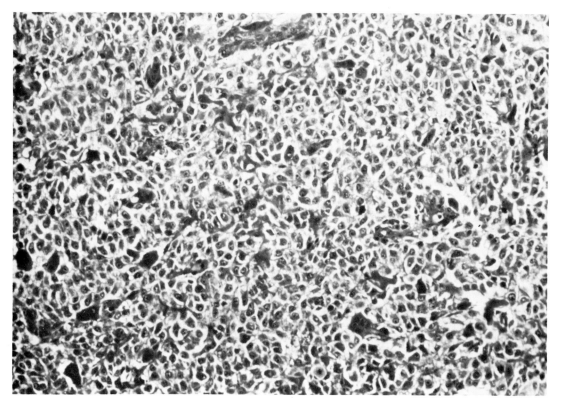

Figure 5–4. Osteogenic sarcoma with an osteoblastic pattern. (Hematoxylin-eosin stain. Magnification ×40.)

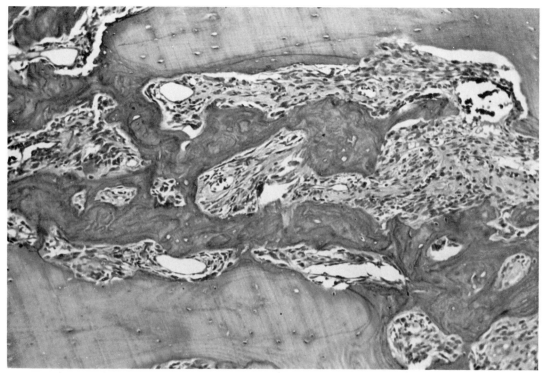

Figure 5–5. Osteogenic sarcoma of the sclerotic type with heavy bone formation. (Hematoxylin-eosin stain. Magnification ×40.)

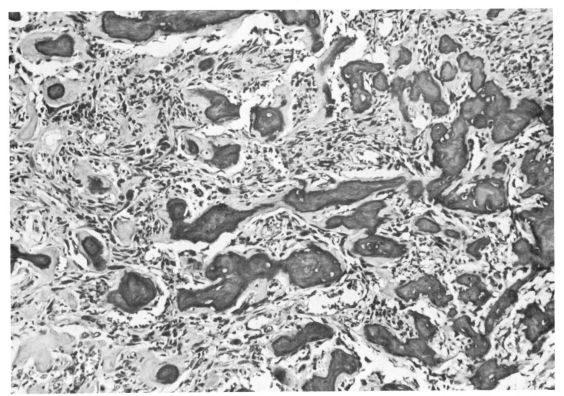

Figure 5–6. Osteogenic sarcoma of the sclerotic type with marked calcified osteoid production. (Hematoxylin-eosin stain. Magnification ×40.)

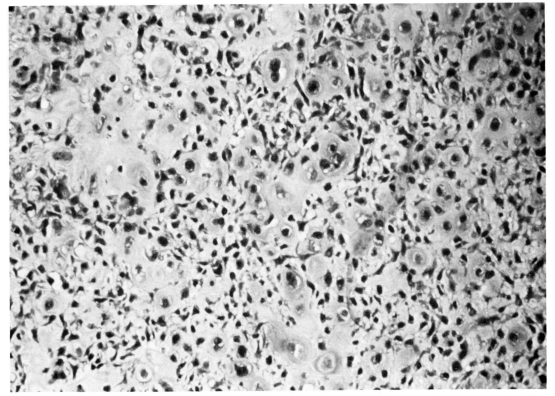

Figure 5–7. Osteogenic sarcoma of the chondrosarcomatous type. (Hematoxylin-eosin stain. Magnification ×40.)

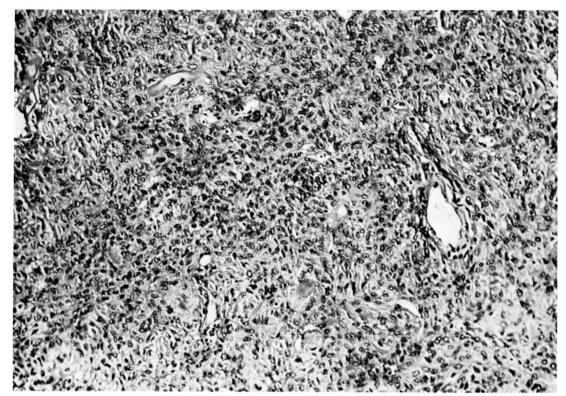

Figure 5–8. Osteogenic sarcoma with a prominent fibrosarcomatous component. (Hematoxylin-eosin stain. Magnification ×40.)

prognosis for either groups of lesions or individual cases.

1. Broders' grading system was originally meant for only epidermoid carcinomas and later for fibrosarcomas.[28]

2. Not all tumors are microscopically homogenous; tissues taken from different areas may give different impressions of the degree of malignancy.

3. It is unrealistic to grade small biopsies.

4. Estimation of proliferative activity depends on prompt and effective fixation for the proper preservation of mitoses.

5. Tumors of identical histologic pattern frequently vary in their clinical behavior according to their location.

TABLE 5–4. Five Year Survival Rates in Osteogenic Sarcoma According to the Predominant Histologic Make-up

	Dahlin and Coventry[69]	Price[304]
Osteoblastic	17.1%	37%
Chondrosarcomatous (Chondroblastic)	22.3%	8%
Fibrosarcomatous (Fibroblastic)	25.5%	33%
Overall survival rate	20.3%	15%

TABLE 5–5. The Prognostic Significance of Grading in Osteogenic Sarcoma

		Number of patients	Five year survival rate	
Grade	I	2	50.0%	Dahlin and
	II	63	27.0%	Coventry[69]
	III	218	19.7%	
	IV	128	17.2%	
Grade	I	12	67.0%	Price[304]
	II	52	17.0%	
	III	24	—	

Grading according to Broders' method.[28]

6. Histologic grading by individual pathologists rarely, if ever, can be reliably and consistently reproduced by others.

Several attempts have been made to relate the presence and degree of lymphocytic infiltration of the osteogenic sarcoma tissue to prognosis.[114, 237] Those investigators considered the presence of lymphocytes associated with this type of tumor to be evidence that an intact host immune system is actively engaged in resisting the "common sarcoma antigen."

A marked variation in the histologic appearance can be seen in different areas of each tumor, from spindle-shaped fibroblastic stromal pattern forming osteoid to lacunar-type cells embedded in a chondromyxoid matrix. The number of mitoses, the degree of cellular anaplasia, and pleomorphism greatly vary within each tumor. In an intensive study by Scranton and associates of a multitude of histologic parameters, like vascularity, number of mitoses, pleomorphism, cellularity, and so on, no direct correlation could be ascertained between the presence or absence of the vast majority of these characteristics and the prognosis.[347]

The making of osteoid (primitive bone) may be extremely limited to microscopic areas or it may be quite prominent. If one has difficulty in finding minute amounts of osteoid, by slicing the larger specimens (especially amputation specimens) suspicious areas of calcification may be seen on radiographic review. These are the areas to select for sectioning using fine grain films. Since not all osteoid is calcified to become bone, this method is not fail-safe.

The recognition of osteoid is not always easy and clear-cut. Often, well-differentiated fibrosarcomas may show foci of homogenous, afibrillar, eosinophilic material that is, in fact, hyalinized collagen. In an apparently radiologically and histologically typical fibrosarcoma, the finding of elevated alkaline phosphatase values in practice rules out this diagnosis and helps one suspect the presence of immature and mature bone formation, i.e., points to osteogenic sarcoma.

During the process of ossification, the

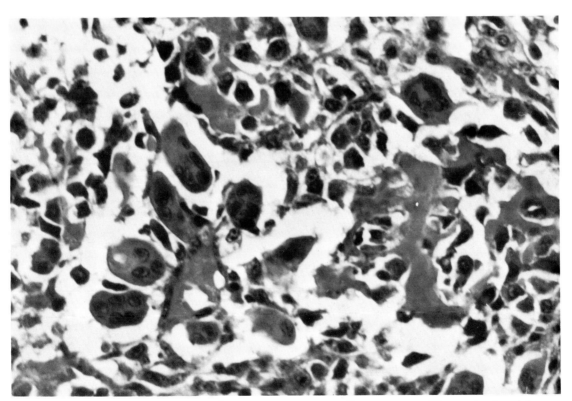

Figure 5–9. Osteogenic sarcoma with a prominent giant cell component. Clear-cut osteoid formation is present. (Hematoxylin-eosin stain. Magnification ×80.)

sarcomatous stromal cells initially become enmeshed in intercellular matrix; in these areas, sheets and trabeculae of tumor osteoid can be seen. The appearance of small blood vessels heralds the breaking up of tumor osteoid in addition to deposition of intercellular calcium with the formation of actual tumor bone. In areas in which the initially plump sarcomatous stromal cells become surrounded by tumor osteoid and bone, they appear smaller and sparser. The process of incorporating sarcomatous stromal cells to serve as the osteocytes of tumor bone is referred to as "normalization."[290]

Benign multinucleated giant cells, morphologically indistinguishable from those seen in giant cell tumors of bone, can dominate the histologic picture in an otherwise typical osteogenic sarcoma (Fig. 5–9). This may give rise to confusion and a mistaken diagnosis of giant cell tumor being rendered.[397] These benign-appearing giant cells may be seen in the telangiectatic variety of osteogenic sarcoma and are usually associated with vascular spaces and hemorrhages. Another area of confusion and diagnostic difficulty relates to the primary malignant giant cell tumor of bone. In this tumor, in addition to the benign-appearing multinucleated giant cells, a malignant, usually fibroblastic, stroma is present but no osteoid is formed directly by the stromal sarcomatous tumor cells. At Memorial Hospital, we have seen several examples of well-documented osteogenic sarcomas with large numbers of giant cells arising in the fingers.

TELANGIECTATIC OSTEOGENIC SARCOMA

In 1854, Sir James Paget briefly mentioned, but did not illustrate, a bone lesion under the designation of "medullary cancer of bone with an excessive development of blood vessels."[286] Whether this was the first description of telangiectatic osteogenic sarcoma is hard to tell. Gaylord, in

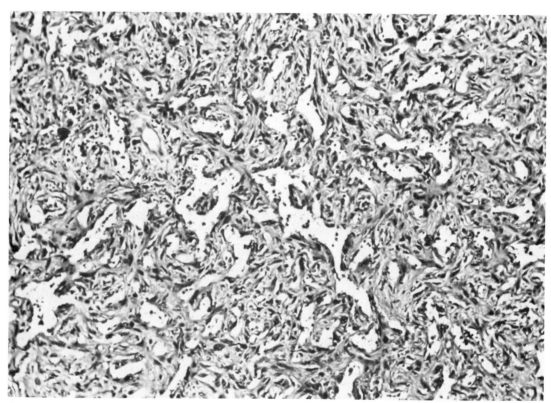

Figure 5–10. Telangiectatic osteogenic sarcoma showing prominent vascular pattern. (Hematoxylin-eosin stain. Magnification ×40.)

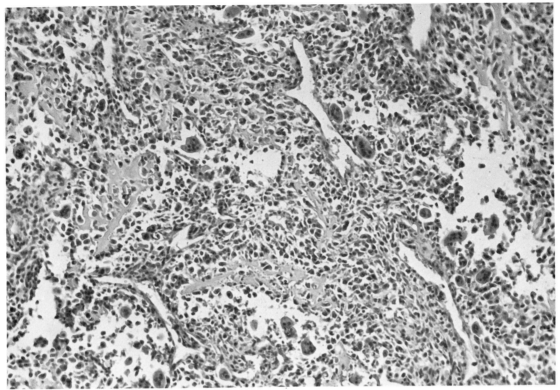

Figure 5–11. Telangiectatic osteogenic sarcoma demonstrating not only prominent vascularity but also an abundance of giant cells. (Hematoxylin-eosin stain. Magnification ×40.)

1903, referred to this tumor as a malignant bone aneurysm.[118] Ewing, in 1922 (and in 1939), considered it for the first time to be a variant of osteogenic sarcoma.[88, 90]

The criteria for the diagnosis of telangiectatic osteogenic sarcoma include the following: (1) a predominantly lytic, destructive lesion of bone with only minimal lesional sclerosis on roentgenograms; (2) a soft, cystic cavity–like tumor on gross examination; (3) histologically single or multiple aneurysmally dilated spaces containing blood or degenerated tumor cells lined or traversed by septa containing anaplastic sarcoma cells with numerous mitoses. Osteoid formation by these sarcoma cells is scanty and has a thin, lacelike filigree pattern (Figs. 5–10 and 5–11).

The radiographic diagnosis of telangiectatic osteogenic sarcoma is hampered by the lack of agreement as to what constitutes the absolute criteria for making such a diagnosis (Fig. 5–12). Matsuno and his coworkers define it as a lytic, destructive lesion with no appreciable areas of sclerosis.[246] Others, like Campanacci and Pizzoferrato[43] and Farr and his associates,[92] feel that a minimal amount of sclerosis within the lesion does not preclude the diagnosis of telangiectatic osteogenic sarcoma. In the series by the Italian authors, one third of the lesions showed some sclerosis.

The rapidly fatal progression in 25 cases of telangiectatic osteogenic sarcoma reported by Matsuno and his coworkers,[246] suggests that this type of osteogenic sarcoma has a worse outlook than the conventional type. Although this may be true, three aspects prove this conclusion to be unsubstantiated: (1) Many cases were initially misdiagnosed and, as such, inadequately treated. (2) the treatment of 10 of the patients dates back to before 1945. The first case was treated in 1912. (3) "In five lesions, unmistakable osteoid was not seen on multiple sections." In a report by Farr and associates, the prognosis was not found to be worse if only those patients who received adequate treatment were considered in the survival statistics.[92]

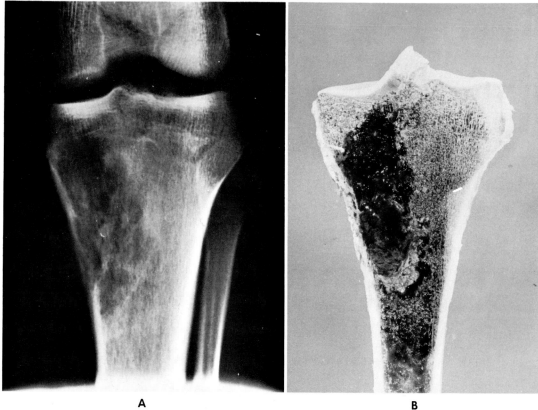

A   **B**

Figure 5–12. *A*, Telangiectatic osteogenic sarcoma of the proximal tibia with ill-defined, large, lytic destructive process. *B*, Cross section of the specimen reveals a blood-filled cavity with rough irregular outlines and brittle friable consistency.

ULTRASTRUCTURE

Several recent *ultrastructural studies* of osteogenic sarcoma outlined the wide cellular spectrum present in these neoplasms.[218] The malignant osteoblastic cells exhibit an extensive network of dilated, interanastomosing, rough endoplasmic reticulum, often containing finely granular or flocculent condensed material appearing in dilated cisternae.[120, 189, 288, 421] Focal collections of slender needle-shaped hydroxyapatite crystals measuring 20 to 40Å in width and 200 to 500Å in length are often seen obscuring underlying collagen fibers.[421] The true nature of the branched material is only postulated and is probably abnormal matrix protein.[29] Intercellular tight junctions connecting tumor cells are seen. These junctions (the zonulae occludentes) serve as intercellular transport of nutrients and electrolytes and have been noted both in human and in canine osteogenic sarcomas.[288, 295]

BIOPSY TECHNIQUES

In order to obtain the maximal diagnostic benefit from a *biopsy*, the technique should be either a core of needle biopsy or an incisional biopsy. Preferably, the tissue removed should include the infiltrating edge of the tumor (Fig. 5–13).

In the histologic interpretation of a biopsy specimen, one is hampered by the fact that the tissue under scrutiny is from the most peripheral portion of the lesion. The advancing edge of an osteogenic sarcoma is the most undifferentiated aspect in which osteoid production may be limited or even entirely absent. Examination of the deeper portions of the lesional tissue, unless it is necrotic, will readily reveal osteoid; elevated tissue alkaline phosphatase values will help one steer away from an erroneous impression of a fibrosarcoma, malignant fibrous histiocytoma, or spindle and giant cell sarcomas.

Aspiration needle biopsy of osteogenic

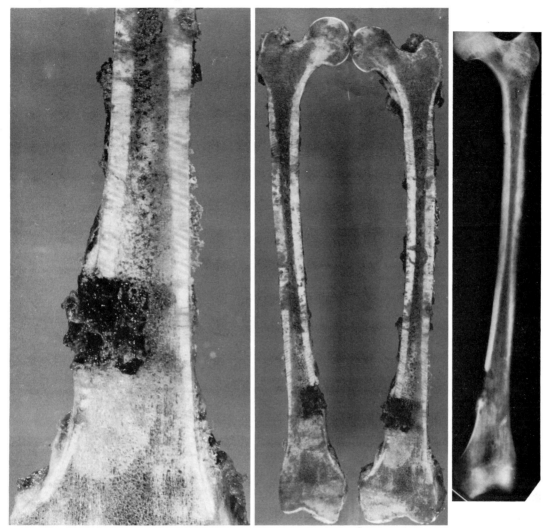

Figure 5–13. Osteogenic sarcoma of distal portion of femur in a 17-year-old boy. The tumor involves the medulla and the cortex and extends into periosteal soft tissues. The hemorrhagic area shows the site of the properly placed biopsy.

sarcomas, or other suspected sarcomas of bone, is a useful technique, especially for those who are experienced by virtue of training and understanding of the morphologic variability. The accuracy of a needle biopsy, when positive, is almost 100 per cent in expert hands, with no false positives.[137] This technique, however, gives a false negative result in 25 per cent of the cases. In such instances, an open biopsy is the next choice.

A definite opinion may be given by examining a frozen section of the biopsy specimen. The cryostat has markedly improved the quality of the frozen section technique and, unless the tumor is heavily calcified and ossified, a definitive diagnosis on frozen section is feasible. In cases of reasonable doubt, it may be necessary to withhold the diagnosis until paraffin-embedded tissue can be examined.

METASTATIC PATTERN

The presumption that there is a straight relationship between the size of the lesion and its capability to metastasize, although most often true, may on occasion be entirely without merit. The radiographic

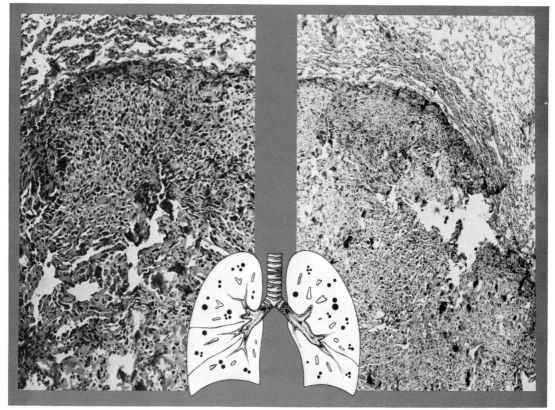

Figure 5–14. Metastatic osteogenic sarcoma nodules in lungs. (Hematoxylin-eosin stain. Magnification ×40.)

demonstration of a small lesion of benign appearance may, in turn, show a rapidly progressive lethal course.[83, 165]

Osteogenic sarcoma has the tendency to metastasize by the hematogenous route primarily to the lungs, and, at the time of autopsy, multiple pulmonary deposits are invariable findings (Fig. 5–14). In spite of solitary or even multiple pulmonary metastases, lung resection in selected instances are of definite benefit since the pulmonary lesions are more often than not the only metastatic sites[127, 157, 224, 335] (Fig. 5–15). Liver and brain metastases may be demonstrated associated with heavy bone formation.[141] Lymph node metastases were already noted in osteogenic sarcoma in 1933.[31] Skin metastases were demonstrated in 1924.[99] Cardiac metastases were shown by Laurain in 1957[207] and by Dorfman and Michaels in 1966.[75] Dorfman and Michaels described the necropsy findings of a solitary metastatic osteogenic sarcoma in the heart without lung involvement.

Regional lymph node metastases at the time of major amputation for osteogenic sarcoma of an extremity were noted in 4 of 35 patients (11.4 per cent). These patients survived for 2, 10, and 11 months respectively, with another patient surviving without evidence of disease more than five years.[37]

The possibility and the expected frequency of lymph node involvement are not generally recognized in the spread of osteogenic sarcoma.[314, 351] In a series of retrospective postmortem examinations at Memorial Hospital, McKenna and his associates found regional lymph node involvement in 32 per cent of the cases. Regional lymph node metastases were found in 6 of 194 patients (3.1 per cent) who underwent surgical ablation. None of these patients survived for five years.[252] In reviewing the Bristol Bone Tumour Registry cases, Hill found 4 patients out of 31 with distal femoral lesions to have ilioinguinal lymph node metastases.[149] Other well-documented

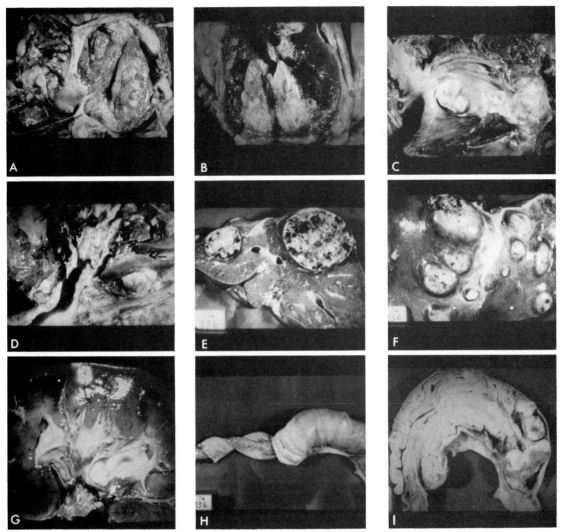

Figure 5–15. Widely disseminated osteogenic sarcoma in a 12-year-old boy at autopsy showing metastases to *A*, pericardium, *B*, left ventricle, *C*, foramen ovale, *D*, lung with bronchial involvement, *E*, liver, *F*, subcapsular liver, *G*, kidney, *H* and *I*, small intestine, resulting in intussusception.

case reports of regional lymph node metastases have been recorded.[213, 417] Sometimes, these metastases are highly ossified and appear to be radiopaque on radiographic examination.[213, 406]

At autopsy, the most frequent metastatic sites are the lungs (95 per cent), bones (50 per cent), and kidneys (12 per cent).[184, 306] The radiographic demonstration of kidney metastases while the patient is still alive is rare unless they are symptomatic and heavily calcified.[131] Two other reports describe solitary or large localized renal metastasis in living patients.[240, 276]

OSTEOGENIC SARCOMA INDUCED BY VIRUSES AND VARIOUS CHEMICAL AGENTS

In the laboratory of Peyton Rous and his coworkers at the Rockefeller Institute, it was established that bone tumors can be induced by a virus.[331, 332] In subsequent years, osteogenic sarcomas were induced by a variety of DNA and RNA viruses.[206] For instance, the SE polyoma, a DNA virus, can produce osteogenic sarcoma in mice,[373] and the SV40 virus (also a DNA virus) does the same after injection at very high doses in Syrian golden hamsters.[73] The various RNA murine sarcoma viruses, which have a C-type virus particle morphology, most often require that the virus be administered to an animal species different from the one that originally supplied it in order to produce an osteogenic sarcoma; they also induce various other mesenchymal tumors.[115, 143, 360] The murine bone sarcoma viruses, like the FBJ and FBR osteosarcoma viruses obtained from CFI and X/GF mice respectively, are quite oncogenic in specific strains. They induce rapidly growing, infiltrating osteogenic sarcomas with a lethal progression.[98]

Is there any evidence for human malignant bone tumor viruses? Cell-free extracts of more than 100 human osteogenic sarcomas injected into Syrian hamsters produced a considerable number of various malignant mesenchymal tumors in addition to osteogenic sarcomas.[98] Additional supporting evidence that the hamster lesions were produced by the human cell-free bone tumor extracts was provided by immunofluorescence assays[310, 315] and cytotoxicity tests.[311]

Interesting experiments with FBJ virus–induced bone tumors in Swiss mice yielded periosteal bone tumors with close gross and microscopic resemblance to human juxtacortical osteogenic sarcoma.[413]

The injection of Moloney murine sarcoma virus into the metaphyseal region of the tibial medullary cavity induces a highly malignant, metastasizing osteogenic sarcoma at the injection site in several strains of neonatal rats. The average latent period for the development of these tumors is 10 days.[67, 109, 110, 162, 284]

Thorotrast-Induced Bone Sarcomas

Malignant bone and soft tissue tumors may arise in patients who receive injections of Thorotrast, a radioactive contrast medium containing a 25 per cent colloidal thorium dioxide suspension (an alpha emitter). In 1956, Zak and his associates reported the appearance of a fibrosarcoma in the ninth thoracic vertebra that developed 21 years after the patient had received 75 ml of Thorotrast.[432] Tsuya and his coworkers noted a pelvic osteogenic sarcoma in a 68-year-old Japanese man

who had received 50 to 75 ml of intravenous Thorotrast 18 years previously.[398] Schajowicz and his colleagues reported an extraskeletal low-grade chondrosarcoma in a patient who had had a Thorotrast brachial arteriogram 22 years previously to demonstrate a hemangioma of the forearm.[339] In a report by Altner and associates, a case was presented of a 16-year-old girl who developed a right tibial osteogenic sarcoma some 15 years after administration of 75 ml of Thorotrast.[5]

To establish a causal relationship between the Thorotrast injection and the bone cancer, the following criteria have been promulgated by Altner and associates: (1) Presence of Thorotrast particles within the tumor or in its immediate vicinity. (2) A sufficiently long period of latency (17.1 years average duration for soft tissue tumors). (3) Exposure to sufficiently high dosages of radiation. (4) Absence of other pre-existent or tumor-inducing factors.

A single local injection of zinc beryllium silicate into the tibial or femoral epiphysis of rabbits caused osteogenic sarcoma in 70 per cent of the 100 animals so treated by Mazabraud.[249] Similar results have been obtained with beryllium oxide.[80, 152, 175, 197]

RADIOGRAPHIC FINDINGS

It is of major importance to consider both the radiologic findings and the pathologic examination in order to arrive at the proper diagnosis of osteogenic sarcoma.[68]

An osteogenic sarcoma may exhibit little, moderate, or much ossification. The more ossification one finds, the easier the correct recognition and the radiographic diagnosis will be. Heavy ossification, e.g., sclerosis, is represented by dense radiopaque areas of bone involvement. In such cases, the extracortical spread of the tumor is at least partly radiopaque. Slight ossification within the lesional tissue enhances the diagnostic difficulties, resulting in an ambiguous radiographic presentation.

The extracortical soft tissue extension of a highly ossified osteogenic sarcoma may display transverse or radiating striations emanating from the involved cortex in a characteristic "sunburst" perpendicular configuration (Fig. 5–16). On histologic

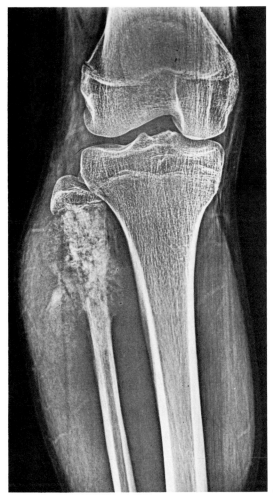

Figure 5–16. Xeroradiograph of a fibular osteogenic sarcoma in an 18-year-old boy, demonstrating enhanced details of tumor destruction and soft tissue extension.

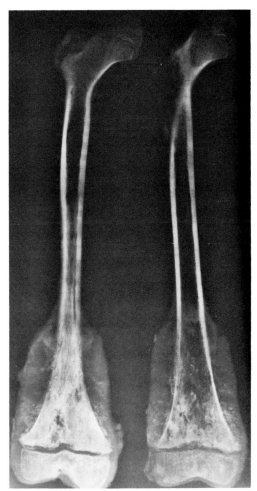

Figure 5–17. Specimen radiograph of a distal femoral sclerotic osteogenic sarcoma with extensive (11.5 cm) proximal shaft involvement not demonstrable on routine roentgenograms. Also note the rare epiphyseal involvement by tumor.

study, such striations or spicules reveal osseous trabeculae traversing the less calcified and less ossified extracortical tumor tissue.

The radiographic appearance of osteogenic sarcoma is characterized by the interrelationship of three aspects, namely destruction of the pre-existent cortical or medullary bone (osteolysis), calcification and bone production, and finally, periosteal new bone formation (Fig. 5–17).

The earliest recognizable radiographic changes include minimal irregular periosteal new bone formation in the metaphysis, with the underlying bone exhibiting a localized mottled radiolucent or radiopaque area (Fig. 5–18). The earliest periosteal reactions may appear as a fine "sun-

burst" or as a single vertical periosteal layer.[151] Although these changes already suggest a malignant tumor, a diagnosis of Ewing's sarcoma is often entertained (Fig. 5–19). The more advanced changes feature definite cortical destruction and breakthrough. The central localized areas within the tumor show a radiolucent, radiopaque, or even mixed pattern of mottling. Characteristic features also include periosteal elevation, the so-called Codman's triangle, and spicule formation (Fig. 5–20). In some cases, markedly sclerotic lesions are observed, while in others, purely lytic forms are seen. Periosteal bone formation may be entirely lacking (Fig. 5–21). The majority of the lesions are

Text continued on page 72

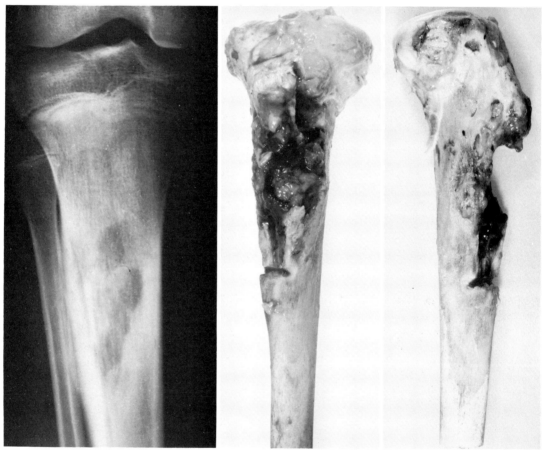

Figure 5–18. Predominantly lytic osteogenic sarcoma of upper tibia in a 13-year-old boy with erosive cortical destruction.

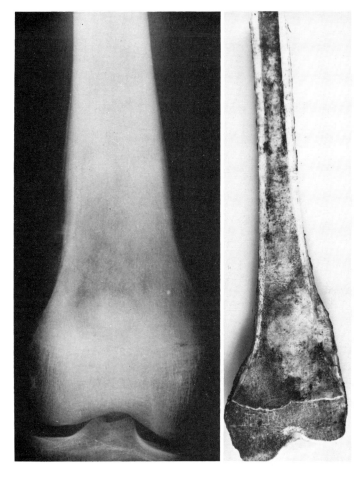

Figure 5–19. Osteogenic sarcoma of the distal femur in a 14-year-old boy with a permeative destructive radiographic pattern and onionskin periosteal layering.

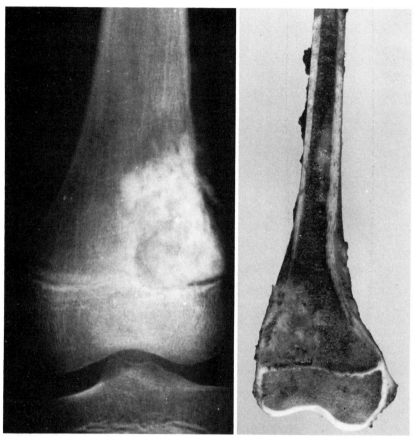

Figure 5–20. Typical sclerotic osteogenic sarcoma of distal femur with periosteal spiculation in a 9½-year-old boy.

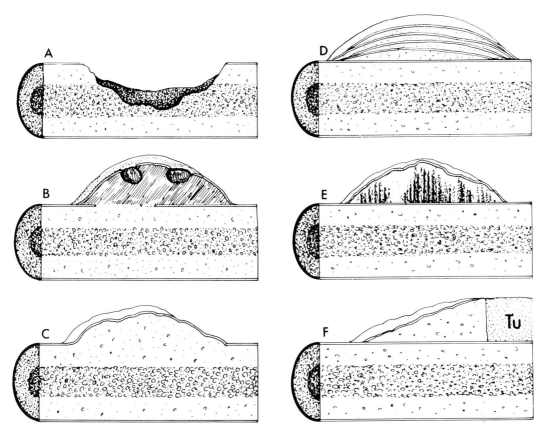

Figure 5–21.   Cortical and periosteal radiographic patterns in osteogenic sarcoma. *A*, Erosive type of cortical loss due to tumor invasion and destruction. *B*, Diffuse, densely calcified, cortical tumor bone deposition in which the underlying cortex can be traced by a narrow radiolucent zone. This "string" sign is characteristic of juxtacortical osteogenic sarcoma. *C*, Diffuse, heavily calcified, cortical tumor deposition seen in tumor extension into adjacent soft tissues. *D*, The "onionskin" type of periosteal bone deposition that is the result of repeated separation and formation of osseous layers. This phenomenon is usually characteristic of Ewing's sarcoma. *E*, Bony spicule formation by the periosteum perpendicular to the cortex. *F*, Codman's triangle represents a periosteal detachment from the cortex characterized by a wedge-shaped bone formation.

purely metaphyseal and eccentric, but some may extend into the epiphysis and destroy the epiphyseal plate. These alterations are usually associated with a large, densely ossified, soft tissue mass. The articular cartilage is very resistant to tumor invasion, and joint space involvement, even in very advanced cases, is rarely encountered.

In a correlative histologic and roentgenographic study of 245 patients with osteogenic sarcoma of the extremities, the following distinct radiographic patterns were found by von Ronnen.[410] The most frequent was the mixed pattern of radiologic bone formation and bone destruction with a poorly defined, irregular border and periosteal spicule or Codman's triangle formation (135 patients). The purely cystic, lytic types and the periosteal variants were relatively uncommon (11 and 9 patients respectively). The predominantly osteosclerotic type was slightly more common (28 patients). In a fairly large number of cases (62 patients), no distinctive characteristics could be observed.

Codman's triangle is a manifestation of extreme periosteal elevation forming an acute angle with the cortex. The periosteal new bone formation is a reactive response to the lifting of the periosteum and is not specific for osteogenic sarcoma since it may be seen, for instance, in Ewing's tumor as well.

In a series of 345 osteogenic sarcomas from the Rizzoli Clinic in Bologna, 43 per cent were predominantly osteolytic and 47 per cent were sclerotic. About 10 per cent presented a mixed osteolytic and sclerotic pattern. No significant differences in survival were noted between the various types.[125] Nevertheless, it is generally assumed, and taught, that osteogenic sarcomas that run a slower, more benign clinical course are generally sclerotic, whereas the purely osteolytic types seem to behave in a virulently fatal manner.[58] In his study of peripheral osteogenic sarcomas, von Ronnen found a relatively more favorable clinical outcome for patients with the rare subperiosteal and cystic types of osteogenic sarcomas. The amount and the composition of the extracortical tumor calcification and periosteal reaction were studied by measuring the spicular bone formation and the onionskin type of periosteal new bone

formation along the cortical bone.[411] Cohen found a statistically significant relationship between more spicule and periosteal bone formation and an improved three and five year survival. According to this study, the composition of the extracortical appearance of the osteogenic sarcoma appears to be more important as far as the ultimate prognosis is concerned.[53]

Occasionally, osteogenic sarcoma may present with radiologic features that are considered benign. The lesions may show small or moderately sized dense intramedullary fluffs. Other benign radiologic appearances can include expansile cyst-like or well-delimited lytic lesions that show neither a soft tissue extension nor a significant degree of periosteal reaction. Any sclerotic intramedullary lesion with rounded fluffy outlines (termed "cumulus cloud appearance" by Freiberger) is an osteogenic sarcoma, regardless of its small size or innocent look.

Differential Diagnosis

Confusing radiographic pictures may result if the tumor is in an atypical location. For instance, destruction of the sacrum by an obviously malignant tumor with dense radiopacity will suggest a chondrosarcoma to most. Osteolytic lesions, although clearly showing indications of malignancy characterized by bone destruction with ill-defined borders, will often result in a diagnosis other than osteogenic sarcoma. Cystic osteolytic and expansile lesions in the presence of periosteal elevation may suggest a giant cell tumor of bone, especially in younger persons. It is good to remember that telangiectatic osteogenic sarcoma, an almost purely lytic destructive lesion, may be misdiagnosed as a giant cell tumor on the one hand or as an aggressive aneurysmal bone cyst on the other. Brodie's abscess with a poorly defined radiolucent lesion, in the absence of marginal sclerosis, may be misinterpreted as an osteogenic sarcoma. Large, ill-defined, lytic lesions with cortical irregularity and diffuse bone destruction may imitate a fibrosarcoma. Osteolytic honeycomb-like cortical destruction with occasional islands of sclerosis and a fine sunburst periosteal spicule formation may also be seen with Ewing's sarcoma. Occasionally, osteogenic sarcoma may be located in the mid-shaft, presenting as a localized osteolytic area. Such instances are hard to differentiate from metastatic carcinoma or an eosinophilic granuloma. Large oval, purely osteolytic, osteogenic sarcomas in the metaphyseal region that show irregular destruction of cortical bone should arouse suspicion; they may, in fact, be metastatic renal carcinoma or, although it is less likely, a solitary manifestation of a plasma cell myeloma.

In acute *osteomyelitis* involving long tubular bones, cortical thickening in addition to medullary reactive new bone formation is noted. The roentgenographic appearance of such an osteomyelitic process may seriously raise the likelihood of an osteogenic sarcoma diagnosis.[54, 82, 372]

In occasional cases of *osteogenesis imperfecta tarda*, exuberant callus formation, usually in the femur, may be present. The roentgenographic picture of this radiopaque massive callus may be misinterpreted as an osteogenic sarcoma.[10, 12, 25, 91, 343]

Angiography

The role of selective angiography in the diagnosis and management of osteogenic sarcoma is a positive one. The less microscopic evidence there is of bone formation within the tumor, the more marked and irregular the vascularity associated with the lesion is. The angiographic demonstration of this vascularity provides useful confirmatory evidence of the roentgenologic diagnosis.[74, 156, 202, 248, 338, 409, 430] Often, the angiogram indicates to the surgeon the exact location and the range of the inapparent soft tissue extension of the osteogenic sarcoma, thereby occasionally suggesting the optimal site for a biopsy specimen. Others, however, deny that there is any practical benefit in determining the biopsy site.[159] Experience at Memorial Hospital has shown that the selection of the optimal area for biopsy is determined by the accessibility to the surgeon, the proposed surgical procedure, and the presence of pathologic fracture. The highly vascular portion of an osteogenic sarcoma is often seen to extend further than would be expected from the plain roentgenologic examination. The most reliable sign of malignancy in these tumors seems to be that the irregular, pathologic vessels of the tumor are fre-

quently filled with contrast medium at an early arterial phase or that an abnormally early venous filling, a sign of rapid arteriovenous shunting, is demonstrated. Often, an overall increase in density of the lesion, the so-called tumor "staining," is present, which is caused by the accumulation of contrast medium in innumerable thin-walled vascular channels.[138]

Angiography may be significant in helping to establish operability of the patients by accurately outlining the extent of the tumor. Angiographic delineation of the tumor facilitates the performance of limited but radical local *en bloc* resection instead of amputation in osteogenic sarcoma.[230] By revealing the extent of soft tissue tumor extension, the operation may become an amputation instead of a local resection.[159]

Angiographic studies in spontaneous animal osteogenic sarcomas demonstrated accumulation of contrast media in the distal portion of the tumor with a central light window ("spot") formation. There was also a longer period of contrast media retention in comparison with adjacent normal tissues.[7]

Bone Scans in the Diagnosis of Osteogenic Sarcoma

Until the 1970's, bone-seeking radiopharmaceuticals had not been regularly employed for the differential diagnosis of primary bone tumors in children or young adults owing to fear of high radiation doses.[374] The short-lived radioisotopes like technetium (Tc^{99m})-labelled compounds do not provoke this objection. Scintillation scanning, however sensitive, is not a reliable means of differentiating benign from malignant bone lesions.[250, 292, 412] Bone-seeking radioisotopes were found to concentrate selectively in pulmonary metastases of osteogenic sarcoma,[255] making it feasible to demonstrate these lesions prior to detection by routine radiographic means.[101]

Most osteogenic sarcomas tend to concentrate radiostrontium (^{85}S) well, and the scans usually show an abnormal area somewhat larger than that demonstrated radiographically but often smaller in volume than the pathologic specimen.[289]

In the surgical management of osteogenic sarcoma, a preoperative determination of the extent and regional involvement of the tumor is highly desirable. Radioisotopic bone scans may be of help in establishing whether "skip" areas of involvement or multicentric presentation are on hand or whether pulmonary metastases may be present. It was found in a study of 13 patients with osteogenic sarcoma, however, that by using technetium (Tc[99m]) polyphosphate or diphosphonate bone scans in no case did the isotope scan demonstrate more extensive intramedullary tumor involvement than the routine radiographic study.[128] Despite good correlation between radiograph, scan, and pathologic evaluation of the local extension of tumor in the area of surgery, subsequent local recurrences were noted in at least three instances. This study casts doubt on the efficacy of technetium scans to reliably demonstrate "skip" areas of bone involvement. It also supports the notion that these areas may be a serious consideration indeed, since in 3 of 13 patients, local recurrence was noted after less than total amputation.

It should be noted that falsely abnormal radioisotopic uptake at the ends of the tumor-bearing long bones may be demonstrated by employing ^{99m}Tc-labelled bone-scanning agents.[129] The recognition of this phenomenon may be of clinical significance since the augmented radioactivity may be mistaken for hematogenous metastases of an osteogenic sarcoma to bone or "skip" bony involvement.

Xeroradiography

Xeroradiography has received less than wide acclaim in the diagnosis of bone tumors in general and of osteogenic sarcomas in particular.[126] However, this technique demonstrates enhanced details of bone destruction, intratumoral bone production, and periosteal reaction as well as soft tissue extension by tumor.[423, 424] Several studies compare the advantages and disadvantages of xeroradiography and conventional roentgenography, each technique having certain preferences over the other.[45, 150] Because of superior "edge enhancement" by the xeroradiographic process, bone tumors are extremely well delineated, and details that are scarcely apparent by conventional radiographic techniques may be demonstrated here (Fig. 5–16).

TREATMENT OF OSTEOGENIC SARCOMA EMPLOYING MAJOR AMPUTATION AND COMBINED WITH CHEMOTHERAPY

As recently as 1965, it was stated that osteogenic sarcoma "is a tumor that always proves fatal regardless of what kind of therapy is employed."[2] In 1970, Trifaud formulated the following therapeutic pessimism concerning osteogenic sarcoma: "Not one of us can make this diagnosis without a sinking of the heart. We undertake treatment, but our minds are distressed because we know we have no weapons adequate to the task. We know that we are no more than instruments in a tragic lottery. And when death comes, we can only admit our utter powerlessness and blame a malign fate." (Trifaud[394] as translated by E. S. Lee)

The level of amputation is a problem of "as much as necessary, but as little as possible." (Thomas Stephen Cullen) "From a practical point of view it should be remembered that the medulla may be affected not only at the immediate seat of the tumor but at some distance beyond . . . the line of practice to be followed is to amputate as far as possible from the seat of the disease as may be consistent with the patient's safety."[134]

Direct extension of osteogenic sarcoma occurs through the medullary marrow cavity (data partly derived from Upshaw and his colleagues).[404] Medullary extension of an osteogenic sarcoma can exist to a considerable length without radiographic evidence of its presence (Fig. 5–17). On thorough microscopic examination, the medullary extension of an osteogenic sarcoma usually proves to be greater than it was on gross inspection. About 40 per cent of osteogenic sarcomas reveal medullary extension for about 1 to 3 inches or more beyond the cortical limit of the lesion. One case extended 8 cm beyond the area seen.[348] The osteoblastic osteogenic sarcoma displays the greatest propensity, the fibroblastic the next greatest propensity, and the chondroblastic the least propensity for spreading through the medullary canal. Proximal extension up the marrow cavity is always greater in distal femoral lesions than distal spread down the medullary cavity in proximal tibial locations.

According to Salzer and Salzer-

TABLE 5–6. Results of Treatment Following Amputation or Disarticulation in
Osteogenic Sarcoma*

Author(s)	Country or hospital	Year	Number of cases reported	Five year survival in per cent
Meyerding	U.S.A.	1938	166	23.4
Geschickter and Copeland	U.S.A.	1949	268	19.0
Hellner	Goettingen, W. Germany	1951	35	11.7
Tracey et al.	U.S.A.	1957	13	15.4
Mondolfo et al.	Argentina	1960	72	13.3
Cederlöf et al.	Karolinska Institute, Stockholm	1960	27	11.0
Lindbom et al.	Sweden	1961	78	16.6
Tudway	England	1961	51	22.0
Weinfeld and Dudley	Massachusetts General Hospital	1962	79	16.5
McKenna et al.	Memorial Hospital, New York	1966	82	20.8
Dahlin and Coventry	Mayo Clinic	1967	282	25.0
Denoix et al.	Institut Gustave-Roussy, Paris	1970	80	20.8
Marcove et al.	Memorial Hospital, New York	1971	145	17.4
Sweetnam et al.	England	1971	61	23.0
Neumann and Fleissner	Leipzig, E. Germany	1974	22	18.0

*Data modified from Trifaud and Meary[396]

Kuntschik, the amputation should be performed approximately 2 inches (5 cm) above the most proximal radiologic demonstration of tumor.[337] At Memorial Hospital, upper tibial osteogenic sarcomas are removed through thigh amputations. For distal femoral lesions, the recommended levels of transection vary from high thigh transmedullary amputation to hip disarticulation. Functional, esthetic, and mechanical disadvantages favor the former approach, but the fear of stump recurrence makes one show partiality toward disarticulation.

Phillips and Higinbotham showed a 31 per cent five year survival in 26 patients with osteogenic sarcoma of the distal femur who underwent hip disarticulation, whereas only an 8 per cent survival was noted in 24 transfemoral amputations.[291]

Results in most series in which these data were analyzed show inferior survival of those patients in whom transfemoral amputation was performed for distal femoral osteogenic sarcoma. In general, it can be stated that transection through bone containing the lesion will have poorer results, since this amputation may occasionally cut through an area of direct medullary extension or "skip" area of marrow involvement undetected at the time of surgery. Modern bone scanning techniques may sharpen the diagnostic acumen to better delineate the degree of marrow involvement.

Experience at Memorial Hospital reveals a 15 per cent stump recurrence following through-the-thigh amputation for femoral osteogenic sarcoma.[252]

In Sweetnam's series of transfemoral amputations for osteogenic sarcoma of the distal femur, 7 of 38 patients (16 per cent)

TABLE 5-7. Local Recurrence Following
Radical Surgery for Osteogenic
Sarcoma ("Stump Recurrence")

McKenna et al.	1966	15%
Dahlin and Coventry	1967	10 of 332 patients
Moore et al.	1973	2 of 62 patients
Sweetnam	1973	18%

showed local recurrence in the femoral stump.[385] Even if "skip" lesions within the medullary cavity of a bone are demonstrated by radiologic examination, it does not preclude the probability that there is an unossified nonmineralized direct extension between the two separate areas of dense bone.

The exact rates of stump recurrences are difficult to substantiate (Table 5-7). A retrospective review of 31 patients from the Bristol Bone Tumour Registry material who had distal femoral osteogenic sarcoma and who were treated by a through-the-femur amputation revealed two stump recurrences manifesting at 11 and 19 months respectively. In addition, in four instances, metastases in the ilioinguinal region were noted. A hip disarticulation presumably would have eliminated these occurrences.[149] The Mayo Clinic's experience with "skip" areas of femoral involvement shows them to be extremely rare.[69] However, Enneking and Kagan, using preoperative tetracycline "tagging," demonstrated a 25 per cent frequency of "skip" metastases in a prospective study of 40 cases.[85, 86] On the other hand, a retrospective pathologic examination of 20 disarticulation and transmedullary amputation specimens of osteogenic sarcoma by Lewis and Lotz failed to reveal "skip" areas in the marrow cavity.[214] Similarly, Upshaw and associates were unable to identify such "skip" areas in studying 70 osteogenic sarcomas.[404] According to these authors, transmedullary amputation through the involved bone is a rational surgical alternative. "Skip" involvement in this context is defined as a grossly or microscopically discontinuous secondary involvement of the same bone by the tumor.

Preoperative and postoperative radiotherapy with total scapulectomy and preservation of the acromioclavicular joint for a scapular osteogenic sarcoma resulted in a 10 year disease-free follow-up.[336] Some,

like Marcove, however, feel that scapulectomy for a fully malignant bone or soft tissue tumor is usually a poor operation.[226]

Another surgical method for treating upper extremity and scapular osteogenic sarcoma, the Tikhoff-Linberg operation, has become popular. This involves total scapulectomy and partial resection of the clavicle and the upper humerus while retaining the neurovascular bundle in the axilla. Details of this operation with subsequent results have been summarized.[230]

The treatment approach for children and young adults with osteogenic sarcoma of long bones who have no clinically or radiographically demonstrable pulmonary or bony metastases is quite variable among the major medical centers specializing in treating such tumors. This is partly due to the demonstrated success of each of the several adjuvant therapy regimens available to forestall the appearance of metastatic lesions and to increase the disease-free survival past the two year mark (Table 5-8).

The foremost principle in the treatment of osteogenic sarcoma is that the result of the curative attempt should be the complete control of the primary lesion. This can be achieved by immediate amputation

TABLE 5-8. Outline of Therapeutic Regimen
in the Treatment of Osteogenic Sarcoma
at Memorial Hospital, New York

I. *No clinical evidence of lung metastases*
  1. Preoperative chemotherapy
  2. Amputation or *en bloc* resection of primary tumor with or without prosthetic bone replacement
  3. Adjuvant chemotherapy
  4. Eventual lung metastases are treated by lung resection and chemotherapy

II. *Clinically evident lung metastases present*
  1. Preoperative chemotherapy
  2. Amputation or *en bloc* resection of primary tumor with or without prosthetic bone replacement
  3. Resections of pulmonary metastases
  4. Adjuvant chemotherapy
    (Resections and chemotherapy [several cycles] continued until lungs are clear of metastases.)

III. *Inoperable primary tumor or widespread metastases*
  1. Chemotherapy with or without palliative amputation or
  2. Chemotherapy with radiation therapy

or by preoperative and postoperative multidrug multicycle chemotherapy coupled with *en bloc* resection of the primary tumor. High dose chemotherapy may control clinically undetectable micrometastases in the lungs or other organs and may shrink the already established, clinically provable, metastases, especially in the lungs. Multiple pulmonary wedge resections to remove metastases proved to be highly successful in prolonging life or even yielding long-term cure in selected patients.[14, 233, 241, 242]

Major amputation of a limb still remains the definitive treatment in primary osteogenic sarcoma. New developments in the approach for management of such patients are in the offing and may change this.[192, 285, 305, 349]

If the primary osteogenic sarcoma is relatively small, the patient is otherwise operable, and the lesion arose in the distal femur or the proximal tibia, the entire bone giving rise to the tumor is excised *en bloc* with adjacent knee joint, including adequate soft tissue surgical lines of resection. The removed bone and joint structures are then replaced by a made-to-measure Vitallium or Guepar alloy prosthesis that includes a Walldius type of total knee.[228, 320, 324]

Bone and joint homografts may be a useful adjunct following resection and chemotherapy of osteogenic sarcoma. A case of distal femoral osteogenic sarcoma with a successful joint homograft following subtotal surgical resection of the tumor-bearing bone was reported by Mastragostino.[244]

RADIATION THERAPY

In 1951, Sir Stanford Cade proposed a large field high-dose rate megavoltage therapy for the control of primary osteogenic sarcoma in the absence of pulmonary metastases.[38] Accordingly, 186 patients were treated at Westminster Hospital in London, with the following results:

1. Satisfactory control of the tumour could almost always be obtained for a few months, but
2. Total tumour destruction, though attainable in some cases, was unreliable and unpredictable at our dose of around 6000 rad in six weeks.
3. Increasing the dose much above this level

TABLE 5–9. Results of Radiation Therapy With or Without Subsequent Amputation*

	Date reported	Five year survival in per cent	Number of patients reported and survivors
K. Francis et al.	1954	26.0	9 out of 34
Ferguson	1959	50.0	8 out of 16
Lee and Mackenzie	1964	21.9	41 out of 187
Farrel and Raventos	1964	31.0	5 out of 16
Phillips and Higinbotham	1965	21.0	4 out of 19
Papillon and Dutou	1967	29.7	9 out of 30
Poppe and Liverud	1969	15.5	14 out of 90
Sweetnam et al.	1971	27.5	22 out of 80
Calle and Mazabraud	1971	17.6	8 out of 45

*Data modified from Trifaud and Meary[396]

brought tissue damage disproportionate to the increased tumour kill. Hence

4. Surgical ablation after some seven to eight months in metastasis-free patients seemed essential to safe management.
5. Most significantly, the salvage rate was just about the same, around 20 per cent of the cases, as after surgery: unfortunately no better, but certainly no worse.[210]

Radiation therapy of osteogenic sarcoma has not been found to be successful in either reliably controlling local recurrence or preventing the appearance of pulmonary metastases, even with doses that exceed normal tissue tolerance. In 72 patients treated by megavoltage radiation therapy with or without surgery reported from Johannesburg, a five year survival of 33.3 per cent has been achieved.[71]

Price and his coworkers have shown that in 125 children the five year survival following immediate amputation was 21 per cent, in contrast to 23.8 per cent when irradiation with or without subsequent amputation was employed.[309] Similar results, with an average of 15.2 months survival following preoperative radiotherapy with subsequent amputation, were noted in 30 patients reported by Korolev and Ivanovsky.[200]

Several possible theories concerning local tumor recurrence or persistence following standard radiation fractions and total doses have been suggested. (1) Hypoxic, relatively radio-resistant tumor cells may be embedded in the dense primitive bone and in the osteoid produced by the osteogenic sarcoma. (2) The cellular repair and recovery of radiation damage may, in fact, be more complete in osteogenic sarcoma than in other tumors, resulting in the wide "shoulder" demonstrated in cell survival curves in murine osteogenic sarcomas, thus rendering the usual 200 to 250 rad fractions relatively ineffective in completely eradicating the tumor cells.[408]

In patients with osteogenic sarcoma of the long tubular bones treated solely by radiation therapy, only those who received orthovoltage therapy showed any long-term therapeutic benefits yielding five year survivors (Brzakovic).[32] At the University of California, San Francisco, between 1950 and 1974, 21 patients received only irradiation for osteogenic sarcoma because of tumor location or extent, refusal of recommended surgery, or presence of metastatic disease. The investigators conclude that primary irradiation in the absence of adjunctive modern chemotherapy offers no palliation or increased survival in patients who do not undergo radical surgery.[15]

A five year disease-free survival of about 20 per cent can be obtained by first irradiating the primary osteogenic sarcoma to about 6500 to 7500 rads in seven to eight weeks and then after about six months amputating the extremity, provided pulmonary metastases are not present. In this set-up, the only therapeutic gain seemed to be the marked reduction of patients actually undergoing amputation. Further follow-up of these patients, however, revealed local recurrence in the irradiated area of bone in some, in addition to pulmonary metastases, necessitating palliative amputations.[297]

Since the aggressive chemotherapeutic approach combined with surgery is the primary treatment of choice, radiation therapy is recommended only for surgically nonresectable lesions located among others in the pelvic girdle or in the vertebral column. In occasional well-documented patients, disease-free survival 10 years or more after aggressive radiation therapy has been reported.[211, 297]

CHEMOTHERAPY

Chemotherapy started with a poor reputation, but this has changed recently with the introduction of new cytotoxic agents and the demonstrated efficacy of aggressive multidrug multicycle chemotherapy against osteogenic sarcoma in children and young adults.[33, 34, 61-63, 76, 77, 167, 168, 320-328, 379]

Although it seems to be evident that small pulmonary metastases may be successfully eliminated solely by aggressive chemotherapy, there are those who maintain that immediate, radical, surgical removal of the primary tumor followed by multidrug multicycle adjuvant chemotherapy is of critical importance.[76, 77]

The prophylactic adjuvant chemotherapy employing a sequential administration of high-dose methotrexate with calcium leucovorin rescue (citrovorum factor; calcium folinade) and doxorubicin hydrochloride (Adriamycin) yields a prolonged disease-free survival in the majority of patients who undergo amputation for osteogenic sarcoma. Current fair estimates for disease-free survival in the three to four year bracket appear in the over 50 per cent level (70–80 per cent). Five year survival rates by surgery alone in published series range from 5 to 23 per cent[209, 215, 222, 229, 234, 263, 283, 346, 383, 387] (Table 5–6).

At Memorial Hospital, this five year survival rate after major surgery was at 17.4 per cent with less than 7.9 months median time for the onset of pulmonary metastases.[235]

Previously reported studies have demonstrated that chemotherapy was effective, not only reducing the size of the primary osteogenic sarcoma but also, on occasion, entirely eradicating small tumors.[325-328]

Aggressive chemotherapy along these lines strongly suggests that although the efficacy of treatment is only temporarily palliative in the presence of an initially large tumor, it may be permanently curative when there is only a minimal, microscopic tumor. The determining factor in successful treatment appears to be the "minimal tumor load."[33, 34]

What are some of the many theoretical considerations in selecting the proper sequence and dosage schedules for the drugs employed in the treatment of osteogenic sarcoma? Experimental considerations and clinical observations suggest selective toxic tissue reactions following methotrexate administration to be controlled by carrier-mediated cell membrane transport.[21, 130, 190]

Cell membranes of osteogenic sarcoma cells quite likely do not possess proper carrier transport sites, which hinders favorable therapeutic responses following low doses of methotrexate. On the other hand, a high-dose therapeutic regimen of this drug may indeed infiltrate the cells by mere concentration gradient alone in sufficient quantity to completely destroy them. Leucovorin in physiologic doses would enter only normal cells with active folate transport mechanisms. This transport mechanism appears to be identical for all plates, i.e., leucovorin and methotrexate. Vincristine is employed prior to the administration of methotrexate since it has been demonstrated in experimental model systems that this enhances cell concentration or methotrexate by its interference with the efflux from the cell.[116] Inhibition of DNA, RNA, and protein synthesis appear to be the three major biochemical effects of methotrexate. Its most important achievement seems to be related to the inhibition of thymidine monophosphate and DNA synthesis.[107, 158, 182, 188]

At the cellular level, the antineoplastic effects of doxorubicin are in its binding to DNA by intercalation among base pairs and inhibition of DNA-dependent RNA synthesis.[16, 17, 19, 111] The important chemotherapeutic trials by Rosen and associates,[327, 328] Cortes and associates,[63] and Jaffe and associates[170, 171] strongly suggest that the intensive multidrug multicycle chemotherapy of patients with large, bulky, primary osteogenic sarcomas will yield only temporarily successful palliation that ultimately entails a higher risk of local recurrence and subsequent pulmonary metastases in the absence of amputation. The currently popular preamputation chemotherapy administered at weekly intervals instead of triweekly seems to be more effective (Table 5–10).[171]

Methotrexate is significantly toxic in high doses. If not monitored very carefully, patients may develop progressive severe leukopenia and die of intercurrent infection. Renal toxicity in addition to hepatic cell injury has been encountered. Skin lesions may also be seen. In drug-resistant osteogenic sarcoma, the dose of methotrexate is escalated or the frequency intervals at which the doses are administered are shortened or a combination of the two is used. These, by necessity, heighten the possibility of fatal complications.

The long-term toxic effect of Adriamycin with current high-dosage schedules is the potentially very serious cardiomyopathy. Previous irradiation to the chest to control pulmonary metastases may intensify the cardiotoxic effects of this drug.

THE TREATMENT OF PULMONARY METASTASES IN OSTEOGENIC SARCOMA

In patients who had definitive major amputation for primary osteogenic sarcoma, the median time for the appearance of pulmonary metastases was 8.5 months. If the pulmonary metastases were left untreated, the median time for survival after the onset of these deposits was 2.9 months. Only 5 per cent of the patients were alive three years after developing pulmonary metastases.[229, 233]

These are some of the indications for the resection of pulmonary metastases in osteogenic sarcoma: (1) the primary lesion is completely resected surgically; (2) the pulmonary lesions are surgically resectable; (3) no other metastases are demonstrable; (4) the patient is otherwise operable. Some emphasize the advisability of only excising solitary pulmonary metastases, while others advocate attempting to remove multiple nodules as well. When pulmonary metastases are apparently inoperable or when an unsuccessful thoracotomy attempt has already been made, aggressive chemotherapy may then render the patients successfully operable.[169, 322] In patients who underwent single or multiple pulmonary wedge resection for metastatic osteogenic sarcoma, 45 per cent three year and 27 per cent five year survivals were achieved.[14, 233, 242] There were six patients apparently free of disease following single or multiple unilateral or bilateral pulmonary nodule resection; the longest follow-up was more than 20 years. Of 15 patients who survived with disease or who died, 12 (80 per cent) developed metastatic osteogenic sarcoma in extrapulmonary sites, i.e., in bones and so forth. This paradoxical metastatic phenomenon appears to be the single most important factor in the ultimate failure of multiple pulmonary resections.

The natural history of osteogenic sarcoma treated primarily by major amputation seems to be materially modified by multidrug multicycle adjuvant chemotherapy. The use of chemotherapeutic agents markedly extends the median time to the expect-

TABLE 5–10.   T-7 Chemotherapy for Osteogenic Sarcoma (Revised) as devised by
Dr. G. Rosen, Memorial Hospital (From Ref. 323)

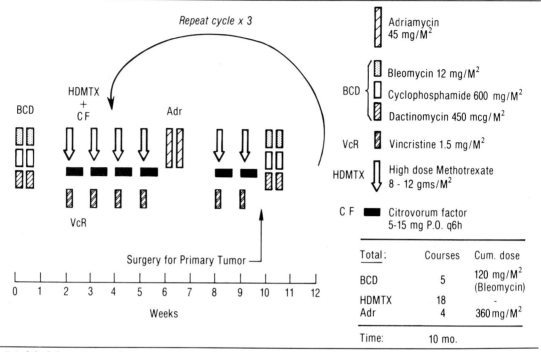

(Modified from Rosen, G., Huvos, A. G., Marcove, R. C., et al.: Primary osteogenic sarcoma: the rationale for treatment with preoperative chemotherapy and delayed surgery. Cancer, in press.)

ed detection of pulmonary metastases. Microscopic pulmonary metastases may be eradicated by adjuvant chemotherapy. In those patients who developed pulmonary metastases, the appearance of these was delayed and the number of metastatic deposits was reduced in some.[299]

Prospective randomized clinical trials of prophylactic total lung irradiation (1700 rads in 10 fractions over two weeks) in Europe and in the United States seem to be inconclusive or without definite demonstrable therapeutic benefits.[312] Elective whole lung irradiation in conjunction with adjuvant chemotherapy shows some promise in improving the survival of patients with osteogenic sarcoma.[39] The subsequent clinically significant and occasionally fatal postirradiation pneumonitis with interstitial fibrosis should be seriously considered.

The management of pulmonary metastasis in osteogenic sarcoma is influenced by whether the metastasis was present at the time of initial diagnosis of the primary tumor or whether it developed subsequently.

In the first instance, aggressive multidrug multicycle chemotherapy is instituted in the hope that the pulmonary lesions will clear; at that time, amputation is performed for the primary lesion. If pulmonary metastases develop following preoperative chemotherapy and surgical treatment of the primary tumor, an attempt is made to resect the pulmonary metastatic nodules if it is surgically feasible.

About two thirds of patients with osteogenic sarcoma have pulmonary metastases, and, in most instances, these metastatic deposits are multiple.[306]

It has been shown by calculating the growth rate of pulmonary metastases in osteogenic sarcoma, and by extrapolating retrospectively, that in four out of five cases the tumor had already metastasized many months previously to the time the patient initially presented.[26, 56, 368, 369]

The growth rate, i.e., the doubling time, is assumed to be constant and of exponential character. Others found the growth rates of individual metastases to vary in range. The ranges for doubling times varied from 2 to 962 days,[368, 369] 11 to 74 days,[11] and 11 to 360 days.[185] The mean doubling times were 42 to 44 days. These average values are probably lower in clinical practice, since the survival of osteogenic sarcoma patients with pulmonary spread is 243 days or 8.1 months.[327] In a more recent study from Ljubljana, Yugoslavia, it was found that pulmonary metastases with diameters of less than 20 mm statistically grew significantly faster (27.1 days) than those with diameters measuring more than 20 mm (37.0 days).[293]

In about 90 per cent of cases, the growth rate decreased with the increase in volume of pulmonary metastases. This decrease in the rate of growth seemed to occur when the metastatic nodule reached the size of 20 mm. In about 10 per cent of all metastases, the growth rate was quite low from the very onset and not strictly determined by the size. The determination of subsequent therapy thus may be influenced by the proper estimation of the doubling times.

Mechanisms of Pneumothorax Secondary to Metastatic Osteogenic Sarcoma

Pneumothorax due to progressive invasion of pulmonary parenchyma may be explained by rapidly expanding metastatic pulmonary lesions, or lesion, outstripping their own blood supply, with subsequent necrosis, slough, and resultant bronchopleural fistula. The metastatic growth may also cause a ball-valve type of pulmonary obstruction or disrupt the normal alveolar architecture, facilitating release of air into the interstitium resulting in lateral or central dissection and finally rupturing into the pleural space.[176, 382]

IMMUNOTHERAPY

In many instances, osteogenic sarcoma has an unpredictable outcome. In two patients who had delayed amputation for advanced and aggressive osteogenic sarcoma, for instance, unexpectedly long-term survival was noted.[350] In another patient, sustained disappearance of pulmonary metastases was achieved by palliative lung irradiation.[103] In these and similar cases, an unspecific immunologic response or the patient's resistance to the tumor may be the explanation.[345]

In attempting to devise a more effective control of sarcomas in general and osteogenic sarcomas in particular, efforts to utilize host-stimulating immunotherapy to destroy blood-borne tumor cells or incipient metastases have recently begun. The agents being used include BCG, various bacterial toxins like *Corynebacterium parvum* and Coley's toxin, as well as others. Coley's toxin consists of a heat-killed mixture of *Streptococcus pyogenes* and *Serratia marcescens*. The first case of osteogenic sarcoma involving the ilium treated by Coley's toxin occurred in 1894.[274] Coley's toxins were administered to 91 patients following definitive therapy for osteogenic sarcoma and 20 patients survived. The investigators, Coley and Pool, however, admitted that it was difficult to ascribe this profound therapeutic benefit to the toxins alone, though they did claim beneficial effect in the prevention of pulmonary metastases.[55]

Since 1963, Marcove and his colleagues have been administering an autogenous lysed cell tumor vaccine, prepared from the patient's own tumor, for a considerable length of time following ablative surgery. The five year survival rate from this adjuvant therapy is approximately 40 per cent.[225]

Marsh and associates considerably increased the expected survival rate in a small series of adolescent patients with osteogenic sarcoma by using autogenous lymphocytes sensitized against the patients' tumors. The lymphocyte infusion was given after the resection of the primary tumor.[237, 238]

Fudenberg has noted a beneficial effect of transfer factor in reducing the incidence of pulmonary metastases in osteogenic sarcoma. This factor is obtained from leukocytes of patients undergoing amputation for osteogenic sarcoma. In a short-term study of only one year follow-up, the injection of transfer factor provided promising but still very preliminary results.[36, 112, 164]

It is difficult to foresee at this time what permanent role, if any, immunotherapy will play in the treatment of osteogenic sarcoma. It is suggested by some[275] that the time adjuvant chemotherapy is administered to the patient would be the logical period to give immunotherapy, either intermittently between the chemotherapy courses or subsequent to chemotherapy when tumor burden is low. There is controversy as to whether this mode of adjuvant therapy has indeed any specific or nonspecific effect on the immune system, whether the recipient receives a tumor implant or *in vitro* cultured tumor cells. Skin tests may suggest transfer of immunity. It seems, however, that the overall "immune" response is nonspecific.[400] On the positive side, it should be emphasized that no intensified tumor growth has been observed while the patient has been undergoing immunotherapy trials.

The agents of experimental immunotherapy vary widely. Autogenous tumor with BCG followed by allogeneically cultured osteogenic sarcoma cells was used at Roswell Park Memorial Institute.[77] A similar therapeutic regimen at the UCLA Medical School, Los Angeles, yielded a prolonged median disease-free interval in patients with localized skeletal and soft tissue sarcomas following surgery and in those patients who experienced recurrence of their sarcomas.[392]

REFERENCES

1. Abbatucci, J. S., Quint, R., Brune, D., et al.: Place de la radiothérapie dans le traitement des métastases pulmonaires irradiation de nécessité et irradiation systématique précoce. J. Radiol. Electrol. Med. Nucl., 51:525–529, 1970.
2. Acchiappati, G., Randelli, G., and Randelli, M.: Observations on osteogenous-osteogenic sarcoma. Arch. Ortop., 78:57–156, 1965.
3. Ackerman, A. J.: Multiple osteogenic sarcoma. Report of 2 cases. Am. J. Roentgenol. Radium Ther. Nucl. Med., 60:623–632, 1948.
4. Alonson deSantos, L., and Goldstein, H. M.: Ultrasonography in tumors arising from the spine and bony pelvis. Am. J. Roentgenol. Radium Ther. Nucl. Med., 129:1061–1064, 1977.
5. Altner, P. C., Simmons, D. J., Lucas, H. F., Jr., et al.: Osteogenic sarcoma in a patient injected with Thorotrast. J. Bone Joint Surg. [Am.], 54:670–675, 1972.
6. Amitani, K., and Nakata, Y.: Establishment and alkaline phosphatase activity of clonal cell lines of murine osteosarcomas. A preliminary study. Clin. Orthop., 113:164–167, 1975.
7. Amosov, I. S., Dolya, A. N., and Terekhov, P. F.: Concerning vascularization of spontaneous osteogenic sarcomas. Vopr. Onkol., 19:65–71, 1973.
8. Amstutz, H. C.: Multiple osteogenic sarcomata — metastatic or multicentric? Report of 2 cases and review of literature. Cancer, 24:923–931, 1969.
9. Anderson, R. L., Jr., Popowitz, L., and Li, J. K.: An unusual sarcoma arising in a solitary osteochondroma. J. Bone Joint Surg. [Am.], 51:1199–1204, 1969.
10. Baker, S. L.: Hyperplastic callus simulating sarcoma in two cases of fragilitas ossium. J. Pathol. Bacteriol., 58:609–623, 1946.
11. Band, P. R., and Kocandrle, C.: Growth rate of pulmonary metastases in human sarcomas. Cancer, 36:471–474, 1975.
12. Banta, J. V., Schreiber, R. R., and Kulik, W. J.: Hyperplastic callus formation in osteogenesis imperfecta simulating osteosarcoma. J. Bone Joint Surg. [Am.], 53:115–122, 1971.
13. Bartkowski, S., and Kleczynski, A.: A case of sarcoma developing in the course of chronic non specific osteitis. Pol. Przegl. Chir., 46:783–785, 1974.
14. Beattie, E. J., Jr., Martini, N., and Rosen, G.: The management of pulmonary metastases in children with osteogenic sarcoma with surgical resection combined with chemotherapy. Cancer, 35:618–621, 1975.
15. Beck, J. C., Wara, W. M., Bovill, E. G., Jr., et al.: The role of radiation therapy in the treatment of osteosarcoma. Radiology, 120:163–165, 1976.
16. Benjamin, R. S., Wiernik, P. H., and Bachur, N. R.: Adriamycin chemotherapy — efficacy, safety, and pharmacologic basis of an intermittent single high-dose schedule. Cancer, 33:19–27, 1974.
17. Benjamin, R. S., Wiernik, P. H., and Bachur, N. R.: Adriamycin: a new effective agent in the therapy of disseminated sarcomas. Med. Pediatr. Oncol., 1:63–76, 1975.
18. Beutel, A., and Tänzer, A.: Frühveränderungen bei Knochensarkomen. Strahlentherapie, 90:307–313, 1953.
19. Blum, R. H., and Carter, S. K.: A new anticancer drug with significant clinical activity. Ann. Intern. Med., 80:249–259, 1974.
20. Bodansky, O.: Biochemistry of Human Cancer. New York, Academic Press, 1975.
21. Borsa, J., and Whitmore, G. F.: Cell killing studies on the mode of action of methotrexate on L-cells in vitro. Cancer Res., 29:737–744, 1969.
22. Bovill, E. G., Silva, J. F., and Subramanian, N.: An epidemiologic study of osteogenic sarcoma in Malaysia. Incidence in urban as compared with rural environments and in each of 3 separate racial groups, 1969–1972. Clin. Orthop., 113:119–127, 1975.
23. Bowers, G. N., Jr., and McComb, R. B.: Measurement of total alkaline phosphatase activity in human serum. Clin. Chem., 21:1988–1995, 1975.
24. Braddock, G. T. F., and Hadlow, V. D.: Osteosarcoma in enchondromatosis (Ollier's disease). Report of a case. J. Bone Joint Surg. [Br.], 48:145–149, 1966.
25. Brailsford, J. F.: Osteogenesis imperfecta. Br. J. Radiol., 16:129–136, 1943.
26. Breur, K.: Growth rate and radiosensitivity of human tumours. I. Growth rate of human tumours. Eur. J. Cancer, 2:157–171, 1966.
27. Breur, K.: Prophylactic irradiation of the lungs in bone tumor cases. Yearbook Cancer Res. (Amsterdam), 22:27–33, 1973.
28. Broders, A. C., Hargrave, R., and Meyerding, H. W.: Pathological features of soft tissue fibrosarcoma. With special reference to the grading of its malignancy. Surg. Gynecol. Obstet., 69:267–280, 1939.
29. Brown, G. A., Cooper, R. R., Maynard, J. A., et al.; Endoplasmic reticulum size and morphology in

bone disorders: relation to protein synthesis and malignancy. Clin. Orthop., *101*:278–285, 1974.

30. Brozmanová, E., and Škrovina, B.: Serum alkaline phosphatase in malignant bone tumours (osteosarcoma, chondrosarcoma, fibrosarcoma, Ewing's sarcoma). Neoplasma, *20*:419–425, 1973.

31. Brunschwig, A., and Harmon, P. H.: Studies in bone sarcoma. I. Malignant osteoblastomata as evidence for the existence of true osteoblasts. Surg. Gynecol. Obstet., *57*:711–718, 1933.

32. Brzaković, P., Savić, L., Barjaktarović, M., et al.: Radiotherapie dans le traitement des sarcomes osteogènes des os longs. Radiobiol. Radiother., *16*:267–270, 1975.

33. Burchenal, J. H.: A giant step forward — if. . . . Editorial. N. Engl. J. Med., *291*:1029–1031, 1974.

34. Burchenal, J. H.: From wild fowl to stalking horses: alchemy in chemotherapy. Cancer, *35*:1121–1135, 1975.

35. Busso, M. G., and Schajowicz, F.: Sarcoma osteogénico a localización múltiple. Rev. Ortop. Traum., *15*:85–96, 1945.

36. Byers, V. S., Levin, A. S., LeCam, L., et al.: Discussion paper: tumor-specific transfer factor therapy in osteogenic sarcoma: a two-year study. Ann. N.Y. Acad. Sci., *277*:621–627, 1976.

37. Caceres, E., Zaharia, M., and Tantalean, E.: Lymph node metastasis in osteogenic sarcoma. Surgery, *65*:421–422, 1969.

38. Cade, S.: Malignant Disease and Its Treatment by Radium. Vol. 4. 2nd ed. Bristol, Wright, 1951.

39. Caldwell, W. L.: Elective whole lung irradiation. Radiology, *120*:659–666, 1976.

40. Calle, R., and Mazabraud, A.: Association radio-chirurgicale dans le traitement des sarcomes ostéogènes des os longs. A propos de 51 observations. Rev. Chir. Orthop., *57*:271–277, 1971.

41. Campanacci, M.: Manifestazioni atipiche dell'osteosarcoma. Chir. Organi Mov., *59*:346–348, 1971.

42. Campanacci, M., and Cervellati, G.: Osteosarcoma. A review of 345 cases. Ital. J. Orthop. Traum., *1*:5–22, 1975.

43. Campanacci, M., and Pizzoferrato, A. Osteosarcoma emorragico. Chir. Organi Mov., *60*:409–421, 1971.

44. Campbell, C. J., Cohen, J., and Enneking, W. F.: New therapies for osteogenic sarcoma. Editorial. J. Bone Joint Surg. [Am.], *57*:143–144, 1975.

45. Campbell, C. J., Roach, J., and Grisolia, A.: Comparative study of xeroroentgenography and routine roentgenography in the recording of roentgen images of bone specimens. J. Bone Joint Surg. [Am.], *39*:577–582, 1957.

46. Cancer Incidence in Sweden, 1959–1965. The National Board of Health and Welfare. Stockholm, The Cancer Registry, 1971.

47. Caron, A. S., Hajdu, S. I., and Strong, E. W.: Osteogenic sarcoma of the facial and cranial bones. A review of forty-three cases. Am. J. Surg., *122*:719–725, 1971.

48. Carroll, R. E.: Osteogenic sarcoma in the hand. J. Bone Joint Surg. [Am.], *39*:325–331, 1957.

49. Cederlöf, S., Hiertonn, T., and Salén, E.: A follow-up study of osteogenic sarcoma. Acta. Orthop. Scand., *30*:107–114, 1960.

50. Chambers, R. G., and Mahoney, W. D.: Osteogenic sarcoma of the mandible: current management. Am. Surg., *36*:463–471, 1970.

51. Chang, P.: Progress in the treatment of osteosarcoma. Med. Clin. North Am., *61*:1027–1038, 1977.

52. Chigot, P.-L., and Thuilleux, G.: Sarcomes ostéogéniques, ostéolytiques, ostéoplastiques ostéofibrosarcomes. Rev Prat (Paris), *19*:2397–2412, 1969.

53. Cohen, P.: Röntgenbeeld en prognose bij osteosarcoma. Yearbook Cancer Res. (Amsterdam), *22*:11–15, 1973.

54. Cohn, L. C.: Non-suppurative osteomyelitis. Radiology, *16*:187–197, 1931.

55. Coley, B. L., and Pool, J. L.: Factors influencing the prognosis in osteogenic sarcoma. Ann. Surg., *112*:1114–1228, 1940.

56. Collins, V. P., Loeffler, R. K., and Tivey, H.: Observations on growth rate of human tumors. Am. J. Roentgenol. Radium Ther. Nucl. Med., *76*:988–1000, 1956.

57. Cook, S. A., Lalli, A. F., and Wilde, A. H.: Multifocal osteosarcoma. A case report. Ohio State Med. J., *69*:838–840, 1973.

58. Copeland, M. M.: Primary malignant tumors of bone. Evaluation of current diagnosis and treatment. Cancer, *20*:738–746, 1967.

59. Cortes, E. P., Chu, T. M., Wang, J. J., et al.: Carcinoembryonic antigen in osteosarcoma. J. Surg. Oncol., *9*:257–265, 1977.

60. Cortes, E. P., Holland, J. F., and Glidewell, O.: Surgery and adriamycin for primary osteogenic sarcoma: a 5 year assessment. *In* Salmon, S. E., and Jones, S. E. (eds.): Adjuvant Therapy of Cancer. Amsterdam, Elsevier, 1977, pp. 407–423.

61. Cortes, E. P., Holland, J. F., Wang, J. J., et al.: Doxorubicin in disseminated osteosarcoma. J.A.M.A., *221*:1132–1138, 1972.

62. Cortes, E. P., Holland, J. F., Wang, J. J., et al.: Chemotherapy of advanced osteosarcoma *In* Price, C. H. G., and Ross, F. G. M. (eds.): Bone — Certain Aspects of Neoplasia. Philadelphia, F. A. Davis (Butterworths), 1973, pp. 265–280.

63. Cortes, E. P., Holland, J. F., Wang, J. J., et al.: Amputation and adriamycin in primary osteosarcoma. N. Engl. J. Med., *291*:998–1000, 1974.

64. Cortes, E. P., Holland, J. F., Wang, J. J., et al.: Adriamycin (NSC-123127) in 87 patients with osteosarcoma. Cancer Chemother. Rep., *6*:305–313, 1975.

65. Coventry, M. B., and Dahlin, D. C.: Osteogenic sarcoma. A critical analysis of 430 cases. J. Bone Joint Surg. [Am.], *39*:741–757, 1957.

66. Cremin, B. J., Heselson, N. G., and Webber, B. L.: The multiple sclerotic osteogenic sarcoma of early childhood. Br. J. Radiol., *49*:416–419, 1976.

67. Czitrom, A. A., Pritzker, K. P. H., Langer, F., et al.: Virus-induced osteosarcoma in rats. J. Bone Joint Surg. [Am.], *58*:303–308, 1976.

68. Dabska, M., and Buraczewski, J.: The problem of complex diagnosis of osteogenic sarcoma. Nowotwory, *24*:157–166, 1974.

69. Dahlin, D. C., and Coventry, M. B.: Osteogenic sarcoma. A study of 600 cases. J. Bone Joint Surg. [Am.], *49*:101–110, 1967.

70. Davidson, J. W., Chacha, P. B., and James, W.: Multiple osteosarcomata. Report of a case. J. Bone Joint Surg. [Br.], *47*:537–541, 1965.

71. de Moor, N. G.: Osteosarcoma. A review of 72 cases treated by megavoltage radiation therapy, with or without surgery. S. Afr. J. Surg., *13*:137–146, 1975.

72. Denoix, P., Genin, J., Kissous, J., et al.: Considérations sur le traitement des sarcomes ostéogéniques (à propos de 80 observations). Chirurgie, *96*:63–67, 1970.

73. Diamandopoulos, G. T.: Induction of lymphocytic leukemia, lymphosarcoma, reticulum cell sarcoma, and osteogenic sarcoma in the Syrian golden hamsters by oncogenic DNA Simian virus 40. J. Natl. Cancer Inst., *50*:1347–1365, 1973.

74. Diethelm, L., Fischer, W., Habighorst, L. V., et al.: Angiographische und szintigraphische Untersuchungen an einigen seltenen Knochentumoren. Radiologe, *9*:311–317, 1969.

75. Dorfman, H. D., and Michaels, G. L.: Cardiac metastasis in osteogenic sarcoma. Bull. Hosp. Joint Dis., *27*:1–8, 1966.

76. Douglass, H. O., Jr.: Management of osteogenic sarcoma. Letter to the Editor. N. Engl. J. Med., *292*:431–432, 1975.

77. Douglass, H. O., Jr., Wang, J., Takita, H., et al.: Improvement in the results of treatment of osteogenic sarcoma. Surg. Gynecol. Obstet., *140*:693–700, 1975.

78. Drompp, B. W.: Bilateral osteosarcoma in the phalanges of the hand. A solitary case report. J. Bone Joint Surg. [Am.], *43*:199–204, 1961.

79. Dunn, D., and Dehner, L. P.: Metastatic osteosarcoma to lung. A clinicopathologic study of surgical biopsies and resections. Cancer, *40*:3054–3064, 1977.

80. Dutra, F. R., and Largent, E. J.: Osteosarcoma induced by beryllium oxide. Am. J. Pathol., *26*:197–209, 1950.

81. Ehrenhaft, J. L., Lawrence, M. S., and Sensenig, D. M.: Pulmonary resections for metastatic lesions. Arch. Surg., *77*:606–612, 1958.

82. Elliott, G. R.: Chronic osteomyelitis presenting distinct tumor formation simulating clinically true osteogenic sarcoma. J. Bone Joint Surg., *16*:137–144, 1934.

83. Ellman, H., Gold, R. H., and Mirra, J. M.: Roentgenographically "benign" but rapidly lethal diaphyseal osteosarcoma. A case report. J. Bone Joint Surg. [Am.], *56*:1267–1269, 1974.

84. Enneking, W. F., and Kagan, A.: "Skip" metastases in osteosarcoma. Cancer, *36*:2192–2205, 1975.

85. Enneking, W. F., and Kagan, A.: The implications of "skip" metastases in osteosarcoma. Clin. Orthop., *111*:33–41, 1975.

86. Enneking, W. F., and Springfield, D. S.: Osteosarcoma. Orthop. Clin. North Am., *8*:785–803, 1977.

87. Epstein, L. I., Bixler, D., and Bennett, J. E.: An incident of familial cancer. Including 3 cases of osteogenic sarcoma. Cancer, *25*:889–891, 1970.

88. Ewing, J.: A review and classification of bone sarcomas. Arch. Surg., *4*:483–533, 1922.

89. Ewing, J.: Bulkley lecture; modern attitude toward traumatic cancer. Arch. Pathol., *19*:690–728, 1935.

90. Ewing, J.: A review of the classification of bone tumors. Bull. Am. Coll. Surg., *24*:290–295, 1939.

91. Fairbank, H. A. T., and Baker, S. L.: Hyperplastic callus formation, with or without evidence of a fracture, in osteogenesis imperfecta. Br. J. Surg., *36*:1–16, 1948.

92. Farr, G. H., Huvos, A. G., Marcove, R. C., et al.: Telangiectatic osteogenic sarcoma: a review of twenty-eight cases. Cancer, *34*:1150–1158, 1974.

93. Farrel, C., and Raventos, A.: Experiences in treating osteosarcoma at the Hospital of the University of Pennsylvania. Radiology, *83*:1080–1083, 1964.

94. Feci, A., and Barile, L.: Il sarcoma osteogenico sclerosante a localizzazione multipla (descrizione di un caso). Arch. Putti Chir. Organi Mov., *26*:1–8, 1971.

95. Ferguson, A. B.: The present trend in the treatment of osteogenic sarcoma. Clin. Orthop., *14*:63–69, 1959.

96. Fielding, J. W., Fietti, V. G., Jr., Hughes, J. E. O., et al.: Primary osteogenic sarcoma of the cervical spine. A case report. J. Bone Joint Surg. [Am.], *58*:892–894, 1976.

97. Fineschi, G.: Il sarcoma osteogenico-osteolitico. Arch. Putti Chir. Organi Mov., *8*:9–59, 1957.

98. Finkel, M. P., Reilly, C. A., Jr., and Biskis, B. O.: Pathogenesis of radiation and virus-induced bone tumors. *In* Grundmann, E. (ed.): Malignant Bone Tumors. New York, Springer-Verlag, 1976, p. 97.

99. Finnerud, C. W.: Ossifying sarcoma of the skin metastatic from ossifying sarcoma of the humerus. Arch. Dermatol., *10*:56–62, 1924.

100. Fitzgerald, R. H., Jr., Dahlin, D. C., and Sim, F. H.: Multiple metachronous osteogenic sarcoma. Report of 12 cases with 2 long-term survivors. J. Bone Joint Surg. [Am.], *55*:595–605, 1973.

101. Flowers, J. M., Jr.: ^{99m}Tc-polyphosphate uptake within pulmonary and soft-tissue metastases from osteosarcoma. Radiology, *112*:377–378, 1974.

102. Fornasier, V. L.: Osteoid: an ultrastructural study. Hum. Pathol., *8*:243–254, 1977.

103. Francis, K. C., Hutter, R. V. P., Phillips, R. K., et al.: Osteogenic sarcoma. Sustained disappearance of pulmonary metastases after only palliative irradiation. N. Engl. J. Med., *266*:694–699, 1962.

104. Francis, K. C., Phillips, R. K., Nickson, J. J., et al.: Massive preoperative irradiation in the treatment of osteogenic sarcoma in children. A preliminary report. Am. J. Roentgenol. Radium Ther. Nucl. Med., *72*:813–818, 1954.

105. Fraumeni, J. F., Jr.: Stature and malignant tumors of bone in childhood and adolescence. Cancer, *20*:967–973, 1967.

106. Frei, E., III, Jaffe, N., Skipper, H. E., et al.: Adjuvant chemotherapy of osteogenic sarcoma: progress and prospectives. *In* Salmon, S. E., and Jones, S. E. (eds.): Adjuvant Therapy of Cancer. Amsterdam, Elsevier, 1977, pp. 49–64.

107. Frei, E., III, Jaffe, N., Tattersall, M. H. N., et al.: New approaches to cancer chemotherapy with methotrexate. N. Engl. J. Med., 292:846–851, 1975.

108. Freiberger, R. H.: Personal communication.

109. Friedlaender, G. E., and Mitchell, M. S.: A laboratory model for the study of the immunobiology of osteosarcoma. Cancer, 36:1631–1639, 1975.

110. Friedlaender, G. E., and Mitchell, M. S.: A virally induced osteosarcoma in rats. A model for immunological studies of human osteosarcoma. J. Bone Joint Surg. [Am.], 58:295–302, 1976.

111. Friedman, M. A., and Carter, S. K.: The therapy of osteogenic sarcoma: Current status and thoughts for the future. J. Surg. Oncol., 4:482–510, 1972.

112. Fudenberg, H. H.: An admittedly biased view of the role of immunology in human bone cancer. Front. Rad. Ther. Onc., 10:63–72, 1975.

113. Fudenberg, H. H.: Dialyzable transfer factor in the treatment of human osteosarcoma: an analytic review. Ann. N.Y. Acad. Sci., 277:545–557, 1976.

114. Fudenberg, H. H., Levin, A. S., Spitler, L. E., et al.: The therapeutic uses of transfer factor. Hosp. Pract., 9(1):95–104, 1974.

115. Fujinaga, S., Poel, W. E., and Dmochowski, L.: Light and electron microscope studies of osteosarcomas induced in rats and hamsters by Harvey and Moloney sarcoma viruses. Cancer Res., 30:1698–1708, 1970.

116. Fyfe, M. J., and Goldman, D.: Characteristics of the VCR-induced augmentation of MTX uptake in Ehrlich ascites tumor cells. J. Biol. Chem., 248:5067–5073, 1973.

117. Gasparini, M., Fossati-Bellani, F., Gennari, L., et al.: Effects of adriamycin in the adjuvant treatment of osteosarcoma. In Salmon, S. E., and Jones, S. E. (eds.): Adjuvant Therapy of Cancer. Amsterdam, Elsevier, 1977, pp. 425–430.

118. Gaylord, H. R.: On the pathology of so-called bone aneurism. Ann. Surg., 37:834–847, 1903.

119. Geschickter, C. F., and Copeland, M. M.: Tumors of Bone. 3rd ed. Philadelphia, J. B. Lippincott Co., 1949.

120. Ghadially, F. N., and Mehta, P. N.: Ultrastructure of osteogenic sarcoma. Cancer, 25:1457–1467, 1970.

121. Glass, A. G., and Fraumeni, J. F., Jr.: Epidemiology of bone cancer in children. J. Natl. Cancer Inst., 44:187–199, 1970.

122. Gliedman, M. L., Horowitz, S., and Lewis, F. J.: Lung resection for metastatic cancer. Twenty-nine cases from the University of Minnesota and a collected review of 264 cases. Surgery, 42:521–532, 1957.

123. Goes, M.: Statistischer Beitrag zum Sarkomproblem. Strahlentherapie, 85:409–434, 1951.

124. Goes, M.: Knochenwachstum und osteogenes Sarkom. Strahlentherapie, 89:194–210, 1952.

125. Goidanich, I. F., Battaglia, L., Lenzi, L., et al.: Osteogenic sarcoma. Analysis of factors influencing prognosis in 100 cases. Clin. Orthop., 48:209–222, 1966.

126. Gold, R. H.: Standard radiography, arteriography, xeroradiography and xeroarteriography in the evaluation of primary bone tumors. Front. Rad. Ther. Onc., 10:82–107, 1975.

127. Goldenberg, R. R.: Osteogenic sarcoma of the tibia with pulmonary metastasis. Report of a case with 10-year survival. J. Bone Joint Surg. [Am.], 39:1191–1197, 1957.

128. Goldman, A. B., Becker, M. H., Braunstein, P., et al.: Bone scanning — osteogenic sarcoma. Correlation with surgical pathology. Am. J. Roentgenol. Radium Ther. Nucl. Med., 124:83–90, 1975.

129. Goldman, A. B., and Braunstein, P.: Augmented radioactivity on bone scans of limbs bearing osteosarcomas. J. Nucl. Med., 16:423–424, 1975.

130. Goldman, I. D.: The characteristics of the membrane transport of amethopterin and the naturally occurring folates. Ann. N.Y. Acad. Sci., 186:440–422, 1971.

131. Goldstein, C., Ambos, M. A., and Bosniak, M. A.: Multiple ossified metastases to the kidney from osteogenic sarcoma. Am. J. Roentgenol. Radium Ther. Nucl. Med., 128:148–149, 1977.

132. Gravanis, M. B., and Whitesides, T. E., Jr.: The unreliability of prognostic criteria in osteosarcoma. Am. J. Clin. Pathol., 53:15–20, 1970.

133. Green, A. A., Pratt, C., Webster, R. G., et al.: Immunotherapy of osteosarcoma patients with virus-modified tumor cells. Ann. N.Y. Acad. Sci., 277:396–411, 1976.

134. Gross, S. W.: Sarcoma of the long bones; based upon a study of 165 cases. Am. J. Med. Sci., 78:17–57, 338–377, 1879.

135. Gutman, A. B., and Kasabach, H.: Paget's disease (osteitis deformans). Analysis of 116 cases. Am. J. Med. Sci., 191:361–380, 1936.

136. Guy, E.-P., Hourtoulle, F.-G., and Loisillier, F.: Ostéosarcomes ossifiants multicentriques des os. Bull. Cancer (Paris), 43:258–265, 1956.

137. Hajdu, S. I.: Aspiration biopsy of primary malignant bone tumors. Front. Rad. Ther. Onc., 10:73–81, 1975.

138. Halpern, M., and Freiberger, R. H.: Arteriography in orthopedics. Am. J. Roentgenol. Radium Ther. Nucl. Med., 94:194–206, 1965.

139. Halpern, M., and Freiberger, R. H.: Arteriography as a diagnostic procedure in bone disease. Radiol. Clin. North Am., 8:277–288, 1970.

140. Halpert, B., Russo, P. E., and Hackney, V. C.: Osteogenic sarcoma with multiple skeletal and visceral involvement. Cancer, 2:789–792, 1949.

141. Harding, W. G., II, and Courville, C. B.: Bone formation in metastases of osteogenic sarcoma. Report of case with metastases to the brain. Am. J. Cancer, 21:787–794, 1934.

142. Harmon, T. P., and Morton, K. S.: Osteogenic sarcoma in four siblings. J. Bone Joint Surg. [Br.], 48:493–498, 1966.

143. Harvey, J. J.: Replication of murine sarcoma virus-Harvey (MSV-H) in tissue cultures of virus induced sarcomas. J. Gen. Virol., 3:327–336, 1968.

144. Hastrup, J., and Jensen, T. S.: Osteogenic sarcoma arising in a non-osteogenic fibroma of bone. Acta Pathol. Microbiol. Scand., 63:493–499, 1965.

145. Hatteland, K.: Osteosarcom ven osteogenesis imperfecta. Tidsskr. Nor. Laegeforen., 77:70–73, 1957.

146. Hayles, A. B., Dahlin, D. C., and Coventry, M. B.:

Osteogenic sarcoma in children. J.A.M.A., *174*:1174–1177, 1960.

147. Hellner, H.: Die Knochensarkome und ihre Behandlung. Zentralbl. Chir., 76:615–616, 1951.

148. Higginson, J. F.: A study of excised pulmonary metastatic malignancies. Am. J. Surg., 90:241–252, 1955.

149. Hill, P.: Local recurrence in primary osteosarcoma of the femur. Br. J. Surg., *60*:40–41, 1973.

150. Hills, T. H., Stanford, R. W., and Moore, R. D.: Xeroradiography. II. Present medical applications. Br. J. Radiol., *28*:545–551, 1955.

151. Hingorani, C. B., and Sharma, O. P.: Osteosarcoma — a roentgenographic study. Indian J. Cancer, *10*:285–294, 1973.

152. Hoagland, M. B., Grier, R. S., and Hood, M. B.: Beryllium and growth. I. Beryllium-induced osteogenic sarcomata. Cancer Res., *10*:629–635, 1950.

153. Höffken, K., and Schmidt, C. G.: Neuere Aspekte in der Therapie des Osteosarkoms. Dtsch. Med. Wochenschr., *101*:251–258, 1976.

154. Hoffmann, D. C., and Brooke, B. N.: Familial sarcoma of bone in a polyposis coli family. Dis. Colon Rectum, *13*:119–120, 1970.

155. Holmes, E. C., and Morton, D. L.: Pulmonary resection for sarcoma metastases. Orthop. Clin. North Am., 8:805–810, 1977.

156. Honkomp, J., and Schomacher, P. H.: Angiographische Differentialdiagnose von Knochentumoren. Chirurg., *44*:167–170, 1973.

157. Hood, R. T., Jr., McBurney, R. P., and Clagett, O. T.: Metastatic malignant lesions of the lungs treated by pulmonary resection. A report of 43 cases. J. Thorac. Cardiovasc. Surg., *30*:81–89, 1955.

158. Hryniuk, W. M.: Purineless death as a link between growth rate and cytotoxicity by methotrexate. Cancer Res., *32*:1506–1511, 1972.

159. Hudson, T. M., Haas, G., Enneking, W. F., et al.: Angiography in the management of musculoskeletal tumors. Surg. Gynecol. Obstet., *141*:11–21, 1975.

160. Hughes, S. P. F., Benson, M. K. D., Ell, P. J., et al.: The use of ⁹⁹ᵐTc-EHDP as a scanning agent in the detection of metastases from osteosarcoma. Fortschr. Geb. Roentgenstr. Nuklearmed., *126*:551–555, 1977.

161. Huvos, A. G., Rosen, G., and Marcove, R. C.: Primary osteogenic sarcoma. Pathologic aspects in 20 patients after treatment with chemotherapy, en bloc resection and prosthetic bone replacement. Arch. Pathol. Lab. Med., *101*:14–18, 1977.

162. Ikemoto, K., and Yamamoto, T.: Induction of rat osteosarcoma by inoculation of murine sarcoma virus into bone marrow. Gann, *63*:141–142, 1972.

163. Ishihara, T., Ideka, T., Yamazaki, S., et al.: Treatment for pulmonary metastasis arising from osteogenic sarcoma. Keio J. Med., *20*:195–202, 1971.

164. Ivins, J. C., Ritts, R. E., Jr., Pritchard, D. J., et al.: Transfer factor versus combination chemotherapy: a preliminary report of a randomized postsurgical adjuvant treatment study in osteogenic sarcoma. Ann. N.Y. Acad. Sci., *277*:558–574, 1976.

165. Jaffe, H. L.: Osteogenic sarcoma of bone. Clin. Orthop., 7:27–39, 1956.

166. Jaffe, H. L.: Intracortical osteogenic sarcoma. Bull. Hosp. Joint Dis., *21*:189–197, 1960.

167. Jaffe, N.: Recent advances in the chemotherapy of metastatic osteogenic sarcoma. Cancer, *30*:1627–1631, 1972.

168. Jaffe, N.: Progress report on high-dose methotrexate (NSC–740) with citrovorum rescue in the treatment of metastatic bone tumors. Cancer Chemother. Rep., 58:275–280, 1974.

169. Jaffe, N.: Metastases in malignant childhood tumors — the role of "adjuvant" therapy and the utility of multidisciplinary treatment. Semin. Oncol., *4*:177–226, 1977.

170. Jaffe, N., Frei, E., III, Traggis, D., et al.: Adjuvant methotrexate and citrovorum-factor treatment of osteogenic sarcoma. N. Engl. J. Med., *291*:994–997, 1974.

171. Jaffe, N., Frei, E., III, Traggis, D., et al.: Weekly high-dose methotrexate-citrovorum factor in osteogenic sarcoma. Pre-surgical treatment of primary tumor and of overt pulmonary metastases. Cancer, *39*:45–50, 1977.

172. Jaffe, N., Traggis, D., Cassady, J. R., et al.: Multidisciplinary treatment for macrometastatic osteogenic sarcoma. Br. Med. J., *2*:1039–1041, 1976.

173. Jaffe, N., Traggis, D., Cassady, J. R., et al.: The role of high-dose methotrexate with citrovorum factor "rescue" in the treatment of osteogenic sarcoma. Int. J. Radiat. Oncol. Biol. Physiol., *2*:261–266, 1977.

174. Jaffe, N., and Watts, H.: Multidrug chemotherapy in primary treatment of osteosarcoma: an editorial commentary. J. Bone Joint Surg. [Am.] . 58:634–635, 1976.

175. Janes, J. M., Higgins, G. M., and Herrick, J. F.: Beryllium-induced osteogenic sarcoma in rabbits. J. Bone Joint Surg. [Br.], *36*:543–552, 1954.

176. Janetos, G. P., and Ochsner, S. F.: Bilateral pneumothorax in metastatic osteogenic sarcoma. Am. Rev. Respir. Dis., 88:73–76, 1963.

177. Jeffree, G. M.: Enzymes in fibroblastic lesions. A histochemical and quantitative survey of alkaline and acid phosphatase, β-glucuronidase, non-specific esterase and leucine aminopeptidase in benign and malignant fibroblastic lesions of bone and soft tissue. J. Bone Joint Surg. [Br.], *54*:535–546, 1972.

178. Jeffree, G. M., and Price, C. H. G.: Bone tumours and their enzymes. A study of the phosphatases, non-specific esterase and beta-glucuronidase of osteogenic and cartilaginous tumors, fibroblastic and giant-cell lesions. J. Bone Joint Surg. [Br.], *47*:120–136, 1965.

179. Jeffree, G. M., Price, C. H. G., and Sissons, H. A.: The metastatic patterns of osteosarcoma. Br. J. Cancer, *32*:87–107, 1975.

180. Jensen, R. D., and Miller, R. W.: Retinoblastoma — epidemiologic characteristics. N. Engl. J. Med., *285*:307–311, 1971.

181. Jewell, F. C., and Lofstrom, J. E.: Osteogenic sarcoma occurring in fragilitas ossium. A case report. Radiology, *34*:741–743, 1940.

182. Johns, D. G., and Bertino, J. R.: Folate antagonists. *In* Holland, J. F., and Frei, E., III (eds.): Cancer Medicine. Philadelphia, Lea & Febiger, 1973, pp. 739–754.

183. Johnson, L. C., Vetter, H., and Putschar, W. G. J.: Sarcoma arising in bone cysts. Virchows Arch. [Pathol. Anat.], *335*:428–451, 1962.

184. Johnson, R., Bonfiglio, M., and Cooper, R.: Osteosarcoma. Clin. Orthop., 78:314–322, 1971.
185. Joseph, W. L., Morton, D. L., and Adkins, P. C.: Prognostic significance of tumor doubling time in evaluating operability in pulmonary metastatic disease. J. Thorac. Cardiovasc. Surg., 61:23–32, 1971.
186. Kahn, L. B., Wood, F. W., and Ackerman, L. V.: Fracture callus associated with benign and malignant bone lesions and mimicking osteosarcoma. Am. J. Clin. Pathol., 52:14–24, 1969.
187. Karlen, A.: Osteogenic sarcomatosis or multifocal osteogenic sarcoma. Acta Pathol. Microbiol. Scand. [A], 55:1–7, 1962.
188. Karnovsky, D. A., and Clarkson, B. D.: Cellular effects of anticancer drugs. Annu. Rev. Pharmacol., 3:357–428, 1963.
189. Kay, S.: Ultrastructure of an osteoid type of osteogenic sarcoma. Cancer, 28:437–445, 1971.
190. Kessel, D., Hall, T. C., Roberts, D., et al.: Uptake as a determinant of methotrexate response in mouse leukemias. Science, 150:752–754, 1965.
191. Keyl, W., and Hör, G.: Angiographie, Szintigraphie und Thermographie bei Knochentumoren. Münch. Klin. Wochenschr., 116:307–314, 1974.
192. Kinney, T. R., and Chung, S. M. K.: Advances in the treatment of tumors arising in bone. Semin. Oncol., 1:47–55, 1974.
193. Kitchin, F. D., and Ellsworth, R. M.: Pleiotropic effects of the gene for retinoblastoma. J. Med. Genet., 11:244–246, 1974.
194. Klenerman, L., Ockenden, B. G., and Townsend, A. C.: Osteosarcoma occurring in osteogenesis imperfecta. Report of two cases. J. Bone Joint Surg. [Br.], 49:314–323, 1967.
195. Knudson, A. G., Jr.: Mutation and cancer — statistical study of retinoblastoma. Proc. Natl. Acad. Sci., 68:820–823, 1971.
196. Knudson, A. G., Jr.: Mutation in human cancer. Adv. Cancer Res., 17:317–352, 1973.
197. Komitowski, D.: Beryllium induced experimental bone sarcomas. Verh. Dtsch. Ges. Pathol., 58:438–440, 1974.
198. Konstantinović, M., Talijančić, B., Palčić, S., et al.: Rare case of a gigantic osteogenic sarcoma. Libri Oncol., 4:209–213, 1975.
199. Koppers, B., Rakow, D., and Schmid, L.: Osteogenic sarcoma combined with non-ossifying fibroma in one bone. Roentgenblaetter, 30:261–266, 1977.
200. Korolev, V. I., and Ivanovsky, G. L.: The combined treatment of patients with osteogenic sarcoma. Vopr. Onkol., 22:17–20, 1976.
201. Kumar, A. P. M., Wrenn, E. L., Jr., Fleming, I. D., et al.: Transmedullary amputation and resection of metastases in combined therapy of osteosarcoma. J. Pediatr. Surg., 12:427–435, 1977.
202. Lagergren, C., and Lindbom, Å.: Angiography of peripheral tumors. Radiology, 79:371–377, 1962.
203. Lagergren, C., Lindbom, Å. and Söderberg, G.: The blood vessels of osteogenic sarcomas. Histologic, angiographic and microradiographic studies. Acta Radiol., 55:161–176, 1961.
204. Larsson, S. E., and Lorentzon, R.: The geographic variation of the incidence of malignant primary bone tumors in Sweden. J. Bone Joint Surg. [Am.], 56:592–600, 1974.
205. Lascari, A. D., and Eveloff, A. R.: Osteogenic sarcoma in a patient with aplastic anemia. South. Med. J, 70:874–875, 1977.
206. Latarjet, R.: On the viral aetiology of certain osteogenic osteosarcomas. A critical review. Bull. Cancer, 58:277–286, 1971.
207. Laurain, A. R.: Intracardial tumor culture of osteogenic sarcoma with fatal tumor embolism. Report of a case. Am. J. Clin. Pathol., 27:664–671, 1957.
208. Laurent, H.-R., Reboul, J., Picot, A., et al.: Multicentric osteogenic sarcoma. Bordeaux Med., 17:2685–2694, 1973.
209. Lee, E. S.: Treatment of bone sarcoma. Proc. R. Soc. Med., 64:1179–1180, 1971.
210. Lee, E. S.: Osteosarcoma: A reconnaissance. Clin. Radiol., 26:5–25, 1975.
211. Lee, E. S., and Mackenzie, D. H.: Osteosarcoma: a study of the value of preoperative megavoltage radiotherapy. Br. J. Surg., 51:252–274, 1964.
212. Lejeune, F. and Gompel, C.: Sarcomas of the osteogenic series. Value of prognosis criteria. Ann. Anat. Pathol., 14:185–194, 1969.
213. Le Treut, A., Dilhuydy, M. H., Denepoux, R., et al.: Ossified lymph node metastases due to osteosarcoma. Report of two cases. J. Radiol. Electrol. Med. Nucl., 55:317–320, 1974.
214. Lewis, R. J., and Lotz, M. J.: Medullary extension of osteosarcoma. Implications for rational therapy. Cancer, 33:371–375, 1974.
215. Lindberg, R. D., Martin, R. G., and Romsdal, M. M.: Surgery and postoperative radiotherapy in the treatment of soft tissue sarcomas in adults. Am. J. Roentgenol. Radium Ther. Nucl. Med., 123:123–129, 1975.
216. Lindbom, Å., Söderberg, G., and Spjut, H. J.: Osteosarcoma. A review of 96 cases. Acta Radiol., 56:1–19, 1961.
217. Litvinov, N. N., and Soloviev, Yu.N.: Tumours of the bone. In Turusov, V. S. (ed.): Pathology of Tumours in Laboratory Animals. Vol. I. Tumours of the Rat, Part I. Lyon, IARC, 1973.
218. Litvinova, L. V.: Electron-microscopic investigation of cell elements and interstitial substance of osteogenic sarcoma. Arkh. Patol., 38(12):36–40, 1976.
219. Lockshin, M. D., and Higgins, I. T. T.: Bone metastasis in osteogenic sarcoma. Arch. Intern. Med., 118:203–204, 1966.
220. Lockshin, M. D., and Higgins, I. T. T.: Prognosis in osteogenic sarcoma. Clin. Orthop., 58:85–103, 1968.
221. Lowbeer, L.: Multifocal osteosarcomatosis, a rare entity. Bull. Pathol., 9:52–53, 1968.
222. MacDonald, I., and Budd, J. W.: Osteogenic sarcoma: I. A modified nomenclature and a review of 118 five-year cures. Surg. Gynecol. Obstet., 76:413–421, 1943.
223. Malpas, J. S.: Advances in the treatment of osteogenic sarcoma. Editorials and Annotations. J. Bone Joint Surg. [Br.], 57:267–268, 1975.
224. Mannix, E. P., Jr.: Resection of multiple pulmonary metastases 14 years after amputation for osteochondrogenic sarcoma of tibia; apparent freedom from recurrence 2 years later. J. Thorac. Surg., 26:544–549, 1953.
225. Marcove, R. C.: A clinical trial of autogenous vaccines in the treatment of osteogenic sarcoma. In Mathé, G., and Weiner, R. (eds.): Investigation

and Stimulation of Immunity in Cancer Patients. New York, Springer-Verlag, 1974, pp. 488–495.

226. Marcove, R. C.: New trends in the treatment of osteogenic sarcoma. Orthop. Dig., 3:11–14, 1975.

227. Marcove, R. C.: En bloc resection for osteogenic sarcoma. Can. J. Surg., 20:521–528, 1977.

228. Marcove, R. C., and Jensen, M. J.: Radical resection for osteogenic sarcoma of fibula with preservation of the limb. Clin. Orthop., 126:173–176, 1977.

229. Marcove, R. C., and Lewis, M. M.: Prolonged survival in osteogenic sarcoma with multiple pulmonary metastases. J. Bone Joint Surg. [Am.], 55:1516–1520, 1973.

230. Marcove, R. C., Lewis, M. M., and Huvos, A. G.: En bloc upper humeral interscapulo-thoracic resection. The Tikhoff-Linberg procedure. Clin. Orthop., 124:219–228, 1977.

231. Marcove, R. C., Lewis, M. M., Rosen, G., et al.: Total femur and total knee replacement. A preliminary report. Clin. Orthop., 126:147–152, 1977.

232. Marcove, R. C., Lewis, M. M., Rosen, G., et al.: Total femur replacement. Compr. Ther., 3:13–19, 1977.

233. Marcove, R. C., Martini, N., and Rosen, G.: The treatment of pulmonary metastasis in osteogenic sarcoma. Clin. Orthop., 111:65–70, 1975.

234. Marcove, R. C., Miké, V., Hajek, J. V., et al.: Osteogenic sarcoma under the age of twenty-one. A review of 145 operative cases. J. Bone Joint Surg. [Am.], 52:411–423, 1970.

235. Marcove, R. C., Miké, V., Hajek, J. V., et al.: Osteogenic sarcoma in childhood. N. Y. State J. Med., 71:855–859, 1971.

236. Marroum, M.-C., Huvos, A. G., and Rosen, G.: Pathologic aspects of chemotherapy response in the treatment of osteogenic sarcoma. An analysis of two cases. Oncology, 34:273–280, 1977.

237. Marsh, B., Flynn, L., and Enneking, W.: Immunologic aspects of osteosarcoma and their applications to therapy. A preliminary report. Part 1. Antigen isolation, anti-body specificity and immunization in patients with osteosarcoma. J. Bone Joint Surg. [Am.], 54:1367–1379, 1972.

238. Marsh, B., Flynn, L., and Enneking, W.: Immunologic aspects of osteosarcoma and their applications to therapy. A preliminary report. Part 2. Passive transfer of cellular immunity to patients with osteosarcoma. J. Bone Joint Surg. [Am.], 54:1379–1397, 1972.

239. Marsh, H. O., and Choi, C.-B.: Primary osteogenic sarcoma of the cervical spine originally mistaken for benign osteoblastoma. A case report. J. Bone Joint Surg. [Am.], 52:1467–1471, 1970.

240. Marshall, D., and Drake, E.: Transthoracic nephrectomy for metastatic osteogenic sarcoma of the kidney. J. Maine Med. Assoc., 41:320–323, 1950.

241. Martini, N., Bains, M. S., Huvos, A. G., et al.: Surgical treatment of metastatic sarcoma to the lung. Surg. Clin. North Am., 54:841–848, 1974.

242. Martini, N., Huvos, A. G., Miké, V., et al.: Multiple pulmonary resections in the treatment of osteogenic sarcoma. Ann. Thorac. Surg., 12:271–280, 1971.

243. Mason, T. J., and McKay, F. W.: U. S. Cancer Mortality by County. Washington, D. C., DHEW Publication No. (NIH) 74–615, 1974.

244. Mastragostino, S.: Massive joint homograft in a case of osteosarcoma of the femur with better than five years survival. Gaslini 6:9–18, 1974.

245. Matejovsky, Z.: Familial occurrence of osteosarcoma. Acta Chir. Orthop. Traumatol. Cech., 44:24–27, 1977.

246. Matsuno, T., Unni, K. K., McLeod, R. A., et al.: Telangiectatic osteogenic sarcoma. Cancer, 38:2538–2547, 1976.

247. Mauck, R. H., and Carpenter, E. B.: Multiosseous occurrence of sclerosing type osteogenic sarcoma. South. Med. J., 52:858–860, 1959.

248. Maurer, H.-J.: Zur arteriographischen Diagnostik von Knochensarkomen. Radiol. Clin. Biol., 38:293–308, 1969.

249. Mazabraud, A.: Production expérimentale de sarcomes osseux chez le lapin par injection unique locale de Béryllium. Bull. Cancer, 62:49–58, 1975.

250. McCready, V. R.: Bone scanning. In Price, C. H. G., and Ross, F. G. M. (eds.): Bone — Certain Aspects of Neoplasia. Philadelphia, F. A. Davis (Butterworths), 1973.

251. McKenna, R. J., Schwinn, C. P., and Higinbotham, N. L.: Osteogenic sarcoma in children. Calif. Med., 103:165–170, 1965.

252. McKenna, R. J., Schwinn, C. P., Soong, K. Y., et al.: Sarcomata of the osteogenic series (osteosarcoma, fibrosarcoma, chondrosarcoma, parosteal osteogenic sarcoma, and sarcomata arising in abnormal bone). Analysis of 552 cases. J. Bone Joint Surg. [Am.], 48:1–26, 1966.

253. McMaster, J. H.: Carbohydrate metabolism in osteosarcoma. Int. Orthop., 1:19–21, 1977.

254. McMaster, J. H., Scranton, P. E., Jr., and Drash, A. L.: Growth and hormone control mechanisms in osteosarcoma. Evidence for a new therapeutic approach. Clin. Orthop., 106:366–376, 1975.

255. McNeil, F. J., Cassaday, J. R., and Geiser, C. F.: Scintigraphy in children with osteosarcoma or Ewing sarcoma. Radiology, 109:627–631, 1973.

256. Meyer, P. C.: The histologic identification of osteoid tissue. J. Pathol., 71:325–333, 1956.

257. Meyerding, H. W.: Results of treatment of osteogenic sarcoma. J. Bone Joint Surg., 20:933–948, 1938.

258. Miller, C. W., and McLaughlin, R. E.: Osteosarcoma in siblings. Report of two cases. J. Bone Joint Surg. [Am.], 59:261–262, 1977.

259. Miller, R. W., and Dalager, N. A.: U. S. childhood cancer deaths by cell type, 1960–68. J. Pediatr., 85:664–668, 1974.

260. Mirra, J. M., Bullough, P. G., Marcove, R. C., et al.: Malignant fibrous histiocytoma and osteosarcoma in association with bone infarcts. Report of four cases, two in caisson workers. J. Bone Joint Surg. [Am.], 56:932–940, 1974.

261. Mondolfo, S., Schajowicz, F., and Derqui, J. C.: Results in the treatment of bone sarcomas. Rev. Ortop. Traum., 2:157–166, 1960.

262. Mookherjee, P. K.: A case of osteogenic sarcoma invading a paired bone. Br. J. Radiol., 44:393–395, 1971.

263. Moore, G. E., Gerner, R. E., and Brugarolas, A.:

Osteogenic sarcoma. Surg. Gynecol. Obstet., *136*:359–366, 1973.

264. Mori, M., Fukuda, M., Tsukamoto, S., et al.: Enzyme histochemistry of osteogenic sarcoma, chondrosarcoma, and giant-cell lesions in jawbones. Oral Surg., *26*:103–117, 1968.

265 Morse, D., Jr., Reed, J. O., and Bernstein, J.: Sclerosing osteogenic sarcoma. Am. J. Roentgenol. Radium Ther. Nucl. Med., *88*:491–495, 1962.

266. Morton, D. L., Eilber, F. R., Townsend, C. M., Jr., et al.: Limb salvage from a multidisciplinary treatment approach for skeletal and soft tissue sarcomas of the extremity. Ann. Surg., *184*:268–278, 1976.

267. Moseley, J. E., and Bass, M. H.: Sclerosing osteogenic sarcomatosis. A radiologic entity. Radiology, *66*:41–45, 1956.

268. Mosende, C., Gutierrez, M., Caparros, B., et al.: Combination chemotherapy with bleomycin, cyclophosphamide and dactinomycin for the treatment of osteogenic sarcoma. Cancer, *40*:2779–2786, 1977.

269. Mulvihill, J. J., Gralnick, H. R., Whang-Peng, J., et al.: Multiple childhood osteosarcomas in an American Indian family with erythroid macrocytosis and skeletal anomalies. Cancer, *40*:3115–3122, 1977.

270. Munzenrider, J. E., Emami, B., Tchakarova, I., et al.: Combined therapy of osteosarcoma: preoperative irradiation, surgery, and chemotherapy. Radiology, *125*:497–502, 1977.

271. Murphy, W. K., Benjamin, R. S., Eyre, H. J., et al.: Adjuvant chemotherapy in osteosarcoma of adults. *In* Salmon, S. E., and Jones, S. E. (eds.): Adjuvant Therapy of Cancer. Amsterdam, Elsevier, 1977, pp. 399–406.

272. Nakakuki, K., Shimokawa, K., Yamauchi, H., et al.: A spontaneous transplantable osteogenic sarcoma in AKR/Ms mice. Gann, *67*:513–521, 1976.

273. Natarajan, M., Balakrishnan, D., and Srinivasan, V.: Solitary osteochondroma causing spinal cord compression. Int. Surg., *61*:494–495, 1976.

274. Nauts, H. C.: Osteogenic sarcoma: End results following immunotherapy with bacterial vaccines, 165 cases or following bacterial infections, inflammation or fever, 41 cases. New York, Cancer Research Institute Monograph #15, 1975.

275. Neff, J. R., and Enneking, W. F.: Adoptive immunotherapy in primary osteosarcoma. An interim report. J. Bone Joint Surg. [Am.], *57*:145–148, 1975.

276. Nelson, J. A., Clark, R., and Palubinskas, A. J.: Osteogenic sarcoma with calcified renal metastasis. Br. J. Radiol., *44*:802–804, 1971.

277. Nessi, R., and Giuliani, F.: Xeroradiographic evaluation of murine osteosarcoma. Tumori, *63*:339–345, 1977.

278. Neumann, H. W., and Fleissner, H. K.: Behandlungsergebnisse bei Osteosarkomen, Chondrosarkomen und Fibrosarkomen. Beitr. Orthop. Traumatol., *21*:559–568, 1974.

279. Nielsen, S. W.: Comparative pathology of bone tumors in animals, with particular emphasis on the dog. *In* Grundmann, E. (ed.): Malignant Bone Tumors. New York, Springer-Verlag, 1976, pp. 3–16.

280. Nirenberg, A., Mosende, C., Mehta, B. M., et al.: High-dose methotrexate with citrovorum factor rescue: predictive value of serum methotrexate concentrations and corrective measures to avert toxicity. Cancer Treat. Rep., *61*:779–783, 1977.

281. Nosanchuk, J. S., Weatherbee, L., and Brody, G. L.: Osteogenic sarcoma. Prognosis related to epiphyseal closure. J.A.M.A., *208*:2439–2441, 1969.

282. O'Hara, J. M., Hutter, R. V. P., Foote, F. W., Jr., et al.: An analysis of thirty patients surviving longer than ten years after treatment for osteogenic sarcoma. J. Bone Joint Surg. [Am.], *50*:335–354, 1968.

283. Ohno, T., Abe, M., Tateishi, A., et al.: Osteogenic sarcoma: A study of 113 cases. J. Bone Joint Surg. [Am.], *57*:397–404, 1975.

284. Olson, H. M., and Capen, C. C.: Virus-induced animal model of osteosarcoma in the rat. Morphologic and biochemical studies. Am. J. Pathol., *86*:437–458, 1977.

285. Osteosarcoma — new hope? Editorial. Br. Med. J., *1*:355, 1975.

286. Paget, J.: Lectures on Surgical Pathology. Philadelphia, Lindsay & Blackiston, 1854, p. 486.

287. Papillon, J., and Dutou, L.: Traitement par cobalt[60] des sarcomes osteogeniques. *In* Jelliffe, A. M., and Strickland, B. (eds.): Symposium Ossium. Edinburgh, E. & S. Livingstone, 1970, pp. 133–134.

288. Paschall, H. A., and Paschall, M. M.: Electron microscopic observations of 20 human osteosarcomas. Clin. Orthop., *111*:42–56, 1975.

289. Pearlman, A. W.: Clinical applications of bone and joint scanning in orthopaedics — a review. Bull. Hosp. Joint Dis., *32*:178–180, 1972.

290. Phemister, D. B.: A study of the ossification in bone sarcoma. Radiology, *7*:17–23, 1926.

291. Phillips, R., and Higinbotham, N. L.: Radiotherapy of skeletal tumors in children. Prog. Radiol., *92*:1537–1545, 1969.

292. Piaszek, L., Tiedjen, K. U., and Strötges, M. W.: Aims and limits of nuclear medicine methods in investigation of malignant and benign bone lesions. Radiologe, *16*:29–37, 1976.

293. Plesničar, S., Klanjšček, G., Modic, S., et al.: The significance of doubling time values in patients with pulmonary metastases of osteogenic sarcoma. Cancer Letters, *1*:351–358, 1976.

294. Pohle, E. A., Stovall, W. D., and Boyer, H. N.: Concurrence of osteogenic sarcoma in two sisters. Radiology, *27*:545–548, 1936.

295. Pool, R. R., and Wolf, H. G.: An unusual case of canine osteosarcoma. Cancer, *34*:771–779, 1974.

296. Poppe, E., and Liverud, K.: Osteosarcoma. *In* Jelliffe, A. M., and Strickland, B. (eds.): Symposium Ossium. Edinburgh, E. & S. Livingstone, 1970, pp. 135–137.

297. Poppe, E., Liverud, K., and Efskind, J.: Osteosarcoma. Acta Chir. Scand., *134*:549–556, 1968.

298. Pratt, C. B., Rivera, G., and Shanks, E.: Osteosarcoma during pregnancy. Obstet. Gynecol., *50*(Supplement):24s–26s, 1977.

299. Pratt, C. B., Shanks, E., Hustu, O., et al.: Adjuvant multiple drug chemotherapy for osteosarcoma of the extremity. Cancer, *39*:51–57, 1977.

300. Price, C. H. G.: The grading of osteogenic sarcoma. Br. J. Cancer, *6*:46–68, 1952.

301. Price, C. H. G.: Osteogenic sarcoma; an analysis

of the age and sex incidence. Br. J. Cancer, 9:558–574, 1955.

302. Price, C. H. G.: The grading of osteogenic sarcoma, and its bearing upon survival and prognosis. J. Fac. Radiol., 7:237–241, 1956.

303. Price, C. H. G.: Primary bone-forming tumours and their relationship to skeletal growth. J. Bone Joint Surg. [Br.], 40:574–593, 1958.

304. Price, C. H. G.: The prognosis of osteosarcoma. Br. J. Radiol., 39:181–188, 1966.

305. Price, C. H. G.: Osteosarcoma — new hope. Letter to the editor. Br. Med. J., 1:683, 1975.

306. Price, C. H. G., and Jeffree, G. M.: Metastatic spread of osteosarcoma. Br. J. Cancer, 28:515–524, 1973.

307. Price, C. H. G., and Truscott, D. E.: Multifocal osteogenic sarcoma. Report of a case. J. Bone Joint Surg. [Br.], 39:524–533, 1957.

308. Price, C. H. G., and Truscott, D. E.: Osteogenic sarcoma — an analysis of survival and its relationship to histologic grading and structure. J. Bone Joint Surg. [Br.], 43:300–313, 1961.

309. Price, C. H. G., Zhuber, K., Salzer-Kuntschik, M., et al.: Osteosarcoma in children. A study of 125 cases. J. Bone Joint Surg. [Br.], 57:341–345, 1975.

310. Pritchard, D. J., Reilly, C. A., Jr. and Finkel, M. P.: Evidence for a human osteosarcoma virus. Nature [New Biol.], 234:126–127, 1971.

311. Pritchard, D. J., Reilly, C. A., Jr., Finkel, M. P., et al.: Cytotoxicity of human osteosarcoma sera to hamster sarcoma cells. Cancer, 34:1935–1939, 1974.

312. Rab, G. T., Ivins, J. C., Childs, D. S., Jr., et al.: Elective whole lung irradiation in the treatment of osteogenic sarcoma. Cancer, 38:939–942, 1976.

313. Raina, V.: Normal osteoid tissue. J. Clin. Pathol., 25:229–232, 1972.

314. Rao, R. S., and Rao, D. N.: Prognostic significance of the regional lymph nodes in osteosarcoma. J. Surg. Oncol., 9:123–130, 1977.

315. Reilly, C. A., Jr., Pritchard, D. J., Biskis, B. O., et al.: Immunologic evidence suggesting a viral etiology of human osteosarcoma. Cancer, 30:603–609, 1972.

316. Rella, W., Kotz, R., Arbes, H., et al.: Tumor-specific immunity in sarcoma patients. Oncology, 34:219–223, 1977.

317. Robbins, R.: Familial osteosarcoma. Fifth reported occurrence. Letter to the editor. J.A.M.A., 202:1055, 1967.

318. Roberts, C. W., and Roberts, C. P.: Concurrent osteogenic sarcoma in brother and sisters. J.A.M.A., 105:181–185, 1935.

319. Rockwell, M. A., and Enneking, W. F.: Osteosarcoma developing in solitary enchondroma of the tibia. J. Bone Joint Surg. [Am.], 53:341–344, 1971.

320. Rosen, G.: The development of an adjuvant chemotherapy program for the treatment of osteogenic sarcoma. Front. Rad. Ther. Oncol., 10:115–133, 1975.

321. Rosen, G.: Management of malignant bone tumors in children and adolescents. Pediatr. Clin. North Am., 23:183–213, 1976.

322. Rosen, G., Huvos, A. G., Mosende, C., et al.: Chemotherapy and thoracotomy for metastatic os-teogenic sarcoma: a model for adjuvant chemotherapy and the rationale for the timing of thoracic surgery. Cancer, 41:841–849, 1978.

323. Rosen, G., Huvos, A. G., Marcove, R. C., et al.: Primary osteogenic sarcoma: the rationale for treatment with preoperative chemotherapy and delayed surgery. Cancer (in press).

324. Rosen, G., Murphy, M. L., Huvos, A. G., et al.: Chemotherapy, en bloc resection, and prosthetic bone replacement in the treatment of osteogenic sarcoma. Cancer, 37:1–11, 1976.

325. Rosen, G., Suwansirikul, S., Kwon, C., et al.: High-dose methotrexate with citrovorum factor rescue and Adriamycin in childhood osteogenic sarcoma. Cancer, 33:1151–1163, 1974.

326. Rosen, G., Tan, C., Exelby, P., et al.: Vincristine, high dose methotrexate with citrovorum factor rescue, cyclophosphamide and Adriamycin cyclic therapy following surgery in childhood osteogenic sarcoma. Proc. Am. Assoc. Cancer Res., 15:172, 1974.

327. Rosen, G., Tan, C., Sanmaneechai, A., et al.: The rationale for multiple drug chemotherapy in the treatment of osteogenic sarcoma. Cancer, 35:936–945, 1975.

328. Rosen, G., Tefft, M., Martinez, A., et al.: Combination chemotherapy and radiation therapy in the treatment of metastatic osteogenic sarcoma. Cancer, 35:622–630, 1975.

329. Ross, F. G. M.: Osteogenic sarcoma. Br. J. Radiol., 37:259–276, 1964.

330. Roth, A., Kolaric, K., Potrebica, V., et al.: Treatment of metastatic osteogenic sarcoma with combination chemotherapy — a preliminary report. Libri Oncol., 4(2):99–102, 1975.

331. Rous, P.: Transmission of a malignant new growth by means of a cell free filtrate. J.A.M.A., 56:198, 1911.

332. Rous, P., Murphy, J. B., and Tytler, W. H.: A filterable agent the cause of a second chickentumor, an osteochondrosarcoma. J.A.M.A., 59:1793–1795, 1912.

333. Roy-Camille, R., Roy-Camille, M., Saillant, G., et al.: The treatment of osteogenic osteosarcoma. Presse Méd., 79:1455–1458, 1971.

334. Royster, R. L., King, E. R., Ebersole, J., et al.: High dose, preoperative supervoltage irradiation for osteogenic sarcoma. Am. J. Roentgenol. Radium Ther. Nucl. Med., 114:536–543, 1972.

335. St. James, A. T.: Resection of multiple metastatic pulmonary lesions of osteogenic sarcoma. J.A.M.A., 169:943–944, 1959.

336. Salmon, M.: Ostéosarcome de l'omoplate chez une enfant. Radiothérapie — scapulectomie — resultat de 10 ans. Chirurgie, 99:887–897, 1973.

337. Salzer, M. and Salzer-Kuntschik, M.: Vergleichende röntgenologisch-pathologische-anatomische Untersuchungen von Osteosarkomen im Hinblick auf die Amputationshöhe. Arch. Orthop. Unfallchir., 65:322–326, 1969.

338. Salzer, M., and Zaunbauer, W.: Über Angiographie bei Extremitätentumoren. Wien. Med. Wochenschr., 77:930–932, 1965.

339. Schajowicz, F., DeFilippi-Novoa, C. A., and Firpo, C. A.: Condrosarcoma de heuco axilar inducido por Thorotrast. Bol. Soc. Argentina Ortop. Traumatol., 30:199–210, 1965.

340. Schimke, R. N., Lowman, J. T., and Cowan, G. A. B.: Retinoblastoma and osteogenic sarcoma in siblings. Cancer, 34:2077–2079, 1974.

341. Schnitzler, M.: Das multiple osteogene Sarkom. Fortschr. Med., 93:657–659, 1975.

342. Schroder, J.: Osteosarcoma of the axial skeleton in a dog. J. S. Afr. Vet. Assoc., 47:293–294, 1976.

343. Schwarz, E.: Hypercallosis in osteogenesis imperfecta. Am. J. Roentgenol. Radium Ther. Nucl. Med., 85:645–648, 1961.

344. Schweitzer, G., and Pirie, D.: Osteosarcoma arising in a solitary osteochondroma. S. Afr. Med. J., 45:810–811, 1971.

345. Schwencke, K.: Ungewöhnlicher Verlauf einer Erkrankung an osteogenem Sarkom. Chirurg., 45:511–513, 1974.

346. Schwinn, C. P., and McKenna, R. J.: The biologic behavior of osteosarcoma. In American Cancer Society, Inc., and National Cancer Institute (eds.): Proceedings. National Cancer Conference, Seventh. Philadelphia, J. B. Lippincott Co., 1972, pp. 925–939.

347. Scranton, P. E., Jr., DeCicco, F. A., Totten, R. S., et al.: Prognostic factors in osteosarcoma. A review of 20 years' experience at the University of Pittsburgh Health Center Hospitals. Cancer, 36:2179–2191, 1975.

348. Seydel, H. G., Kim, Y. H., and Inouye, W.: Intramedullary extension of osteogenic sarcoma. Letter to the editor. J.A.M.A., 224:903, 1973.

349. Shaeffer, J., El-Mahdi, A. M., and Constable, W. C.: Treatment of metastatic osteosarcoma by cyclophosphamide and radiotherapy. Radiology, 111:467–469, 1974.

350. Sherman, M., and Irani, R. N.: Osteogenic sarcoma. Two cases of unexpectedly long survival. J. Bone Joint Surg. [Am.], 44:561–566, 1962.

351. Shrikhande, S. S., and Rao, R. S.: Histopathological study of regional lymph nodes in osteosarcoma. J. Surg. Oncol., 9:371–377, 1977.

352. Siegal, G. P., Dahlin, D. C., and Sim, F. H.: Osteoblastic osteogenic sarcoma in a 35-month-old girl. Report of a case. Am. J. Clin. Pathol., 63:886–890, 1975.

353. Silverman, G.: Multiple osteogenic sarcoma. Arch. Pathol., 21:88–95, 1936.

354. Simmons, C. C.: Bone sarcoma: factors influencing prognosis. Surg. Gynecol. Obstet., 68:67–75, 1939.

355. Singleton, E. B., Rosenberg, H. S., Dodd, G. D., et al.: Sclerosing osteogenic sarcomatosis. Am. J. Roentgenol. Radium Ther. Nucl. Med., 88:483–490, 1962.

356. Skoog, L., Nordenskjöld, B., Humla, S., et al.: Effects of methotrexate on deoxyribonucleotide pools and nucleic acid synthesis in human osteosarcoma cells. Eur. J. Cancer, 12:839–845, 1976.

357. Škrovina, B., Červeňanský, J., Kossey, P., et al.: Primary osteosarcoma. A clinical evaluation of 73 cases. Neoplasma, 18:377–393, 1971.

358. Skurzak, H., and Sawadro-Rochowska, M.: Immunology of osteogenic sarcoma. Nowotwory, (Supplement):21–31, 1976.

359. Slullitel, J. A., Schajowicz, F., and Slullitel, J.: Ostéochondrome solitaire avec dégénérescence maligne vers un sarcome osteogenique. Rev. Chir. Orthop., 57:471–478, 1971.

360. Soehner, R. L., and Dmochowski, L.: Induction of bone tumours in rats and hamsters with murine sarcoma virus and their cell-free transmission. Nature, 224:191–192, 1969.

361. Sokolova, I. N., and Litvinova, L. V.: Localization of alkaline phosphatase in subcellular structures of human osteogenic sarcomas. Folia Histochem. Cytochem. (Krakow), 14(4):239–241, 1976.

362. Soloviev, Yu.N.: On the relationship between the rate of skeleton growth and occurrence of primary osteogenic sarcoma. Vopr. Onkol., 15(5):3–7, 1969.

363. Soloviev, Yu.N., and Ponomarkov, V. I.: Clinicomorphological analysis of spontaneous bone sarcoma in dogs. Arkh. Patol., 33(8):36–41, 1971.

364. Spanos, P. K., Payne, W. S., Ivins, J. C., et al.: Pulmonary resection for metastatic osteogenic sarcoma. J. Bone Joint Surg. [Am.], 58:624–628, 1976.

365. Spiers, F. W., King, S. D., and Beddoe, A. H.: Measurements of endosteal surface areas in human long bones: relationship to sites of occurrence of osteosarcoma. Br. J. Radiol., 50:769–776, 1977.

366. Spiess, H., and Mays, C. W.: Bone cancers induced by ^{224}Ra (Th X) in children and adults. Health Phys., 19:713–729, 1970.

367. Spratt, J. S., Jr.: The rates of growth of skeletal sarcomas. Cancer, 18:14–24, 1965.

368. Spratt, J. S., Jr., and Spratt, J. A.: The prognostic value of measuring the gross linear radial growth of pulmonary metastases and primary pulmonary cancers. J. Thorac. Cardiovasc. Surg., 71:274–278, 1976.

369. Spratt, J. S., Jr., and Spratt, T. L.: Rates of growth of pulmonary metastases and host survival. Ann. Surg., 159:161–171, 1964.

370. Spyra, S.: Osteogenic sarcoma in chronic osteitis. Chir. Narzadow Ruchu Ortop. Pol., 41:99–100, 1976.

371. Stein, J. J.: Osteogenic sarcoma (osteosarcoma): Results of therapy. Am. J. Roentgenol. Radium Ther. Nucl. Med., 123:607–613, 1975.

372. Stewart, G. A.: The report of five cases of subacute osteomyelitis of the femur resembling sarcoma. Radiology, 16:271–277, 1931.

373. Stewart, S. E.: The polyoma virus. In Smith, K. M., and Lauffer, M. A. (eds.): Advances in Virus Research. Vol. 7. New York, Academic Press, 1960, p. 61.

374. Subramanian, G., and McAfee, J. G.: A new complex of ^{99m}Tc for skeletal imaging. Radiology, 99:192–196, 1971.

375. Suit, H. D.: Radiotherapy in osteosarcoma. Clin. Orthop., 111:71–75, 1975.

376. Sutow, W. W.: Combination chemotherapy with adriamycin (NSC-123127) in primary treatment of osteogenic sarcoma. Cancer Chemother. Rep., 6:315–317, 1975.

377. Sutow, W. W.: Inferences and projections regarding current clinical capabilities for the control of osteogenic sarcoma. In Sinks, L. F., and Godden, J. O. (eds.): Conflicts in Childhood Cancer. An Evaluation of Current Management. New York, Alan R. Liss, Inc., 1975.

378. Sutow, W. W., Gehan, E. A., Vietti, T. J., et al.: Multidrug chemotherapy in primary treatment

of osteosarcoma. J. Bone Joint Surg. [Am.], 58:629–633, 1976.

379. Sutow, W. W., Sullivan, M. P., and Fernbach, D. J.: Adjuvant chemotherapy in primary treatment of osteogenic sarcoma. Proc. Am. Assoc. Cancer Res., 15:20, 1974.

380. Sviridov, S. A., Zvekotkina, L. S., Kuznetsova, I. P., et al.: Some roentgenological manifestations of osteogenic sarcomas of the long bones. Vestn. Rentgenol. Radiol., 51(3):14–18, 1976.

381. Swaney, J. J.: Familial osteogenic sarcoma. Clin. Orthop., 97:64–68, 1973.

382. Swaney, J. J., and Cangir, A.: Spontaneous pneumothorax in metastatic osteogenic sarcoma. Letter to the editor. J. Pediatr., 82:165–166, 1973.

383. Sweetnam, R.: Amputation in osteosarcoma. Disarticulation of the hip or high thigh amputation for lower femoral growths? J. Bone Joint Surg. [Br.], 5:189–192, 1973.

384. Sweetnam, R.: Surgical aspects of metastatic and residual sarcoma. In Price, C. H. G., and Ross, F. G. M. (eds.):Bone — Certain Aspects of Neoplasia. Philadelphia, F. A. Davis (Butterworths), 1973, pp. 297–302.

385. Sweetnam, R.: The surgical management of primary osteosarcoma. Clin. Orthop., 111:57–64, 1975.

386. Sweetnam, R., Knowelden, J., and Seddon, H.: Bone sarcoma: treatment by irradiation, amputation, or a combination of the two. Br. Med. J., 2:363–367, 1971.

387. Sweetnam, R., and Ross, K.: Surgical treatment of pulmonary metastases from primary tumours of bone. J. Bone Joint Surg. [Br.], 49:74–79, 1967.

388. Tateishi, A., Sekine, K., Ohno, T., et al.: Perfusion chemotherapy of osteosarcoma. A clinical study on 75 cases. Panminerva Med., 18:22–25, 1976.

389. Tavernier, L., and Rousselin, L.: Ostéosarcomes ossifiants, limités, à evolution lente, improprement dits ostéomes. Lyon Chir., 45:741–744, 1950.

390. Tjalma, R. A. Canine bone sarcoma: Estimation of relative risk as a function of body size. J. Natl. Cancer Inst., 36:1137–1150, 1966.

391. Tokunaga, M., Sato, K., Funayama, K., et al.: Rothmund Thomson syndrome associated with osteosarcoma. J. Jpn. Orthop. Assoc., 50:287–293, 1976.

392. Townsend, C. M., Jr., Eilber, F. R., and Morton, D. L.: Skeletal and soft tissue sarcomas. Treatment with adjuvant immunotherapy. J.A.M.A., 236:2187–2189, 1976.

393. Tracey, J. F., Brindley, H. H., and Murray, R. A.: Primary malignant tumors of bone. J. Bone Joint Surg. [Am.], 39:554–560, 1957.

394. Trifaud, A.: Symposium sur ostéosarcome. Introduction. Chirurgie, 96:37–40, 1970.

395. Trifaud, A., Groulier, P., and Roux, G.: Le pronostic pulmonaire des ostéosarcomes. Chirurgie, 96:73–74, 1970.

396. Trifaud, A., and Meary, R.: Pronostic et Traitement des Sarcomes Ostéogéniques. Paris, Masson & Cie, 1972.

397. Troup, J. B., Dahlin, D. C., and Coventry, M. B.: The significance of giant cells in osteogenic

sarcoma: do they indicate a relationship between osteogenic sarcoma and giant cell tumor of bone? Mayo Clin. Proc., 35:179–186, 1960.

398. Tsuya, A., Tanaka, T., Mori, T., et al.: Four cases of Thorotrast injury and estimation of absorbed tissue dose in critical organs. J. Radiat. Res., 4:126–145, 1963.

399. Tudway, R. C.: Radiotherapy for osteogenic sarcoma. J. Bone Joint Surg. [Br.], 43:61–67, 1961.

400. Twomey, P. L., and Chretien, P. B.: Impaired lymphocyte responsiveness in osteosarcoma. J. Surg. Res., 18:551–554, 1975.

401. Uehlinger, E.: Fibulaschaftfraktur mit hyperplastischer Kallusbildung, röntgenologisch ein Osteosarkom vortäuschend. Arch. Orthop. Unfallchir., 87:129–131, 1977.

402. Uehlinger, E.: Osteoplastisches Osteosarkom der distalen Femurmetaphyse. Arch. Orthop. Unfallchir., 87:361–363, 1977.

403. Unni, K. K., Dahlin, D. C., McLeod, R. A., et al.: Intraosseous well-differentiated osteosarcoma. Cancer, 40:1337–1347, 1977.

404. Upshaw, J. E., McDonald, J. R., and Ghormley, R. K.: Extension of primary neoplasms of bone to bone marrow. Surg. Gynecol. Obstet., 89:704–714, 1949.

405. Uribe-Botero, G., Russell, W. O., Sutow, W. W., et al.: Primary osteosarcoma of bone. A clinicopathologic investigation of 243 cases, with necropsy studies in 54. Am. J. Clin. Pathol., 67:427–435, 1977.

406. Van de Voort, P. L. M., and Rosenbusch, G.: Ossifizierende Lymphknotenmetastasen eines Osteosarkoms. Fortschr. Geb. Roentgenstr. Nuklearmed., 126:492–494, 1977.

407. van Hinsbergh, W. C. M., and Hoogbergen, A. J. M.: Two primary osteosarcomas in the same patient? Ned. Tijdschr. Geneeskd., 118:708–712, 1974.

408. Van Putten, L. M.: Tumor reoxygenation during fractionated radiotherapy: studies with transplantable mouse osteosarcoma. Eur. J. Cancer, 4:173–182, 1968.

409. Voegeli, E., and Fuchs, W. A.: Arteriography in bone tumours. Br. J. Radiol., 49:407–415, 1976.

410. von Ronnen, J. R.: Histological and radiographical classification of osteosarcoma in relation to therapy. A review of 245 cases located in the extremities. J. Belge Radiol., 51:215–221, 1968.

411. von Ronnen, J. R.: Radiologic diagnosis of osteosarcoma. Classification of radiologic types. Reliability of radiologic diagnosis. Can the radiologic examination replace biopsy? Ann. Radiol., 13:465–482, 1970.

412. Wanken, J. J., Eyring, E. J., and Samuels, L. D.: Diagnosis of pediatric bone lesions: correlation of a clinical roentgenographic, SR^{87m} scans and pathologic diagnosis. J. Nucl. Med., 14:803–806, 1973.

413. Ward, J. M., and Young, D. M.: Histogenesis and morphology of periosteal sarcomas induced by FBJ virus in NIH Swiss mice. Cancer Res., 36:3985–3992, 1976.

414. Weichselbaum, R. R., Cassady, J. R., Jaffe, N., et al.: Preliminary results of aggressive multimo-

dality therapy for metastatic osteosarcoma. Cancer, 40:78–83, 1977.

415. Weichselbaum, R., Epstein, J., and Little, J. B.: A technique for developing established cell lines from human osteosarcomas. In Vitro, 12:833–836, 1976.

416. Weinfeld, M. S., and Dudley, H. R., Jr.: Osteogenic sarcoma. A follow-up study of the 94 cases observed at the Massachusetts General Hospital from 1920 to 1960. J. Bone Joint Surg. [Am.], 44:269–276, 1962.

417. Weitzner, S.: Osteosarcoma of humerus with axillary lymph node metastases. Clin. Orthop., 90:233–235, 1973.

418. Werner, R.: Mehrfaches Vorkommen einer Neigung zu Knochenbrüchen und Sarkomentwicklung in einer Familie. Z. Krebsforsch., 32:40–42, 1930.

419. White, J. R.: A case of multiple pulsating bone tumours. Br. J. Surg., 9:458–461, 1922.

420. Wilimas, J., Barrett, G., and Pratt, C.: Osteosarcoma in two very young children. Clin. Pediatr., 16:548–551, 1977.

421. Williams, A. H., Schwinn, C. P., and Parker, J. W.: The ultrastructure of osteosarcoma. A review of twenty cases. Cancer, 37:1293–1301, 1976.

422. Witt, A. N.: Das Osteosarkom. Munch. Med. Wochenschr., 119:635–636, 1977.

423. Wolfe, J. N.: Xeroradiography of the bones, joints and soft tissues. Radiology, 93:583–587, 1969.

424. Wolfe, J. N.: Xeroradiography. Image content and comparison with film roentgenograms. Am. J. Roentgenol. Radium Ther. Nucl. Med., 117:690–695, 1973.

425. Wolke, R. E., and Nielsen, S. W.: Site incidence of canine osteosarcoma. J. Small Anim. Pract., 7:489–492, 1966.

426. Wolman, L.: Sclerosing osteogenic sarcomatosis. J. Clin. Pathol., 14:109–114, 1961.

427. Woodard, H. Q., and Higinbotham, N. L.: The correlation between serum phosphatase and roentgenographic type in bone disease. Am. J. Cancer, 31:221–237, 1937.

428. Woods, C. G.: Diagnostic Orthopedic Pathology. Philadelphia, F. A. Davis, 1972, p. 178.

429. Wright, F. W.: Spontaneous pneumothorax and pulmonary malignant disease — a syndrome sometimes associated with cavitating tumours. Report of nine new cases, four with metastases and five with primary bronchial tumours. Clin. Radiol., 27:212, 1976.

430. Yaghmai, I.: Angiographic features of osteosarcoma. Am. J. Roentgenol. Radium Ther. Nucl. Med., 129:1073–1081, 1977.

431. Yaghmai, I., Shamsa, A. Z., Shariat, S., et al.: Value of arteriography in the diagnosis of benign and malignant bone lesions. Cancer, 27:1134–1147, 1971.

432. Zak, F., Stryhal, F., Sosna, A., et al.: Permanent damage of the human organism by Thorotrast. Univ. Carolina Med., 2:325–364, 1956.

6

JUXTACORTICAL OSTEOGENIC SARCOMA

DEFINITION

Juxtacortical, or parosteal, osteogenic sarcoma is a distinctive type of malignant bone tumor that originates on the external surface of a bone specifically in relation to the periosteum or the immediate parosteal connective tissue or both.

INCIDENCE

This type of malignant bone tumor is a relatively uncommon lesion representing approximately 3 to 4 per cent of all osteogenic sarcomas and about 1 per cent of all bone tumors. It was originally described in 1951 by Geschickter and Copeland, who named it "parosteal osteoma," recognizing both benign and malignant forms.[6, 7, 11] As a result of the numerous subsequent studies by these and other authors, it became well established that this lesion is exclusively a malignant tumor with a high degree of structural differentiation, limited growth potential, and good over-all prognosis.[1, 3, 4, 8, 10, 12, 14, 15, 18, 19, 21, 22, 27, 35, 37, 40, 42, 43, 45, 46, 47] In due course, it also became evident that some of the tumors, al-

though parosteally located, differed appreciably in their histologic pattern from those of the classic description with a fully malignant clinical progression of the disease.[1, 10, 16, 19]

AGE AND SEX DISTRIBUTION

Juxtacortical osteogenic sarcoma occurs most frequently in the third decade of life and slightly less frequently in the second and fourth decades. Most patients are over 20 years; the average age is about 5 to 10 years more than that of patients with central (conventional) osteogenic sarcoma (Fig. 6–1). In the Memorial Hospital series, the age range was from 12 to 43 years;[1] in the Mayo Clinic series, the range was from 12 to 58 years.[40] In most series, the sex distribution is nearly equal or shows slightly more females.

SIGNS AND SYMPTOMS

The presenting complaint is swelling or a mass, occasionally interfering with joint function, dull aching pain, or local tenderness. The duration of these insidious

JUXTACORTICAL OSTEOGENIC SARCOMA

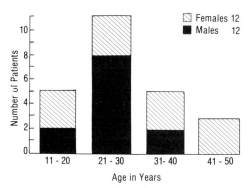

Figure 6–1. Age and sex distribution in 24 patients. (From Ahuja, S. C., Villacin, A. B., Smith, J., et al.: Juxtacortical (parosteal) osteogenic sarcoma. Histological grading and prognosis. J. Bone Joint Surg. [Am.], 59:632–647, 1977.)

symptoms varies from two weeks to eight years, with about half the patients having symptoms for at least one year before seeking medical attention.

SKELETAL LOCATION

In over 50 per cent of the reported cases, the distal end of the femur in its posterior aspect at or near the metaphysis is the site (Fig. 6–2). Other locations, in descending order of frequency, are the humerus, the tibia, the radius, and the ulna (Fig. 6–3). Unusual sites of occurrence are the foot,[1, 31] the clavicle,[28] the scapula,[16] the metacarpal bones,[34, 41] the phalanges,[35] the mastoid,[11] and the mandible.[13, 26, 32, 33]

GROSS FEATURES

Most of these bulky, oval, or spherical tumors are quite large, varying in size from 3 to 25 cm with an average of 10 cm. At the site of origin, these lesions are more sessile, rarely pedunculated, with a curious and often noted propensity to encircle the cortex of the bone (Fig. 6–4). In most cases, the tumor is in direct continuity with the underlying cortex, but occasionally a periosteal fibrous tissue layer separates the tumor mass from the cortical surface, which is often sclerotic. Regional cortical tumor involvement or medullary canal invasion may be demonstrated on gross examination of the cut section in approximately 50 per cent of all cases. The exposed cut surface is grayish white and variegated with the base of the tumor usually densely ossified, as compared to

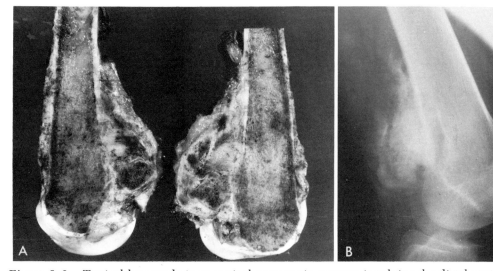

Figure 6–2. Typical low-grade juxtacortical osteogenic sarcoma involving the distal posterior aspect of femur. *A,* Cross section reveals a large hard bony mass attached to the cortical surface with focal cortical erosion. *B,* Radiograph outlines this lesion, exhibiting a cleavage plane, a periosteal lucency at the base. (From Ahuja, S. C., Villacin, A. B., Smith, J., et al.: Juxtacortical (parosteal) osteogenic sarcoma. Histological grading and prognosis. J. Bone Joint Surg. [Am.], 59:632–647, 1977.)

**JUXTACORTICAL
OSTEOGENIC SARCOMA**

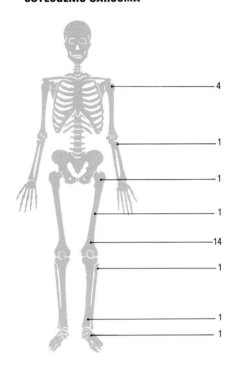

Figure 6–3. Skeletal location in 24 patients. (From Ahuja, S. C., Villacin, A. B., Smith, J., et al.: Juxtacortical (parosteal) osteogenic sarcoma. Histological grading and prognosis. J. Bone Joint Surg. [Am.], 59:632–647, 1977.)

Figure 6–4. Bulky juxtacortical osteogenic sarcoma, Grade II, of the femur in a 42-year-old woman. The lesion, measuring 11 by 7 by 5 cm encircles the cortex without invading it. (From Ahuja, S. C., Villacin, A. B., Smith, J., et al.: Juxtacortical (parosteal) osteogenic sarcoma. Histological grading and prognosis. J. Bone Joint Surg. [Am.], 59:632–647, 1977.)

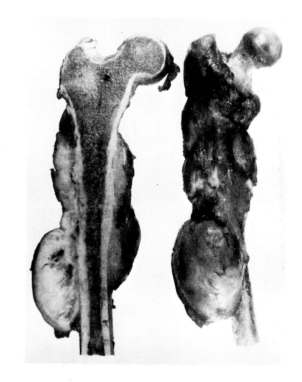

the periphery, where the bony spicules are divided by the fibrous or cartilaginous components.

MICROSCOPIC FEATURES

There is considerable difficulty in histologically assessing well-differentiated osseous neoplasms, the paradigm of which is low-grade juxtacortical osteogenic sarcoma. Characteristically, tissue removed for biopsy purposes is quite hard to evaluate, and the actual sarcomatous appearance present is usually underestimated. At the periphery, the lesions are more likely to show increased cellularity, thereby facilitating definitive diagnosis. In a detailed clinicopathologic analysis of juxtacortical osteogenic sarcoma, three histologic grades of malignancy were identified and correlated with subsequent prognosis (Fig. 6–5).

Evaluation of *Grade I* (classic, low-grade) lesions reveals proliferating atypical trabecular bone with irregular cement lines intermingled with focal collections of well-differentiated cartilage cells. The fibrous stroma appears quite innocuous in its pattern of growth and does not have the obvious appearance of a sarcoma, but the proliferation resembles that seen in "fibromatosis" (Fig. 6–6). The cartilage component in these low-grade lesions does not appear in caplike arrangement and shows varying degrees of endochondral ossification (Fig. 6–7). In *Grade II* (intermediate degree of malignancy) lesions, the fibroblastic stroma becomes more cellular and the cells show a moderate degree of anaplasia with mitotic figures. (Fig. 6–8). The woven bone pattern becomes more pronounced, and irregular deposits of new bone formation and plump hyperchromatic osteoblasts can be recognized. Crowding and anaplasia with occasional mitosis char-

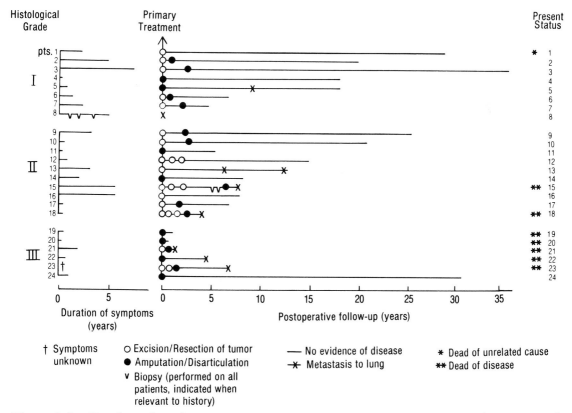

Figure 6–5. Histological grade, type of treatment, and survival in 24 patients with juxtacortical osteogenic sarcoma. (From Ahuja, S. C., Villacin, A. B., Smith, J., et al.: Juxtacortical (parosteal) osteogenic sarcoma. Histological grading and prognosis. J. Bone Joint Surg. [Am.], 59:632–647, 1977.)

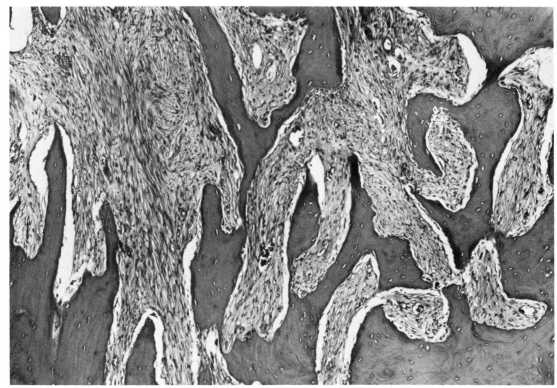

Figure 6–6. Typical Grade I juxtacortical osteogenic sarcoma showing the deceptively innocuous fibroblastic stroma and the trabeculae composed of organized lamellar bone. (Hematoxylin-eosin stain. Magnification × 180.) (From Ahuja, S. C., Villacin, A. B., Smith, J., et al.: Juxtacortical (parosteal) osteogenic sarcoma. Histological grading and prognosis. J. Bone Joint Surg. [Am.], 59:632–647, 1977.)

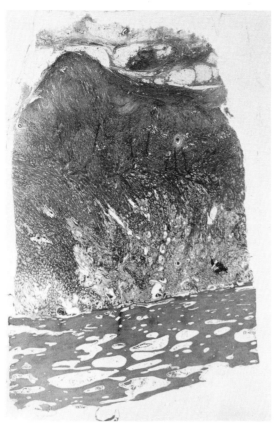

Figure 6–7. Full thickness microscopic section of a typical juxtacortical osteogenic sarcoma. Note arrangement of cartilage component adjacent to cortex and not in a caplike fashion. (Hematoxylin-eosin stain. Magnification × 20.)

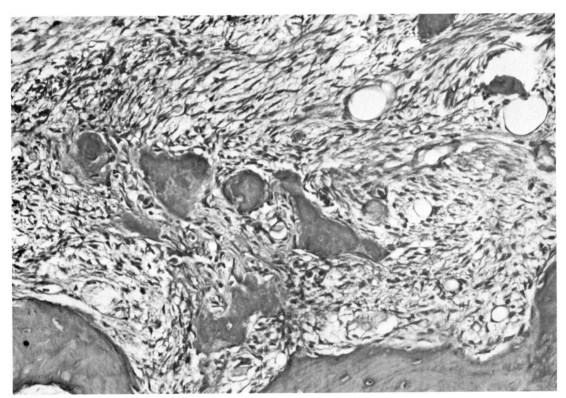

Figure 6–8.   Loosely cellular fibrous stroma and islands of irregular osteoid formation in a Grade II juxtacortical osteogenic sarcoma. (Hematoxylin-eosin stain. Magnification ×180.) (From Ahuja, S. C., Villacin, A. B., Smith, J., et al.: Juxtacortical (parosteal) osteogenic sarcoma. Histological grading and prognosis. J. Bone Joint Surg. [Am.], 59:632–647, 1977.)

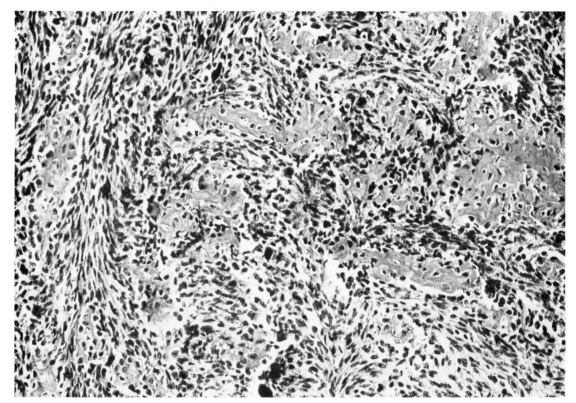

Figure 6–9. Obviously malignant fibrous stroma, frequent mitoses, and large areas of osteoid formation in a Grade III juxtacortical osteogenic sarcoma. (Hematoxylin-eosin stain. Magnification ×180.) (From Ahuja, S. C., Villacin, A. B., Smith, J., et al.: Juxtacortical (parosteal) osteogenic sarcoma. Histological grading and prognosis. J. Bone Joint Surg. [Am.], 59:632–647, 1977.)

acterize the cartilage component in these lesions. In *Grade III* (high-grade, fully malignant) tumors, the sarcomatous fibrous stroma directly forms new bone (osteoid) similar to a conventional osteogenic sarcoma (Fig. 6–9). The cartilage is obviously malignant, as demonstrated by markedly anaplastic nuclei and numerous double-nucleated chondrocytes appearing in the lacunae.

Since in an occasional case the various tissue components may show a discrepancy (a Grade I fibrous stroma may accompany a Grade II osseous or cartilaginous constituent part), the component with the highest grade of malignancy determines the ultimate tumor grade and subsequent prognosis.

From a practical standpoint, a high-grade lesion can be diagnosed by the pathologist with relative assurance, even when only little but well-oriented biopsy material is available, and thus prompt radical surgical treatment may be carried out.

An obviously low-grade tumor can also be properly diagnosed, even in limited biopsy tissue, and wide resection with adequate surgical margins can be recommended to the surgeon. The exact histologic grade of the lesion, i.e., whether it is Grade I or Grade II, can be evaluated after thorough sampling of the removed tumor. The treatment in these cases (Grades I and II) is essentially identical.

The danger of diagnostic indecision and therapeutic procrastination is vividly emphasized by the case of a 22-year-old man whose progressively enlarging left distal femoral lesion was biopsied and interpreted microscopically in 1971 as either a low-grade juxtacortical osteogenic sarcoma or myositis ossificans (Fig. 6–10). The patient refused treatment, even in the face of marked gradual increase in the size of the tumor, and rebiopsy in 1974 again revealed an aggressive fibro-osseous lesion. By 1975, roentgenograms of the chest revealed lung metastases (Fig. 6–11).

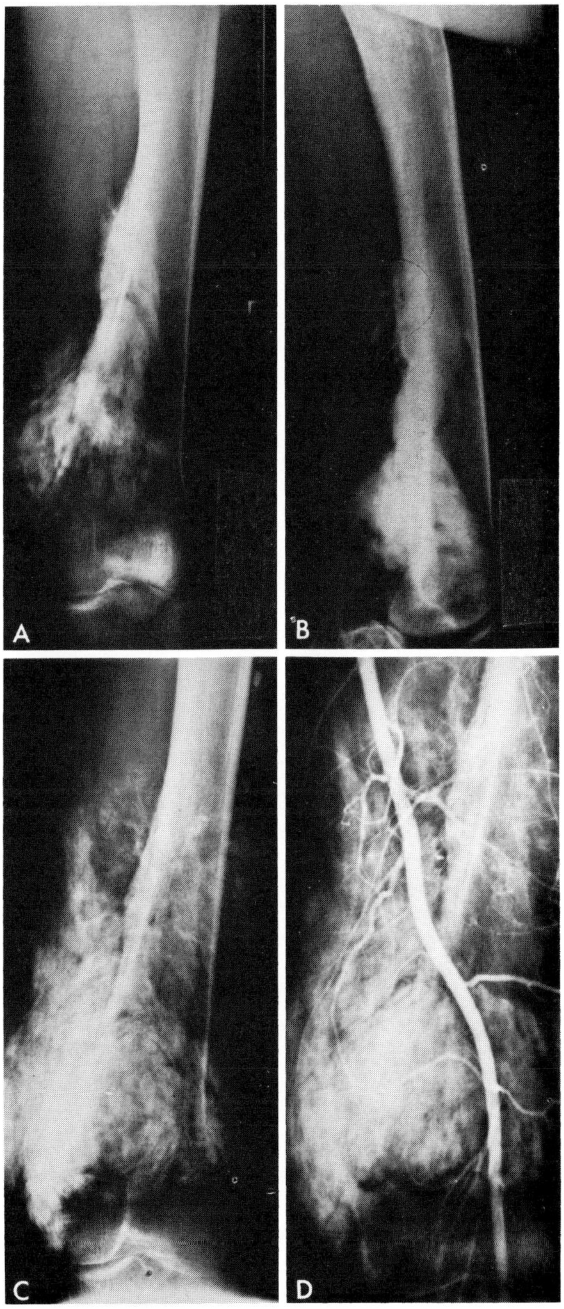

Figure 6–10. A and B, Radiographs showing a low-grade, densely ossified juxtacortical osteogenic sarcoma of the distal femur in a 22-year-old man (1972). The tumor is lobulated with an extremely long base and linear extensions along the periosteum into the soft tissues. C and D, In the absence of therapy, by 1974 the tumor had grown to a huge size.

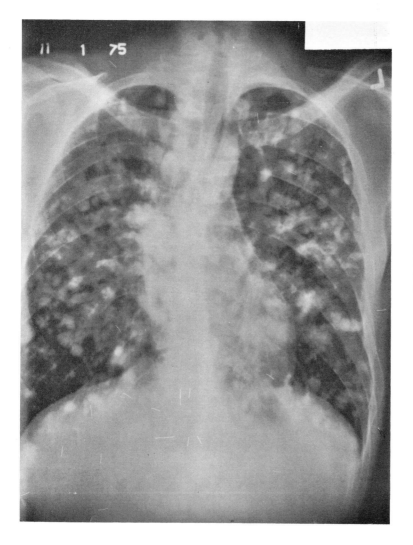

Figure 6–11. In November, 1975, multiple metastatic nodules to both lungs were noted.

Adequate sampling of the specimen is obviously very important before any attempt is made to establish exact diagnosis and to determine the histologic grade of the tumor. It is more than likely that limited amounts of tissue in a poorly oriented biopsy will fail to achieve these purposes.

RADIOGRAPHIC APPEARANCE

On radiographic examination, the lesion appears as an irregular, lobulated, densely radiopaque tumor. In about one third of the cases, one can establish truly smooth margins without serrations or linear extensions into adjacent soft tissues. The heavy ossification of the tumor is rarely uniform throughout (in only 27 per cent of cases), and areas of irregularity and radiolucency are commonly observed. At the site of the broad tumor base, the cortical bone is densely sclerotic but does not signify bony invasion. The thin periosteal lucency (about 1 to 3 mm in width), the so-called "string sign," which separates the tumor from the subjacent cortex, is quite characteristic and diagnostic for this lesion but is only present in about 30 per cent of the cases (Fig. 6–2B). Tomograms and oblique views may increase the likelihood of finding this periosteal lucency, but bulky circumferential lesions obliterate this valuable radiographic sign. Smith and his associates were unable to demonstrate clear-cut radiographic evidence of cortical bony destruction, even in those closely studied instances in which subsequent gross examination proved this to be the case. Nor did they find any correlation between the histologic grade of the sarcoma and the roentgen features.[31] Periosteal reaction manifested by lamellation or spiculation was not seen; the presence of lamellae or spicules would have strongly suggested a conventional osteogenic sarcoma with periosteal extension.

Reports by Probst[24] and Ranniger and Altner[25] described the *angiographic findings* in four examples of juxtacortical sarcoma. They found, similarly to angiographic studies at Memorial Hospital, that no abnormal vascularity was associated with any of the low-grade juxtacortical lesions.[31] Blood vessels appeared to be displaced by the tumor mass but were not encased by it (Fig. 6–10D).

The true significance of angiographic studies seems to be in the exact evaluation of the intimate relationship between tumor and blood vessels in order to better assess the feasibility of local or *en bloc* resection instead of amputation. Abnormal tumor vascularity may be associated with high-grade, fully malignant, juxtacortical osteogenic sarcoma. Furthermore, arteriography may be of great help in evaluating the presence or absence of medullary cavity involvement in classic juxtacortical osteogenic sarcoma The advancing intramedullary portion of the lesion will be more vascular and can be easily visualized angiographically.[17] This was not our experience at Memorial Hospital, however.[31]

RADIOGRAPHIC DIFFERENTIAL DIAGNOSIS

Osteochondroma of the sessile variety may indeed cause diagnostic confusion with juxtacortical osteogenic sarcoma. These types of osteocartilaginous exostoses tend to be not as densely radiopaque, are better outlined, and fail to show circumferential presentation. The occurrence of calcification in the cartilage cap of an osteochondroma is absent in juxtacortical osteogenic sarcoma.

Myositis ossificans, which in soft tissues is clearly separate from bone, does not pose real diagnostic problems. If, however, in rare instances it becomes attached to adjacent periosteum, the separation of the two entities may become quite difficult. New bone formation, frequently extensive, is the dominant feature of conventional roentgen examination in myositis ossificans. This newly deposited osseous tissue may be situated in the immediate proximity of the skeleton, thereby masquerading as a juxtacortical osteogenic sarcoma. In heterotopic ossification, on the radiographs bone production is more regular and the trabecular bony pattern is more distinct, with the zoning phenomenon (i.e., increased peripheral density) being present. In the same condition, angiography reveals a large number of fine blood vessels as well as an accumulation of contrast material. The rich vascularity differs in great measure from the paucity of blood vessels reported in juxtacortical osteogenic sarcoma.[24] In exceptional circumstances, soft

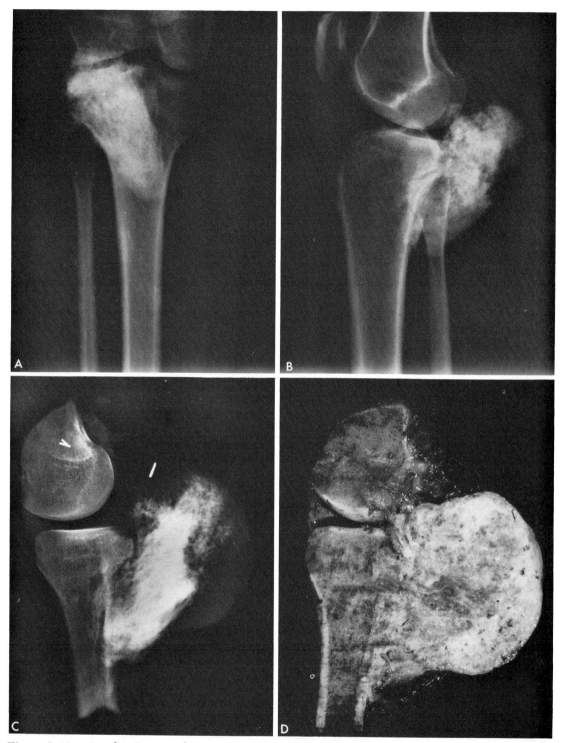

Figure 6–12.   A and B, Low-grade juxtacortical osteogenic sarcoma in a 32-year-old woman. The non-homogenously calcified 8 cm mass arising from the posterolateral aspect of the proximal tibia extends into soft tissues of the popliteal space. Extension into underlying medullary canal is present. C and D, The *en bloc* resection radiograph and specimen reveal the extent of lesion. A total knee prosthesis was immediately inserted. (Courtesy of Dr. R. C. Marcove.)

tissue osteogenic sarcoma may extend and invade the neighboring bone, masquerading as a primary juxtacortical osteogenic sarcoma.

Recently, Unni and associates proposed subdividing juxtacortical osteogenic sarcoma into parosteal and periosteal variants.[39, 40] The periosteal types presented as small, predominantly radiolucent lesions most often on the surface of the upper tibial shaft with perpendicular bony spicule formation and chondroblastic, relatively high-grade, sarcomatous traits. In spite of these malignant histologic features, the periosteal lesions proved to have a relatively more favorable prognosis than those of the conventional osteogenic sarcoma. There is, however, considerable doubt as to whether periosteal osteogenic sarcoma is a truly separate clinicopathologic entity.

The prognostic significance of medullary involvement at the time of presentation remains unsettled. Stevens and his coworkers suggested that such occurrence had no bearing on the prognosis,[36] whereas Unni and his associates, in their recent study from the same medical center, concluded that medullary extension does indicate a worse outcome.[40] Regional cortical and medullary invasion was seen in 46 per cent of the tumors studied at Memorial Hospital, including low- and high-grade lesions. Careful study of these patients showed that medullary involvement does not necessarily imply a worse prognosis with low-grade lesions, although it may do so in those patients with high-grade tumors.[1] It should be emphasized that even on retrospective examination of the routine roentgenograms, focal medullary tumor extension could not be predicted and identified.

TREATMENT

In the past, recommended surgical treatment has varied from local excision to radical amputation, but no clear-cut relationship has emerged between the method of treatment and the ultimate postoperative survival. The histologic grading system as proposed by Farr and Huvos,[10] and further developed by Ahuja and his coworkers,[1] seems to provide a reliable and reproducible histologic assessment of the tumor. These histologic criteria help to identify patients with the best and the worst prognoses, thus assisting in the selection of the most appropriate surgical treatment. When technically feasible, Grades I and II juxtacortical osteogenic sarcomas may be amenable to *en bloc* resection, assuming the tumor can be removed in its entirety with an adequate surgical margin including soft tissues and underlying bone (Fig. 6–12). Local recurrence will be evident in about half of the low- and intermediate-grade lesions if the surgical resection does not encompass underlying bone. Tomography may be of assistance in determining the adequacy of the bony surgical resection line. Since high-grade lesions can be diagnosed preoperatively with great confidence by histologic examination, early radical ablative surgery is clearly indicated despite the poor prognosis. Postoperative adjuvant high-dose multidrug, multicycle therapy is recommended for Grade III lesions, whereas Grades I and II tumors should be treated by surgical means exclusively.

REFERENCES

1. Ahuja, S. C., Villacin, A. B., Smith, J., et al.: Juxtacortical (parosteal) osteogenic sarcoma. Histological grading and prognosis. J. Bone Joint Surg. [Am.], 59:632–647, 1977.
2. Bloodgood, J. C.: Bone tumors: sarcoma. Periosteal group. Ossifying type. Benign ossifying periostitis and myositis. J. Radiol., 4:119–127, 1923.
3. Calandriello, B.: Ancora sul sarcoma parostale ossificante. Arch. Putti Chir. Organi Mov., 9:371–382, 1957.
4. Campanacci, M., and Giunti, A.: Periosteal osteosarcoma. Review of 41 cases, 22 with long-term follow-up. Ital. J. Orthop. Traum., 2:23–35, 1976.
5. Coley, B. L.: Neoplasms of Bone and Related Conditions. Etiology, Pathogenesis, Diagnosis and Treatment. 2nd ed. New York, Paul B. Hoeber, Inc., 1960, pp. 305–307.
6. Copeland, M. M.: Parosteal osteoma: Differential diagnosis and treatment. *In* Tumors of Bone and Soft Tissues. Anderson Hospital and Tumor Institute. Chicago, Year Book Medical Publishers, 1965, pp. 201–218.
7. Copeland, M. M., and Geschickter, C. F.: The treatment of parosteal osteoma of bone. Surg. Gynecol. Obstet., 108:537–548, 1959.
8. Dwinnell, L. A., Dahlin, D. C., and Ghormley, R. K.: Parosteal (juxtacortical) osteogenic sarcoma. J. Bone Joint Surg. [AM.], 36:732–744, 1954.
9. Edeiken, J., Farrell, C., Ackerman, L. V., et al.:

Parosteal sarcoma. Am. J. Roentgenol. Radium Ther. Nucl. Med., *111*:579–583, 1971.

10. Farr, G. H., and Huvos, A. G.: Juxtacortical osteogenic sarcoma. An analysis of fourteen cases. J. Bone Joint Surg. [Am.], *54*:1205–1216, 1972.

11. Geschickter, C. F., and Copeland, M. M.: Parosteal osteoma of bone: a new entity. Ann. Surg., *133*:790–807, 1951.

12. Harkess, J. W.: Parosteal osteosarcoma. Am. Surg., *30*:730–736, 1964.

13. Hoffman, W. B.: Osteogenic sarcoma of the mandible. Arch. Otolaryngol., *84*:439–440, 1966.

14. Hupfauer, W.: Juxtacortical osteosarcoma. Arch. Orthop. Unfallchir., *84*:291–297, 1976.

15. Jacobson, S. A.: Early juxtacortical osteosarcoma (parosteal osteoma). J. Bone Joint Surg. [Am.], *40*:1310–1328, 1958.

16. Jaffe, H. L.: Tumors and Tumorous Conditions of the Bones and Joints. Philadelphia, Lea & Febiger, 1958, pp. 279–297.

17. Lagergren, C., Lindbom, A., and Söderberg, G.: The blood vessels of osteogenic sarcomas. Histologic, angiographic, and microradiographic studies. Acta Radiol., *55*:161–176, 1961.

18. Laurence, G.: Sarcomes juxta-corticaux. Rev. Prat. (Paris), *19*:2461–2465, 1969.

19. Lichtenstein, L.: Tumors of periosteal origin. Cancer, *8*:1060–1069, 1955.

20. McKenna, R. J., Schwinn, C. P., Soong, K. Y., et al.: Sarcomata of the osteogenic series (osteosarcoma, fibrosarcoma, chondrosarcoma, parosteal osteogenic sarcoma, and sarcomata arising is abnormal bone). An analysis of 552 cases. J. Bone Joint Surg. [Am.], *48*:1–26, 1966.

21. Merle d'Aubigné, R., Meary, R., and Mazabraud, A.: Sarcome ostéogénique juxtacortical. Rev. Chir. Orthop., *45*:873–884, 1959.

22. Merle d'Aubigńe, R., and Thomine, J. M.: A propos de 9 cas de sarcomes juxta-corticaux. Chirurgie, *96*:45–49, 1970.

23. Murashkovski, M. A.: Parosteal osteosarcoma with soft tissue metastasis. Vestn. Rentgenol. Radiol., *3*:86–88, 1977.

24. Probst, F. P.: Angiography in juxtacortical osteosarcomas. Case report with special reference to the differential diagnosis. Acta Radiol. [Diagn.](Stockh.), *11*:49–56, 1971.

25. Ranniger, K., and Altner, P. C.: Parosteal osteoid sarcoma. Radiology, *86*:648–651, 1966.

26. Roca, A. N., Smith, J. L., and Jina, B.: Osteosarcoma and parosteal osteogenic sarcoma of the maxilla and mandible: study of 20 cases. Am. J. Clin. Pathol., *4*:625–636, 1970.

27. Sammons, B. P., Sarkisian, S. S., and Krepela, M. C.: Juxtacortical osteogenic sarcoma. Am. J. Roentgenol. Radium Ther. Nucl. Med., *79*:592—597, 1958.

28. Sanchis Olmos, V., Ferrer Torrelles, M., and Fernández Criado, M.: Osteoma parostal de clavicula. Acta Ortop. Traumatol. Iber., *4*:471–486, 1956.

29. Scaglietti, O., and Calandriello, B.: Ossifying parosteal sarcoma. Parosteal osteoma or juxtacortical osteogenic sarcoma. J. Bone Joint Surg. [Am.], *44*:635–647, 1962.

30. Sirsat, M. V., and Doctor, V. M.: Parosteal (juxta-

cortical) osteogenic sarcoma: an emphasis on histopathology. J. Postgrad. Med., *11*:191–197, 1965.

31. Smith, J., Ahuja, S. C., Huvos, A. G., et al.: Parosteal (juxtacortical) osteogenic sarcoma — a roentgenological study of 30 patients. J. Can. Assoc. Radiol, in press.

32. Solomon, M. P., Biernacki, J., Slippen, M., et al.: Parosteal osteogenic sarcoma of the mandible. Existence masked by diffuse periodontal inflammation. Arch. Otolaryngol., *101*:754–760, 1975.

33. Som, M., and Peimer, R.: Juxtacortical osteogenic sarcoma of the mandible. Arch. Otolaryngol., *74*:532–536, 1961.

34. Stark, H. H., Jones, F. E., and Jernstrom, P.: Parosteal osteogenic sarcoma of a metacarpal bone. A case report. J. Bone Joint Surg. [Am.], *53*:147–153, 1971.

35. Steinhauser, J., and Michel, R.: Langzeitbeobachtung eines juxtakortikalen Osteosarkoms der Mittelfingergrundphalanx. Handchirurgie, *9*:37–38, 1977.

36. Stevens, G. M., Pugh, D. G., and Dahlin, D. C.: Roentgenographic recognition and differentiation of parosteal osteogenic sarcoma. Am. J. Roentgenol. Radium Ther. Nucl. Med., *78*:1–12, 1957.

37. Tseshkovsky, M. S., and Soloviev, Yu.N.: Parosteal osteogenic sarcoma (clinical, roentgenological and morphological characteristics). Vestn. Rentgenol. Radiol., *3*:13–21, 1977.

38. Unni, K. K., Dahlin, D. C., and Beabout, J. W.: Periosteal osteogenic sarcoma — an entity distinct from parosteal osteogenic sarcoma. Abstract. Lab. Invest., *32*:438–439, 1975.

39. Unni, K. K., Dahlin, D. C., and Beabout, J. W.: Periosteal osteogenic sarcoma. Cancer, *37*:2476–2485, 1976.

40. Unni, K. K., Dahlin, D. C., Beabout, J. W., et al.: Parosteal osteogenic sarcoma. Cancer, *37*:2466–2475, 1976.

41. Val Bernal, J. F., and Garijo Ayensa, M. F.: Juxtacortical osteogenic sarcoma of the skeleton of the hand. Patologia, *6*:189–196, 1973.

42. van der Heul, R. O.: Het periostale ossificerende fibrosarcoom en de gradering van osteosarcomen. Thesis. Leiden, 1962, pp. 132–135.

43. van der Heul, R. O., and von Ronnen, J. R.: Juxtacortical osteosarcoma. Diagnosis, differential diagnosis, treatment, and an analysis of eighty cases. J. Bone Joint Surg. [Am.], *49*:415–439, 1967.

44. Vuletin, J. C.: Myofibroblasts in parosteal osteogenic sarcoma. Letter to the editor. Arch. Pathol. Lab. Med., *101*:272, 1977.

45. Weston, W. J., Reid, J. D., and Saunders, J. H.: Parosteal osteogenic sarcoma of bone. Report of a case. J. Bone Joint Surg. [Br.], *40*:722–729, 1958.

46. Witwicki, T., Dziak, A., and Daniluk, A.: Juxtacortical sarcoma. Chir. Narzadow Ruchu Ortop. Pol., *39*:89–97, 1974.

47. Wolfel, D. A., and Carter, P. R.: Parosteal osteosarcoma. Am. J. Roentgenol., *105*:142–148, 1969.

7

OSTEOGENIC SARCOMA OF THE CRANIOFACIAL BONES

DEVELOPMENTAL AND ANATOMIC PECULIARITIES OF CRANIOFACIAL BONES

The bones of the cranial vault and most of the facial bones are not developed from preformed cartilage. In these anatomic structures, the mesenchyme initially forms a primitive connective tissue membrane instead of precartilage or cartilage. This membrane gives rise to the differentiating connective tissue cells, like osteoblasts, heralding early osteogenesis. The bones of the cranial vault and most of the facial bones are referred to as "membrane bones," since they develop by intramembranous ossification. The maxilla develops by way of this type of bone formation in close proximity to the nasal capsular cartilage. The mandible arises as an intramembranous bone lateral to Meckel's cartilage; the latter disappears without any contribution to the mandibular development except for a small area lateral to the midline that subsequently shows endochondral ossification. Although secondary cartilaginous growth centers are present during mandibular development, only the one located at the condylar process, where endochondral ossification takes longer than in any other part of the bony framework, appears to be of significance. Notwithstanding the fact that the mandible is not bone preformed in cartilage but is instead a "membrane bone," cartilaginous tumors may develop from it, since fibrous tissue, cartilage, and bone may be produced from preformed connective tissue. Bones of the base of the skull are preformed in cartilage and are commonly referred to as "cartilage preformed bone."

The tubular mandibular bone presents an outer cortical plate within which there are trabeculae of bone similar to the long tubular bones of the appendicular skeleton. The maxilla has thin cortical plates enclosing cancellous bone structured more similarly to the flat bones of the axial skeleton.

INCIDENCE AND ASSOCIATED DISEASES

Osteogenic sarcoma afflicts the bones of the craniofacial regions relatively infrequently. The incidence varies somewhat in the larger series available. The Mayo

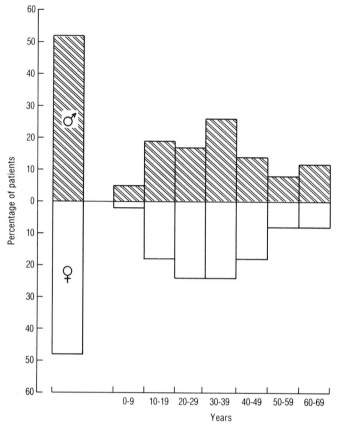

Figure 7–1. Osteogenic sarcoma of craniofacial bones: age and sex distribution in 412 patients. (Data from the literature.)

Clinic reports 63 cases among 650 (9.7 per cent).[13] At Memorial Hospital, 43 patients were noted among 605 (7 per cent).[6] In the estimate of Garrington and associates, approximately 6.5 per cent of all osteogenic sarcomas arise in the jaw. These authors calculate the occurrence of the lesions to be about 0.07 cases per 100,000 people a year in the United States.[24] The pertinent literature on this subject contains approximately 412 published cases, as summarized in Figures 7–1 and 7–2.

Osteogenic sarcomas of the cranial vault are the rarest of cranial tumors. Thompson and his coworkers found 7 of the 14 cases of calvarial sarcomas to be associated with Paget's disease of the skull.[69]

In a review of 24 cases in which Paget's disease involved the jaw, Tillman noted sarcoma to be associated in three instances.[70] Eight of the 43 patients with os-

teogenic sarcoma involving the craniofacial bones showed evidence of Paget's disease in the Memorial Hospital series.[6] Osteogenic sarcoma of the craniofacial bones may also be induced by preoperative or postoperative irradiation for treatment of other head and neck cancers.[2] (See Chapter 9).

In a survey of 314 cases of canine osteogenic sarcoma, accumulated from the literature by Wolke and Nielsen,[76] only 33 (10.5 per cent) developed in the skull.[34, 49]

The much discussed human mandibular fragment from Kanam, East Africa, discovered by Leakey and described by Lawrence, dates from the Lower or Middle Pleistocene Epoch.[41] This paleopathologic find, commonly referred to as the "Kanam mandible," reveals an asymmetric osseous enlargement involving the lingual and labial surfaces of the mandible adja-

Osteogenic Sarcoma of Craniofacial Bones

Location of 412 Lesions
(data from literature)

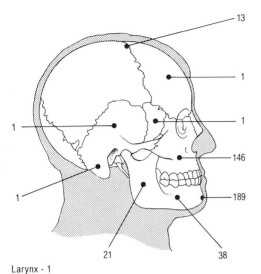

Larynx - 1

Figure 7–2. Osteogenic sarcoma of craniofacial bones: location of 412 lesions. (Data from the literature.)

cent to the symphysis. It is probably the earliest example of a human mandibular osteogenic sarcoma. Some, however, doubt this interpretation and suggest instead that the swelling is due to callus formation following a fracture.[59, 66, 67] The large tumor of the skull of an elderly pre-Columbian male Peruvian from Paucarcancha originally was diagnosed as an osteogenic sarcoma of the skull.[45] However, the heavily ossified and radiating spicules of bone of this large hyperostotic cranial lesion may more likely be due to a slowly evolving meningioma.

CLINICAL PRESENTATION AND SIGNS AND SYMPTOMS

None of the presenting signs or symptoms are characteristic enough specifically for osteogenic sarcoma, since all of them can be produced by benign tumors and nonneoplastic conditions as well. Symptoms are of relatively short duration, most of the patients having had complaints for three months or less, and rarely for more than a year, before diagnosis. The most common complaint noted by patients was painful swelling in approximately 50 per cent of cases, although painless swelling was reported by 35 per cent.[6] As patients often believe their symptoms to be due to dental structures, dentists and oral surgeons are frequently the first to be consulted and to diagnose these rare tumors. In 40 to 50 per cent of maxillary or mandibular lesions, an initial extraction of the teeth was performed. In a study of 17 patients, Richards and Coleman noted that 12 had dental extractions in the area of tumor, and in 8 of these, this extraction took place within one year of the establishment of the osteogenic sarcoma diagnosis.[54]

The serum alkaline phosphatase values may be elevated in the presence of osteogenic sarcoma of the craniofacial bones. In 6 of 22 patients in whom such determinations were performed, elevated levels were obtained.[6]

In neurosurgical clinical practice, one occasionally encounters cranial osteogenic sarcomas presenting with symptoms of a primary brain tumor.[38]

AGE AND SEX DISTRIBUTION

A summary of most of the reported cases in which this information was available reveals an average age of 32 years with a range from 4 to 82 years (Fig. 7–1). The average age of patients with osteogenic sarcoma at all skeletal sites was 27 years, in contrast to 39 years for those with craniofacial presentation in the Memorial Hospital series.[6] The peak frequency for patients with craniofacial lesions is in the second, third, and fourth decades of life, with the 30 to 39 year age group being most commonly affected. It should be noted, however, that craniofacial osteogenic sarcoma can occur in children and adolescents. Seven per cent of the patients were under the age of 10, and 37 per cent were known to be between 10 and 19 years of age. In general, patients with mandibular lesions were slightly younger than those with maxillary presentation, an average age of 35 to 37 years. The oldest patients were those with cranial involvement, the average age being 46 years.[6] In the M.D. Anderson Hospital series of 24 cases, the age relationship was completely reversed; patients with mandibular lesions were approximately 10 years older than those with maxillary tumors.[18]

Among the 411 cases in which sex was noted, males showed a slight but nonsignificant predominance (215:196). This corresponds with other previous reports.[20, 30]

LOCATION OF TUMORS

Mandibular presentation is more common than maxillary (Fig. 7–2). Among the 412 cases reported in the literature, 248 occurred in the mandible and 146 in the maxilla. The body of the mandible is most commonly involved and then, in descending order of frequency, the symphysis, angle, and ascending ramus. Any portion of the maxilla may give rise to osteogenic sarcoma; most frequently, however, these lesions present along the alveolar ridge or within the maxillary antrum. In large lesions, it is quite often impossible to assign the exact site of origin in the maxilla. Several instances of typical juxtacortical presentation in the mandible have been reported.[32, 57, 63, 64]

RADIOGRAPHIC APPEARANCE

Osteogenic sarcomas arising in the mandible show no specific radiographic changes other than those demonstrated by similar lesions springing from long bones (Fig. 7–3).

Roentgenologic identification of new tumor bone formation is best visualized when the lesion extends into soft tissues; this is one of the most helpful findings in osteogenic sarcoma of jaws.[18] Curtis and associates,[12] however, point to the finding of Meyer,[48] who demonstrated osteoid to be entirely radiolucent, thereby questioning the diagnostic value of this radiographic finding. Characteristic "sunburst" or "sunray" types of spiculation extending from the cortex into soft tissues similar to the lesions in long bones may be seen. This sunburst pattern, however, may also be encountered in examples of metastatic carcinoma, well-advanced Ewing's sarcoma, tuberculosis, and various inflammatory osseous diseases. The radiographic appearance, in general, may be predominantly osteolytic or osteoblastic (sclerotic) or a mixed pattern may be evident. Typically, the lesions cause destruction of the mandible with indefinite margins or sclerosis with heightened radiopacity or an intermixture of these appearances can be demonstrated. The main feature of the sclerosing type of osteogenic sarcoma presents as a dense, structureless, ivory-like bony tumor. The lytic type, however, presents extensive osseous destruction predominating over bone production without any radiopacity.

Symmetrical widening of the periodontal ligament involving one or more teeth has been shown to represent a manifestation of incipient osteogenic sarcoma or chondrosarcoma of the mandible.[23, 24] Others have failed to substantiate these findings, however.[57] In our own experience, the presence of this radiographic sign is useful and should raise the suspicion that osteogenic sarcoma is a real possibility. It has also been noted that malignant jaw tumors are less likely to result in root resorption than benign lesions.[15] The presence of root resorption of a permanent erupted tooth would be most unusual for an osteogenic sarcoma and, therefore, would be more likely to be the result of an inflammatory process, benign tumor, or tumorous condition.[15, 18]

Sinus opacification of the maxillary sinus with various grades of bone destruction is the usual finding of an osteogenic sarcoma. Both carcinomas and other sarcomas, however, may present with such roentgenographic features without showing ostensible tumor matrix formation.

If an early osteogenic sarcoma retains the normal contours of the maxillary antrum and there is only minimal or no osseous destruction, the diagnosis will be in doubt. Once the normal contours become distorted by heavily radiopaque merging areas of new bone formation, the diagnosis of an osteogenic sarcoma is considerably easier. Calcific mineralization of a destructive mass within the maxillary sinus or nasal fossa should raise the possibility of an osteogenic sarcoma or chondrosarcoma.

The most consistently helpful radiographic features of a mandibular osteogenic sarcoma, based on the cases at Memorial Hospital, were found to be the following: medullary origin, asymmetric location

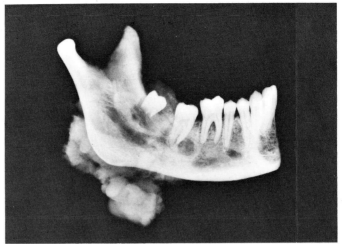

Figure 7–3. Specimen radiograph of a mandibular osteogenic sarcoma in an 18-year-old girl reveals a permeative and destructive lesion in the superior portion of the posterior mandibular alveolar ridge. Grossly, the 4 cm tumor predominantly occupies the molar triangle and destroys the posterior half of the horizontal ramus. Considerable lingual plate expansion is noted. (Courtesy of Dr. E. W. Strong.)

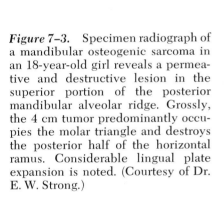

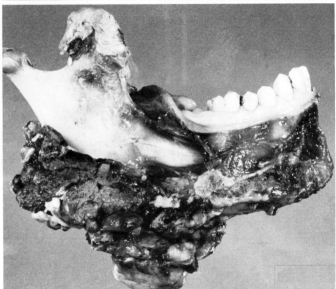

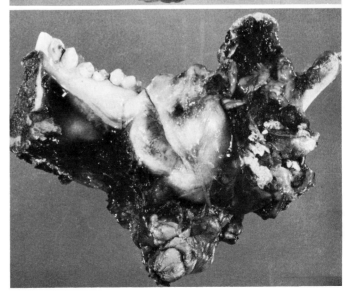

within the bone, medullary and cortical destruction, periosteal reaction, ill-defined borders, oval or pear shape, soft tissue mass, and disorganized internal structural pattern.[62]

Differential Diagnosis

The radiographic differential diagnosis in sclerosing osteogenic sarcoma should include metastatic prostatic carcinoma, which may closely mimic it. Metastatic osseous disease, however, is generally widespread by the time craniofacial involvement is present. The lytic form of osteogenic sarcoma frequently has a less specific roentgen presentation, and accordingly, the differential considerations are more complex: cancer secondarily invading bone; metastatic lesions like neuroblastoma, for instance; or primary non-Hodgkin's lymphoma of bone. In most cases of lytic osteogenic sarcoma, the radiologist must be satisfied with an unspecific diagnosis of a malignant tumor affecting the jaw.[62] Osteomyelitis, syphilis, and so on rarely may resemble the lytic form of mandibular osteogenic sarcoma.

MICROSCOPIC APPEARANCE

The histologic criteria for diagnosing osteogenic sarcomas of the craniofacial bones do not differ in any way from those for diagnosis of this tumor in any other osseous site. It is, therefore, quite remarkable how often the lesion is misdiagnosed, at least initially, because the location in the maxilla or mandible makes the pathologist consider primarily an odontogenic neoplasm. Basically, osteogenic sarcoma is defined as a tumor of bone in which the malignant spindle cell stroma directly forms osteoid or primitive bone. The proliferation of tumor cells may be predominantly osteoblastic, chondroblastic, or fibroblastic. Occasionally, the pattern may be dominated by aneurysmally dilated vascular channels with multinucleated giant cells and scanty osteoid formation, the so-called telangiectatic variant. The rare examples arising in the cranial vault are usually heavily bone-forming neoplasms with dense radiopacity due to calcified bone production. Those osteogenic sarcomas that involve the bones of the facial area and the mandible tend to show a more mixed (fibroblastic, chondroblastic, or osteoblastic) microscopic gradient. In the series of 56 cases reported by Garrington and his colleagues, there was no correlation between the histologic appearance of the tumor and the eventual prognosis of the case.[24]

Differential Diagnosis

As a result of dental infections, the maxilla and mandible are quite commonly involved by sclerosing osteomyelitis and other reactive osseous lesions, and it is of considerable importance to rule out such lesions microscopically before a final diagnosis of osteogenic sarcoma is made. Rare cellular odontogenic tumors may produce considerable amounts of mineralized odontogenic tissue, thereby causing diagnostic difficulties. Unusual bone tumors, like rapidly growing ossifying fibroma, osteoblastoma, or even an occasional osteoid osteoma, should also be considered. Paget's disease of bone showing areas of increased cellularity may also be confused with osteogenic sarcoma when the abnormal cement lines of the so-called mosaic pattern are not visualized. The widened periodontal ligament space, described by Garrington and associates,[24] and Gardner and Mills,[23] is considered by many to be a useful sign of early osteogenic sarcoma of the jaw. This occurrence is caused by sarcoma cell invasion of the periodontal ligament, since this structure presents less resistance to the advancing tumor than the neighboring alveolar bone.

The histologic criteria for diagnosis do not differ in any significant way from those arising in other bones of the appendicular or axial skeleton.

About two thirds of osteogenic sarcomas arising in the craniofacial bones are of the osteoblastic type, demonstrating ample dense tumor bone formation. There was no correlation between the histologic characteristics and ultimate prognosis of cases.[24]

TREATMENT AND PROGNOSIS

Practically all treatment modalities have been recommended for these tumors. Radical surgery, irradiation, cautery, and chemotherapy have all been tried.

Radiation therapy prior to radical surgical resection of osteogenic sarcoma of the jaw bone is recommended by Suit.[68] The basis for this approach, according to this radiotherapist, is the experience that the most important reason for therapeutic failure following a straight surgical mandibular resection seems to be local recurrence. For instance, in 8 of 17 patients (47 per cent) with mandibular osteogenic sarcoma, local recurrence was noted.[6] The local recurrence rate was even higher in maxillary lesions (80 per cent) and in skull tumors (75 per cent).

Radium implants in a mandibular lesion have been recommended by Gomez and his coworkers, delivering from 7000 to 11,040 rads of calculated tumor dose followed by a hemimandibulectomy within a day. This particular patient was alive without disease 13 months after treatment.[28] Chambers and Mahoney reported a series of osteosarcomas of the craniofacial bones treated by radical dose radiation therapy (external beam) or with interstitial radium implantation, delivering an estimated tumor dose of 10,000 to 16,000 rads immediately and followed by radical surgery in four days with primary closure and delayed reconstruction.[9] This combined treatment modality afforded 22 of 30 patients (75 per cent) five or more years of survival. Twenty-two of the 27 patients (82 per cent) treated with curative intent were alive for five or more years. The overall disease-free survival rate of this series of 33 patients was 76 per cent.

The clinical preoperative examination of a mandibular osteogenic sarcoma does not yield a consistently reliable estimate of the full extent of the lesion because microscopic tumor involvement of surgical margins may still be present after wide local excision. Because of this possibility, some advocate hemimandibulectomy with intraoperative frozen section examination of surrounding tissues and marrow curettings or smears from the cut edge of the mandible to establish adequate surgical lines of resection.[51]

The primary or delayed restoration of function after resection of the jaws and prosthetic closure of maxillary defects, the principles behind it, the timing, and the various methods are very important con-

siderations in the treatment of osteogenic sarcomas of these sites but are beyond the scope of this chapter.

Osteogenic sarcoma in the craniofacial bones has a better prognosis than it has in the long bones. A tendency to remain localized, late systemic spread in spite of frequently delayed primary treatment, and relatively low average histologic grade of malignancy, as concluded by Kragh and associates,[37] may be some of the factors that contribute to better prognosis and successful therapy. Mortality is often due to locally persistent tumor or intracranial extension. The best five year survival rates vary from 31 per cent[37] to 35 per cent.[24] The five year survival at Memorial Hospital was found to be better (33.3 per cent) in those patients whose lesion formed in the maxilla, as compared to those with sarcomas of the mandible (23.6 per cent). The average survival with maxillary presentation was 80 months, with a median of only 17 months. In comparison, a 51.5 month average survival was noted in patients with a mandibular lesion, with a median survival of 21 months.[6]

Osteogenic sarcomas arising in the skull have an extremely poor prognosis. Of the 11 patients treated at Memorial Hospital, only one (9 per cent) survived for five years. An average survival in skull lesions of only 20.4 months with a median of five months after treatment was achieved.[6] A compilation of survival data from several reports by Curtis and his colleagues yielded only a 25.8 per cent five year survival in patients with maxillary lesions. In patients with mandibular osteogenic sarcomas, a 34.8 per cent five year survival rate was computed by the same authors.[12]

About one third of the patients with craniofacial osteogenic sarcomas will develop distant metastases within an average of two years after initial treatment. Once such metastases were detected, the survival averaged six months in the pre–aggressive multidrug multicycle chemotherapy era.[6]

In analyzing the metastatic pattern of mandibular osteogenic sarcoma, Schwartz and Alpert found a 13 per cent incidence of metastases predominantly involving the lungs.[61] Occasionally, upper cervical lymph node metastases may also be encountered, necessitating a radical neck dissection.[44]

REFERENCES

1. Andrade, J., Del Pilar Canseco, M., and Chavolla, N.: Fibroblastic variety of osteogenic sarcoma of the mastoid process. Case presentation. Rev. Med. Hosp. Gen. (Mex.), 36:631–641, 1973.
2. Arlen, M., Shah, I. C., Higinbotham, N., et al.: Osteogenic sarcoma of head and neck induced by radiation therapy. N.Y. State J. Med., 72:929–934, 1972.
3. Bennett, J. E., Tignor, S. P., and Shafer, W. G.: Osteogenic sarcoma of the facial bones. Am. J. Surg., 116:538–541, 1968.
4. Boyer, C. W., Jr., Brickner, T. J., Jr., Perry, R. H., et al.: Interstitial radiation in the management of malignant disease of the facial structures. Am. J. Roentgenol. Radium Ther. Nucl. Med., 105:14–19, 1969.
5. Boyer, C. W., Jr., Brickner, T. J., Jr., and Wratten, G. P.: The treatment of osteogenic sarcoma of the mandible. Am. J. Roentgenol. Radium Ther. Nucl. Med., 99:326—332, 1967.
6. Caron, A. S., Hajdu, S. I., and Strong, E. W.: Osteogenic sarcoma of the facial and cranial bones. A review of 43 cases. Am. J. Surg., 122:719–725, 1971.
7. Caron, J., Perreau, P., Verger, P., et al.: Ostéosarcome de la voûte crânienne. J. Radiol. Electrol. Med. Nucl., 53:285–286, 1972.
8. Cernéa, P., Payen, J., and Brochériou, Cl.: Bone sarcoma affecting the jaw. An analysis of 41 cases. Bull. Cancer, 61:151–160, 1974.
9. Chambers, R. G., and Mahoney, W. D.: Osteogenic sarcoma of the mandible: current management. Am. Surg., 36:463–471, 1970.
10. Cocke, W. M., Jr., and Wade, W. M., Jr.: Osteogenic sarcoma of the mandible. Oral Surg., 30:601–606, 1970.
11. Courville, C. B., Deeb, P., and Marsh, C.: Notes on the pathology of cranial tumors. 7. Osteogenic sarcomas of the cranial vault with particular reference to those associated with osteitis deformans (Paget's disease) and their tendency to involve dura and brain. Bull. Los Angeles Neurol. Soc., 27:57–74, 1962.
12. Curtis, M. L., Elmore, J. S., and Sotereanos, C.: Osteosarcoma of the jaws: report of case and review of the literature. J. Oral Surg., 32:125–130, 1974.
13. Dahlin, D. C.: Bone Tumors. 2nd ed. Springfield, Illinois, Charles C Thomas, 1967, p. 157.
14. Daramola, J. O., Aghadiuno, P. U., Ajagbe, H. A., et al.: Osteogenic sarcoma of the jaws in Ibadan, Nigeria. Br. J. Oral Surg., 14:23–30, 1976.
15. Davidoff, S. M.: A method for early and differential diagnosis of central tumours of the jaws. Int. Dent. J., 18:753–758, 1968.
16. Dechaume, M., and Baclesse, F.: Ostéosarcome du maxillaire inférieur. Presse Méd., 59:386–388, 1951.
17. De Lathouwer, C., Lerinck, P. L., Mayer, R., et al.: Two cases of osteogenic sarcoma of the mandible. Indications for immediate reconstruction. Acta Chir. Belg., 73:49–58, 1974.
18. Finkelstein, J. B.: Osteosarcoma of the jaw bones. Radiol. Clin. North Am., 8:425–443, 1970.
19. Fontaine, R., Warter, P., Champy, M., et al.: Ostéosarcome du maxillaire supérieur. J. Radiol. Electrol. Med. Nucl., 46:233–236, 1965.

20. Friedberg, M. J., Serlin, O., Orlean, S. L., et al.: Osteosarcoma of the maxilla: surgical removal and reconstruction of defect by a dental prosthesis. Report of a case. Oral Surg., 15:883–891, 1962.
21. Fu, Y.-S., and Perzin, K. H.: Non-epithelial tumors of the nasal cavity, paranasal sinuses, and nasopharynx: a clinicopathologic study. II. Osseous and fibro-osseous lesions, including osteoma, fibrous dysplasia, ossifying fibroma, osteoblastoma, giant cell tumor, and osteosarcoma. Cancer, 33:1289–1305, 1974.
22. Gaillard, J., Bernard, P. A., Dumolard, P., et al.: Sarcoma ostéogénique du maxillaire supérieur. J. Fr. Otorhinolaryngol., 20:1163–1164, 1971.
23. Gardner, D. G., and Mills, D. M.: The widened periodontal ligament of osteosarcoma of the jaws. Oral Surg., 41:652–656, 1976.
24. Garrington, G. E., Scofield, H. H., Cornyn, J., et al.: Osteosarcoma of the jaws. Analysis of 56 cases. Cancer, 20:377–391, 1967.
25. Geschickter, C. F.: Tumors of the jaws. Am. J. Cancer, 24:90–126, 1935.
26. Geschickter, C. F.: Primary tumors of the cranial bones. Am. J. Cancer, 26:155–180, 1936.
27. Ginapolous, H., Khan, F. R., and Nickson, J. J.: A case of osteogenic sarcoma of maxillary antrum cure by radiation therapy. J. Radiol. Electrol. Med. Nucl., 56:429–431, 1975.
28. Gomez, A. C., Youmans, R. D., and Chambers, R. G.: Osteogenic sarcoma of the mandible. A method of treatment. Am. J. Surg., 100:613–616, 1960.
29. Halmoš, J., and Sadko, I.: Fibrosarcoma and osteosarcoma of jaws. Cesk. Stomatol., 72:350–355, 1972.
30. Harris, H. H., Muller, D. J., and Greenberg, S. D.: Primary osteogenic sarcoma of the maxillary sinus. Report of two cases. Laryngoscope, 73:429–445, 1963.
31. Hendee, R. W., Jr.: Primary osteogenic sarcoma of the calvaria. Case report. J. Neurosurg., 45:334–337, 1976.
32. Hoffman, W. B.: Osteogenic sarcoma of the mandible. Arch. Otolaryngol., 84:439–440, 1966.
33. Horn, R. C., Jr.: Osteogenic sarcoma, maxilla. In Proceedings. 26th Seminar of the American Society of Clinical Pathologists, September 30, 1960, pp. 23–26.
34. Johnson, T. C.: Osteosarcoma of the canine skull (a case report). Vet. Med. Small Anim. Clin., 71:629–631, 1976.
35. Jung, H., and Gutjahr, P.: Primäre Sarkome der Schädelknochen beim Kind. Laryngol. Rhinol. Otol., 54:762–771, 1975.
36. Kleinsasser, O., and Albrecht, H.: Zur Kenntnis der Osteosarkome des Stirn- und Keilbeines. Arch. Ohr. Heilk., 170:595–603, 1957.
37. Kragh, L. V., Dahlin, D. C., and Erich, J. B.: Osteogenic sarcoma of the jaws and facial bones. Am. J. Surg., 96:496–505, 1968.
38. Kretschmer, H.: Tumoren der Schädelknochen mit Hirntumorsymptomatik. Zentralbl. Neurochir., 31:247–271, 1970.
39. Krolls, S. O.: Case for diagnosis. Milit. Med., 138:649, 668, 1973.
40. Lachard, J., Gola, R., Zattara, H., et al.: Ostéosarcomes de la mandibule. A propos de quatre cas. Rev. Stomatol. Chir. Maxillofac., 76:56–58, 1976.

41. Lawrence, J. W. P.: Appendix A. *In* Leakey, L. S. B.: Stone Age Races of Kenya. New York, Oxford University Press, 1935.

42. LiVolsi, V. A.: Osteogenic sarcoma of the maxilla. Arch. Otolaryngol., *103*:485–488, 1977.

43. Long, D. M., Kieffer, S. A., and Chou, S. N.: Tumorous lesions in the skull. *In* Youmans, J. R. (ed.): Neurological Surgery. Vol. 3. Philadelphia, W. B. Saunders Co., 1973, pp. 1231–1274.

44. Looser, K. G., and Kuehn, P. G: Primary tumors of the mandible. A study of 49 cases. Am. J. Surg., *132*:608–614, 1976.

45. MacCurdy, G. G.: Human skeletal remains from the highlands of Peru. Am. J. Phys. Anthropol., 6:217–329, 1923.

46. Madhavan, M., Aurora, A. L., and Sen, S. B: Osteogenic sarcoma of the maxilla. J. Laryngol. Otol., 88:1125–1129, 1974.

47. McDonald, R. C., and Fredricks, W. H.: Osteogenic sarcoma of maxilla. Report of a case. Oral Surg., 26:736–741, 1968.

48. Meyer, P. C.: The histological identification of osteoid tissue. J. Pathol., 71:325–333, 1956.

49. Miller, W. A.: Osteosarcoma of the mandible in a dog: a case report. J. Small Anim. Pract., 16:185–191, 1975.

50. Morley, A. R., Cameron, D. S., and Watson, A. J.: Osteosarcoma of the larynx. J. Laryngol. Otol., 87:997–1005, 1973.

51. Pease, G. L., Maisel, R. H., and Cantrell, R. W.: Surgical management of osteogenic sarcoma of the mandible. Arch. Otolaryngol., 101:761–762, 1975.

52. Potdar, G. G.: Osteogenic sarcoma of the jaws. Oral Surg., 30:381–389, 1970.

53. Prowler, J. R: Osteogenic sarcoma of the maxilla. Report of a case. Oral Surg., 28:141–148, 1969.

54. Richards, W. G., and Coleman, F. C.: Osteogenic sarcoma of the jaw. Oral Surg., 10:1156–1165, 1957.

55. Ries Centeno, G., Yoel, J., and Barros, R. E: Osteosarcoma osteolítico de mandíbula. Rev. Asoc. Odontol. Argent., 56:396–399, 1968.

56. Rintala, A., Gylling, U., Lahti, A., et al.: Malignant mesenchymal tumours of the mandible. Duodecim, 86:1158–1166, 1970.

57. Roca, A. N., Smith, J. L., Jr., and Jing, B.-S.: Osteosarcoma and parosteal osteogenic sarcoma of the maxilla and mandible. Am. J. Clin. Pathol., 54:625–636, 1970.

58. Rowe, N. H., and Hungerford, R. W.: Osteosarcoma of the mandible. J. Oral Surg., 21:42–49, 1963.

59. Sandison, A. T.: Kanam mandible's tumour. Letter to the editor. Lancet, 1:279, 1975.

60. Schwartz, D. T., and Alpert, M.: The clinical course of mandibular osteogenic sarcoma. Oral Surg., 16:769–776, 1963.

61. Schwartz, D. T., and Alpert, M.: The malignant transformation of fibrous dysplasia. Am. J. Med. Sci., 247:1–20, 1964.

62. Sherman, R. S., and Melamed, M.: Roentgen characteristics of osteogenic sarcoma of the jaw. Radiology, 64:519–527, 1955.

63. Solomon, M. P., Biernacki, J., Slippen, M., et al.: Parosteal osteogenic sarcoma of the mandible. Existence masked by diffuse periodontal inflammation. Arch. Otolaryngol., 101:754–760, 1975.

64. Som, M., and Peimer, R.: Juxtacortical osteogenic sarcoma of the mandible. Arch. Otolaryngol., 74:532–536, 1961.

65. Spiessl, B., and Prein, J.: Zur Klinik und Morphologie der Kiefersarkome. Dtsch. Zahnaerztl. Z., 26:1243–1249, 1971.

66. Stathopoulos, G.: Kanam mandible's tumour. Letter to the editor. Lancet, 1:165, 1975.

67. Steinbock, R. T.: Paleopathological Diagnosis and Interpretation. Bone Diseases in Ancient Human Populations. Springfield, Illinois, Charles C Thomas, 1976, p. 370.

68. Suit, H. D.: Radiotherapy in osteosarcoma. Clin. Orthop., *111*:71–75, 1975.

69. Thompson, J. B., Patterson, R. H., Jr., and Parsons, H.: Sarcomas of the calvaria. Surgical experience with 14 patients. J. Neurosurg., 32:534–538, 1970.

70. Tillman, H. H.: Paget's disease of bone. A clinical, radiographic, and histopathologic study of twenty-four cases involving the jaws. Oral Surg., 15:1225–1234, 1962.

71. Vandenberg, H. J., Jr., and Coley, B. L.: Primary tumors of the cranial bones. Surg. Gynecol. Obstet., 90:602–612, 1950.

72. Vernino, D. M., Lock, F. L., and Anderson, A. G.: Osteogenic sarcoma of the mandible. Problems associated with its diagnosis and treatment. Oral Surg., 15:129–135, 1962.

73. Ward, G. E., and Hendrick, J. W.: Diagnosis and Treatment of Tumors of the Head and Neck. Baltimore, Williams & Wilkins, 1950, pp. 359–361.

74. Wilcox, J. W., Dukart, R. C., Kolodny, S. C., et al.: Osteogenic sarcoma of the mandible: review of the literature and report of case. J. Oral Surg., 31:49–52, 1973.

75. Wolfowitz, B. L.: Osteosarcoma and chondrosarcoma of the maxilla. J. Laryngol. Otol., 87:409–416, 1973.

76. Wolke, R. E., and Nielsen, S. W.: Site incidence of canine osteosarcoma. J. Small Anim. Pract., 7:489–492, 1966.

8

TUMORS ASSOCIATED WITH PAGET'S DISEASE OF BONE

DEFINITION AND INCIDENCE

Paget's disease is a benign but precancerous condition affecting the mesenchymal cells of the bones and resulting in the activation of new groups of functional osseous tissue cells.[6, 56] Both bone resorption and formation of bone are increased, represented by elevated urinary hydroxyproline excretion and serum alkaline phosphatase concentration respectively.[87] In progressively active Paget's disease, woven bone replaces cortical lamellar bone and the haversian system is obliterated by bone of chaotic structural traits. Not only is increased woven bone formation demonstrated but the newly produced osteoid volume is also augmented.

In a detailed autopsy study of 650 unselected human skeletons aged 40 years or older, Paget's disease of bone was noted in 24 (3.7 per cent).[12] This disease is exceptionally rare under the age of 40 years and is uncommon between the ages of 40 and 55 years.[22, 33, 82] In general, it occurs slightly more frequently in men than in women. The most common anatomic sites

of involvement, in descending order of frequency, are as follows: lumbar vertebrae, sacrum, skull, pelvic bones, femur, tibia, clavicle, humerus, and ribs.[17] Only rarely does it appear in the bones of the hand or foot. In about 10 per cent of cases, Paget's disease is solitary (monostotic); that is, a single bone in whole or in part is involved.[22]

FREQUENCY

As far back as 1933, Jaffe suggested that the markedly increased proliferative capacity of the osseous tissue involved in Paget's disease might be the basic stimulus for tumor formation.[33]

Estimates differ widely as to the frequency with which tumors complicate Paget's disease.[20, 23, 55] The lowest incidence figure comes from the Mayo Clinic data. Among 1753 patients with this osseous affliction, only 16 cases (0.9 per cent) were complicated by sarcoma. This series includes asymptomatic cases discovered on routine radiographic examina-

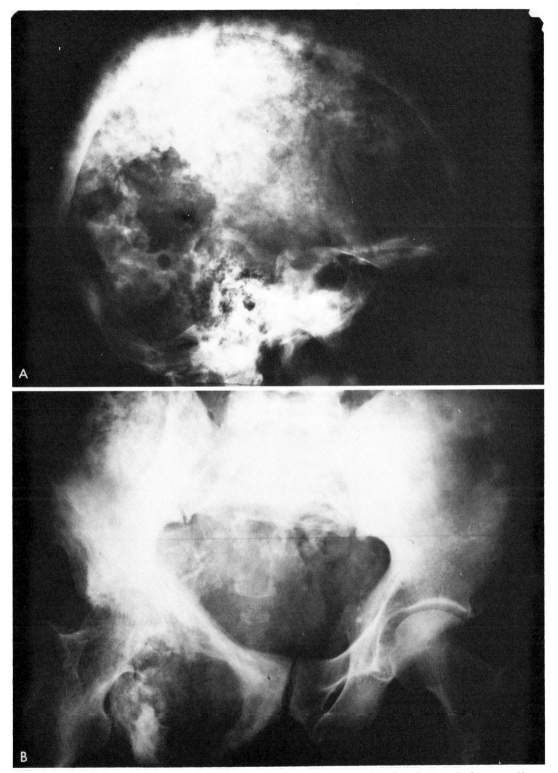

Figure 8–1. Radiographs show multifocal osteogenic sarcoma associated with Paget's disease of bone in a 48-year-old male. The Paget's sarcoma involves the skull, right pelvis, and L$_2$ vertebra simultaneously.

tion.[52] Considerably higher figures have been reported by Kirschbaum[39] (12.5 per cent), Packard and associates[48] (7.5 per cent), and Bird[5] (11 per cent), but these estimates were based on cases with advanced skeletal involvement while numerous asymptomatic or uncomplicated instances of Paget's disease remained unreported and undetected. Barry calculates the frequency to be 2 per cent, which is probably the fairest estimate.[3, 4]

In a series reported from Memorial Hospital of 33 patients with Paget's sarcoma, 22 (67 per cent) had polyostotic and 11 (33 per cent) had monostotic Paget's disease.[42]

In many instances, advanced Paget's disease need not be present before sarcoma develops.[59] Sarcoma may complicate this disease even if only one bone is involved to a limited degree (focal monostotic involvement). When a sarcoma appears in one bone in a patient with fully developed and widespread Paget's disease, other synchronous foci of sarcoma are occasionally present (Fig. 8–1).

Sarcomas superimposed on Paget's disease of bone possess a definite predilection for synchronous or metachronous multiple bone involvement. In a series of 148 cases, at least 23 of the patients (16 per cent) showed multifocal osseous affection.[62] Whether this represents a true multicentric propensity of Paget's sarcoma or is due to early and widespread metastatic dissemination of a highly virulent form of cancer is not always easy to decide with certainty. The "metastases" may indeed appear in bones unaffected by Paget's disease, although in the majority of instances, "pagetoid" bones are the preferred sites of tumor. Histologic examination of the lesions reveals an identical microscopic appearance. For these and other reasons, as discussed by McKenna and his colleagues, these foci are favored to be metastases rather than multicentric primary sites.[42] In all fairness, it must be stated that others, like Jaffe,[34, 35] prefer the latter possibility.

LOCATION OF PAGET'S SARCOMA

Sarcomas superimposed on Paget's disease follow a pattern of distribution similar to the most common osseous sites of uncomplicated Paget's disease (femur, humerus, craniofacial bones, pelvis, and tibia) (Fig. 8–2). Two exceptions to this rule appear to be the relatively high frequency of humeral Paget's sarcoma and the rarity of vertebral sarcomas. Hauw and his coworkers found nine reported sarcomas associated with Paget's disease of the vertebral column and summarized four additional cases of their own.[29] Eleven of the patients were over 60 years of age, and two were under 60 years. The male to female ratio was 11:2.

In a study from England of 148 cases of Paget's sarcoma, the femur was the most commonly affected bone (39 per cent), with the ilium (15 per cent), humerus (14.5 per cent), and tibia (11 per cent) involved less frequently.[62]

When Paget's sarcoma involves the long bone, neither the diaphysis nor the metaphysis is predilected. The midportion of the shaft is more frequently involved than in ordinary osteogenic sarcomas.

AGE AND SEX DISTRIBUTION

There is no basic difference in the age distribution of patients with uncomplicated Paget's disease and with Paget's sarcoma. The age varies from 32 to 79 years, with an average age of about 60 years. Paget's sarcoma is extremely rare under the age of 40 years and only two or three such cases have been reported.[42, 52] Each large series of reported cases demonstrates an approximate male to female ratio of 2:1.

The discovery of a sarcoma in a bone of an individual older than 40 years should instigate a roentgenographic survey of the entire skeleton for Paget's disease, since in this age group, the sarcoma is frequently based on Paget's disease.[11] The frequency of Paget's sarcoma in Britain is estimated to be 30 per cent of all primary malignant bone tumors developing in persons after the age of 40 years, although this group of patients makes up only 3 per cent of the population.[53, 73]

SIGNS AND SYMPTOMS

The cardinal clinical features of sarcomas associated with Paget's disease are severe disabling pain and often pulsatile

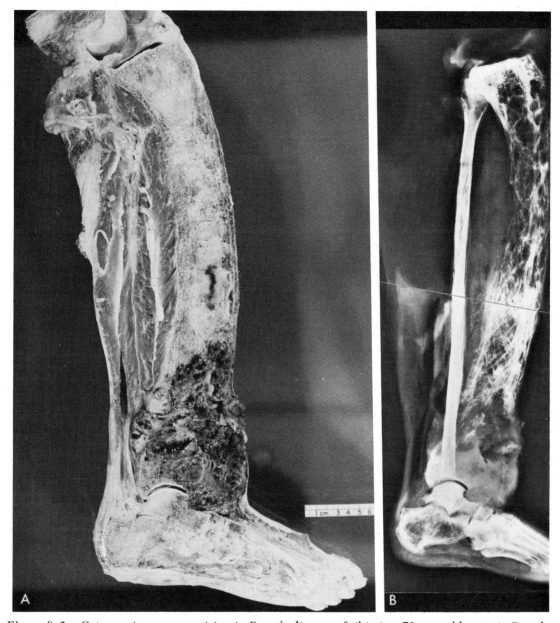

Figure 8–2. Osteogenic sarcoma arising in Paget's disease of tibia in a 72-year-old man. *A,* Grossly, there is marked cortical thickening with a large hemorrhagic tumor distally. *B,* The specimen radiograph shows extreme bony expansion with a coarse trabecular pattern. The tumor is lytic and ill-defined and extends into soft tissues, with fracture of the tibia.

local swelling. The onset of pain in a patient known to have Paget's disease should seriously suggest the development of a sarcoma, but the pain usually precedes the radiologic changes of a developing tumor. In some instances, the pain is intractable, necessitating immediate ablative surgery, irradiation, or cordotomy. Especially with tumors in the skull, little pain may be experienced. Approximately 75 per cent of patients seek medical attention within an average of four to five months of the onset of symptoms, and very few delay consultation longer than a year.[42] The average interval from onset of symptoms to definite diagnosis is 7.8 months, with a median duration of seven months.

Spontaneous or pathologic fractures due to minimal trauma are striking features in patients with Paget's disease, both in the early and in the late phases. In our experience, 40 per cent of patients with Paget's sarcoma arising in long bones had a pathologic fracture occurring either before or after the development of the sarcoma.

A rare cauda equina syndrome due to Paget's sarcoma with lumbosacral location may be encountered.[36, 71]

SERUM ALKALINE PHOSPHATASE

In 1959, Woodard in her classic study emphasized the gradual increase in the serum alkaline phosphatase values in patients with uncomplicated Paget's disease of bone.[86] This ultimately unremitting rise, however, is marred by unpredictable fluctuations. A rapidly rising phosphatase value not only is compatible with a virulent clinical progression to an early onset osteogenic sarcoma but also is consistent with a rampant, but otherwise uncomplicated, Paget's disease.

Serum alkaline phosphatase values are, almost without exception, markedly elevated in polyostotic Paget's disease, and therefore it is not feasible to correlate the onset of Paget's sarcoma with additionally increased values. In some instances, the occurrence of sarcoma is accompanied by only slight or moderate phosphatase rise. Apparently, there is no predictive value in serum alkaline phosphatase findings to pinpoint which patient with monostotic or polyostotic Paget's disease will eventually develop sarcoma.

As reported by McKenna and associates from Memorial Hospital,[42] alkaline phosphatase values varied from 3.4 to 111.0 Bodansky units (normal is 1.5–5.0 B.U.) in patients with Paget's sarcomas, with a mean of 31.8 units. On the average, individuals with polyostotic disease had higher phosphatase levels than those with monostotic involvement did. Resection or amputation resulted in approximately a 50 per cent decrease in the alkaline phosphatase values. No prognostic value could be ascertained between preoperative alkaline phosphatase levels and length of survival. Serum calcium and phosphorus values are within normal limits at all times, even in the presence of severe, generalized disease. Urinary hydroxyproline excretion also represents an accurate index of skeletal involvement and the degree of activity of the disease.[38]

RADIOGRAPHIC FINDINGS

The features of the earliest radiographically recognizable changes of an osteogenic sarcoma superimposed on Paget's disease include a small focus of subcortical bone destruction associated with cortical erosion.[72] The cortical erosion dominates the picture in advanced cases, and occasionally, the cortical bone destruction outstrips the medullary bone disruption. Periosteal reactions, such as Codman's triangles, are quite rare in this disease, but soft tissue extension of the tumor is relatively common.[84, 85]

Radiographic examination of Paget's sarcoma of the long bones reveals an ill-defined, usually fusiform mass of predominantly lytic, sclerotic, or mixed type. The lytic variety usually lacks internal structure, and only occasionally can one identify foci of calcification, thin wavy lines, osseous ridge, or septum formation.[2] Often, an ossified soft tissue mass is demonstrated. The sclerotic variants show intense bone production with a dense and irregular structure and disorganized patches of sclerosis and destruction.

Osteogenic sarcomas coexisting with Paget's disease of the cranial vault can be either of the osteolytic type, which is more frequent, or of the sclerotic variety. Even on initial radiographic examination, both the inner and outer tables with the diploë are consistently found to be destroyed. The usually pulsating spherical mass has well-delimited borders and, occasionally, thin sclerotic margins. Wilner and Sherman emphasized the importance of tangential radiographs to highlight the destroyed tables and the extent of soft tissue involvement. Otherwise, small sarcomatous lesions of the skull, on anteroposterior or posteroanterior views, are difficult to separate from radiolucent foci of uncomplicated Paget's disease.[84, 85]

RADIOGRAPHIC DIFFERENTIAL DIAGNOSIS

It is well nigh impossible to roentgenologically distinguish between sarcomatous transformation in Paget's disease and metastatic carcinoma.[78]

Osteoblastic skeletal metastases of prostatic carcinoma may mimic the sclerotic lesions of Paget's disease. Determination of serum alkaline and acid phosphatase values will help to arrive at the proper diagnosis. The coexistence of Paget's disease of bone and metastatic prostatic carcinoma in the same bone, although rare, may occur.[1] One such case is illustrated in Figure 8–3. Wilner and Sherman illustrated several well-documented cases in which a coexistence of metastatic carcinoma and Paget's disease was encountered. The primary sites of these metastatic carcinomas, in addition to the prostate, which was the most common, included the breast, colon, kidneys, and lungs.[84, 85]

On occasion, radiologically sinister-looking lesions of bone associated with Paget's disease develop, but on histologic examination, they prove to be benign. Two such *pseudomalignant lesions*, one with a juxtacortical soft tissue mass in a

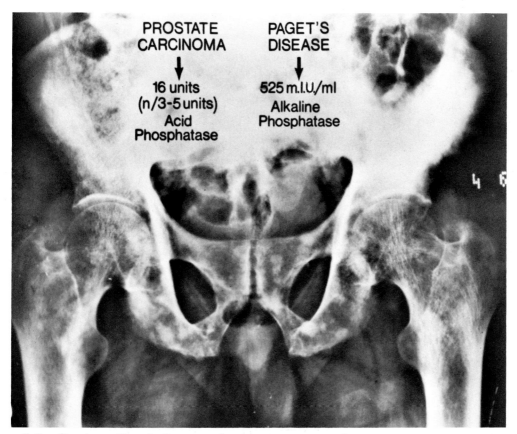

Figure 8–3. Coexistent Paget's disease and osseous metastases of a prostatic carcinoma in a 74-year-old man with pelvic pain of many months duration. Radiograph shows diffuse osteoporosis and sclerosis. Total alkaline phosphatase was 525 m.I.U./ml, with the following isoenzymes: liver and intestinal isoenzymes normal; bone isoenzyme elevated. Thermostabile fraction: 18 per cent. The clinical impression was Paget's disease of bone. Acid phosphatase was 16 units (normal 3–5 units). Biopsy showed both Paget's disease and metastatic prostatic carcinoma.

distal femur and another with a radiolucent midtibial lesion, have been reported by Bowerman and associates.[7]

PATHOLOGIC FINDINGS

The gross appearance and microscopic characteristics of Paget's sarcoma are no different from those of osteogenic sarcoma arising in a bone unaffected by Paget's disease.[15]

The type of malignant tumor formation present in Paget's disease is not necessarily an osteogenic sarcoma.[21, 32, 45, 47, 63, 68, 75, 77, 80, 88] Snapper was perhaps the first to describe a chondrosarcoma forming in Paget's disease.[74] In a study of 148 cases collected from three different bone tumor registries in England, 60 per cent of the Paget's sarcomas were classified as osteogenic sarcomas and 19 per cent were fibrosarcomas.[62] In 14 per cent of the cases, the type of sarcoma was unspecified, an example of the difficulty in exact classification of Paget's sarcomas. In the Memorial Hospital series of 33 patients reported by McKenna and his colleagues, 23 were classified as osteogenic sarcomas, 8 were fibrosarcomas, and 2 were chondrosarcomas.[42] Among 68 patients with chondrosarcoma studied by Thomson and Turner-Warwick, six were associated with Paget's disease.[79]

Periosteal, juxtacortical sarcomas are not found to occur in association with Paget's disease.

The coexistence of multiple myeloma and Paget's disease has been reported by several investigators.[13, 25, 27, 28, 43, 57, 60, 69, 70]

The association of giant cell tumors with Paget's disease of bone is a well-recognized clinical, radiographic, and pathologic entity.[8, 24, 26, 30, 66] One should not take it for granted, therefore, that all tumors complicating Paget's disease are malignant.[31] Approximately 20 to 25 cases of giant cell tumors associated with Paget's disease have been noted in the literature.[44] The majority occur in the craniofacial bones, and only occasional cases have been encountered in the ilium, humerus, tibia, and innominate bone (Fig. 8–4). Those arising in long bones do not involve the epiphyseal end of the bone. One coincidental example of a localized nodular tenosynovitis (giant cell tumor of tendon

sheath origin) occurred in the patellar tendon of a 44-year-old woman and was associated with Paget's disease.[40] True giant cell tumors in the craniofacial bones are extremely rare, and therefore it is surprising to note the predilection of these bones for giant cell tumors based on Paget's disease. Hutter and coworkers[31] also noted that ilial and innominate bone presentation is most uncommon (less than 5 per cent) with giant cell tumors uncomplicated by Paget's disease. The age distribution of giant cell tumors of bone uncomplicated by Paget's disease is distinctly different from that of giant cell tumors superimposed on this condition. The former occur in patients between 20 and 40 years of age, and the latter appear in those older than 40 years.

Several examples of malignant tumors with abundant giant cells, reported in the literature and analyzed by McKenna and associates[42] as well as Hutter and associates,[31] proved to be either malignant giant cell tumors or pleomorphic osteogenic sarcomas with a prominent giant cell component.[39]

PROGNOSIS AND TREATMENT

Paget's original patient developed a sarcoma, and four other early cases that he collected were patients who also died from secondary malignant transformation.[49-51] Schatzki and Dudley reported three patients with Paget's sarcoma who survived amputation without evidence of disease for 8, 9, and 17 years respectively.[67]

In a careful and painstaking analysis of the well-documented 212 patients with Paget's sarcoma in the pertinent literature, McKenna and his coworkers found that only four survived more than five years without recurrence or metastases after appropriate treatment, usually amputation. Ten of 33 patients at Memorial Hospital had metastases at the time of diagnosis, and most patients died within two years.[42] Accordingly, the conclusion that any treatment for Paget's sarcoma is ineffective, whether radical ablative surgery or radiation therapy, seems justified. Radiation therapy reduces the ever-present pain in approximately half of the patients but does

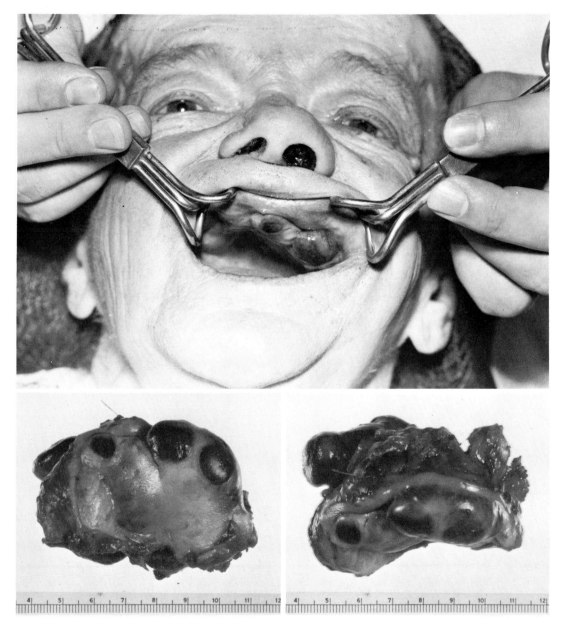

Figure 8–4. Giant cell tumor of maxilla associated with Paget's disease of long standing in a 75-year-old woman. The 7 cm, soft, spongy tumor mass obstructs the left nasal cavity and involves the left upper alveolus from the bicuspid to the third molar with medial extension to the midline.

not alter the ultimate outcome of the disease, nor does it appreciably diminish the tumor size. In contrast to the dismal prognosis for Paget's sarcoma, patients with giant cell tumors associated with Paget's disease have an excellent prospect, and virtually none will die from causes directly related to the tumor.[8, 24, 31, 44, 66] On the other hand, the malignant giant cell tumors are fatal within a short time.[31, 64, 79]

It has been suggested that the poor prognosis for bone sarcoma arising in Paget's disease may be due to the extreme vascularity of the bone in this condition that allows tumor cells easy access to vascular dissemination.[67] In an interesting study by Demmler, it was established that even in the early stages of Paget's disease of bone there is a marked increase in the number of arterial capillaries that rises with the duration and severity of the disease.[16] The venous system does not participate, at least initially, in this disease process. The circulation of blood in the active phase of Paget's disease closely mimics arteriovenous fistula formation, but in none of the reported studies could such major arteriovenous shunting be demonstrated.[14, 18, 58, 65, 76]

Treatment with salmon calcitonin had no apparent effect on the course of osteogenic sarcoma arising in Paget's disease of bone.[83]

REFERENCES

1. Agha, F. P., Norman, A., Hirschl, S., et al.: Paget's disease. Coexistence with metastatic carcinoma. N.Y. State J. Med., 76:734–735, 1976.
2. Anderson, J. T., and Dehner, L. P.: Osteolytic form of Paget's disease. Differential diagnosis and pathogenesis. J. Bone Joint Surg. [Am.], 58:994–1000, 1976.
3. Barry, H. C.: Sarcoma in Paget's disease of bone in Australia. J. Bone Joint Surg. [Am.], 43:1122–1134, 1961.
4. Barry, H. C.: Paget's disease of bone. Baltimore, Williams & Wilkins, 1969.
5. Bird, C. E.: Sarcoma complicating Paget's disease of bone: Report of 9 cases, 5 with pathologic verification. Arch. Surg., 14:1187–1208, 1927.
6. Bordier, P., Rasmussen, H., and Dorfmann, H.: Effectiveness of parathyroid hormone, calcitonin and phosphate on bone cells in Paget's disease. Am. J. Med., 56:850–857, 1974.
7. Bowerman, J. W., Altman, J., Hughes, J. L., et al.: Pseudomalignant lesions in Paget's disease of bone. Am. J. Roentgenol. Radium Ther. Nucl. Med., 124:57–61, 1975.
8. Brooke, R. I.: Giant cell tumor in patients with Paget's disease. Oral Surg., 30:230–241, 1970.
9. Burgener, F. A., and Perry, P. E.: Solitary renal cell carcinoma metastasis in Paget's disease simulating sarcomatous degeneration. Am. J. Roentgenol. Radium Ther. Nucl. Med., 128:853–855, 1977.
10. Cattaneo, E.: Considerazioni istogenetiche su un caso di sarcoma mandibolare a peculiare morfologia insorto su malattia di Paget. Riv. Ital. Stomatol., 22:1341–1352, 1967.
11. Coley, B. L., and Sharp, G. S.: Paget's disease. A predisposing factor to osteogenic sarcoma. Arch. Surg., 23:918–936, 1931.
12. Collins, D. H.: Paget's disease of bone. Incidence and subclinical forms. Lancet, 2:51–57, 1956.
13. Copelan, H. L.: Coexistence of multiple myelo-

ma and Paget's disease of bone. Calif. Med., 101:118–120, 1964.
14. De Marneffe, R.: Données actuelles concernant la vascularisation osseuse dans la maladie de Paget. Acta Cardiol. (Brux.), 8:181–188, 1953.
15. Dehner, L. P., Anderson, J. T., and Brown, D.: Orthopedic and pathologic aspects of Paget's disease. Minn. Med., 60:422–430, 1977.
16. Demmler, A.: Die Vaskularisation des Paget-Knochens. Dtsch. Med. Wochenschr., 99:91–95, 1974.
17. Dickson, D. D., Camp, J. D., and Ghormley, R. K.: Osteitis deformans: Paget's disease of the bone. Radiology, 44:449–470, 1945.
18. Edholm, E. G., Howarth, S., and McMichael, J.: Heart failure and bone blood flow in osteitis deformans. Clin. Sci., 5:249–260, 1945.
19. Fölsch, S.: Ostitis deformans Paget und sarkomatöse Entartung. Langenbecks Arch. Chir., 321:359–369, 1968.
20. Freydinger, J. E., Duhig, J. T., and McDonald, L. W.: Sarcoma complicating Paget's disease of bone. Arch. Pathol., 75:496–500, 1963.
21. Gerstel, G., and Janker, R.: Über die Entwicklung eines Spindelzellsarkoms auf dem Boden einer monostotischen Ostitis deformans Paget. Dtsch. Z. Chir., 238:577–603, 1933.
22. Goldenberg, R. R.: The skeleton in Paget's disease. Bull. Hosp. Joint Dis., 12:299–255, 1951.
23. Goldenberg, R. R.: Neoplasia in Paget's disease of bone. Bull. Hosp. Joint Dis., 22:1–38, 1961.
24. Goldstein, B. H., and Laskin, D. M.: Giant cell tumor of the maxilla complicating Paget's disease of bone. J. Oral Surg., 32:209–213, 1974.
25. Grader, J., and Moynihan, J. W.: Multiple myeloma and osteogenic sarcoma in a patient with Paget's disease. J.A.M.A., 176:685–687, 1961.
26. Griffey, L. E., and Tedeschi, L. G.: Giant cell tumor of ethmoid: Complication of Paget's disease of bone. Arch. Otolaryngol., 87:615–617, 1968.
27. Gross, R. J., and Yelin, G.: Multiple myeloma complicating Paget's disease. Am. J. Roentgenol. Radium Ther. Nucl. Med., 65:585–589, 1951.
28. Hanisch, C. M.: Paget's disease complicated by multiple myeloma. Bull. Hosp. Joint Dis., 11:43–47, 1950.
29. Hauw, J. J., Henin, D., Chomette, G., et al.: Bone sarcoma developing on spinal localisations of Paget's disease. Report of 4 cases. Arch. Anat. Pathol., 21:241–249, 1973.
30. Hilton, G.: Osteoclastoma associated with generalised bone disease. Br. J. Radiol., 23:437–439, 1950.
31. Hutter, R. V. P., Foote, F. W., Jr., Frazell, E., et al.: Giant cell tumors complicating Paget's disease of bone. Cancer, 16:1044–1056, 1963.
32. Immenkamp, M.: Die sekundären Knochensarkome. Orthopäde, 5:116–124, 1976.
33. Jaffe, H. L.: Paget's disease of bone. Arch. Pathol., 15:83–131, 1933.
34. Jaffe, H. L.: Tumors and Tumorous Conditions of the Bones and Joints. Philadelphia, Lea & Febiger, 1958, pp. 463–473.
35. Jaffe, H. L.: Metabolic, Degenerative, and Inflammatory Diseases of Bones and Joints. Philadelphia, Lea & Febiger, 1972, pp. 264–268.

36. Julien, J., Vallat, J. M., Lunel, G., et al.: A case of the cauda equina syndrome caused by sarcomatous degeneration of the sacrum with Paget's disease. Bordeaux Med., 7/8:1191–1198, 1974.

37. Karpawich, A. J.: Paget's disease with osteogenic sarcoma of maxilla. Oral Surg., 11:827–834, 1958.

38. Khairi, M. R. A., Wellman, H. W., Robb, J. A., et al.: Paget's disease of bone (osteitis deformans): symptomatic lesions and bone scan. Ann. Intern. Med., 79:348–351, 1973.

39. Kirschbaum, J. D.: Fibrosarcoma of the skull in Paget's disease. Arch. Pathol., 36:74–79, 1943.

40. Levine, H. A., and Enrile, F.: Giant cell tumor of patellar tendon coincident with Paget's disease. J. Bone Joint Surg. [Am.], 53:335–340, 1971.

41. Maldonado, A., Abdenour, G., and Hodes, P. P.: The masquerading effect of Paget's disease. Rev. Interam. Radiol., 1:31–34, 1976.

42. McKenna, R. J., Schwinn, C. P., Soong, K. Y., et al.: Osteogenic sarcoma arising in Paget's disease. Cancer, 17:42–66, 1964.

43. Mehbod, H., and Sweeney, W. M.: Multiple myeloma in Paget's disease. To the editor. J.A.M.A., 177:531, 1961.

44. Miller, A. S., Cuttino, C. L., Elzay, R. P., et al.: Giant cell tumor of the jaws associated with Paget disease of bone. Report of 2 cases and review of the literature. Arch. Otolaryngol., 100:233–236, 1974.

45. Miner, I. E.: Sarcoma in Paget's disease of bone. Bull. Hosp. Joint Dis., 11:26–42, 1950.

46. Morlock, G., Sany, J., and Serre, H.: Sarcomas associated with Paget's disease. Rev. Rhum. Mal. Osteoartic., 42:669–679, 1975.

47. Neuner, O.: Ein Sarkom des Oberkiefers auf dem Boden einer Ostitis deformans (Paget). Öst. Z. Stomatol., 53:655–665, 1956.

48. Packard, F. A., Steele, D. J., and Kirkbride, T. S.: Osteitis deformans. Am. J. Med. Sci., 122:552–569, 1901.

49. Paget, J.: On a form of chronic inflammation of bones (osteitis deformans). Trans. R. Med.-Chir. Soc. Lond., 60:37–63, 1877.

50. Paget, J.: Additional cases of osteitis deformans. Trans. R. Med.-Chir. Soc. Lond., 65:225–236, 1882.

51. Paget, J.: Remarks on osteitis deformans. Illustrated Med. News, 2:181–182, 1889.

52. Porretta, C. A., Dahlin, D. C., and Janes, J. M.: Sarcoma in Paget's disease of bone. J. Bone Joint Surg. [Am.], 39:1314–1329, 1957.

53. Price, C. H. G.: The incidence of osteogenic sarcoma in South-West England and its relationship to Paget's disease of bone. J. Bone Joint. Surg. [Br.], 44:366–376, 1962.

54. Price, C. H. G.: Myeloma occurring with Paget's disease of bone. Skeletal Radiol., 1:15–19, 1976.

55. Price, C. H. G., and Goldie, W.: Paget's sarcoma of bone. A study of 80 cases from the Bristol and the Leeds Bone Tumour Registries. J. Bone Joint Surg. [Br.], 51:205–224, 1969.

56. Rasmussen, H., and Bordier, P.: The Physiological and Cellular Basis of Metabolic Bone Disease. Baltimore, Williams & Wilkins, 1974, pp. 292–302.

57. Reich, C., and Brodsky, A. E.: Coexisting multiple myeloma and Paget's disease of bone treated with Stilbamidine. J. Bone Joint Surg. [Am.] , 30:642–646, 1948.

58. Rhodes, B. A., Greyson, N. D., Hamilton, C. R., Jr., et al.: Absence of anatomic arteriovenous shunts in Paget's disease of bone. N. Engl. J. Med., 287:686–689, 1972.

59. Roca, D. J.: Degeneracion sarcomatosa en la enfermedad de Paget del hueso. Univ. Med. Jav., Apr.-June:91–99, 1973.

60. Rosenkrantz, J. A., and Gluckman, E. C.: Coexistence of Paget's disease of bone and multiple myeloma. Case reports of 2 patients. Am. J. Roentgenol. Radium Ther. Nucl. Med., 78:30–38, 1957.

61. Rosenmertz, S. K., and Schare, H. J.: Osteogenic sarcoma arising in Paget's disease of the mandible. Review of the literature and report of a case. Oral Surg., 28:304–309, 1969.

62. Ross, F. G. M., Middlemiss, J. H., and Fitton, J. M.: Paget's sarcoma in bone — a radiological study. In Price, C. H. G., and Ross, F. G. M. (eds.): Bone — Certain Aspects of Neoplasia. Philadelphia, F. A. Davis (Butterworths), 1973, pp. 41–62.

63. Rubens-Duval, A.: Histological aspects of sarcomatous degeneration of bone affected by Paget's disease. Rev. Rhum. Mal. Osteoartic., 42:663–668, 1975.

64. Russell, D. S.: Malignant osteoclastoma and association of malignant osteoclastoma with Paget's osteitis deformans. J. Bone Joint Surg. [Br.], 31:281–290, 1949.

65. Rutishauser, E., Veyrat, R., and Rouiller, Ch.: La vascularisation de l'os Pagétique: étude anatomo-pathologique. Presse Méd., 62:654–657, 1954.

66. Schajowicz, F., and Slullitel, I.: Giant-cell tumor associated with Paget's disease of bone. A case report. J. Bone Joint Surg. [Am.], 48:1340–1349, 1966.

67. Schatzki, S. E., and Dudley, H. R.: Bone sarcoma complicating Paget's disease: A report of 3 cases with long survival. Cancer, 14:517–523, 1961.

68. Schwamm, H. A.: Case for diagnosis. Milit. Med., 136:895, 903, 1971.

69. Scurr, J. A.: Myeloma occurring in Paget's disease. Proc. R. Soc. Med., 65:725, 1972.

70. Serre, H., and Simon, L.: Maladie osseuse de Paget et myélome plasmocytaire multiple. Rev. Rhum. Mal. Osteoartic., 26:347–353, 1959.

71. Shannon, F. T., and Hopkins, J. S.: Paget's sarcoma of the vertebral column with neurological complications. Acta Orthop. Scand., 48:385–390, 1977.

72. Sherman, R. S., and Soong, K. Y.: A roentgen study of osteogenic sarcoma developing in Paget's disease. Radiology, 63:48–58, 1954.

73. Sissons, H. A.: Epidemiology of Paget's disease. Clin. Orthop., 45:73–79, 1966.

74. Snapper, I.: Maladies osseuses et parathyroides. Ann. Med., 29:201–221, 1931.

75. Stern, W. E.: Malignant "degeneration" (osteogenic sarcoma) occurring in pre-existing Paget's disease of the skull. A new case report with supplemental tabulation of recent cases. Bull. Los Angeles Neurol. Soc., 34:221–232, 1969.

76. Stortsteen, K. A., and Janes, J. M.: Arteriography

and vascular studies in Paget's disease of bone. J.A.M.A., *154*:472–474, 1954.

77. Summey, T. J., and Pressly, C. L.: Sarcoma complicating Paget's disease of bone. Ann. Surg., *123*:135–153, 1946.

78. Sutherland, C. G.: The differentiation of osteitis deformans and osteoplastic metastatic carcinoma. Radiology, *10*:150–152, 1928.

79. Thomson, A. D., and Turner-Warwick, R. T.: Skeletal sarcoma and giant-cell tumour. J. Bone Joint Surg. [Br.], *37*:266–303, 1955.

80. Venturoli, L., and Brusori, G.: L'evoluzione sarcomatosa, insolita e grave complicanza della malattia di Paget. Minerva Med., *67*:694–696, 1976.

81. Villiaumey, J., Di Menza, C., Rotterdam, M., et al.: A new observation on the sarcomatous degeneration of the spine affected by Paget's disease. Rev. Rhum. Mal. Osteoartic., *42*:687–691, 1975.

82. Wagner, M.: Report of a case of Paget's disease in an 18 year old male, with a review of the literature. Wis. Med. J., *46*:1093–1107, 1947.

83. Walton, I. G., and Strong, J. A.: Calcitonin and osteogenic sarcoma. Letter to the editor. Lancet, *1*:887–888, 1973.

84. Wilner, D., and Sherman, R. S.: Bone sarcoma associated with Paget's disease. CA, *16*:238–244, 1966.

85. Wilner, D., and Sherman, R. S.: Roentgen diagnosis of Paget's disease (Osteitis deformans). The usual. The unusual. The complications. Med. Radiogr. Photogr., *42*:35–78, 1966.

86. Woodard, H. Q.: Long term studies of blood chemistry in Paget's disease of bone. Cancer, *12*:1226–1237, 1959.

87. Woodhouse, N. J. Y.: Paget's disease of bone. Clin. Endocrinol. Metabol., *1*:125–141, 1972.

88. Zichner, L.: Sarcomatous transformation in Paget's disease. Langenbecks Arch. Chir., *336*:57–65, 1974.

9

RADIATION AS AN ONCOGENIC AGENT IN SARCOMA OF BONE

INCIDENCE

Considering the extent to which radiation has been used in the treatment of osseous and soft tissue lesions, in addition to incidental irradiation of adjacent normal tissues, the frequency of postirradiation sarcoma is very low (0.03 per cent of radiated cases).[102] In part, it may be that in the past only a few patients with cancer survived long enough to develop radiation-induced sarcomas.[19] Since there has been a definite trend in the treatment of cancer toward employing radiation for more favorable cases, in addition to technical improvements in the administration of radiotherapy, e.g., more modern equipment, survival data may have been altered considerably in many malignant tumors.[64] Accordingly, more radiation-induced tumors may be encountered in the future. Tefft and his colleagues estimated that a second primary tumor was likely to develop in 5 per cent of all children who survive for more than two years after receiving radiotherapy in a dose exceeding 100 rads.[103, 139, 140] In 1967, Castro and asso-

ciates collected only 93 cases of radiation-induced bone sarcoma that were published in the literature.[24] By now, about 200 cases of well-documented radiation-induced bone sarcomas have been reported.[92, 107] Between the years 1931 and 1970, approximately 50 cases of radiation-induced sarcomas of bone were seen at Memorial Hospital.[5, 6, 19, 30, 72]

It has afflicted people in all age groups, and practically every location has been involved by radiation-induced bone sarcoma.[142] Ages of the patients at Memorial Hospital varied from 9 to 75 years at the time the secondary bone sarcoma developed. There was no sexual predominance. These lesions followed a great variety of radiation doses. Orthovoltage was usually utilized, but occasionally, some tumors developed following supervoltage radiation. Calcified tissues preferentially absorb low-energy high-dose orthovoltage radiation with great efficiency.[114] Patients with these bone tumors received a radiation dose of 1000 to 3000 R or more. The actual dose may have been much higher since radiation equipment of 100 to 250 Kv used in

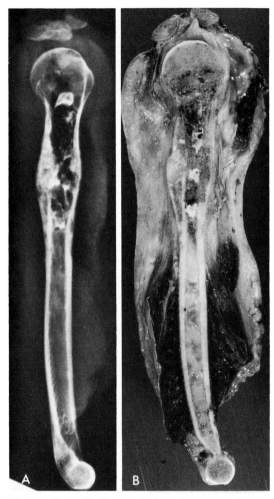

Figure 9–1. Radiation-induced osteogenic sarcoma of humerus with epiphyseal and soft tissue involvement in a 25-year-old woman. The patient received 5400 rads radiation therapy for a biopsy-proved Ewing's sarcoma of the same site 12 years previously. *A,* Specimen radiograph; *B,* forequarter amputation specimen.

of experimental atomic bomb explosions.[57, 88, 127, 131, 148]

The following *criteria* should be present before a lesion can be classified as a *postradiation sarcoma* of bone following treatment of benign osseous tumor. There should be microscopic confirmation that a benign tumor existed, that irradiation was indeed administered, that the sarcoma that subsequently formed was in the area included within the radiation field, and that a relatively long asymptomatic latent period elapsed before clinical manifestations of sarcoma, and this diagnosis must be confirmed histologically. Sarcomas arising after irradiation for malignant tumors of bone, provided there is a histologic delineation between the primary and secondary lesions, would also qualify (e.g., osteogenic sarcoma following radiation for Ewing's sarcoma) (Fig. 9–1).

LATENT PERIOD

At Memorial Hospital, the interval between irradiation and the appearance of sarcoma has varied between 4 and 27 years, with a median of 11.5 and a mean of 12.4 years.[72] In general, a 20 year mean after ionizing beam therapy and a 10 year mean after orthovoltage therapy are fair estimates. It is suggested that at least 3000 rads and about a three to four year "latent period" will provide a universally acceptable cause and effect relationship between radiation and tumor. It is of interest that bone tumors have been induced in children in one year after treatment with ^{224}Ra for tuberculosis, gout, arthritis, syphilis, and other diseases.[81, 82, 132, 133] The latent period extended up to 39 years.

"Latent period" refers to the time interval between exposure to radiation and detection of, or death from, tumor. This incubation period is a well-recognized but controversial characteristic of bone cancer induction by external or internal irradiation. The discussion centers around the dose sufficient to produce cancer and the time period between the exposure and the appearance of tumor. The radiation is usually delivered as a therapeutic measure for benign or malignant tumors of nonosseous origin or for essentially benign lesions of bone (giant cell tumor, fibrous

these cases resulted in an extremely intense local scatter of the radiation density. The radiobiologic effect of irradiation is chiefly determined by the magnitude of the absorbed dose (rad). Soft tissues within bone or adjacent to bone receive more radiation since these tissues are also irradiated by secondary electrons generated in the mineral matrix.

A possible increase in the incidence of bone sarcomas in children and adolescents may be expected after accidental exposure to and deposition of the radioactive fission product strontium as a result dysplasia, and so forth).[6] For instance, a patient with carcinoma of the cervix was treated by an intracavitary radium source and 14 years later developed a sarcoma of the pelvis.[14, 45, 112] Another patient was treated by external irradiation for a mammary carcinoma, and 18 years later she developed a chondrosarcoma of the scapula in the field of irradiation.[152] Bhansali and Desai reported the occurrence of a chondrosarcoma following radiation therapy for a Ewing's sarcoma eight years previously.[12] Occasionally, the history of previous irradiation is so distant that the patient fails to recall it: a bone sarcoma arose in the field of irradiation delivered 26 years previously for a hematoma of the thigh.[60]

It is commonly assumed that, as in experimental carcinogenesis, the "latent period" is inversely proportional to the radiation dose and may be longer than the normal life span of an individual if very small doses are delivered. Radiation data carefully analyzed at Memorial Hospital dispute these assumptions and indicate that the latent period for patients receiving less than the median radiation dose is shorter than for those receiving more than the median. At Memorial Hospital, no radiation-induced bone sarcomas were seen at doses below 1100 rets (3000 rads in three weeks).[72] The inverse relationship may only be applicable to low-dose levels of radiation exposure. At the high therapeutic levels of cancericidal radiation doses, i.e., more than 4000 rads in four weeks, not only the number of the potentially transformable cells will be greatly reduced but the proliferative activity of these transformed cells will also be impeded by poor vascular supply and increased fibrosis.

Postradiation sarcoma may occur in any bone. The bone may have been normal at the time of treatment, the radiation having been instituted for a soft tissue lesion, such as an epidermoid carcinoma of the gingiva[30, 70] or cervicofacial actinomycosis[69] or for the control of keloids.[74, 115]

In other instances, there have been lesions in the bones themselves. Osteogenic sarcoma has followed irradiation for fibrous dysplasia or giant cell reparative granuloma, giant cell tumor, and so on.[19, 35, 115, 134]

Secondary bone sarcoma, with or without preceding radiotherapy for fibrous dysplasia of bone, is a recognized but rare complication.[33, 66, 137] The risk of malignant transformation complicating this condition is increased, regardless of whether treated by low- or high-dose radiation therapy.

About 10 to 15 per cent of patients with giant cell tumors of bone treated by irradiation will develop bone sarcoma in the area included within the therapeutic beam.[33, 65, 67, 135] Five of the 12 radiation-induced bone sarcomas reported by Steiner developed 4 to 30 years following irradiation of giant cell tumor of bone.[136] In Campbell and Bonfiglio's series of 218 patients with giant cell tumors, 46 had radiation but only three demonstrated malignant transformation 9, 13, and 31 years respectively after this mode of therapy. The radiation doses given were 6300, 13,400, and 7400 R respectively.[20] Eight of 28 cases of radiation-induced sarcoma of bone reported by Arlen and associates from Memorial Hospital followed such treatment for giant cell tumor of bone.[5]

Radiation therapy for other benign bone tumors may result in a transmutation to a sarcoma. Such instances include the development of chondrosarcoma after treatment for chondroblastoma.[65a, 67]

After radiation treatment for ankylosing spondylitis and bursitis, at least three bone sarcomas developed in patients followed for 5 to 25 years. These individuals generally received less than 4000 rads.[29, 41, 53] A fibrosarcoma of the tibia developed eight years after an intra-articular injection of 10 mg of radium chloride for chronic arthritis of the knee.[97]

It is estimated that approximately 1 in 100 to 400 patients treated by heavy doses of irradiation for breast carcinoma will develop a bone sarcoma of the chest wall if followed for 10 to 20 years.[123, 124, 152] This incidence will vary considerably depending on the radiation dose, the type of equipment, and the size of the irradiated field[59] (Fig. 9–2).

There are approximately 36 cases of orbital sarcomas following radiotherapy for retinoblastoma, only 19 of which were diagnosed as osteogenic sarcoma.[51, 78, 116, 129, 138] One of the cases, for instance, studied histologically at Memorial Hospital, proved to be a highly malignant fibrous histiocytoma of bone. It is estimat-

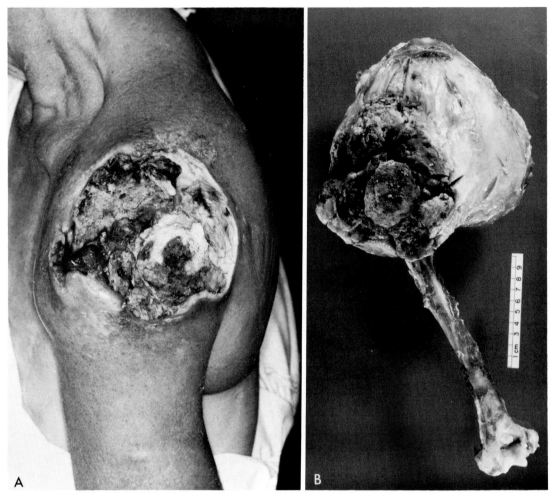

Figure 9–2. Radiation-induced osteogenic sarcoma of the shoulder girdle in a 55-year-old woman who, 11 years previously, underwent radical mastectomy followed by radiation therapy of 4000 rads in 16 treatments and an additional 2700 rads in 11 treatments to the chest wall, the supraclavicular fossa, and the shoulder girdle.

ed that approximately 5 per cent of the irradiated retinoblastoma patients will develop sarcomas in the field of irradiation. An excessively high incidence of osteogenic sarcoma of the femur, unassociated with any radiation treatment, seems to be prevalent with bilateral or familial retinoblastoma.[73] (See Chapter 5.) The hazard of orbital sarcoma developing after radiotherapy is increased when the retinoblastoma is bilateral or familial, as compared to those patients who have only unilateral tumors of sporadic incidence.[91] Patients with retinoblastoma followed by orbital sarcoma received, on the average, 4000 to 5000 rads, with an occasional patient receiving dose levels of 6000 to 7000 rads.

Nasopharyngeal carcinoma and medulloblastoma of the posterior fossa are commonly and successfully treated with radiotherapy, the well-recognized hazard of which is the development of craniofacial bone sarcoma in the field of irradiation.[101, 151]

The long-term analysis of bone sarcomas, as of April, 1974, in approximately 700 radium dial–painters (^{226}Ra and ^{228}Ra) represents a classic epidemiologic study in occupational medicine, whereby 25 employees with malignant bone tumors have already been identified[7, 131, 146] (Table 9–1).

There is still considerable uncertainty with regard to the actual radiation dose involved in producing bone sarcomas in the

TABLE 9–1.　The More Important Bone-Seeking Radionuclides and Their Potential to Induce Bone Sarcoma or Leukemia

	Half-life	Bone Seeker Surface	Volume	Bone Sarcoma	Leukemia
Ra-226	1,622 years	++	++	++	+−
Ra-224	3.6 days	+++	+−	+++	+
Sr-90	28 years	++	++	++	+
Sr-89	53 days	++	+	++	?
P-32	14 days	++	++	++	?
Th⟨228	1.9 years	0	0	+	+++
Th⟨232	10 years	0	0	+	+++
Pu-239	24,300 years	+++	0	+++	?
S-35	87 days	+−	+−	?	+++
Fe-55	2.7 years	+++	+−	+++	+++

*Data compiled by Dr. H. Q. Woodard.

radium dial–painters (luminizers) or in workers in the luminous paint industry.[32, 43, 81, 82, 150] The first cases of bone sarcoma among those employees who ingested radium and mesothorium were described in the 1920's by Martland and his coworkers.[23, 62, 86, 87] Histologic examination of about 50 malignant bone lesions in these individuals revealed an equal frequency of fibrosarcoma and osteogenic sarcoma. Examples of malignant hemangioendotheliomas of bone were not encountered, and only two cases of chondrosarcoma were recognized.[94] There was no preferential site of localization. The high incidence of fibrosarcoma was an unexpected finding.[47]

The therapeutic trial to treat osseous tuberculosis with Peteosthor ([224]Ra), a short-range alpha-emitting radionuclide, ended in disaster (Table 9–1). Between the years 1944 and 1951, about 2000 patients were treated with doses calculated to range from 6 to 5750 rads over the entire skeleton. Forty-seven of the 815 patients followed developed bone sarcomas: 35 of these had treatment before the age of 21 years and 15 were adults.[132, 133] Children are about twice as sensitive per rad dose as compared to adults in their propensity to develop radiation-induced bone tumors.[68] This radionuclide ([224]Ra) is still used in the treatment of ankylosing spondylitis.[29, 41]

A relatively low radiation dose is delivered to the skeleton in Thorotrast instillation in humans, and this is the reason why only a few cases of Thorotrast-induced bone tumors have been reported[90] (Table 9–1). An extraosseous chondrosarcoma in the left axillary region has developed approximately 22 years after an intravenous but partially extravasated Thorotrast injection.[117, 118] Extraosseous soft tissue osteogenic sarcomas or chondrosarcomas have also been known to develop after external irradiation.[1, 8, 15, 16]

Not only malignant but also benign bone tumors may be induced by radiation. There was a definite increase in the incidence of osteochondroma within the field of the x-ray beam in children who were irradiated for "status thymicolymphaticus" (thymic enlargement) with doses less than 1000 R.[104, 143] None developed bone sarcomas, but in several, an acute leukemia became apparent. Atypical osteoblastoma and osteocartilaginous exostosis have also been found to develop after irradiation for neuroblastoma, Wilms' tumor, eosinophilic granuloma, and hemangioma.[27, 28, 44, 71, 96, 101, 105]

HISTOLOGIC FEATURES

The histologic appearance of a radiation-induced bone sarcoma does not give a good clue as to whether it was an "induced" or a "spontaneous" bone cancer or whether it was produced by a specific bone-seeking radionuclide or external irradiation.[78, 80, 144, 145]

About 200 cases of bone sarcomas induced by external irradiation have been reported.[2, 5, 6, 36, 38, 50, 52, 58, 69, 98, 100, 102, 107, 109, 115, 121, 122, 126, 130, 134, 141, 149, 153] Approximately 60 per cent of these were diagnosed as osteogenic sarcomas, 30 per cent as fibrosarcomas, and 10 per cent as chondrosarcomas. One to two per cent of these sarcomas were not further classified histologically.

Osteogenic sarcomas or fibrosarcomas arising in bones that have been subjected to previous irradiation or those that develop following radiotherapy for giant cell tumor occasionally may exhibit a minor, or infrequently a major, component microscopically indistinguishable from a malignant fibrous histiocytoma.

RADIOGRAPHIC FEATURES

The radiographically detectable osseous changes at the periphery of radiation-induced bone sarcomas include trabecular coarsening and thickening (dense bone necrosis), areas of rarefaction (osteoporosis), and transverse radiopaque lines at the growth plates in children and are similar to changes in chronic lead poisoning and fractures.[7, 128] It must be stated that bone sarcomas can occur after documented radiation therapy without gross radiologic evidence of pre-existent osseous changes of so-called "radiation osteitis."

Pre-existent radiation osteitis is usually demonstrable on radiologic examination preceding the development of bone sarcomas or at the periphery of the already developed tumor.[99] Histologically, the radiation osteitis in the immediately adjacent bone was manifested by the lack of osteocytes in the osseous tissue, as well as by disintegration of the bony trabeculae. The intertrabecular marrow was replaced, in foci, by fibrous tissue or appeared to be necrotic.[4] Such changes were seen in about half of the cases at Memorial Hospital[5, 6] and in most of the instances studied by Steiner.[136]

TREATMENT AND RESULTS

Major surgical intervention has remained the cornerstone of treatment in radiation-induced sarcomas of bone, but not all are amenable to radical surgery. Maxillectomy, orbital exenteration, and mandibulectomy were carried out for most of the tumors arising in the craniofacial bones.[6] For sarcomas developing in the appendicular skeleton, interscapulothoracic amputation and hemipelvectomy were performed.[5]

The overall five year disease-free survival rate in the Memorial Hospital series of cases was 28 per cent. The survival rate was much more unfavorable in tumors arising in the craniofacial bones, and only one of seven patients survived for five or more years. The best results were noted among those patients whose sarcomas were superimposed on primary osseous conditions, mainly giant cell tumor. Once local recurrence of the sarcoma after definitive therapy intervened, or pulmonary metastases were demonstrated, the survival rate ranged from three to seven months. Radiation therapy aimed at the recurrent tumor resulted in some diminution in its size. In none of the cases was modern multicyclic multidrug therapy employed as a primary treatment.

EXPERIMENTAL INDUCTION OF BONE TUMORS IN ANIMALS AND THE MECHANISM OF CANCER INDUCTION BY IONIZING RADIATION

In bone tumors experimentally induced by various radioactive isotopes, it is mandatory to separate those induced by a single administration of the radionuclide from those induced by continuous feeding (Table 9–1). There seem to be differences in the types of tumor induced by single and by continuous administration. The character of the radiation dose obtained by the tissues is different under the two methods of administration. The single administration results in the skeletal distribution of the radionuclide to be unevenly transmitted. Following continuous administration of a radionuclide, the entire skeleton will be irradiated and labelled in a relatively even pattern.[26] In none of the animal experiments has it been possible to pinpoint exactly the smallest radiation dose in terms of the absorbed energy necessary for bone tumor induction, the "practical threshold," because radionuclides do not localize uniformly in the skeleton and they diminish in amount with time.[42, 43] Evans and colleagues, in an extensive survey of radiation-induced osteogenic sarcomas in animals, found a "practical threshold." In their opinion, no osteogenic sarcomas arose in bones that had received less than 1000 rads.[43] Five hundred rads delivered to the endosteal surface of a mouse femur by external irradiation is known to result in osteogenic sarcoma. The exact time when irreversible neoplastic transformation takes place has not been determined. The mechanism of cancer-induction by radiation is also not clear. Studies by radionuclides and cell-free extracts of virus-induced bone tumors revealed interactions pointing to the possibility that radiation induces cancer by inactivating a viral inhibitor or a latent cancer virus.[49] The support of this thesis has been the demonstration in neutralization tests of the occurrence of an antigen, very closely related to FBJ virus, in some ^{90}Sr-induced animal osteogenic sarcomas.[48, 110] Another currently popular hypothesis maintains that ionizing events occurring at the time radiation is absorbed in the tissues results in changes in the genes and chromosomes of one or more cells. This initiating event is frequently referred to as a point mutation.[31] During the extended latent period, secondary factors may play an important role. Hormones and chronic chemical irritants, for instance, may promote cellular unrest during this period.

It is generally believed that the average period of latency, i.e., interval between exposure to irradiation and discovery of tumor, is inversely proportional to the amount of radionuclide administered; the less radioactive source applied, the longer the incubation period. A careful re-evaluation of data, however, points to this assumption as probably being incorrect, at least in the reported animal experiments. It seems the inverse relationship of dose and latent period applies only to extremely high radiation dosages and is due to the fact that increased dosage elicits an increased incidence of bone tumors with the likelihood becoming greater that the osseous lesion appears earlier. The inverse relationship accordingly is considered to be erroneous, and the time required for tumor induction seems to be independent of the radiation dose.[49, 113]

The shortest latent periods following internal irradiation by bone-seeking nuclides are 143 days for mice, 186 days for rats, 153 days for rabbits, 274 days for cats, and 547 days for dogs.[49]

The earliest detectable roentgenographic changes following administration of bone-seeking radionuclides are manifested by alterations in the metaphyseal ends of the distal femur and proximal tibia. The normal trabecular bony pattern here becomes mottled and irregular, with alternating areas of increased and decreased bone densities.[40, 108, 146]

Osteogenic sarcomas were induced by intraperitoneal injections of ^{32}P in female rats. Except in one case, which was an intramedullary fibrosarcoma, the tumors showed osteoblastic activity and osteoid formation with an occasional area of tumor cartilage production.[26] A high metastatic rate in 50 per cent of the animals was noted.

In ^{90}Sr-induced bone tumors in CBA/H mice, instead of the expected osteogenic sarcomas, a high incidence of malignant hemangioendotheliomas and "lymphoreticular sarcomas" was found.[83, 84] An increased incidence (over 40 per cent) of malignant hemangioendotheliomas of bone was noted in beagles with internally deposited radionuclides.[11, 106] Strontium (^{90}Sr) induces a pleomorphic osteogenic sarcoma in rabbits, with marked regional variation in microscopic structure.[22, 39, 63, 75] Thorium (^{228}Th) is known to have induced 33 osteogenic sarcomas and one hemangioendothelioma in dogs.[145]

Plutonium-239, a surface-seeking alpha-emitter radionuclide retained in the body for prolonged periods, causes osteogenic sarcomas in beagles[37, 89] and rabbits.[13] The average cumulative skeletal dose was about 60 rads.

An increased incidence of osteogenic sarcoma was reported by Warren and Chute in externally irradiated parabiotic rats exposed to 1000 rad whole-body radiation.[147] Baserga and associates irradiated the legs of male rats to 3000 rads of gamma radiation and produced an incidence of 29 per cent for osteogenic sarcomas. The control animals developed no such bone tumors at all.[9]

REFERENCES

1. Alpert, L. I., Abaci, I. F., and Werthamer, S.: Radiation-induced extraskeletal osteosarcoma. Cancer, *31*:1359–1363, 1973.
2. Amine, A. R. C., and Sugar, O.: Suprasellar os-

teogenic sarcoma following radiation for pituitary adenoma. Case report. J. Neurosurg., *44*:88–91, 1976.

3. Anderson, W. A. D., Zander, G. E., and Kuzma, J. F.: Cancerogenic effects of Ca⁴⁵ and Sr⁸⁹ on bones of CF₁ mice. Arch. Pathol., *62*:262–271, 1956.

4. Andrä, A., and Beetke, E.: On the osteoradionecrosis of the jaws. Dtsch. Stomatol., *23*:713–721, 1973.

5. Arlen, M., Higinbotham, N. L., Huvos, A. G., et al.: Radiation-induced sarcoma of bone. Cancer, *28*:1087–1099, 1971.

6. Arlen, M., Shah, I. C., Higinbotham, N., et al.: Osteogenic sarcoma of head and neck induced by radiation therapy. N.Y. State J. Med., *72*:929–934, 1972.

7. Aub, J. C., Evans, R. D., Hempelmann, L. H., et al.: The late effects of internally-deposited radioactive materials in man. Medicine, *31*:221–329, 1952.

8. Auerbach, O., Friedman, M., Weiss, L., et al.: Extraskeletal osteogenic sarcoma arising in irradiated tissue. Cancer, *4*:1095–1106, 1951.

9. Baserga, R., Lisco, H., and Cater, D. B.: The delayed effects of external gamma irradiation on the bones of rats. Am. J. Pathol., *39*:455–472, 1961.

10. Beck, A.: Zur Frage des Röntgensarkoms, zugleich ein Beitrag zur Pathogenese des Sarkoms. Münch. Med. Wochschr., *69*:623–625, 1922.

11. Benjamin, S. A., Hahn, F. F., Chiffelle, T. L., et al.: Occurrence of hemangiosarcomas in beagles with internally deposited radionuclides. Cancer Res., *35*:1745–1755, 1975.

12. Bhansali, S. K., and Desai, P. B.: Ewing's sarcoma: observations on 107 cases. J. Bone Joint Surg. [Am.], *45*:541–553, 1963.

13. Bleaney, B., and Vaughan, J.: Distribution of ²³⁹Pu in the bone marrow and on the endosteal surface of the femur of adult rabbits following injection of ²³⁹Pu(NO₃)₄. Br. J. Radiol., *44*:67–73, 1971.

14. Bloch, C.: Postradiation osteogenic sarcoma. Report of a case and review of the literature. Am. J. Roentgenol. Radium Ther. Nucl. Med., *87*:1157–1162, 1962.

15. Boyer, C. W., Jr., and Navin, J. J.: Extraskeletal osteogenic sarcoma: A late complication of radiation therapy. Cancer, *18*:628–633, 1965.

16. Brenner, R. W., and Garret, R.: Soft tissue chondrosarcoma-like tumor. Tumor arising in an area of radiation injury. Arch. Surg., *86*:471–476, 1963.

17. Brown, J. M.: Linearity vs non-linearity of dose response for radiation carcinogenesis. Health Phys., *31*:231–245, 1976.

18. Cade, S.: Radiation induced cancer in man. Br. J. Radiol., *30*:393–402, 1957.

19. Cahan, W. G., Woodard, H. Q., Higinbotham, N. L., et al.: Sarcoma arising in irradiated bone. Report of eleven cases. Cancer, *1*:3–29, 1948.

20. Campbell, C. J., and Bonfiglio, M.: Aggressiveness and malignancy in giant-cell tumors of bone. *In* Price, C. H. G., and Ross, F. G. M. (eds.): Bone — Certain Aspects of Neoplasia. Philadelphia, F. A. Davis (Butterworths), 1973, pp. 15–38.

21. Carroll, R. E., Godwin, J. T., and Watson, W. L.: Osteogenic sarcoma of phalanx after chronic roentgen-ray irradiation. Cancer, *9*:753–755, 1956.

22. Casarett, G. W., Tuttle, L. W., and Baxter, R. C.: Pathology of imbibed ⁹⁰Sr in rats and monkeys. *In* Dougherty, F. F., Jee, W. S. S., Mays, C. W., et al. (eds.): Some Aspects of Internal Irradiation. New York, Pergamon Press, 1962, pp. 329–336.

23. Castle, W. B., Drinker, K. R., and Drinker, C. K.: Necrosis of jaw in workers employed in applying luminous paint containing radium. J. Industr. Hyg., *7*:371–382, 1925.

24. Castro, L., Choi, S. H., and Sheehan, F. R.: Radiation induced bone sarcomas. Report of five cases. Am. J. Roentgenol. Radium Ther. Nucl. Med., *100*:924–930, 1967.

25. Chilton, A. B.: Linearity of dose response for radiation carcinogenesis. Letter to the editor. Health Phys., *33*:627, 1977.

26. Cobb, L. M.: Radiation-induced osteosarcoma in the rat as a model for osteosarcoma in man. Br. J. Cancer, *24*:294–299, 1970.

27. Cohen, J., and D'Angio, G. J.: Unusual bone tumors after roentgen therapy of children. Two case reports. Am. J. Roentgenol. Radium Ther. Nucl. Med., *86*:502–512, 1961.

28. Cole, A. R. C., and Darte, J. M. M.: Osteochondromata following irradiation in children. Pediatrics, *32*:285–288, 1963.

29. Court-Brown, W. M., and Doll, R.: Mortality from cancer and other causes after radiotherapy for ankylosing spondylitis. Br. Med. J., *2*:1327–1332, 1965.

30. Cruz, M., Coley, B. L., and Stewart, F. W.: Postradiation bone sarcoma. Report of eleven cases. Cancer, *10*:72–88, 1957.

31. Curtis, H. J.: Somatic mutations in radiation carcinogenesis. Radiat. Res., *36*:45–50, 1968.

32. Daels, F.: Beitrag zur experimentellen Hervorrufung von Tumoren mittels Radium. Strahlentherapie, *25*:675–678, 1927.

33. Dahlin, D. C., Ghormley, R. K., and Pugh, D. G.: Giant-cell tumor of bone: differential diagnosis. Mayo Clin. Proc., *31*:31–42, 1956.

34. Dahlin, D. C., and Ivins, J. C.: Fibrosarcoma of bone — a study of 114 cases. Cancer, *23*:35–41, 1969.

35. De Lathouwer, C., and Brocheriou, C.: Sarcoma arising in irradiated jawbones. Possible relationship with previous nonmalignant bone lesions. Report of 6 cases and review of the literature. J. Maxillofac. Surg., *4*:8–20, 1976.

36. De Young, R.: The development of sarcoma in bone subjected to irradiation. A case report. Am. Surg., *18*:816–819, 1952.

37. Dougherty, T. F.: Incidence of bone cancer in internally irradiated dogs. *In* Dougherty, T. F., Jee, W. S. S., Mays, C. W., et al. (eds): Some Aspects of Internal Irradiation. New York, Pergamon Press, 1962, p. 47.

38. Dowdle, J. A., Jr., Winter, R. B., and Dehner, L. P.: Postradiation osteosarcoma of the cervical spine in childhood. A case report. J. Bone Joint Surg. [Am.], *59*:969–971, 1977.

39. Downie, E. D., Macpherson, S., Ramsden, E. N., et al.: The effect of daily feeding of ⁹⁰Sr to rabbits. Br. J. Cancer, *13*:408–423, 1959.

40. Drouet, J., Deloince, R., and Baron, R.: Ultra-structural study of the periosteal response in case of diaphyseal fractures in mice subjected to X-ray exposure. Med. Arm., 2:427–436, 1974.
41. Edgar, M. A., and Robinson, M. P.: Post-radiation sarcoma in ankylosing spondylitis. A report of five cases. J. Bone Joint Surg. [Br.], 55:183–188, 1973.
42. Evans, R. D.: The effect of skeletally deposited alpha-ray emitters in man. Br. J. Radiol., 39:881–895, 1966.
43. Evans, R. D., Keane, A. T., Kolenkow, R. J., et al.: Radiogenic tumors in the radium and mesothorium cases studied at M.I.T. In Mays, C. W., Jee, W. S. S., Lloyd, R. D., et al. (eds: Delayed Effects of Bone-Seeking Radionuclides. Salt Lake City, University of Utah Press, 1969, pp. 157–194.
44. Fanconi, G., and Illig, R.: Beinverkürzung und Entstehung einer solitären cartilaginären Exostose nach gelenknaher Bestrahlung eines Hämangioms im Säuglingsalter. Helv. Paediatr. Acta, 14:425–429, 1959.
45. Fehr, P. E., and Prem, K. A.: Postirradiation sarcoma of the pelvic girdle following therapy for squamous cell carcinoma of the cervix. Am. J. Obstet. Gynecol., 116:192–200, 1973.
46. Feintuch, T. A.: Chondrosarcoma arising in a cartilaginous area of previously irradiated fibrous dysplasia. Cancer, 31:877–881, 1973.
47. Finkel, A. J., Miller, C. E., and Hasterlik, R. J.: Radium-induced malignant tumors in man. In Mays, C. W., Jee, W. S. S., Lloyd, R. D., et al. (eds.): Delayed Effects of Bone-Seeking Radionuclides. Salt Lake City, University of Utah Press, 1969, pp. 195–225.
48. Finkel, M. P., and Reilly, C. A., Jr.: Observations suggesting the viral etiology of radiation-induced tumors, particularly osteogenic sarcomas. In Sanders, C. L., Busch, R. H., Ballou, J. E., et al. (eds.): Radionuclide Carcinogenesis. Proceedings Twelfth Annual Hanford Biology Symposium. U.S. Atomic Energy Commission, 1973, p. 278.
49. Finkel, M. P., Reilly, C. A., Jr., and Biskis, B. O.: Pathogenesis of radiation and virus-induced bone tumors. In Grundmann, E. (ed.): Malignant Bone Tumors. New York, Springer-Verlag, 1976, pp. 92–103.
50. Fitzwater, J. E., Cabaud, H. E., and Farr, G. H.: Irradiation-induced chondrosarcoma. A case report. J. Bone Joint Surg. [Am.], 58:1037–1039, 1976.
51. Friedmann, G., and Kleinsasser, O.: Strahleninduzierte Sarkome des Schädels. Strahlentherapie, 137:33–37, 1969.
52. Gane, N. F. C., Lindup, R., Strickland, P., et al.: Radiation-induced fibrosarcoma. Br. J. Cancer, 24:705–711, 1970.
53. Glicksman, A. S., and Toker, C.: Osteogenic sarcoma following radiotherapy for bursitis. Mt. Sinai J. Med. N.Y., 43:163–167, 1976.
54. Goldman, M., Dungworth, D. L., Bulgin, M. S., et al.: Radiation-induced neoplasms in beagles after administration of ^{90}Sr and ^{226}Ra. In Radiation Induced Cancer. Vienna, International Atomic Energy Agency, 1969, pp. 345–360.

55. Gössner, W., Hindringer, B., Luz, A., et al.: Morphologie und Enzymhistochemie ^{224}Ra-induzierter osteogener Sarkome bei der Maus. Z. Krebsforsch., 78:225–235, 1972.
56. Gössner, W., Hug, O., Luz, A., et al.: Experimental induction of bone tumors by short-lived bone-seeking radionuclides. In Grundmann, E. (ed.): Malignant Bone Tumors. New York, Springer-Verlag, 1976, pp. 36–49.
57. Graf, B., Lafuma, J., Parmentier, C., et al.: Tumeurs osseuses provoquées par le 90 Strontium. Bull. Cancer (Paris), 57:381–396, 1970.
58. Hatcher, C. H.: The development of sarcoma in bone subjected to roentgen or radium irradiation. J. Bone Joint Surg., 27:179–195, 1945.
59. Hatfield, P. M., and Schulz, M. D.: Postirradiation sarcoma. Including five cases after X-ray therapy of breast. Radiology, 96:593–602, 1970.
60. Hellner, H.: Knochensarkom als mittelbare Unfallfolge anerkannt. Monatsschr. Unfallheilkd., 68:101–104, 1965.
61. Hems, G.: The risk of bone cancer in man from internally deposited radium. Br. J. Radiol., 40:506–511, 1967.
62. Hoffman, F. L.: Radium (mesothorium) necrosis. J.A.M.A., 85:961–965, 1925.
63. Howard, E. B., Clarke, W. J., Karagianes, M. T., et al.: ^{90}Sr induced bone tumours in miniature swine. Radiat. Res., 39:594–607, 1969.
64. Hutchison, G. B.: Late neoplastic changes following medical irradiation. Cancer, 37:1102–1107, 1976.
65. Hutter, R. V. P., Worcester, J. N., Jr., Francis, K. C., et al.: Benign and malignant giant-cell tumors of bone. A clinicopathological analysis of the natural history of the disease. Cancer, 15:653–690, 1962.
65a. Huvos, A. G., Higinbotham, N. L., Marcove, R. C., et al.: Aggressive chondroblastoma. Review of the literature on aggressive behavior and metastases with a report of one new case. Clin. Orthop., 126:266–272, 1977.
66. Huvos, A. G., Higinbotham, N. L., and Miller, T. R.: Bone sarcomas arising in fibrous dysplasia. J. Bone Joint Surg. [Am.], 54:1047–1056, 1972.
67. Jaffe, H. L.: Giant-cell tumor (osteoclastoma) of bone: its pathologic delimitation and the inherent clinical implications. Ann. R. Coll. Surg. Engl., 13:343–355, 1953.
68. Jee, W. S. S.: Bone-seeking radionuclides and bones. In Berdjis, C. C. (ed.): Pathology of Irradiation. Baltimore, Williams & Wilkins, 1971, pp. 186–212.
69. Jones, A.: Irradiation sarcoma. Br. J. Radiol., 26:273–284, 1953.
70. Kaae, S., and Glahn, M.: Case of sarcoma in irradiated mandible. Acta Radiol., 31:431–434, 1949.
71. Katzman, H., Waugh, T., and Berdon, W.: Skeletal changes following irradiation of childhood tumors. J. Bone Joint Surg. [Am.], 51:825–842, 1969.
72. Kim, J. H., Woodard, H. Q., Huvos, A. G., et al.: Radiation induced soft tissue sarcoma and bone sarcoma. Radiology (in press).
73. Knudson, A. G., Jr.: Mutation in human cancer. Adv. Cancer Res., 17:317–352, 1973.

74. Kragh, L. V., Dahlin, D. C., and Erich, J. B.: Osteogenic sarcoma of the jaws and facial bones. Am. J. Surg., 96:496–505, 1958.

75. Kuzma, J. F., and Zander, G.: Cancerogenic effects of Ca[45] and Sr[89] in Sprague-Dawley rats. Arch. Pathol., 63:198–206, 1957.

76. Laissue, J. A., Burlington, H., Cronkite, E. P., et al.: Induction of osteosarcomas and hematopoietic neoplasms by [55]Fe in mice. Cancer Res., 37:3545–3550, 1977.

77. Langlands, A. O., Souter, W. A., Samuel, E., et al.: Radiation osteitis following irradiation for breast cancer. Clin. Radiol., 28:93–96, 1977.

78. Lee, W. R., Laurie, J., and Townsend, A. L.: Fine structure of a radiation-induced osteogenic sarcoma. Cancer, 76:1414–1425, 1975.

79. Li, F. P., Cassady, J. R., and Barnett, E.: Cancer mortality following irradiation in infancy for hemangioma. Radiology, 113:177–178, 1974.

80. Litvinov, N. N.: Growth dynamics of bone sarcomas which form under the effect of a radioactive substance. Vopr. Onkol., 2(3):285–294, 1956.

81. Looney, W. B.: Late effects (twenty-five to forty years) of the early medical and industrial use of radioactive materials. Their relation to the more accurate establishment of maximum permissible amounts of radioactive elements in the body. J. Bone Joint Surg. [Am.], 37:1169–1187, 1955.

82. Looney, W. B.: Late effects (twenty-five to forty years) of the early medical and industrial use of radioactive materials. Their relation to the more accurate establishment of maximum permissible amounts of radioactive elements in the body. J. Bone Joint Surg. [Am.], 38:175–218 (Part II); 392–406 (Part III), 1956.

83. Loutit, J. F.: Vasoformative non-osteogenic (angio) sarcomas of bone-marrow stroma due to strontium-90. Int. J. Radiat. Biol., 30:359–383, 1976.

84. Loutit, J. F., Bland, M. R., Carr, T. E. F., et al.: Tumours in bone and bone marrow induced in CBA/H mice by ^{90}Sr and [226]Ra. In Price, C. H. G., and Ross, F. G. M. (eds.): Bone — Certain Aspects of Neoplasia. Philadelphia, F. A. Davis (Butterworths), 1973, pp. 395–407.

85. Martland, H. S.: The occurrence of malignancy in radioactive persons. A general review of data gathered in the study of radium dial painters, with special reference to the occurrence of osteogenic sarcoma and the interrelationship of certain blood diseases. Am. J. Cancer, 15:2435–2516, 1931.

86. Martland, H. S., Conlon, P., and Knef, J. P.: Unrecognized dangers in use and handling of radioactive substances; with especial reference to storage of insoluble products of radium and mesothorium in the reticulo-endothelial system. J.A.M.A., 85:1769–1776, 1925.

87. Martland, H. S., and Humphries, R. E.: Osteogenic sarcoma in dial painters using luminous paint. Arch. Pathol., 7:406–417, 1929.

88. Mays, C. W.: Cancer induction in man from internal radioactivity. Health Phys., 25:585–592, 1973.

89. Mays, C. W., Dougherty, T. F., Taylor, G. N., et al.: Radiation-induced bone cancer in beagles. In Mays, C. W., Jee, W. S. S., Lloyd, R. D., et al. (eds.): Delayed Effects of Bone-Seeking Radionuclides. Salt Lake City, University of Utah Press, 1969, p. 387.

90. Matzen, P., and Giuliani, K.: Peteosthor und Tumorgenese. Zentralbl. Chir., 87:881–886, 1962.

91. Miller, R. W.: Etiology of childhood bone cancer: epidemiologic observations. In Grundmann, E. (ed.): Malignant Bone Tumors. New York, Springer-Verlag, 1976, pp. 50–62.

92. Mindell, E. R., Shah, N. K., and Webster, J. H.: Postradiation sarcoma of bone and soft tissues. Orthop. Clin. North Am., 8:821–834, 1977.

93. Morris, L. L., Cassady, J. R., and Jaffe, N.: Sternal changes following mediastinal irradiation for childhood Hodgkin's disease. Radiology, 115:701–705, 1975.

94. Moskalev, Y. J., Streltsova, V. N., and Buldakov, L. A.: Late effects of radionuclide damage. In Mays, C. W., Jee, W. S. S., Lloyd, R. D., et al. (eds.): Delayed Effects of Bone-Seeking Radionuclides. Salt Lake City, University of Utah Press, 1969, pp. 589–599.

95. Müller, W. A., and Luz, A.: The osteosarcomagenic effectiveness of the short-lived [224]Ra compared with that of the long-lived [226]Ra in mice. Radiat. Res., 70:444–448, 1977.

96. Murphy, F. D., Jr., and Blount, W. P.: Cartilaginous exostoses following irradiation. J. Bone Joint Surg. [Am.], 44:662–668, 1962.

97. Norgaard, F.: The development of fibrosarcoma as a result of the intra-articular injection of radium chloride for therapeutic purposes. A new form of radium poisoning in human beings. Am. J. Cancer, 37:329–342, 1939.

98. Paik, H. H., and Wilkinson, E. J.: Peritoneal osteosarcoma following irradiation therapy of ovarian cancer. Obstet. Gynecol., 47:488–491, 1976.

99. Parker, R. G., and Berry, H. C.: Late effects of therapeutic irradiation on the skeleton and bone marrow. Cancer, 37:1162–1171, 1976.

100. Peimer, C. A., Yuan, H. A., and Sagerman, R. H.: Postradiation chondrosarcoma. A case report. J. Bone Joint Surg. [Am.], 58:1033–1036, 1976.

101. Perez, C. A., Vietti, T., Ackerman, L. V., et al.: Tumors of the sympathetic nervous system in children. An appraisal of treatment and results. Radiology, 88:750–760, 1967.

102. Phillips, T. L., and Sheline, G. E.: Bone sarcomas following radiation therapy. Radiology, 81:992–996, 1963.

103. Pickren, J. W.: Cancer often strikes twice. N.Y. State J. Med., 63:95–99, 1963.

104. Pifer, J. W., Toyooka, E. T., Murray, R. W., et al.: Neoplasms in children treated with X-rays for thymic enlargement. I. Neoplasms and mortality. J. Natl. Cancer Inst., 31:1333–1356, 1963.

105. Pogrund, H., and Yosipovitch, Z.: Osteochondroma following irradiation. Case report and review of the literature. Isr. J. Med. Sci., 12:154–157, 1976.

106. Pool, R. R., Williams, R. J. R., and Goldman, M.: [90]Sr toxicity in beagles. In Goldman, M., and Bustad, L. (eds.): Biomedical Implications

of Radiostrontium Exposure. Oak Ridge, Division of Technical Information, U.S. Atomic Energy Commission, 1972, pp. 277–284.

107. Potdar, G. G., and Shrikhande, S. S.: Post radiation bone sarcoma. Indian J. Cancer, 10:361–365, 1973.

108. Poznanski, T. W., and Frankel, S.: The roentgenographic development (Sr 90) induced osteogenic sarcoma in the rat. J. Bone Joint Surg. [Am.], 47:349–358, 1965.

109. Raventos, A., Gross, S. W., and Pendergrass, E. P.: Sarcoma following radiation injury of skull. Am. J. Roentgenol. Radium Ther. Nucl. Med., 83:145–148, 1960.

110. Reilly, C. A., Jr., and Finkel, M. P.: Evidence of FBJ virus antigen in Sr-induced osteosarcomas. Radiat. Res., 47:252–253, 1971.

111. Rowland, R. E.: The risk of malignancy from internally-deposited radioisotopes. *In* Nygaard, O. F., Adler, H. I., and Sinclair, W. K. (eds.): Radiation Research. Biomedical, Chemical and Physical Perspectives. New York, Academic Press, 1975, pp. 146–155.

112. Rushforth, G. F.: Osteosarcoma of the pelvis following radiotherapy for carcinoma of the cervix. Br. J. Radiol., 47:149–152, 1974.

113. Rushton, M. A., Owen, M., Holgate, W., et al.: The relation of radiation dose to radiation damage in the mandible of weanling rabbits. Arch. Oral Biol., 3:235–246, 1961.

114. Rutherford, H., and Dodd, G. D.: Complications of radiation therapy: growing bone. Semin. Roentgenol., 9:15–27, 1974.

115. Sabanas, A. O., Dahlin, D. C., Childs, D. S., Jr., et al.: Postradiation sarcoma of bone. Cancer, 9:528–542, 1956.

116. Sagerman, R. H., Cassady, J. R., Tretter, P., et al.: Radiation induced neoplasia following external beam therapy for children with retinoblastoma. Am. J. Roentgenol. Radium Ther. Nucl. Med., 105:529–535, 1969.

117. Schajowicz, F., Defilippi-Novoa, C. A., and Firpo, C. A.: Chondrosarcoma of the axilla induced by Thorotrast. Bol. Soc. Argentina Ortop. Traumatol., 30:199–210, 1965.

118. Schajowicz, F., Defilippi-Novoa, C. A., and Firpo, C. A.: Thorotrast induced chondrosarcoma of the axilla. Am. J. Roentgenol. Radium Ther. Nucl. Med., 100:931–937, 1967.

119. Schmitt, G., and Littmann, K.: Contribution to the discussion about the induction of tumors by ionizing radiation. Strahlentherapie, 153:538–542, 1977.

120. Schürch, O., and Uehlinger, E.: Experimentelles Ewing-Sarkom nach Mesothoriumbestrahlung beim Kaninchen. Z. Krebsforsch., 45:240–251, 1937.

121. Schwartz, E. E., and Rothstein, J. D.: Fibrosarcoma following radiation therapy. J.A.M.A., 203:296–298, 1968.

122. Sears, W. P., Tefft, M., and Cohen, J.: Post-irradiation mesenchymal chondrosarcoma. A case report. Pediatrics, 40:254–258, 1967.

123. Senyszyn, J. J., Johnston, A. D., Jacox, H. W., et al.: Radiation-induced sarcoma after treatment of breast cancer. Cancer, 26:394–403, 1970.

124. Seydel, H. G.: The risk of tumor induction in man following medical irradiation for malignant neoplasm. Cancer, 35:1641–1645, 1975.

125. Sim, F. H., Cupps, R. E., Dahlin, D. C., et al.: Postradiation sarcoma of bone. J. Bone Joint Surg. [Am.], 54:1479–1489, 1972.

126. Skolnik, E. M., Fornatto, E. J., and Heydemann, J.: Osteogenic sarcoma of the skull following irradiation. Ann. Otol. Rhinol. Laryngol., 65:915–936, 1956.

127. Skoryna, S. C., and Kahn, D. S.: The late effects of radioactive strontium on bone. Cancer, 12:306–322, 1959.

128. Smith, J., O'Connell, R. S., Huvos, A. G., et al.: Radiation-induced sarcoma in normal bone. Submitted for publication.

129. Soloway, H. B.: Radiation-induced neoplasms following curative therapy for retinoblastoma. Cancer, 19:1984–1988, 1966.

130. Sparagana, M., Eells, R. W., Stefani, S., et al.: Osteogenic sarcoma of the skull: a rare sequela of pituitary irradiation. Cancer, 29:1376–1379, 1972.

131. Spiers, F. W.: Radionuclides and bone — from ^{226}Ra to ^{90}Sr. Br. J. Radiol., 47:833–844, 1974.

132. Spiess, H., and Mays, C. W.: Some cancers induced by ^{224}Ra(Th X) in children and adults. Health Phys., 19:713–729, 1970; addendum, 20:543–545, 1971.

133. Spiess, H., Poppe, H., and Schoen, H.: Strahleninduzierte Knochentumoren nach Thorium-X-Behandlung. Monatsschr. Kinderheilkd., 110:198–201, 1962.

134. Spitz, S., and Higinbotham, N. L.: Osteogenic sarcoma following prophylactic roentgen-ray therapy. Report of a case. Cancer, 4:1107–1112, 1951.

135. Stargardter, F. L., and Cooperman, L. R.: Giant-cell tumour of sacrum with multiple pulmonary metastases and long-term survival. Br. J. Radiol., 44:976–979, 1971.

136. Steiner, G. C.: Postradiation sarcoma of bone. Cancer, 18:603–612, 1965.

137. Tanner, H. C., Jr., Dahlin, D. C., and Childs, D. S., Jr.: Sarcoma complicating fibrous dysplasia. Probable role of radiation therapy. Oral Surg., 14:837–846, 1961.

138. Tebbet, R. D., and Vickery, R. D.: Osteogenic sarcoma following irradiation for retinoblastoma. With report of a case. Am. J. Ophthalmol., 35:811–818, 1952.

139. Tefft, M., Lattin, P. B., Jereb, B., et al.: Acute and late effects on normal tissues following combined chemo- and radiotherapy for childhood rhabdomyosarcoma and Ewing's sarcoma. Cancer, 37:1201–1213, 1976.

140. Tefft, M., Vawter, G. F., and Mitus, A.: Second primary neoplasms in children. Am. J. Roentgenol. Radium Ther. Nucl. Med., 103:800–822, 1968.

141. Tewfik, H., Tewfik, F., Latourette, H., et al.: Radiotherapy-induced rib osteosarcoma after successful treatment of lung cancer. Radiology, 125:503–504, 1977.

142. Thurman, G. B., Mays, C. W., Taylor, G. N., et al.: Skeletal location of radiation-induced and naturally occurring osteosarcomas in man and dog. Cancer Res., 33:1604–1607, 1973.

143. Toyooka, E. T., Pifer, J. W., Crump, S. L., et al.: Neoplasms in children treated with X-rays for thymic enlargement. II. Tumor incidence as a function of radiation dose. J. Natl. Cancer Inst., 31:1357–1377, 1963.

144. Vaughan, J. M.: The effects of skeletal irradiation. Clin. Orthop., 56:283–303, 1968.

145. Vaughan, J. M.: Skeletal tumours induced by internal radiation. In Price, C. H. G., and Ross, F. G. M. (eds.): Bone — Certain Aspects of Neoplasia. Philadelphia, F. A. Davis (Butterworths), 1973, pp. 377–389.

146. Warren, S.: Skeletal and tissue lesions resulting from exposure to radium and fission products. Ann. Clin. Lab. Sci., 5:75–81, 1975.

147. Warren, S., and Chute, R. N.: Radiation-induced osteogenic sarcoma in parabiont rats. Lab. Invest., 12:1041–1045, 1963.

148. Wittig, G., and Wildner, G. P.: Differenzierungspotenzen und Klinik der primären osteogenen Sarkome. Arch. Geschwulstforsch., 30:53–70, 1967.

149. Wolfe, J. J., and Platt, W. R.: Postirradiation osteogenic sarcoma of the nasal bone. Cancer, 2:438–446, 1949.

150. Woodard, H. Q., and Higinbotham, N. L.: Development of osteogenic sarcoma in radium dial painter thirty-seven years after the end of exposure. Am. J. Med., 32:96–102, 1962.

151. Yoneyama, T., and Greenlaw, R. H.: Osteogenic sarcoma following radiotherapy for retinoblastoma. Radiology, 93:1185–1186, 1969.

152. Zimmerman, G.: Chondrosarkom der Skapula nach Ablatio mammae und Roentgenbestrahlung. Kasuistischer Beitrag zur Differentialdiagnose des Stewart-Treves-Syndrom. Munch. Med. Wochenschr., 110:1647–1651, 1968.

153. Zomer-Drozda, J., Buraczewska-Lipinska, H., and Buraczewski, J.: Radiation-induced bone neoplasm in facial cranium. Pol. Przegl. Radiol., 40:392–396, 1977.

Cartilage-forming Tumors — Benign
Chapters 10, 11, and 12

10

SOLITARY AND MULTIPLE OSTEOCHONDROMAS AND ENCHONDROMAS. JUXTACORTICAL CHONDROMA. MAFFUCCI'S DISEASE.

SOLITARY OSTEOCARTILAGINOUS EXOSTOSIS (OSTEOCHONDROMA)

DEFINITION

An osteochondroma (osteocartilaginous exostosis) is a cartilage-capped bony protrusion on the external surface of a bone.

INCIDENCE

This lesion is by far the most common benign tumor of bone, representing approximately 50 per cent of benign bone neoplasms and about 10 to 15 per cent of all primary tumorous skeletal affections. The number of reported cases does not reflect the true incidence of this tumor because uncomplicated, symptomless cases are seldom referred to or seen or treated by physicians. Probably the first person to describe and clearly illustrate exostosis was Sir Astley Cooper, surgeon and anatomist at St. Thomas' and Guy's Hospitals, London, in 1818.[39]

SIGNS AND SYMPTOMS

The osteochondroma is usually symptomless and therefore is only discovered by feeling a painless lump on the involved bone.[33] If pain is present, however, it is not severe and may be caused by mechanical factors like irritation or pressure of surrounding muscles and tendons in the course of normal function. Nerve compression, usually of the popliteal nerve, caused by enlarging osteochondroma may incite symptoms. A false popliteal artery aneurysm has been reported as being induced by direct traumatic fracture of an osteochondroma of the femur[4, 34, 82, 87, 142] or of the proximal tibia.[25] Pseudoaneurysm of the femoral artery caused by an osteochondroma of the femur has also been noted.[180] Pain may also be caused by fracture through the base of the stalk of an exostosis. In general, interference with normal function, limitation of movement, and asymmetry may be noted in the slowly and insidiously growing lesions. An enlarging exostosis of the spinal column may cause an angular kyphosis, or if it is attached to the intervertebral joint, a spondylolisthesis may be encountered.[17] Spinal compression syndrome may also be seen.[19] An odontoid osteochondroma has caused sudden death.[166] These lesions arising in the region of the head and neck may be associated with facial asymmetry and masticatory dysfunction.[108]

AGE AND SEX DISTRIBUTION

Osteochondromas are usually discovered in youth, during adolescence or childhood, and occasionally even in infancy or in a newborn,[174] when the individual and the lesion are still growing. Since many of these tumors never manifest symptoms, they may only be found accidentally at radiologic examination at a much later age. In the total experience of 323 cases at Memorial Hospital, the average age of the patients was 22 years, with female patients being significantly older (averaging 26 years) than male patients (averaging 21 years) (Fig. 10–1). The ages ranged from 5 to 84 years in female patients as compared to a range of 1 to 62 years in male patients. The great majority of the patients of both sexes were in the second decade of life (Fig. 10–1).

Lichtenstein[120] reports no significant difference between sexes, although Jaffe,[94]

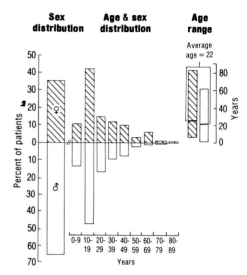

Figure 10–1. Age and sex distribution of 323 patients (211 male and 112 female) at Memorial Hospital with solitary osteochondromas.

Dahlin,[44a] and the Netherlands Committee on Bone Tumours[146] record the number of male patients to be almost twice that of female patients. A similar male to female ratio of 2:1 was demonstrated in patients studied at Memorial Hospital (Fig. 10–1).

LOCATION AND PATHOGENESIS

This tumor only occurs in bones that have developed from cartilage (cartilage preformed bone), most often in the long tubular bones (Fig. 10–2). The lesion starts to grow adjacent to the cortex at or near the epiphyseal cartilage plate, which is the zone of endochondral growth. The exostosis eventually rotates and moves shaftward away from the epiphyseal growth zone. At the lesional site of origin, the cortex is impaired and the osseous portion of the osteochondroma merges imperceptibly with the underlying spongy bone. Lichtenstein and others feel that the basic fault in this condition lies in an anomalous periosteal development that produces displaced nests of cartilage.[120] Continued stimulation of these cartilaginous foci, accompanied by endochondral bone growth, may give rise

SOLITARY OSTEOCHONDROMA
Skeletal Distribution of 323 Cases

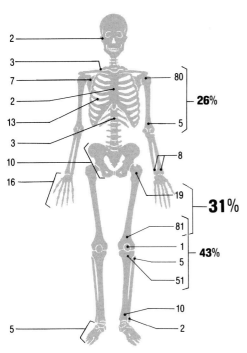

Figure 10–2. Skeletal distribution of 323 lesions of solitary osteochondroma at Memorial Hospital.

to osteocartilaginous exostosis. In fact, experimental implantation of epiphyseal cartilage of young rabbits into the juxtaepiphyseal region of the metaphysis yielded lesions very similar to osteochondromas.[47] Cartilaginous exostosis has been produced by irradiation.[145]

Osteochondroma is considered by many a perversion in the direction of bone growth, not a true neoplasm but rather an enchondromatous hyperplasia, since the lesion is formed by endochondral ossification and the bone substance produced is in every way normal.[2] A congenital anomaly of the diaphyseal blood vessels is postulated as being responsible for the development of osteochondromas.[106]

The most common sites of occurrence are the distal metaphysis of the femur and the proximal metaphysis of the tibia, representing jointly about half of the cases encountered (43 per cent in the experience of Memorial Hospital) (Fig. 10–2). Other sites of predilection include the humerus (proximal end), radius (distal end),

tibia (distal end), and fibula (both ends). Rarely involved are the metatarsal and the metacarpal bones,[67] the scapula,[11, 157, 207] the ribs, and the innominate bone. The incidence is even rarer in the mandibular condyle (condylar process)[31, 54, 103, 132, 202] and the coronoid process[134, 137, 147] or in the spine (the base of the skull included).[17, 99]

In the spine, the lesions are located close to the secondary centers of ossification, near the tip of the spinous process, the vertebral arch, the peduncle, or the costovertebral joint.[91] In the mandibular condyle, the growths arise consistently from the anteromedial surface of the condylar process at the site of attachment of the lateral pterygoid muscle. At the coronoid process, they involve most frequently the medial surface at the site of insertion of the temporal muscle.[162] Osteochondromas may originate anywhere on the surface of the scapula, but the vertebral border of its costal surface is the preferred site. Osteochondromas and chondromas arising in the base of the skull are very rare tumors. They emerge along the basilar synchondroses, where the sphenopetrosal, the petro-occipital and the spheno-occipital synchondroses join in a starlike fashion.[109] They may extend intracranially.[1, 61]

A distinct type of cartilage capped exostosis arises from the distal portion of the terminal phalanx of the toes, from the region of the tuft, expecially from the great toe, and is commonly referred to as a *subungual exostosis* (Fig. 10–3). Very rarely, it may involve the thumb and the fingers. This lesion develops from the tip of the terminal phalanx, and not in a juxtaepiphyseal area like other osteochondromas. Its cap is fibrocartilaginous, in contrast to the hyaline cartilage cap of the usual osteochondroma.[56] They are about twice as common in women as in men. *Ivory exostosis* (osteoma) of the craniofacial bones develops in membrane preformed bones, in contrast to osteochondromas, which arise in bones developing from cartilage (see Chapter 1). The term "epiexostotic chondroma" is employed in the German literature for wide-based metaphyseal osteochondromas of the pelvis and also to describe osteochondromas that have undergone sarcomatous transformation (Fig. 10–4).[14, 50, 131, 203]

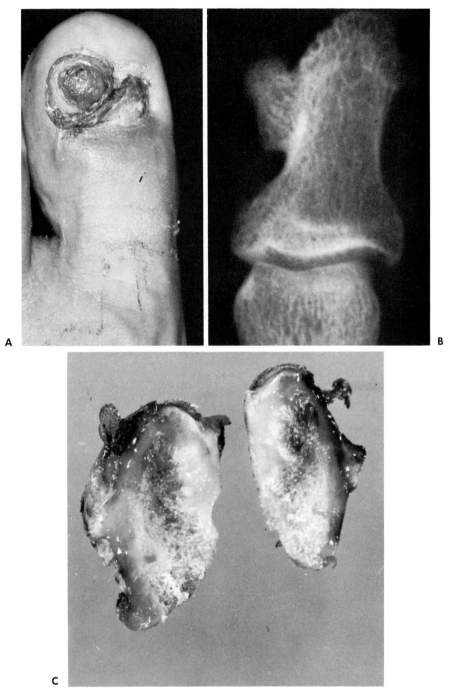

Figure 10–3.   *A*, Typical subungual exostosis of the great toe. *B*, Radiograph shows an outgrowth of trabeculated bone with a cartilage cap. *C*, Specimen reveals the fibrocartilaginous character of the lesion.

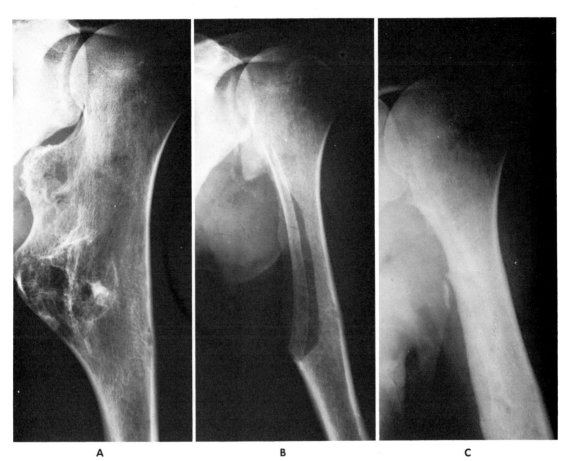

A   B   C

Figure 10–4.   A, Wide-based, sessile, camel hump-like osteochondroma on the medial side of the humerus in a 45-year-old man. B, Extent of resection with bone graft. C, Almost complete healing one year after surgery.

RADIOGRAPHIC APPEARANCE

The roentgen picture is, in most instances, so distinctive that, in general, it does not require histologic confirmation, as it can hardly be diagnosed as any other lesion. Osteochondromas appear as a bony excrescence jutting from the skeleton, merging with the adjacent normal cortex at the peripheral basal portion, and growing away from adjacent joints. Interference with molding of the parent bone frequently causes "flaring" of the cortex at the site of lesional attachment.[135] They may show a flat, sessile, plateau-like protuberance or display a more or less pronounced stalk or tubular projection ending in a hook ("Kleiderhaken") or in spikes (Fig. 10–5). The outlines can vary from even and smooth to irregular but are almost always well-demarcated. In cases in which the cartilaginous cap predominates the lesion, marked calcification and ossification obscure the presence of a stalk (Fig. 10–6). Ossification may appear as linear streaks on radiographs. In the experience of the Netherlands Committee on Bone Tumours,[146] the cortex affected by the hereditary form of this disease may display a bulge at the level of the base of an exostosis. This sign is normally absent in the solitary form of osteochondroma. *Malignant transformation* may be suspected if the demarcation of an osteochondroma is interrupted and a soft tissue mass is present with streaky and blotchy radiopacity. Fluffy amorphous radiopacities, usually considered to be calcifications, however, can also be apparent in benign as well as malignant lesions.[125] Some osteochondromas have been mistaken for enchondromas owing to the radiographic projection of an end-on view of a sessile exostosis.

The most important differential diagnostic considerations concern distinguishing these lesions from malignant bone tumors like peripheral chondrosarcoma, juxtacortical osteogenic sarcoma, as well as myositis ossificans. A large atypical osteochondroma of the sessile type may often be misinterpreted as a juxtacortical osteogenic sarcoma. The latter are usually more densely radiopaque with less distinct outlines and circumferential presentation (see Chapter 6). In cases of radiographic diagnostic uncertainty, a biopsy or excision of the lesion is required. In peripheral (eccentric) chondrosarcomas, small or large, spotty, irregular radiopacities are present, with the borderline between the tumor and the surrounding soft tissue being quite indistinct. The cortex underlying the chondrosarcoma may show radiolucencies caused by the invasive growth of the tumor. In cases of myositis ossificans clearly related to bone, the radiopaque lesions lack normal bone stucture and have no homogenously dense architecture. The demarcation toward the soft tissue is sharp and lobulated. Slight periosteal reaction may be present.

GROSS APPEARANCE

Osteochondromas vary greatly in size, ranging up to more than 10 cm in greatest diameter. The largest, which arose in the scapula, was described by Jones, measured 30 by 40 by 45 cm, and weighed 5250 gm.[100] Another, mentioned by Harsha, weighed 2150 gm.[80] On removing the covering periosteum from a sessile or stalked osteochondroma, one encounters a bulging surface partially or totally topped by a bluish-white hyaline cartilage cap, usually only a few millimeters thick (average 6 mm; range 1 mm–3 cm). The younger the patient, the thicker, the more regular and smooth the overlying cartilaginous layer. Occasionally, this cap is irregular, broken up, and bosselated. Slender elongated lesions exhibit small amounts of cartilage at the tip, the rest of the tubular surface being entirely osseous. If the thickness of the cartilage cap exceeds 1 cm, serious consideration should be given to the likelihood of the lesion becoming, or already being, a chondrosarcoma. The inside bulk of an exostosis consists of spongy bone merging with the underlying normal cancellous bone. On cut section, a yellowish, thin zone of endochondral ossification is noted if the child is still growing. Occasionally, a bursal sac may develop around the base of an exostosis (exostosis bursata).[152, 179] This sac may contain mucinous fluid, fibrin-like rice bodies lying free or attached to the synovium-like lining, and sometimes one or more calcified cartilage bodies.

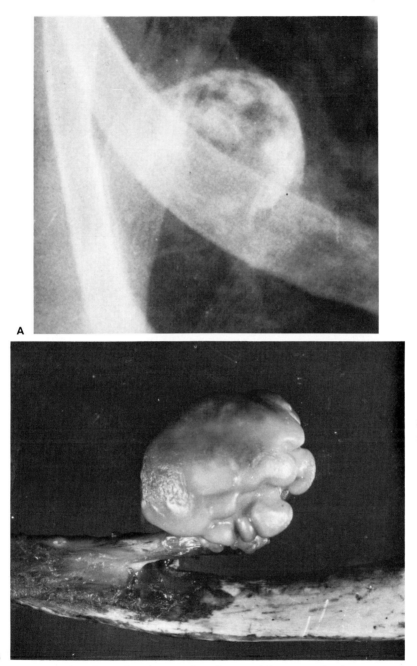

Figure 10–5. A, Typical pedunculated osteochondroma of the seventh rib in a 21-year-old man. B, Thin pedicle with large cartilage cap. (From Marcove, R. C., and Huvos, A. G.: Cartilaginous tumors of the ribs. Cancer, 27:794–801, 1971.)

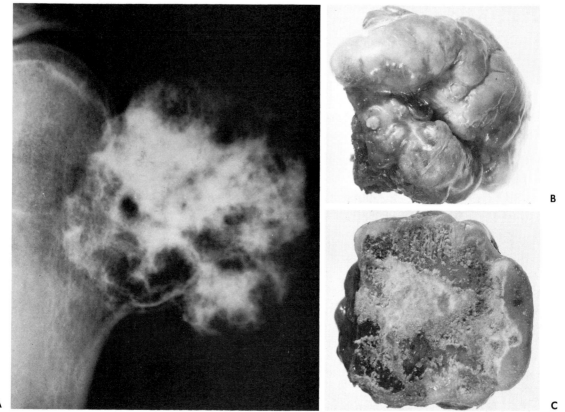

Figure 10–6. *A,* Large sessile osteochondroma of the left upper humerus in a 45-year-old man. *B,* The gross specimen reveals a lobulated ridged surface. *C,* On cut section, central ossification and a peripheral cartilage cap are noted.

MICROSCOPIC APPEARANCE

Examination of the cartilage cap of an osteochondroma in a child reveals endochondral ossification on the basal surface. The hyaline cartilage is cellular, with the chondrocytes arranged in vertical rows (Fig. 10–7). Binucleate chondrocytes may appear in the lacunae. Upon completion of the growth period, the remaining cartilage cap is sealed off by a layer of bone, turns inactive, and may regress almost completely (Fig. 10–8). Residual microscopic foci of cartilage may, however, be identified well into adult life.

Inlays of calcified cartilage and acellular calcific debris may be present deep in the interior of a lesion (Fig. 10–9). They are probably the result of a piled up mass of cartilage matrix caused by a disorderly endochondral ossification process due to inadequate local blood supply within the exostosis.

Chondrosarcoma may arise from either the cartilage cap or its rests. This rare complication, which is estimated to occur in only 1 to 2 per cent, is somewhat more frequent in osteochondromas in the area of the hip joint and usually does not appear before late adulthood. The growth of a chondrosarcoma arising on the basis of an exostosis is quite gradual and slow.[49]

Chondrosarcoma forming in the cap of an osteochondroma often produces a mass that, unless it is quite large, is difficult to appreciate on the roentgenogram. Irregular blotchy calcifications and ossification may be seen. As a rule of thumb, it is important to remember that in cases in which the cartilage cap is irregular and more than a few millimeters thick, it should definitely be suspected of being a chondrosarcoma.[46] Lichtenstein considers the upper limit of the thickness to be 1 cm.[120]

The question of local recurrence following excision of an osteochondroma is not

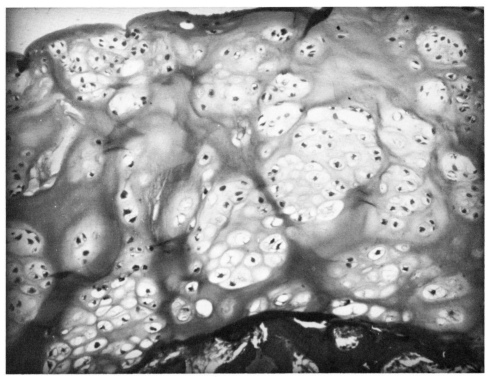

Figure 10–7.   Actively growing cartilaginous cap of an osteochondroma in a child. Note binucleate chondrocytes in the lacunae. (Hematoxylin-eosin stain. Magnification × 180.)

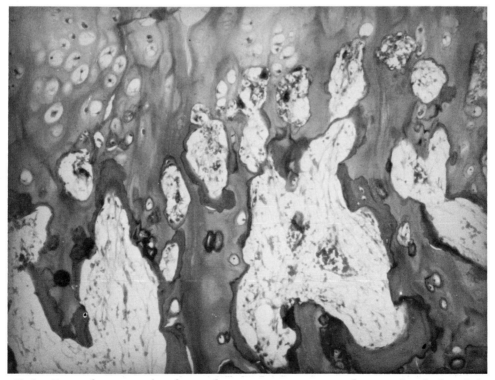

Figure 10–8.   Base of an osteochondroma demonstrating transitional zone of endochondral ossification. (Hematoxylin-eosin stain. Magnification × 180.)

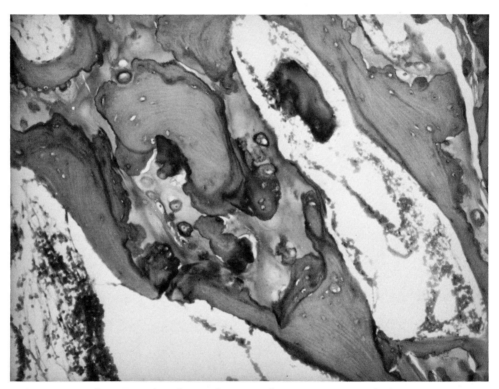

Figure 10–9.   Base of an osteochondroma that ceased growing. Note calcific osseous debris in the interior of the bony trabeculae. (Hematoxylin-eosin stain. Magnification × 180.)

entirely settled in the pertinent literature. Morton, on the basis of two cases, concluded that the reappearance of the tumors following excision represented second independent lesions and were not true recurrences.[139] On the other hand, Schmidt reports two recurrences among 10 cases of sessile solitary osteochondromas.[173]

TREATMENT

The presence or the discovery of a solitary, asymptomatic osteochondroma is not sufficient indication for its mandatory surgical removal. When an exostosis becomes so large as to cause symptoms of pain and disfigurement, it is time to remove it. The gradual enlargement of the lesion tends to slow down as the patient matures, and from then on, no further change in size takes place. Renewed outgrowth of a tumor after cessation of the growth phase should arouse the suspicion that a malignant transformation is taking place, notwithstanding its benign radiographic appearance, i.e., whether or not blotchy calcifications and ossifications are present. At this time, the growing lesion, including periosteum, should be widely excised in order to forestall local recurrence of a more aggressive neoplasm. Fracture, neurologic symptoms like paraplegia,[73] and aneurysm[87, 117, 158, 188] are complications requiring surgical removal. In our experience with benign cartilaginous lesions of the ribs, local resection without radical removal of the underlying pleura and ribs proved to be uniformly curative.[125]

MULTIPLE OSTEOCARTILAGINOUS EXOSTOSIS (HEREDITARY MULTIPLE EXOSTOSIS, DIAPHYSIAL ACLASIS)

INHERITANCE PATTERN

Multiple osteocartilaginous exostosis, originally described in 1814 by Boyer,[20] as observed in both humans and animals, reveals a definite inheritance pattern for a single autosomal dominant gene in which about half the progeny of an affected parent carry the gene and express the trait.[70, 110, 189] Those who do not exhibit the trait do not pass this abnormality on to their offspring. Both sexes are nearly equally susceptible, and the severity of the disease does not increase in successive generations.[182-184] The condition appears to be somewhat less severe in female patients. Chromosome studies failed to reveal persistent numerical or structural irregularities.[70]

PATHOGENESIS

Many divergent theories have been put forward to explain the pathogenetic mechanism in the development of multiple osteocartilaginous exostosis. The first was promulgated by both Virchow[198] and von Recklinghausen,[200] who maintained that both exostoses and enchondromas are derived from the cartilaginous growth plates. Accordingly, small portions of cartilage may become separated from the lateral aspect of the epiphyseal plate and make a right angle turn shaftward, establishing the onset of an exostosis. Müller postulated that exostoses originated in nests of cartilage arising from the disordered osteogenic layer of the periosteum.[143] The concept espoused by Sir Arthur Keith maintains that the most important mechanism in the pathogenesis is related to the defective development of the periosteal ring surrounding the growth plate. According to him, the lack, or the defective deposition, of bone in this area permits the expansion of cartilage preformed bone to grow in anomalous directions precluding normal osseous modeling. This unrestrained growth of bone at the epiphyseal plate "runneth over" onto the outer surface of the bone constituting the exostoses. Keith called this process *diaphysial aclasis,* the term by which the

British literature refers to this condition.[105]

Coley mentions this condition under the term "hereditary deforming dyschondroplasia."[35]

SKELETAL ABNORMALITIES, SYMPTOMS

This condition is first manifested during childhood—the youngest patient in Jaffe's experience was 2 years old—and it is quite likely that the skeleton of an affected newborn child already displays the basic pathologic alterations.[94] In fact, a horse studied by Gardner and associates demonstrated this abnormality at birth.[70] New exostoses do not form in adults. A visible or palpable bump on the surface of a bone draws attention to this condition, and gradually, similar lesions can be seen involving other bones as well. Initially, the patients are completely asymptomatic and have no complaints, but eventually, growth abnormalities like shortness of stature appear, manifested by disparate bony development of the lower and upper extremities. Osseous deformities of the forearms resulting from unequal growth of the radius and ulna with subluxation of the radiohumeral joint may be present in addition to functional disturbances of the joints due to enlarging exostoses.[181] Valgus deformities of the knee and ankle may be produced by tibiofibular growth discrepancy. Spinal cord compression by vertebral exostoses may be seen.[122, 197] Curvature or shortening of the involved phalanges or metacarpals may be demonstrated.

RADIOGRAPHIC AND PATHOLOGIC FEATURES

Both gross and microscopic aspects of this condition are essentially analogous to those seen in the solitary form of disease, although perhaps the lesional changes are more pronounced and the abnormalities more exaggerated. Keith has demonstrated markedly defective molding of bone with resulting broadening and blunting of the metaphyseal regions in the hereditary form of exostosis.

LOCATION

Multiple osteocartilaginous exostoses may occur in either single or multiple bones distributed bilaterally and rather symmetrically (Fig. 10–10A). This disease manifests itself most frequently in the long tubular bones of the appendicular skeleton throughout the skeletal system and appears to be associated with other constitutional syndromes, like the trichorhinophalangeal syndrome.[74] The ribs, the pelvis, and the scapula are the most frequently affected areas, and the vertebral bodies, the patella, and the carpal and tarsal bones are usually unaffected.[182]

AGE AND SEX DISTRIBUTION

In our experience at Memorial Hospital, in 45 cases of hereditary multiple exostosis the average age of the patients was 15 years (Fig. 10–11). In female patients, the ages ranged from 20 months to 48 years, as compared to a range of 7 to 62 years in male patients. The great majority of the patients of both sexes were in the first decade of life (Fig. 10–11). This study reveals the number of male patients to be almost three times that of female patients (Fig. 10–11).

PROGNOSTIC SIGNIFICANCE

Exostoses (osteocartilaginous exostoses, osteochondromas) and enchondromas are entirely separate clinicopathologic entities rather than variants of each other.[85] A contrary view existed for some time, and the eponym "Ollier's disease" was employed to signify both conditions. Some used the designation of Ollier's disease only for those cases of enchondromatosis that demonstrated solely unilateral affliction. Ollier himself, by using the term "dyschondroplasia," created considerable confusion.[151] Enchondroma refers to a cartilaginous lesion that involves the interior of a bone. Jaffe has emphasized that the reason for the confusion in the roentgenographic separation of exostoses and enchondromas may be found in the common practice of viewing the affected bone end-on in a sin-

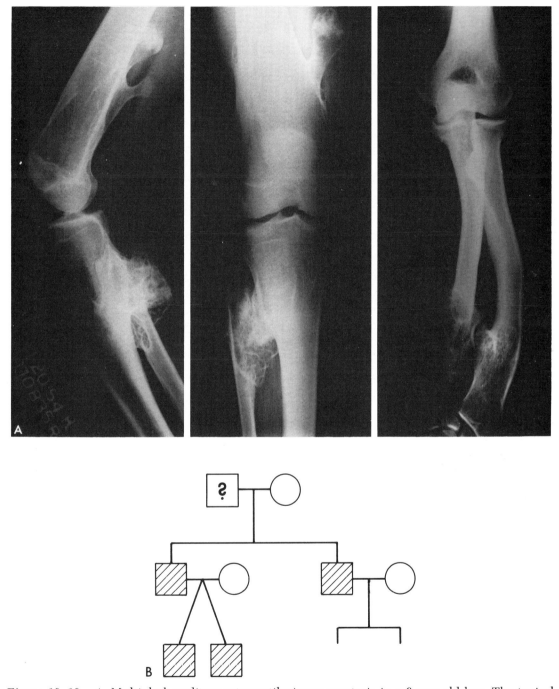

Figure 10–10.   *A,* Multiple hereditary osteocartilaginous exostosis in a 6-year-old boy. The typical lesions involve the right femur, tibia, and fibula as well as the radius and ulna. *B,* Pedigree showing the affected members of this family.

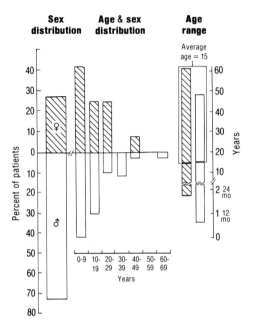

Figure 10–11. Age and sex distribution in 45 patients (33 male and 12 female), at Memorial Hospital with hereditary multiple exostosis (diaphysial aclasis).

gle plane only.[94] In such cases, an exostosis may not be demonstrated to be a projection from the bony surface.

In addition to the hereditary aspects of solitary and multiple exostoses, it is quite important to separate these two conditions on clinical grounds. It is estimated that a secondary chondrosarcoma develops as a complication in about 5 to 25 per cent of the patients with multiple hereditary exostoses.[13, 43, 64, 92, 107, 184, 204] This wide range is due to the patients' age distribution in particular reports, the criteria of diagnosis for chondrosarcoma, and the type of medical center, i.e., whether a primary medical care facility or specialized referral center, from which the incidence is reported.

Most commonly, these secondary chondrosarcomas involve the region of the pelvic or shoulder girdles. These patients are usually mature adults, although malignant transformation of an exostosis may also occur, quite rarely, in teenagers.[13, 49] Pathologic studies of these cases reveal the chondrosarcoma to be arising in the cartilaginous cap or, occasionally, in cartilage rests appearing between the periosteum and the cortex.

TREATMENT

The transformation of hereditary multiple exostosis into chondrosarcoma should be seriously considered if the tumor is large, has an increased degree of calcification in the cartilage cap, or continues to expand progressively following the cessation of the normal growth period or if any other clear clinical radiographic and histologic evidence of malignant change are obtained. Removal of the enlarging lesion, or lesions, is mandatory if it is evolving rapidly, if it is painful, or, in general, if it becomes symptomatic. Occasionally, cosmetic considerations may also play an important role. When the lesions are surgically excised, it is important to include the removal of the adjacent periosteum, not just stripping it back, to forestall recurrence.[92]

Recurrence of the tumor following adequate excision is highly suspicious of an aggressive lesion. The subsequent tumor reappearances show a gradual and progressive change towards malignancy on histologic examination.

SOLITARY ENCHONDROMA

DEFINITION

The solitary enchondroma, also known as central chondroma, is a benign hyaline cartilage growth that develops within the medullary cavity of a single bone.

PATHOGENESIS

Enchondroma probably evolves from heterotopic cartilage rests found frequently in otherwise normal bones. The cartilage cells giving rise to this lesion may be embryonic rests derived from the epiphyseal cartilage plate.[95] In a systematic autopsy study of more than 1000 femoral bones of patients over 25 years of age, 1.7 per cent showed small foci of cartilage rests usually located in the metaphysis.[172] In contrast to an osteocartilaginous exostosis (osteochondroma) that arises by progressive endochondral ossification in a proliferating cartilage cap, an enchondroma is produced by disordered endochondral bone formation that results in the occurrence of a cartilage tumor in the metaphyseal and diaphyseal regions of the shaft.

AGE AND SEX DISTRIBUTION

Both sexes are about equally affected (Fig. 10–12). The tumors arise during the growth period but usually do not manifest clinically until the third or fourth decade of life. Its appearance in preteen children is quite exceptional. The youngest patient seen at Memorial Hospital was 5 years old, the oldest was 79 years old. The average age was 34 years, with the female patients slightly older (36 years) than the male patients (32 years).

SIGNS AND SYMPTOMS

The lesion develops slowly and gradually and is well established before clinical complaints become apparent, resulting in relatively short duration of symptoms. Often, local trauma directs attention to the previously asymptomatic lesion. Pain due to trauma may point to an infraction, but this cause-effect relationship is not always the case, since pain and tenderness may be due to the lesional growth becoming active. Painful lesions without preceding trauma should arouse the suspicion that a malignant transformation is taking place. Due to the scarcity of subjective symptoms, often painless swelling is the first manifestation, giving the phalanx or the metacarpal a fusiform appearance.[124] At times, the discovery of an enchondroma is entirely fortuitous; i.e., roentgenograms performed for completely unrelated reasons will reveal a central asymptomatic chondroma. Lesions appearing at the skull

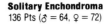

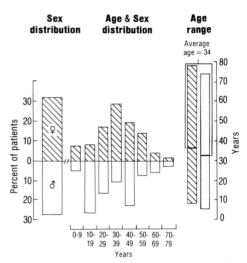

Figure 10–12. Age and sex distribution of 136 patients (64 male and 72 female) at Memorial Hospital with solitary enchondroma.

base or vertebra may cause neurologic symptoms.[61]

LOCATION

The tumors may be situated centrally in a bone (enchondroma) or may lie subperiosteally (periosteal or juxtacortical chondroma). Enchondroma is the most common tumor arising in the hand, and about 35 per cent of all such lesions occur in the small tubular bones of the hands (Fig. 10–13). It is of interest to note that this location is the least significant clinically since it shows only infrequent tendencies to undergo malignant transformation.[44, 135] In the 48 monostotic cases involving the hand in our series, only two were in the thumb (Fig. 10–13). Similar to the findings of Takigawa[191] and Noble and Lamb,[148] the proximal phalanges, the metacarpals, and the middle and distal phalanges, in descending order of frequency, were affected. The femur, humerus, and ribs (about 13 per cent each) are the less commonly affected bones. Those lesions involving the long tubular bones manifest an increased propensity to turn into chondrosarcomas in adult life.[50] This occur-

SOLITARY ENCHONDROMA
Skeletal Distribution in 136 Cases

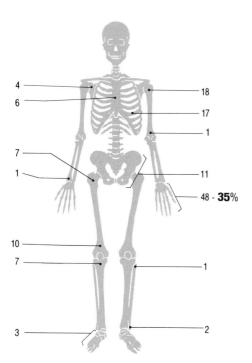

Figure 10–13. Skeletal distribution of 136 lesions of solitary enchondroma at Memorial Hospital.

rence is even more pronounced in lesions arising in the bones of the shoulder and pelvic girdles.[119] Enchondromas in the patella are quite uncommon,[45, 112, 121a] as are lesions at the base of the skull and vertebrae.[61, 171] Several examples of chondromas involving the mandible, the nasal cavity, paranasal sinuses, and nasopharynx have been reported.[9, 31, 59, 68, 161a]

RADIOGRAPHIC APPEARANCE

The lesions present as a well-circumscribed, distinct area of rarefaction that expands and may deform the bone (Fig. 10–14). They may show varying degrees of degeneration and necrosis, producing a degree of calcification from slightly spotty to marked. The intact cortex is expanded, considerably thinned over the lesion, and in rare instances, cortical outlines may be attenuated and not demonstrable. The central location within

the bone permits a considerable size to be reached before clinically appreciable cortical expansion is seen. Slightly eccentric lesions are more prone to thin the overlying cortex sooner, with a greater likelihood of pathologic fracture. While the epiphysis is still open, enchondromas are exclusively located within the shaft; upon completion of the growth period, the fused growth plate may also be involved. The spotty, speckled calcification in a well-circumscribed, expanded, rarefied lesion is the hallmark of enchondromas at any site.

In the carpal bones, the lesions present as radiolucent areas with sclerotic margins that may imitate cystic lesions (Fig. 10–15). Therefore, the radiographic differential diagnosis includes giant cell tumors that may affect the metacarpals and, very infrequently, the phalanges. One must also consider a rare case of skeletal echinococcosis.

Enchondromas involving the long tubular bones of both lower and upper extremities are large; they extensively involve the shaft, with relatively minor cortical swelling owing to the thicker cortical bone. The calcification and ossification within the rarefied lesion result in fine spotty or irregularly blotchy stippling (Fig. 10–16). The lack of calcifications, according to Lichtenstein,[120] makes a definite diagnosis more elusive, especially in long bones, and other possibilities, like monostotic fibrous dysplasia with bulging cortical contours or unicameral bone cyst, should be seriously considered, especially if the proximal humeral shaft is affected. One might also misinterpret an enchondroma as a benign chondroblastoma or even a giant cell tumor.

Radiographs of enchondromas in long bones may occasionally show sharply delimited granular or flocculent deposits of dense calcium without any periosteal reaction. These are referred to as "calcifying enchondromas."[114] These lesions, according to Jaffe, rarely may evolve from the epiphysis rather than from the shaft of a long bone occupying an area between epiphysis and articular cartilage.[94] A heavily calcified enchondroma may have to be differentiated from a bone infarct. In a central cartilage lesion, the radiopacities are small, rounded, and often gathered

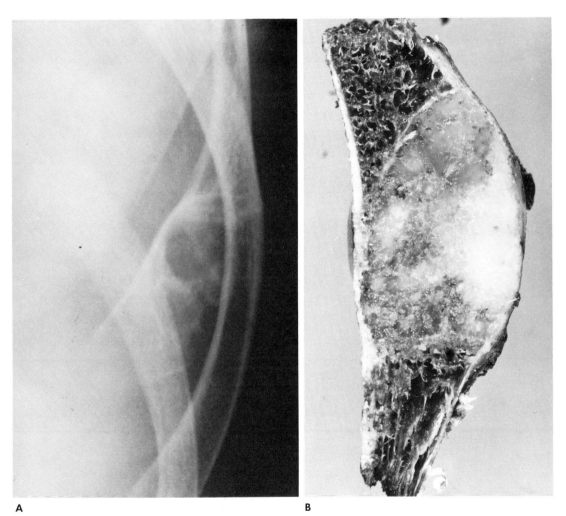

A   B

Figure 10–14.   Enchondroma of the eighth rib in a 13-year-old boy. *A,* Radiograph demonstrates widening with several radiolucent areas in the anterior end of the rib. *B,* Cross section reveals a 2.5 by 2.0 by 1.5 cm lobulated, gray-white, translucent tumor extending from cortex to cortex.

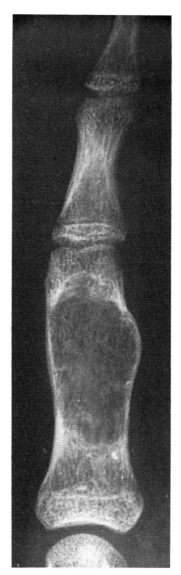

Figure 10–15. Typical location of an enchondroma in a 13-year-old girl. The fifth proximal phalanx shows a radiolucent lesion with a ballooned-out, thin but intact, cortical bone shell.

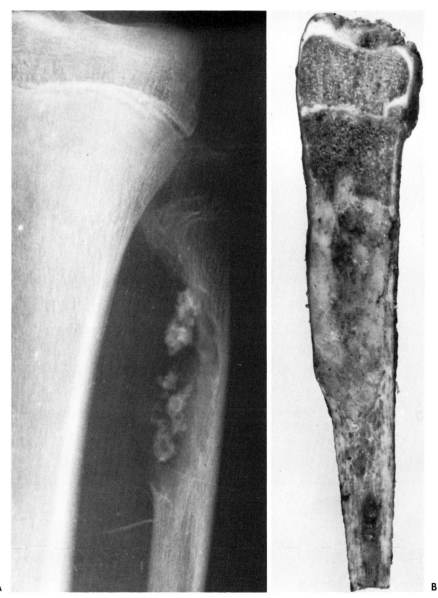

A   B

Figure 10–16.   Enchondroma of proximal fibula in a 14-year-old boy. *A*, Expanding, slightly eccentric, radiolucent lesion with spotty calcifications. *B*, Cross section shows a firm, well-delineated, glassy gray tumor measuring 5.6 by 1.9 cm. The covering periosteum is elevated but intact. Intralesional ossification is noted.

into clusters. The bone infarcts, however, show streaky and curlicued opacities outlining a distinct area of radiolucency.

PATHOLOGIC FEATURES

The separation of an osteochondroma from an enchondroma is largely a gross distinction since bone formation mimicking enchondral osteogenesis is present microscopically to some extent in most central cartilage tumors. *Grossly,* enchondromas show a coarsely lobular or nodular myxomatous structure with a bluish opalescence. The degree of calcification determines the consistency, the grittiness. Portions of the overlying cortical bone removed at curettage may be paper thin if cortical expansion, usually in the small bones of the hands and feet, has taken place, or it may be entirely normal if a cortical bulge, usually in a long tubular bone, has not been demonstrated. Calcification and ossification within the lesional cartilage is more pronounced in adults. These lesions are referred to in the literature as "calcifying enchondromas."[114]

The *histologic diagnosis* of chondromas as being benign or malignant is difficult, especially with those involving the small tubular bones of the extremities. It is quite important not only to study the histologic aspects but also to consider the clinical and radiologic features in order to establish the proper diagnosis.

Microscopic examination reveals the hyaline cartilage lesional tissue to be separated into fields or lobules of differing size divided by cleftlike spaces. These tissue tracts are formed by degeneration of cartilage cells within the lacunae and carry nutrient blood vessels. Calcification and ossification is always in juxtaposition to these blood vessels. The cellularity varies greatly among various enchondromas and also within the same tumor. Limited biopsy specimens thus are of restricted value in assessing the true potential of a tumor. The cartilage cells embedded in the abun-

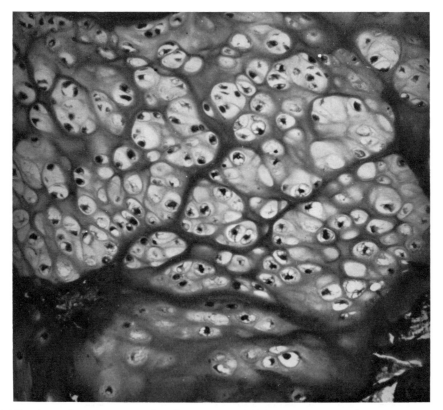

Figure 10–17. Actively growing enchondroma in a child, showing binucleate and slightly atypical chondrocytes as well as increased cellularity. (Hematoxylin-eosin stain. Magnification × 180.)

dant hyaline matrix appear in a lacunar arrangement, usually a solitary cell per lacuna. Since the majority of the lesions develop in individuals who are still growing, the cartilage tumor itself exhibits proliferative activity, represented by increased cellularity with more than one cell, or even a small cluster of cells, within one lacuna (Fig. 10–17). Myxoid degeneration of the lesion may be quite pronounced, giving the impression that one is dealing with a myxoma or a chondromyxoma. In order to properly evaluate the histologic properties of an enchondroma, one should focus on the nuclei of the chondrocytes in areas where the tumor is viable, lacks extensive calcification or ossification, and is removed from sites of infraction. The nucleus of the single chondrocyte, in the vast majority of instances, is uniformly small, rounded, and somewhat pyknotic. The corresponding cytoplasm is vacuolated and vesicular and the cellular borders are indistinct. Mitotic figures are rarely present and do not signify an ominous state.

MALIGNANT TRANSFORMATION

It is certain that, occasionally, malignant cartilage tumors may develop from preexisting solitary enchondromas, especially in long tubular bones, although the majority of chondrosarcomas are clinically malignant from the onset.[44] The transformation of a benign enchondroma to a chondrosarcoma has been traced and well documented histologically.[95] The pathologist's tendency to underdiagnose chondrosarcomas, especially on limited biopsy material, makes evaluation of this contention rather difficult in most cases.[37] The rapid evolution of a chondrosarcoma arising in an enchondroma is quite an exception; this process is most likely to be slow and subtle. The beginning of persistent unrelenting pain or cortical penetration by the tumor without apparent trauma are foreboding signs. Histologic confirmation of malignant transformation is characterized by increased cellularity, more than an occasional binucleate chondrocyte, and appreciable plumpness of the nuclei. Other reliable features include giant cartilage cells with enlarged nuclei and multinucleated forms with coarsely granular nuclei. Roentgenographic features of chondrosarcomatous transformation include poor marginal delimitation within the bone, cortical penetration, focal periosteal reaction, and renewed growth of a previously stable enchondroma.[36, 78] An example of an osteogenic sarcoma developing in a solitary enchondroma of the tibia has been reported.[164]

TREATMENT

Surgical intervention is clearly the preferred treatment.[210] In cases that are still well contained, the procedure is thorough curettage with cryosurgery through the cortex. If the cortex reveals expansion and thinning, then curettage with or without cryosurgery and installation of cancellous bone chips is the treatment of choice.[96, 124] In symptomatic enchondromas involving the phalanges and the metacarpals with extensive loss of bone and cortical involvement or pathologic fractures, an autogenous solid bone graft, usually from the tibia, should be employed, as recommended by Mangini.[124] In uncomplicated cases, bone grafting is not essential, since conservative management of phalangeal lesions with fracture may lead to uneventful healing.[148] The recurrence rate is extremely low after adequate therapy, with uniformly prompt and uncomplicated cure. Irradiation of benign cartilaginous lesions is absolutely contraindicated. Tumors in the long tubular bones and the pelvis usually require primary radical *en bloc* resection with prosthetic bone replacement. Curettage alone will result in local recurrence in a significant number of cases. These recurrences and soft tissue tumor implants may eventually herald a sarcomatous degeneration.

The proper planning of the open biopsy approach in cartilage lesions is quite important for the surgeon, especially in cases in which further major surgical intervention is anticipated. A poorly placed biopsy incision may make the subsequent curative removal of the lesion difficult, since previous operative scars should be excised *en bloc* with the bone tumor. It is noteworthy that cartilage tumors, both benign and malignant, possess a definite propensity to grow in soft tissues at the site of implantation. A limited biopsy specimen obtained by the surgeon often will not provide a definite answer since the zone of malignant transformation in a large chondromatous lesion is often limited.

JUXTACORTICAL (PERIOSTEAL) CHONDROMA

DEFINITION

Juxtacortical chondroma is a benign cartilage growth that forms beneath the periosteum and external to the cortex of bone.

It may erode the underlying bone cortex, producing the effect of saucerization without actually penetrating the medullary cavity. It has also been referred to as "eccentric chondroma" or "periosteal chondroma."

INCIDENCE

This is a rather uncommon tumor with about 50 cases reported in the literature.[38, 66, 75, 93, 116, 121, 127, 133, 149, 165, 170]

LOCATION

The most common location by far is the small bones of the hand and foot, with cases reported to occur in other long bones and ribs[125] (Fig. 10–18). The lesions are not related to the areas of the cartilaginous growth plates but are probably produced by subperiosteal cartilage formation. Rarely, the hyoid bone may also be afflicted.[75]

AGE AND SEX DISTRIBUTION

The lesions occur most often in young adults and measure up to 3 to 4 cm in diameter. There is no apparent sex predilection. In contrast to enchondromas and cartilage-capped exostoses, juxtacortical chondromas sometimes form and continue to grow past skeletal maturity, giving rise to considerable concern about the true nature of the growth. The recognition and awareness of this behavior may help to avoid the mistaken diagnosis of a chondrosarcoma and its subsequent overtreatment.

Clinically, they present as painful, hard, bony protrusions.

RADIOGRAPHIC PRESENTATION

The radiographic presentation is quite typical for this radiolucent lesion. Characteristically, the base of the juxtacortical lesion shows erosion in a saucer-like fashion, with secondary sclerosis of the adjacent cortical bone (Fig. 10–18). There is a localized soft tissue mass with calcification and occasional ossification.

The radiographic differential diagnosis should also consider pigmented villonodular tenosynovitis, nonspecific tenosynovitis, ganglion, glomus tumor, osteochondroma, and finally, chondrosarcoma.

Most importantly, juxtacortical chondroma can be kept apart from a chondrosarcoma in juxtacortical presentation by its relatively limited size, by the presence of a rim of reactive bone deposition beneath the saucer-like cortical erosion, and by the benign histologic picture. The location of the lesion and the age of the patient, in addition, provide useful features to distinguish these tumors.[41]

HISTOLOGIC APPEARANCE

The overall histologic appearance is that of an actively growing lobulated hyaline cartilage lesion with focal peripheral areas of cellular pleomorphism. Foci of calcification and ossification may be present. The cellularity of the lesional tissue and areas of myxoid changes make periosteal chondromas worrisome for the uninitiated. On the whole, these lesions are more cellular than central chondromas, and double nu-

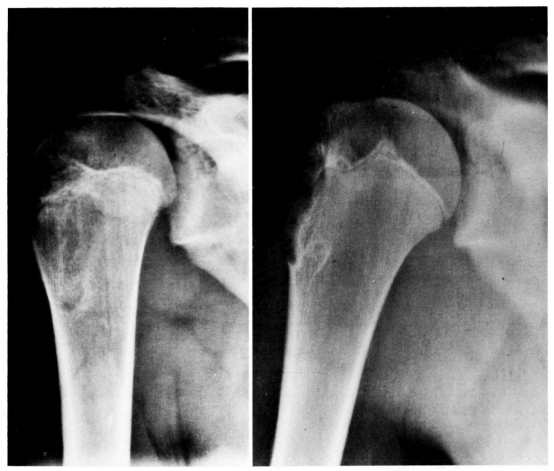

Figure 10–18. Typical juxtacortical chondroma of the humerus in a 15-year-old boy. Radiographs outline a large radiolucent area with concave cortical defect. (Courtesy of Dr. J. M. Lane.)

cleated chondrocytes with cellular pleomorphism are well within the limits seen in juxtacortical chondromas. Familiarity with the clinicopathologic presentation will help to exclude a diagnosis of an eccentric chondrosarcoma.

TREATMENT

The peripheral location and small size permit *en bloc* excision of juxtacortical chondroma with an intact rim of underlying sclerotic cortex.[165] Recurrent lesions are always due to inadequate initial treatment and may require *en bloc* re-excision with bone grafting. These methods of treatment provide a recurrence-free long-term cure and complete healing. Curettage is contraindicated because it raises the likelihood of recurrence and does not provide easily orientable pathologic specimens for microscopic confirmation of the clinical diagnosis.

MULTIPLE ENCHONDROMATOSIS ("OLLIER'S DISEASE")

DEFINITION

Skeletal enchondromatosis (Ollier's disease) is a cartilage dysplasia of bone representing an inborn anomaly of osseous development, a developmental error in endochondral ossification.

PATHOGENESIS

There is no definite evidence for any genetic factor, and nearly all reported cases have been sporadic. A few reports indicated more than one affected sib, suggesting a possible recessive inheritance in rare cases.[209] The epiphyseal cartilage plates are normal and contribute very little, if at all, to the lesional cartilage present in the interior of the affected bone.[185] This cartilage, which according to Jaffe seems to be derived from the cambium layer of the periosteum, penetrates the shaft of the involved long bone and is distributed throughout.[94] These unossified remnants of cartilage in the metaphysis and diaphysis may evolve to form large tumor masses.[81, 126, 129, 140, 175, 194, 201]

HISTORICAL ASPECTS

The eponym "Ollier's disease" originally denoted only the unilateral and monostotic cases, but enchondromatosis is often bilateral, although usually asymmetric, affecting one part of the body more than another. The initial description of this condition was by Ollier, a French physician from Lyon, who beclouded the clear separation of exostoses from enchondromas, with their genetic implication, by coining the term "dyschondroplasia" for reference to both conditions.[150, 151]

The association of Ollier's disease with a functioning ovarian tumor has been reported.[76]

LOCATION

Bones of the hands, especially the phalanges and the metacarpals, are the most common sites of involvement.[60] Among the long tubular bones of the appendicular skeleton, the femur and tibia are most often involved, with the knee region showing the most severe affection (Fig. 10–19). The iliac crest is the most frequently involved flat bone. Vertebral lesions are rare but may result in progressive and debilitating deformity. A base of skull location may cause cranial nerve palsy.[89, 113]

SYMPTOMS

When enchondromas appear close to the epiphysis, they can severely affect the progressive development of a bone. In the hand, for instance, enchondromas may re-

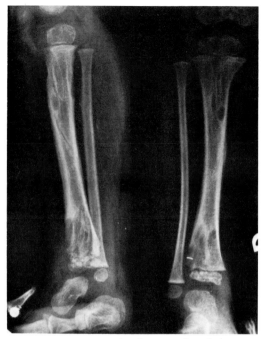

Figure 10–19. Multiple enchondromatosis (Ollier's disease) involving the tibia of a 9-year-old girl. Radiographs show numerous central radiolucent defects associated with deformity of the bone. (Courtesy of Dr. R. C. Marcove.)

radiolucency within the bone to eccentrically placed lesions, which are often difficult to differentiate from exostoses, especially if only an end-on view is available for study. The apparent "exostoses" demonstrated by radiographic examination in Ollier's disease in fact represent an expansion of the overlying cortex by a centrally located enchondroma, confirming the distinction from multiple exostoses (diaphysial aclasis). Sometimes the enchondromas appear to involve the bones more diffusely, displaying bizarre, irregular, central osseous changes (Fig. 10–19). The severity of involvement is variable, from subtle radiographic alterations of a few bones to considerable changes widely involving many bones. In infancy and early childhood, the enchondromas are quite innocuous, presenting as small radiolucent defects. With progressive skeletal growth, the lesions become more evident and characteristic. An interesting analysis of two patients studied by the same authors revealed that the enchondromas observed from birth to adulthood gradually became completely replaced by mature bone.[123]

sult in deviation and failure of proper growth, i.e., distortion in shape and length of the digits, with eventual brachydactyly. The condition is compatible with long life.

MALIGNANT TRANSFORMATION

Chondrosarcoma occurring as a complication of multiple enchondromatosis has been reported on several occasions, although the true incidence is difficult to determine.[42, 129] This event usually occurs in adults and primarily affects the pelvic bones and the shoulder girdle. Jaffe's estimate of about 50 per cent seems to be too high.[94] Osteogenic sarcomas have also been noted in association with enchondromatosis.[21]

RADIOGRAPHIC FINDINGS

The multiple enchondromas may appear to be radiologically similar to the solitary variety. They vary from a single expansile

HISTOLOGIC FEATURES

The microscopic appearance of the lesional cartilage in multiple enchondroma, in general, closely resembles that seen in solitary enchondroma. Some important differences exist, however, and should be mentioned.

The lesional cartilaginous tissue is much more cellular, the nuclei of the chondrocytes are slightly larger, and more binucleate forms are seen than in the corresponding tissue of the solitary form of this disease. The cartilage matrix appears to be less calcified in multiple enchondromatosis. These slight, but definite, microscopic differences may enable the pathologist to suspect that the disease under scrutiny is the multiple form of enchondroma.

DIFFERENTIAL DIAGNOSIS

The diagnosis of enchondromatosis is rarely in doubt, but "metachondromatosis," described in 1971 by Maroteaux, may mimic some of its features. The latter condition may also exhibit enchondromas affecting the small bones of the hands and feet, but an irregularly dominant inheritance pattern and spontaneous regression of the cartilage lesions in metachondromatosis separate the two entities.[128]

Is there any possible relationship between the various metaphyseal dysostoses (metaphyseal chondrodysplasia) and enchondromatosis (Ollier's disease)?[27, 48, 205] Although both skeletal enchondromatosis and metaphyseal dysostosis are well-recognized anomalies of skeletal development, there are a great variety of features that clearly separate the two conditions with respect to site of origin and histologic characteristics of the lesional cartilage present. In metaphyseal dysostosis, the cartilage originates from abnormally altered sites of active endochondral ossification, like the epiphyseal cartilage plate or the costochondral junction. The sites of abnormal enchondral ossification, in fact, become indelibly amalgamated into the lesional cartilage mass present in the affected metaphyseal regions of the distended tubular bones. The epiphyseal cartilage plates in skeletal enchondromatosis, however, contribute very little to the lesional cartilage present within the bone, and the epiphyseal cartilage is normal on radiologic review.

According to Jaffe and Lichtenstein, the cartilage appears to be derived from the cambium layer of the periosteum and may involve the entire diaphysis of the long bone. After the process of skeletal maturation and fusion of the epiphysis with the shaft, cartilage remnants may be seen at the ends of tubular bones. These rests are actually minute extensions of this tissue present in the shaft. The microscopic appearance of the cartilage in enchondromatosis is much more cellular than that in metaphyseal dysostosis.[94, 120]

TREATMENT

Various surgical methods have been employed in the successful treatment of multiple enchondromatosis. Curettage alone, curettage with autogenous or freeze-dried homologous cancellous bone graft, and *en bloc* excision with grafting have all been reported.[18, 71, 96, 140, 191, 192]

REFERENCES

1. Acquaviva, R., Tamic, P. M., Thevenot, C., et al.: Los condromas intracraneales. Revisión de la literatura a propósito de dos casos. Rev. Esp. Otoneurooftalmol. Neurocir., 24:15–34, 1965.
2. Aegerter, E., and Kirkpatrick, J. A., Jr.: Orthopedic Diseases. 4th ed. Philadelphia, W. B. Saunders Co., 1975, p. 498.
3. Allan, J. H., and Scott, J.: Osteochondroma of the mandible.. Oral Surg., 37:556–565, 1974.
4. Anastasi, G. W., Wertheimer, H. M., and Brown, J. R.: Popliteal aneurysm with osteochondroma of the femur. Arch Surg., 87:636–639, 1963.
5. Anderson, R. L., Jr., Popowitz, L., and Li, J. K. H.: An unusual sarcoma arising in a solitary osteochondroma. J. Bone Joint Surg. [Am.], 51:1199–1204, 1969.
6. Angelo, J. J., and Bentzel, G. W. T.: An unusual cartilaginous tumor of the symphysis of the mandible. Plast. Reconstr. Surg., 21:399–404, 1958.
7. Antoni, A. A., Brown, A., and Johnson, J. H.: Osteochondroma of the coronoid process of the mandible: report of case. J. Oral Surg., 16:514–517, 1958.
8. Arlet, J., Pujol, M., Buc, A., et al.: The role of vertebral hyperostosis in cervical myelopathies. Rev. Rhum. Mal. Osteoartic., 43:167–175, 1976.
9. Arwill, T., and Kahnberg, K. E.: Odontogenic keratocyst associated with an intramandibular chondroma. J. Oral Surg., 35:64–67, 1977.
10. Banks, W. C., and Bridges, C. H.: Multiple cartilaginous exostoses in a dog. J. Am. Vet. Med. Assoc., 129:131–135, 1956.
11. Battin, J., Azanza, X., and Héhunstre, J.-P.: Maladie exostosante avec volumineux ostéochondrome de l'omoplate. Arch. Fr. Pediatr., 28:999–1000, 1971.
12. Bell, M. S.: Benign cartilaginous tumours of the spine. A report of one case together with a review of the literature. Br. J. Surg., 58:707–711, 1971.
13. Bennett, G. E., and Berkheimer, G. A.: Malignant degeneration in a case of multiple benign exostoses: with a brief review of the literature. Surgery, 10:781–792, 1941.
14. Bessler, W.: Die malignen Potenzen der Skelettchondrome. Schweiz. Med. Wochenschr., 96:461–466, 1966.
15. Bethge, J. F. J.: Ollier's disease. Pathogenetic problems and therapeutic possibilities. Dtsch. Med. Wochenschr., 87:535–541, 1962.
16. Bethge, J. F. J.: Hereditäre, multiple Exostosen und ihre pathogenetische Deutung. Arch. Orthop. Unfallchir., 54:667–696, 1963.
17. Blaauw, G.: Osteocartilaginous exostosis of the spine. *In* Vinken, P. J., and Bruyn, G. W. (eds.): Handbook of Clinical Neurology. Tumours of the Spine and Spinal Cord. Part I. New York, American Elsevier Publishing Co., Inc., 1975, pp. 313–319.
18. Blauth, W., and Hippe, P.: Enchondromatosis of the hand. Handchirurgie, 5:33–37, 1973.
19. Borne, G., and Payrot, C.: Right lumbo-crural

sciatica due to a vertebral osteochondroma. Neurochirurgie, 22:301–306, 1976.

20. Boyer, A.: Traite des Maladies Chirurgicales. Vol. 3. Paris, Ve. Migneret, 1814, p. 594.

21. Braddock, G. T. F., and Hadlow, V. D.: Osteosarcoma in enchondromatosis (Ollier's disease). Report of a case. J. Bone Joint Surg. [Br.], 48:145–149, 1966.

22. Brailsford, J. F.: An unusual osteochondroma from the coronoid process of the mandible. Br. J. Radiol., 25:555–556, 1952.

23. Brown, I. D., and Shaw, D. G.: Multiple osteochondroses of the feet in a West Indian family. J. Bone Joint Surg. [Br.], 55:864–870, 1973.

24. Burack, P. I.: Ossifying enchondroma of head of humerus. Bull. Hosp. Joint Dis., 1:3–8, 1940.

25. Bussière, J.-L., Missioux, D., Champeyroux, J., et al.: Présentation d'observation d'une exostose agressive. Rev. Rhum. Mal. Osteoartic., 44:183–186, 1977.

26. Callan, J. E., and Wood, V. E.: Spontaneous resolution of an osteochondroma. J. Bone Joint Surg. [Am.], 57:723, 1975.

27. Cameron, J. A. P., Young, W. B., and Sissons, H. A.: Metaphyseal dysostosis; report of a case. J. Bone Joint Surg. [Br.], 36:622–629, 1954.

28. Campanacci, M., Leonessa, C., and Boni, A.: Cartilaginous tumors in the hand bones; report of 112 cases. Chir. Organi Mov., 62:483–490, 1975.

29. Cannon, J. F.: Hereditary multiple exostoses. Am. J. Hum. Genet., 6:419–425, 1954.

30. Cary, G. R.: Juxtacortical chondroma. A case report. J. Bone Joint Surg. [Am.], 47:1405–1407, 1965.

31. Chaudhry, A. P., Robinovitch, M. R., Mitchell, D. F., et al.: Chondrogenic tumors of the jaws. Am. J. Surg., 102:403–411, 1961.

32. Chiurco, A.: Multiple exostoses of bone with fatal spinal cord compression. Neurology, 20:275–278, 1970.

33. Chrisman, O. D., and Goldenberg, R. R.: Untreated solitary osteochondroma. Report of two cases. J. Bone Joint Surg. [Am.], 50:508–512, 1968.

34. Clark, P. M., and Keokarn, T.: Popliteal aneurysm complicating benign osteocartilaginous exostosis. Review of the literature and report of one case. J. Bone Joint Surg. [Am.], 47:1386–1388, 1965.

35. Coley, B. L.: Neoplasms of Bone and Related Conditions. 2nd ed. New York, Paul B. Hoeber, Inc., 1960, p. 110.

36. Coley, B. L., and Higinbotham, N. L.: The significance of cartilage in abnormal locations. Cancer, 2:777–788, 1949.

37. Coley, B. L., and Santoro, A. J.: Benign central cartilaginous tumors of bone. Surgery, 22:411–423, 1947.

38. Cooke, G. M., and Pearce, J. G.: Periosteal chondroma. Report of two cases with atypical radiologic features. J. Can. Assoc. Radiol., 27:301–303, 1976.

39. Cooper, A.: Exostosis. In Cooper, A., and Travers, B. (eds.): Surgical Essays. 3rd ed. London, Cox and Son, 1818, pp. 169–226.

40. Cooper, J. C., and Finch, L. D.: Coronoid osteochondroma presenting as a coronozygomatic ankylosis. A case report. Br. Dent. J., 137:99–102, 1974.

41. Cooper, R. R.: Juxtacortical chondrosarcoma. A case report. J. Bone Joint Surg. [Am.], 47:524–528, 1965.

42. Cowan, W. K.: Malignant change and multiple metastases in Ollier's disease. J. Clin. Pathol., 18:650–653, 1965.

43. Crowell, R. M., and Wepsic, J. G.: Thoracic cord compression due to chondrosarcoma in two cousins with hereditary multiple exostoses. Report of two cases. J. Neurosurg., 36:86–89, 1972.

44. Culver, J. E., Jr., Sweet, D. E., and McCue, F. C.: Chondrosarcoma of the hand arising from a pre-existent benign solitary enchondroma. Case report and pathological description. Clin. Orthop., 113:128–131, 1975.

44a. Dahlin, D. C.: Bone Tumors. 2nd ed. Springfield, Illinois, Charles C Thomas, 1967.

45. Dahlin, D. C.: Osteochondroma of patella. Questions and answers. J.A.M.A., 205:193, 1968.

46. Dahlin, D. C.: Chondrosarcoma and its "variants". In Ackerman, L. V.., Spjut, H. J., and Abell, M. R. (eds.): Bones and Joints. Baltimore, Williams & Wilkins, 1976, pp. 300–311.

47. D'Ambrosia, R., and Ferguson, A. B., Jr.: The formation of osteochondroma by epiphyseal cartilage transplantation. Clin. Orthop., 61:103–115, 1968.

48. de Haas, W. H. D., de Boer, W., and Griffiden, F.: Metaphysial dysostosis: a late follow-up of the first reported case. J. Bone Joint Surg. [Br.], 51:290–299, 1969.

49. Drevon, P., Mourgues, M., and Santamaria, F.: Un cas d'exostose ostéogenique degeneree. J. Radiol. Electrol. Med. Nucl., 31:80–82, 1950.

50. Dreyer, J., Becker, W., and Georgi, P.: Die Problematik des atypisch lokalisierten Chondroms. Arch. Orthop. Unfallchir., 73:25–32, 1972.

51. Ehrenfried, A.: Multiple cartilaginous exostoses, hereditary deforming chondrodysplasia. A brief report on a little known disease. J.A.M.A., 64:1642–1646, 1915.

52. Ehrenfried, A.: Hereditary deforming chondrodysplasia; more cases. Am. J. Orthop., 15:463–478, 1917.

53. Ehrenfried, A.: Hereditary deforming chondrodysplasia; multiple cartilaginous exostoses; a review of the American literature and report of twelve cases. J.A.M.A., 68:502–508, 1917.

54. Eller, D. J., Blakemore, J. R., Stein, M., et al.: Transoral resection of a condylar osteochondroma: report of case. J. Oral Surg., 35:409–413, 1977.

55. Ellis, V. H., and Taylor, J. G.: Diaphyseal aclasis. Report of an unusual case. J. Bone Joint Surg. [Br.], 33:100–105, 1951.

56. Evison, G., and Price, C. II. G.. Subungual exostosis. Br. J. Radiol., 39:451–455, 1966.

57. Faccini, J. M., and Williams, J. L.: Nasal chondroma. J. Laryngol. Otol., 87:811–816, 1973.

58. Fairbank, H. A. T.: Dyschondroplasia. Synonyms: Ollier's disease, multiple enchondroma. J. Bone Joint Surg. [Br.], 30:689–708, 1948.

59. Fairbank, H. A. T.: Diaphyseal aclasis. J. Bone Joint Surg. [Br.], 31:105–113, 1949.

60. Farriaux, J.-P., Renard, V., Samaille, G., et al.:

La dyschondroplasie. Étude d'une observation suivie de l'âge de 18 mois à 7 ans et demi. Presse Méd., 76:1240–1243, 1968.

61. Fassbender, C. W., Häussler, G., and Stössel, H. G.: Schädelbasis-Chondrome mit intrakranieller Ausdehnung. Fortschr. Geb. Roentgenstr. Nuklearmed., 94:718–723, 1961.

62. Fejér, R., and Révay, S.: Exostosis cartilaginea multiplex familiaris. Am. J. Med., 39:296–297, 1965.

63. Fielding, J. W., and Ratzan, S.: Osteochondroma of the cervical spine. J. Bone Joint Surg. [Am.], 55:640–641, 1973.

64. Flatt, A. E.: Chondrosarcoma supervening on diaphysial aclasis. Br. J. Surg., 43:85–87, 1955.

65. Fombeur, J. P., Seguin, D., Desprès, P. H., et al.: Chondroma of the cricoid in a woman of seventy-eight. Ann. Otolaryngol. Chir. Cervicofac., 91:485–490, 1974.

66. Fornasier, V. L., and McGonigal, D.: Periosteal chondroma. Clin. Orthop., 124:233–236, 1977.

67. Freund, E.: Unusual cartilaginous tumor formation of the skeleton. Arch. Surg., 33:1054–1077, 1936.

68. Fu, Y.-S., and Perzin, K. H.: Non-epithelial tumors of the nasal cavity, paranasal sinuses, and nasopharynx: A clinicopathologic study. III. Cartilaginous tumors (chondroma, chondrosarcoma). Cancer, 34:453–463, 1974.

69. Gabrielsen, T. O., and Kingman, A. F., Jr.: Osteocartilaginous tumors of the base of the skull. Am. J. Roentgenol. Radium Ther. Nucl. Med., 91:1016–1023, 1964.

70. Gardner, E. J., Shupe, J. L., Leone, N. C., et al.: Hereditary multiple exostosis. A comparative genetic evaluation in man and horses. J. Hered., 66:318–322, 1975.

71. Giannikas, A. C.: Treatment of metacarpal enchondromata. Report of three cases. J. Bone Joint Surg. [Br.], 48:333–335, 1966.

72. Gilmer, W. S., Jr., Kilgore, W., and Smith, H.: Central cartilage tumors of bone. Clin. Orthop., 26:81–103, 1963.

73. Gokay, H., and Bucy, P. C.: Osteochondroma of the lumbar spine. Report of a case. J. Neurosurg., 12:72–78, 1955.

74. Gorlin, R. J., Cohen, M., and Wolfson, J.: Tricho-rhino-phalangeal syndrome. Am. J. Dis. Child., 118:595–599, 1969.

75. Grayson, A., and Bain, M.: Juxtacortical chondroma of the hyoid bone. Report of a case. Arch. Otolaryngol., 86:679–680, 1967.

76. Grenet, P., Badoual, J., Gallet, J. P., et al.: Dyschondroplasia and ovarian tumour. Ann. Pediatr. (Paris), 19:759–765, 1972.

77. Grislain, J.-R., Mussini, J., de Berranger, P., et al.: Bilateral costal chondroma in the newborn. Ann. Pediatr. (Paris), 15:449–453, 1968.

78. Hamlin, J. A., Adler, L., and Greenbaum, E. I.: Central enchondroma — a precursor to chondrosarcoma? J. Can. Assoc. Radiol., 22:206–209, 1971.

79. Han, S. K., Henein, M. H. G., Novin, N., et al.: An unusual arterial complication seen with a solitary osteochondroma. Am. Surg., 43:471–472, 1977.

80. Harsha, W. N.: The natural history of osteocartilaginous exostoses (osteochondroma). Am. Surg., 20:65–72, 1954.

81. Heckman, J. A.: Ollier's disease. Arch. Surg., 63:861–865, 1951.

82. Hershey, S. L., and Lansden, F. T.: Osteochondromas as a cause of false popliteal aneurysms. Review of the literature and report of two cases. J. Bone Joint Surg. [Am.], 54:1765–1768, 1972.

83. Hirvonen, J., and Heikinheimo, H.: A case of intracerebral chondroma. A case report. Acta Pathol. Microbiol. Scand., 76:19–24, 1969.

84. Hochheim, W.: Malignant evolution of osteochondromatosis type Ollier. Acta Chir. Orthop. Traumatol. Cech., 33:161–163, 1966.

85. Hodges, P. C., and Moseley, R. D., Jr.: Solitary and multiple osteocartilaginous exostoses and enchondromatoses. Postgrad. Med., 26:A-77–A-83, 1959.

86. Hopkins, S. M., and Freitas, E. L.: Bilateral osteochondroma of the ribs in an infant: an unusual cause of cyanosis. J. Thorac. Cardiovasc. Surg., 49:247–249, 1965.

87. Hudson, O. C.: Traumatic aneurysm of the popliteal artery due to osteochondroma. Am. J. Surg., 90:528–530, 1955.

88. Hunter, D., and Wiles, P.: Dyschondroplasia (Ollier's disease), with report of a case. Br. J. Surg., 22:507–519, 1935.

89. Imagawa, K., Toda, I., Hayashi, M., et al.: A case of enchondroma of the skull base: a manifestation of generalized chondromatosis. Neurol. Surg., 5:457–463, 1977.

90. Immenkamp, A.: Die Malignitätsbewertung des Kieferchondroms und des zentralen Kieferfibroms. Fortschr. Kiefer Gesichtschir., 14:70–77, 1970.

91. Inglis, A. E., Rubin, R. M., Lewis, R. J., et al.: Osteochondroma of the cervical spine. Case report. Clin. Orthop., 126:127–129, 1977.

92. Jaffe, H. L.: Hereditary multiple exostosis. Arch. Pathol., 36:335–357, 1943.

93. Jaffe, H. L.: Juxtacortical chondroma. Bull. Hosp. Joint Dis., 17:20–29, 1956.

94. Jaffe, H. L.: Tumors and Tumorous Conditions of the Bones and Joints. Philadelphia, Lea & Febiger, 1958.

95. Jaffe, H. L., and Lichtenstein, L.: Solitary benign enchondroma of bone. Arch. Surg., 46:480–493, 1943.

96. Jewusiak, E. M., Spence, K. F., and Sell, K. W.: Solitary benign enchondroma of the long bones of the hand. Results of curettage and packing with freeze-dried cancellous bone allograft. J. Bone Joint Surg. [Am.], 53:1587–1590, 1971.

97. Johanson, P. H.: Tumors of the patella. Letter to the editor. J.A.M.A., 206:650, 1968.

98. Jokinen, K., Stenbäck, F., Palva, A., et al.: Benign cartilagenous tumour of the temporomandibular joint. J. Laryngol. Otol., 90:299–303, 1976.

99. Jones, H. M.: Cartilaginous tumours of the head and neck. J. Laryngol. Otol., 87:135–151, 1973.

100. Jones, S.: Excision of the scapula for enchondroma. Lancet, 2:665–667, 1868.

101. Katz, J. F.: Osteochondroma of the neck of the femur in Legg-Calvé-Perthes disease. Report of 2 cases. Clin. Orthop., 68:50–54, 1970.

102. Katzman, H., Waugh, T., and Berdon, W.: Skele-

tal changes following irradiation of childhood tumors. J. Bone Joint Surg. [Am.], *51*:825–842, 1969.

103. Keen, R. R., and Callahan, G. R.: Osteochondroma of the mandibular condyle: report of case. J. Oral Surg., 35:140–143, 1977.

104. Keiller, V. H.: Cartilaginous tumors of bone. Surg. Gynecol. Obstet., 40:510–521, 1925.

105. Keith, A.: Studies on the anatomical changes which accompany certain growth disorders of the human body. I. The nature of the structural alterations in the disorder known as multiple exostoses. J. Anat., 54:101–115, 1919–1920.

106. Klümper, A.: Intraosseous angiography in the investigation of the pathogenesis of osteochondromas. Fortschr. Geb. Roentgenstr. Nuklearmed., *127*:142–145, 1977.

107. Knight, J. D. S.: Sarcomatous change in three brothers with diaphysial aclasis. Br. Med. J., *1*:1013–1015, 1960.

108. Koehl, G. L., and Tilson, H. B.: Osteochondromas associated with facial asymmetry and masticatory dysfunction: report of two cases. J. Oral Surg., 35:934–939, 1977.

109. Krayenbühl, H., and Yaşargil, M. G.: Chondromas. Prog. Neurol. Surg., 6:435–463, 1975.

110. Krooth, R. S., Macklin, M. T., and Hilbish, T. F.: Diaphyseal aclasis (multiple exostoses) on Guam. Am. J. Hum. Genet., *13*:340–347, 1961.

111. Labayle, J., Auriat, J., and Dumaine, A.: Infantile chondroma of the cricoid. Description of a case. Ann. Otolaryngol., *91*:51–53, 1974.

112. Lammot, T. R.: Enchondroma of the patella. A case report. J. Bone Joint Surg. [Am.], *14*:1230–1232, 1968.

113. Lapresle, J., Doyon, D., Derome, P., et al.: Maladie d'Ollier avec atteinte multiple des nerfs crâniens par un chondrome de la base du crâne. Nouv. Presse. Med., 5:419–421, 1976.

114. Laurence, W., and Franklin, E. L.: Calcifying enchondroma of long bones. J. Bone Joint Surg. [Br.], 35:224–228, 1953.

115. LeConte, R. G., Lee, W. E., and Belk, W. P.: Enchondroma of the femur with repeated recurrences and ultimate death; report of case. Arch. Surg., *11*:93–99, 1925.

116. Lénárt, G., and Szepesi, K.: An unusual cartilaginous tumour of the finger. Arch. Orthop. Unfallchir., 73:7–10, 1972.

117. Lesser, A. J., and Greeley, C. E.: Femoropopliteal arteriovenous aneurysm caused by fractured osteochondroma of the femur. J.A.M.A., *167*:1830–1833, 1958.

118. Levine, M. H., Chessen, J., and McCarthy, W. D.: Osteochondroma of the coronoid process of the mandible. Report of a case and review of the literature. N. Engl. J. Med., 257:374–376, 1957.

119. Levy, W. M., Aegerter, E. E., and Kirkpatrick, J. A., Jr.: The nature of cartilaginous tumors. Radiol. Clin. North Am., 2:327–336, 1964.

120. Lichtenstein, L.: Bone Tumors. 4th ed. St. Louis, C. V. Mosby Co., 1972.

121. Lichtenstein, L., and Hall, J. E.: Periosteal chondroma. A distinctive benign cartilage tumor. J. Bone Joint Surg. [Am.], *34*:691–697, 1952.

121a. Linscheid, R. L., and Dahlin, D. C.: Unusual lesions of the patella. J. Bone Joint Surg. [Am.], *48*:1359–1366, 1966.

122. Madigan, R., Worral, T., and McClain, E. J.: Cervical cord compression in hereditary multiple exostosis. Review of the literature and report of a case. J. Bone Joint Surg. [Am.], 56:401–404, 1974.

123. Mainzer, F., Minagi, H., and Steinbach, H. L.: The variable manifestations of multiple enchondromatosis. Radiology, 99:377–388, 1971.

124. Mangini, U.: Tumors of the skeleton of the hand. Bull. Hosp. Joint Dis., 28:61–103, 1967.

125. Marcove, R. C., and Huvos, A. G.: Cartilaginous tumors of the ribs. Cancer, 27:794–801, 1971.

126. Marmor, L.: Chondrodysplasia. Case report of Ollier's disease. Am. J. Surg., *108*:733–734, 1964.

127. Marmor, L.: Periosteal chondroma (juxtacortical chondroma). Clin. Orthop., 37:150–153, 1964.

128. Maroteaux, P.: Metachondromatosis. Z. Kinderheilkd., *109*:246–261, 1971.

129. Maroteaux, P., and Lamy, M.: La dyschondroplasie. Chondromatose multiple du squelette. Sem. Hop. Paris, 36:50–61, 1960.

130. McFarland, G. B., Jr., and Morden, M. L.: Benign cartilaginous lesions. Orthop. Clin. North Am., 8:737–749, 1977.

131. Meffert, O., and Peiper, H. J.: Die Knorpelgeschwülste des Skeletts. Chirurg., *47*:392–399, 1976.

132. Melarkey, D. W., Roffinella, J. P., and Kaplan, H.: Osteocartilaginous exostosis (osteochondroma) of the mandibular condyle: report of case. J. Oral Surg., 24:271–275, 1966.

133. Meyer, R.: Juxtacortical chondroma. Br. J. Radiol., *31*:106–107, 1958.

134. Meyer, R. A.: Osteochondroma of coronoid process of mandible: report of a case. J. Oral Surg., 30:297–300, 1972.

135. Middlemiss, J. H.: Cartilage tumours. Br. J. Radiol., 37:277–286, 1964.

136. Minagi, H., and Newton, T. H.: Cartilaginous tumors of the base of skull. Am. J. Roentgenol. Radium Ther. Nucl. Med., *105*:308–313, 1969.

137. Mohnac, A. M.: Bilateral coronoid osteochondromas. J. Oral Surg., 20:500–506, 1962.

138. Monat, Y., and Meary, R.: Chondromes — chondroblastomes — fibromes chondro-myxoides. Rev. Prat., *19*:2177–2184, 1969.

139. Morton, K. S.: On the question of recurrence of osteochondroma. J. Bone Joint Surg. [Br.], *46*:723–725, 1964.

140. Mosher, J. F.: Multiple enchondromatosis of the hand. A case report. J. Bone Joint Surg. [Am.], *58*:717–719, 1976.

141. Moulonguet, P., and Cazala, J. Fr.: Chondromes évolutifs sur exostoses ostéogéniques. Presse Méd., 67:1055 1057, 1959.

142. Mukerjea, S. K.: Traumatic aneurysm of the popliteal artery due to osteochondroma. Br. J. Surg., 54:810–811, 1967.

143. Müller, E.: Über hereditäre multiple cartilaginäre Exostosen und Ecchondrosen. Beitr. Pathol. Anat., 57:232–281, 1913–1914.

144. Murken, J. D.: Zur Haufigkeit und Genetik der multiplen cartilaginären Exostosen (multiple

Osteochondromatose). Z. Kinderchir., 6:563–566, 1969.

145. Murphy, F. D., Jr., and Blount, W. P.: Cartilaginous exostoses following irradiation. J. Bone Joint Surg. [Am.], 44:662–668, 1962.

146. Netherlands Committee on Bone Tumours: Radiological Atlas of Bone Tumours. Vol. 2. Baltimore, Williams & Wilkins, 1973, pp. 5 and 354.

147. Nickerson, J. W., Jr., Grafft, N. L., and Sazima, H. J.: Bilateral coronoid process enlargement: report of a case. J. Oral Surg., 27:885–890, 1969.

148. Noble, J., and Lamb, D. W.: Enchondromata of bones of the hand. A review of 40 cases. Hand, 6:275–284, 1974.

149. Nosanchuk, J. S., and Kaufer, H.: Recurrent periosteal chondroma. Report of two cases and a review of the literature. J. Bone Joint Surg. [Am.], 51:375–380, 1969.

150. Ollier, M.: Exostoses ostéogéniques multiples. Lyon Méd., 88:484–486, 1898.

151. Ollier, M.: Dyschondroplasie. Lyon Méd., 93:23–25, 1900.

152. Orlow, L. W.: Die Exostosis bursata und ihre Entstehung. Dtsch. Z. Chir., 31:293–308, 1890–1891.

153. Owen, L. N., and Bostock, D. E.: Multiple cartilaginous exostoses with development of a metastasizing osteosarcoma in a Shetland Sheepdog. J. Small Anim. Pract., 12:507–512, 1971.

154. Owen, L. N., and Nielsen, S. W.: Multiple cartilaginous exostoses (diaphyseal aclasis) in a Yorkshire terrier. J. Small Anim. Pract., 9:519–521, 1968.

155. Palme, E.: Intracapsullary osteochondroma in the region of the knee joint. Beitr. Orthop. Traumatol., 24:292–296, 1977.

156. Pandey, S.: Hereditary deforming dyschondroplasia. Two case reports followed through four generations of each family. Int. Surg., 54:264–267, 1970.

157. Parsons, T. A.: The snapping scapula and the subscapular exostoses. J. Bone Joint Surg. [Br.], 55:345–349, 1973.

158. Paul, M.: Aneurysm of the popliteal artery from perforation by a cancellous exostosis of the femur. Report of a case. J. Bone Joint Surg. [Br.], 35:270–271, 1953.

159. Petrova, A. S.: Cytological diagnosis of some types of cartilage tissue tumours. Arkh. Patol., 27:25–31, 1965.

160. Phadke, A. R., Tambaku, S. N., and Phadke, S. A.: Osteochondroma of tongue — a case report. Indian J. Cancer, 11:1382–1385, 1974.

161. Pogrund, H., and Yosipovitch, Z.: Osteochondroma following irradiation. Case report and review of the literature. Isr. J. Med. Sci., 12:154–157, 1976.

161a. Potdar, G. G., and Srikhande, S. S.: Chondrogenic tumors of the jaws. Oral Surg., 30:649–658, 1970.

162. Ramon, Y., Horowitz, I., Oberman, M., et al.: Osteochondroma of the coronoid process of the mandible. Oral Surg., 43:692–697, 1977.

163. Ramon, Y., Lerner, M. A., and Leventon, G.: Osteochondroma of the mandibular condyle. Report of a case. Oral Surg., 17:16–21, 1964.

164. Rockwell, M. A., and Enneking, W. F.: Osteosarcoma developing in solitary enchondroma of the tibia. J. Bone Joint Surg. [Am.], 53:341–344, 1971.

165. Rockwell, M. A., Saiter, E. T., and Enneking, W. F.: Periosteal chondroma. J. Bone Joint Surg. [Am.], 54:102–108, 1972.

166. Rose, E. F., and Fekete, A.: Odontoid osteochondroma causing sudden death. Report of a case and review of the literature. Am. J. Clin. Pathol., 42:606–609, 1964.

167. Rowe, N. L.: Bilateral developmental hyperplasia of the mandibular coronoid process. A report of two cases. Br. J. Oral Surg., 1:90–104, 1963.

168. Sarmiento, A., and Elkins, R. W.: Giant intra-articular osteochondroma of the knee. J. Bone Joint Surg. [Am.], 57:560–561, 1975.

169. Sarwar, M., Swischuk, L. E., and Schechter, M. M.: Intracranial chondromas. Am. J. Roentgenol. Radium Ther. Nucl. Med., 127:973–977, 1976.

170. Scaglietti, O., and Stringa, G.: Periosteal myxoma of infancy and periosteal chondroma of adolescence, with local malignancy. Clin. Orthop., 9:147–157, 1957.

171. Schacter, I. B., Wortzman, G., and Noyek, A. M.: The clinical and radiological diagnosis of cartilaginous tumors of the base of the skull. Can. J. Otolaryngol., 4:364–377, 1975.

172. Scherer, E.: Exostosen, Enchondrome und ihre Beziehung zum Periost. Frankf. Z. Pathol., 36:587–605, 1928.

173. Schmidt, W.: Exostoses, osteochondroma and osteochondromatosis. Clinical findings and therapy. Zentralbl. Chir., 94:1515–1524, 1969.

174. Seibert, J. J., Rossi, N. P., and McCarthy, E. F.: A primary rib tumor in a newborn. J. Pediatr. Surg., 11:1031–1032, 1976.

175. Seror, J., Rives, J., and Alexandre, J.: La maladie d'Ollier. Afr. Fr. Chir., 16:299–304, 1958.

176. Shackelford, R. T., and Brown, W. H.: Osteochondroma of the coronoid process of the mandible. Surg. Gynecol. Obstet., 77:51–54, 1943.

177. Shackelford, R. T., and Brown, W. H.: Restricted jaw motion due to osteochondroma of the coronoid process. J. Bone Joint Surg. [Am.], 31:107–114, 1949.

178. Shellito, J. G., and Dockerty, M. B.: Cartilaginous tumors of the hand. Surg. Gynecol. Obstet., 86:465–472, 1948.

179. Smithuis, Th.: Exostosis bursata. Report of a case. J. Bone Joint Surg. [Br.], 46:544–545, 1964.

180. Solhaugh, J. H., and Olerud, S. E.: Pseudoaneurysm of the femoral artery caused by osteochondroma of the femur. A case report. J. Bone Joint Surg. [Am.], 57:867–868, 1975.

181. Solomon, L.: Bone growth in diaphysial aclasis. J. Bone Joint Surg. [Br.], 43:700–716, 1961.

182. Solomon, L.: Hereditary multiple exostosis. J. Bone Joint Surg. [Br.], 45:292–304, 1963.

183. Solomon, L.: Hereditary multiple exostosis. Am. J. Hum. Genet., 16:351–363, 1964.

184. Solomon, L.: Chondrosarcoma in hereditary multiple exostosis. S. Afr. Med. J., 48:671–676, 1974.

185. Speiser, F.: Ein Fall von systematisierter En-

chondromatose des Skeletts. Virchows Arch. [Pathol. Anat.], 258:126–160, 1925.

186. Stark, J. D., Adler, N. N., and Robinson, W. H.: Hereditary multiple exostoses. Radiology, 59:212–215, 1952.

187. Stephenson, W. H.: Enchondroma of patella. Br. J. Radiol., 26:156–157, 1953.

188. Stevenson, C. A., and Zuska, J. J.: Aneurysm of the popliteal artery from perforation by a solitary exostosis of the femur. A case report. J. Bone Joint Surg. [Am.], 39:431–434, 1957.

189. Stocks, P., and Barrington, A.: Hereditary Disorders of Bone Development. Francis Galton Laboratory for National Eugenics, Memoir 22. Cambridge, Cambridge University Press, 1925.

190. Strong, M. L., Jr.: Chondromas of the tendon sheath of the hand. Report of a case and review of the literature. J. Bone Surg. [Am.], 57:1164–1165, 1975.

191. Takigawa, K.: Chondroma of the bones of the hand. A review of 110 cases. J. Bone Joint Surg. [Am.], 53:1591–1600, 1971.

192. Takigawa, K.: Carpal chondroma. Report of a case. J. Bone Joint Surg. [Am.], 53:1601–1604, 1971.

193. Tomich, C. E., and Hutton, C. E.: Chondroma of the anterior nasal spine. J. Oral Surg., 34:911–915, 1976.

194. Trinchieri, P., and Goria-Fazio, M.: Sulla malattia di Ollier. Minerva Med., 47:1195–1203, 1956.

195. Twersky, J., Kassner, E. G., Tenner, M. S., et al.: Vertebral and costal osteochondromas causing spinal cord compression. Am. J. Roentgenol. Radium Ther. Nucl. Med., 124:124–128, 1975.

196. Villiger, K. J.: "Kleiderhaken"-Exostose. Chirurg., 45:480–482, 1974.

197. Vinstein, A. L., and Franken, E. A., Jr.: Hereditary multiple exostoses. Report of a case with spinal cord compression. Am. J. Roentgenol. Radium Ther. Nucl. Med., 112:405–407, 1971.

198. Virchow, R.: Exostosen und Hyperostosen von Extremitäten-knochen des Menschen, im Hinblick auf den Pithecanthropus. Z. Ethnol., 27:787–793, 1895.

199. Vittali, H. P.: Die Osteochondrome bei Jugendlichen. Arch. Orthop. Unfallchir., 52:270–280, 1960.

200. von Recklinghausen, F.: Ein Fall von multiplen Exostosen. Arch. Pathol. Anat. Phys., 35:203–207, 1866.

201. Vykydal, M.: Maladies des chondromes multiples. Rev. Rhum. Mal. Osteoartic., 30:753–756, 1963.

202. Wang-Norderud, R., and Ragab, R. R.: Osteocartilaginous exostosis of the mandibular condyle. Scand. J. Plast. Reconstr. Surg., 9:165–169, 1975.

203. Weber, H. G.: Semimaligne Knochengeschwülste. Chir. Praxis, 13:433–448, 1969.

204. Weber, O.: Zur Geschichte des Enchondroms namentlich in Bezug auf dessen hereditäres Vorkommen und secundäre Verbreitung in inneren Organen durch Embolie. Arch. Pathol. Anat., 35:501–524, 1866.

205. Wekselman, R.: Familial metaphyseal dysostosis. A case report. J. Bone Joint Surg. [Am.], 59:690–691, 1977.

206. Woods, C. G.: Diagnostic Orthopaedic Pathology. Philadelphia, F. A. Davis Co. (Blackwell), 1972, pp. 109–110.

207. Wouters, H. W., Szepesi, K., and Kullmann, L.: Solitary osteochondroma of the scapula. A report on 6 cases. Arch. Chir. Neerl., 26:63–69, 1974.

208. Würdinger, H., Feuerbacher, H. J., and Schneider, G. F.: Zentrales Osteochondrom der Humerusmetaphyse. Fortschr. Geb. Roentgenstr. Nuklearmed., 124:189–190, 1976.

209. Wynne-Davies, R., and Fairbank, T. J.: Fairbank's Atlas of General Affections of the Skeleton. 2nd ed. New York, Churchill Livingstone, 1976, pp. 126–133.

210. Zifko, B.: Behandlung von Frakturen in Chondromen der Hand. Monatsschr. Kinderheilkd., 69:538–543, 1966.

MAFFUCCI'S DISEASE

The association of soft tissue hemangiomas with enchondromatosis was described by Maffucci in 1881.[15] Similarly to Ollier's disease, there is no genetic factor demonstrable. The reported cases are quite rare, and the disease appears to be less frequent than enchondromatosis. The condition afflicts both sexes alike. About one fourth of the cases are congenital or present soon after birth. Practically all bones may be involved, although the hands and feet are the most commonly affected. The distribution of bony abnormalities and soft tissue hemangiomas does not always correspondingly involve the same region of the body.

The tendency toward malignant transformation of enchondroma is greater in Maffucci's disease than it is in Ollier's disease without hemangiomas. The incidence of malignant change in Maffucci's disease is described as 18.6 per cent by Elmore and Cantrell[9] and 15.2 per cent by Lewis and Ketcham.[13]

The radiographic features are identical with the lesions seen in Ollier's disease. In some cases, numerous phleboliths can be seen in the accompanying hemangiomas. On arteriographic study, multiple arteriovenous malformations may be noted.[11]

REFERENCES

1. Aimes, A., and Franchebois, P.: Ostéochondrodysplasies et lésions associées. A propos d'un cas de syndrome de Mafucci. Sem. Hop. Paris, *31*:363–369, 1955.
2. Albores Saavedra, J., Altamirano Dimas, M., Peniche, J., et al.: Sindrome de Maffucci. Rev. Med. Hosp. Gen. (Méx.), *27*:571–578, 1964.
3. Anderson, I. F.: Maffucci's syndrome. Report of a case with a review of the literature. S. Afr. Med. J., *39*:1066–1070, 1965.
4. Andrén, L., Dymling, J. F., Elner, Å., et al.: Maffucci's syndrome. Report of four cases. Acta Chir. Scand., *126*:397–405, 1963.
5. Banna, M., and Parwani, G. S.: Multiple sarcomas in Maffucci's syndrome. Br. J. Radiol., *42*:304–307, 1969.
6. Bean, W. B.: Dyschondroplasia and hemangiomata (Maffucci's syndrome). II. Arch. Intern. Med., *102*:544–550, 1958.
7. Carleton, A., Elkington, J. St. C., Greenfield, J. G., et al.: Maffucci's syndrome (dyschondroplasia with haemangeiomata). Q. J. Med., *11*:203–228, 1942.
8. Cook, P. L., and Evans, P. G.: Chondrosarcoma of the skull in Mafucci's syndrome. Br. J. Radiol., *50*:833–836, 1977.
9. Elmore, S. M., and Cantrell, W. C.: Maffucci's syndrome. Case report with a normal karyotype. J. Bone Joint Surg. [Am.], *48*:1607–1613, 1966.
10. Fernández, C. I., Gascó, J., and Esquerdo, J.: Síndrome de Maffucci. Aportación de un caso. Rev. Esp. Cir. Osteoartic., *9*:59–73, 1974.
11. Howard, F. M., and Lee, R. E., Jr.: The hand in Maffucci syndrome. Arch. Surg., *103*:752–756, 1971.
12. Johnson, J. L., Webster, J. R., Jr., and Sippy, H. I.: Maffucci's syndrome (dyschondroplasia with hemangiomas). Am. J. Med., *28*:864–866, 1960.
13. Lewis, R. J., and Ketcham, A. S.: Maffucci's syndrome: functional and neoplastic significance. Case report and review of the literature. J. Bone Joint Surg. [Am.], *55*:1465–1479, 1973.
14. Loewinger, R. J., Lichtenstein, J. R., Dodson, W. E., et al.: Maffucci's syndrome: a mesenchymal dysplasia and multiple tumour syndrome. Br. J. Dermatol., *96*:317–322, 1977.
15. Maffucci, A.: Di un caso di encondroma ed angioma multiplo. Contribuzione alla genesi embrionale dei tumori. Mov. Med. Chir., *13*:399–412, 1881.
16. Regnier, R., Vlaeminck, J., and Balon, J.: Malignant transformation of a case of Maffucci-Kast syndrome. Acta Chir. Belg., *73*:75–84, 1974.
17. Strang, C., and Rannie, I.: Dyschondroplasia with haemangiomata (Maffucci syndrome). J. Bone Joint Surg. [Br.], *32*:376–383, 1950.
18. Tiwisina, Th.: Dyschondroplasie (Ollier) mit multiplen Haemangiomen und örtlicher maligner Entartung (Chondrosarkom). Bruns' Beitr. Klin. Chir., *188*:8–15, 1954.
19. Trisant, H., Touraine, R., De Funes, P., et al.: Syndrome de Mafucci et angiomes des membres (à propos de deux observations). J. Radiol. Electrol. Med. Nucl., *52*:413–416, 1971.

11

CHONDROBLASTOMA

DEFINITION

Chondroblastoma is a rare primary, usually benign, bone tumor of immature cartilage cell derivation with preferential localization in the epiphysis.

INCIDENCE

Chondroblastoma makes up less than 1 per cent of all primary bone tumors. There are over 500 cases reported in the world literature, many of which are case reports or small series of cases.

HISTORICAL BACKGROUND

In the earliest descriptions of chondroblastoma, this lesion was referred to as a "giant cell tumor variant, a cartilage containing giant cell tumor" by Kolodny in 1927[45] and as a "calcifying giant cell tumor" by Ewing in 1928.[20] In 1931, Codman was the first to describe this tumor in detail, regarding it as an "epiphyseal chondromatous giant-cell tumor."[11] Subsequently, this lesion became known by some as "Codman's tumor." In 1942, Jaffe and Lichtenstein introduced the designa-

tion "benign chondroblastoma," emphasizing that this neoplasm is a distinct clinicopathologic entity clearly separate from giant cell tumor of bone.[41]

HISTOGENESIS

Jaffe and Lichtenstein[41] proposed, in their now classic study, that chondroblastoma is a primary tumor of bone that developed from cells best considered as cartilage germ cells. Valls and associates, in 1951, suggested that this tumor had a reticulohistiocytic origin.[94] Their purported evidence, now known to be mistaken, for this assumption was derived from the use of a silver impregnation technique on histologic material in eight cases. The ultrastructural features of chondroblastoma cells fail to support the theory that they are of reticulohistiocytic derivation and strongly suggest a definite resemblance to immature chondrocytes.[39] Both rapid proliferation and lack of differentiation preclude the formation of lacunae or the production of a cartilage matrix, usually a feature of chondrocytes. Tissue culture studies demonstrate a remarkable similarity between chondroblasts and normal human epiphyseal chondrocytes.

SIGNS AND SYMPTOMS

The symptoms in general are quite non-specific. Pain and swelling in the tumor area, usually lasting several months or even years, is the most characteristic complaint. Pathologic fracture as a primary manifestation is exceedingly rare, and local swelling is present only in less than 10 per cent of cases.[12, 23] Vague symptoms related to joints and articular regions may result in arthrotomy or meniscectomy. Joint effusion was noted by Schajowicz and Gallardo in one third of their cases.[81] Laboratory determination of blood calcium, phosphorus, and alkaline phosphatase levels is nonspecific and not even suggestive of the diagnosis.

AGE AND SEX DISTRIBUTION

The patients vary in age from 3 to 73 years and most are teenagers[59] (Fig. 11–1). The tumor is uncommon in preteen children or adults over 25 years of age. The younger and older patients usually demonstrate lesions involving rare sites: unusual age goes hand in hand with atypical location. Males are predilected in a ratio of approximately 2:1 (Fig. 11–1). The sole reported case of a congenital chondroblastoma of the rib appears to be so "atypical" that it seems to be hardly acceptable.[42]

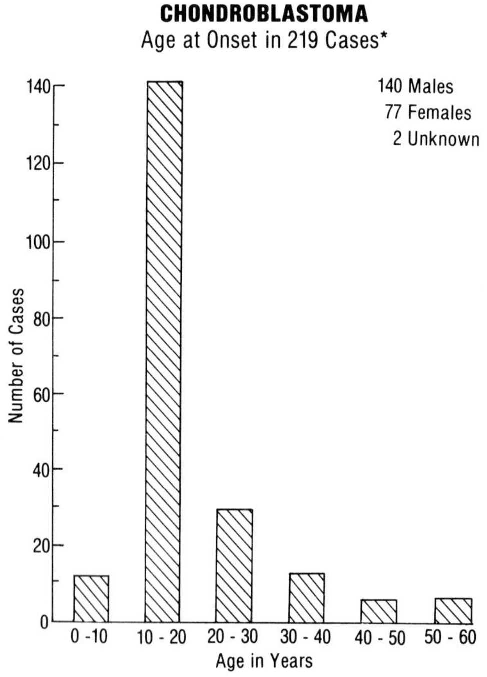

LOCATION

Typically, chondroblastomas form within the epiphyseal region of a long bone, with occasional extension into adjacent metaphysis. Once the metaphysis is affected, the lesion is usually situated eccentrically, thereby resulting in bulging of the cortex. They vary in size from 1 to 6 cm; as a rule, exclusively epiphyseal lesions are smaller than those extending into the metaphysis. The most common locations, in descending order of frequency, are the femur, humerus, tibia, and the tarsal and innominate bones, according to the published cases (Fig. 11–2). These locations represent approximately 75 per cent of all the lesions. No area of the axial or appendicular skeleton is spared as a possible site, however. Chondroblastomas arising in the pelvis have a marked predilection to originate near the triradiate cartilage of the innominate bone.[61]

The exclusiveness of humeral location, originally espoused by Codman in conjunction with his particular interest in shoulder diseases, is no longer held valid. Codman was the first, however, to appreciate the pronounced predilection for the humeral tubercles in contrast to the sparing or rare localization in the capital epiphysis.[11] In the upper end of the femur, the lesion most frequently arises from the greater trochanter.

The occurrence of chondroblastoma in the flat bones of the skeleton is not inconsistent with the maxim that this lesion is of epiphyseal inception, for these bones have multiple primary centers of ossification. Predominantly or exclusively metaphyseal location, with or without a connection to the epiphyseal plate, has been reported.[1, 22, 79, 83] The sites of the tumors are such that they are always associated with either primary or secondary centers

CHONDROBLASTOMA
Age at Onset in 219 Cases*

140 Males
77 Females
2 Unknown

*Mayo Clinic, Latin American Bone Registry, Memorial Hospital

Figure 11–1. Age and sex distribution of 219 patients reported in three larger series of cases. (Data from Huvos, A. G., and Marcove, R. C.: Chondroblastoma of bone. A critical review. Clin. Orthop., 95:300–312, 1973.)

BENIGN CHONDROBLASTOMAS

Location in 458 Cases

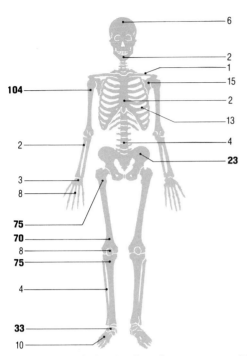

Figure 11–2. Skeletal distribution in 458 cases from the literature. (Data from Huvos, A. G., and Marcove, R. C.: Chondroblastoma of bone. A critical review. Clin. Orthop., 95:300–312, 1973.)

of endochondral ossification. Diaphyseal location is not seen.

RADIOGRAPHIC APPEARANCE

The characteristic radiographic findings in chondroblastoma include a more or less lytic, round or oval area of bone destruction involving the epiphysis or neighboring metaphysis of a long bone, usually while the growth plate is still open (Fig. 11–3).[72, 83] Metaphyseal extension of a lesion results in eccentric location with bulging expansion of the overlying cortex. Varying degrees of central and peripheral, radiopaque, fuzzily stippled or fluffy calcifications with occasional streaky ossification are usually present. Although one might not expect periosteal reaction with a benign tumor, about one third of the cases will show a buttress type of periosteal activity.[83] Prior to treatment, chondroblasto-

mas are apt to be well defined by a narrow line of sclerosis delimiting the lesion from the surrounding normal bone. The clinically early lesions, as determined by the clinical history and presentation, and recurrent tumors display slight peripheral sclerosis (Fig. 11–4). Subsequently, gradual and progressive expansion takes place, with a thickened ring of peripheral sclerosis coupled with the development of central mottled fluffy calcifications (Fig. 11–5A). In the process of reaching complete maturation, more marked peripheral sclerosis occurs, accompanied by central opacification.

Similarly to the experience of those at the Massachusetts General Hospital, our observation at Memorial Hospital confirms the occurrence of healing and cure in the absence of complete curettage or resection; some healing, in fact, has gradually progressed for over 30 years (Fig. 11–5B and C).[10, 38] The increasing microscopically demonstrable calcific encrustation initially manifests peripherally and later centrally. Such advancement of sclerosis and healing is demonstrable in cases observed over a protracted period, during which sequential roentgenograms are taken and examined, even in the absence of bone chips. This centripetal healing and resorption of the lesion is probably expected and is of clear clinical significance. If an originally lytic defect fails to develop this peripheral sclerosis, it serves as a warning signal that the patient has a recurrence. This is especially the case if, in addition to the lack of roentgenographic healing, a clinical resurgence of pain and tenderness at this lytic area is experienced.[38]

Often, the maturation of the epiphyseal growth plate of the involved bone appears to be more advanced than expected for a teenage patient, and occasionally, the epiphysis may be completely fused. This advanced state of growth plate maturation in turn may confuse the diagnostic radiologist, who, as a result, may entertain the diagnosis of a giant cell tumor.

Neuroradiologic investigations in the rare cases of intracranial extension of a temporal bone chondroblastoma should include radioactive technetium scintiscan, since this tumor showed a remarkably high uptake in one reported case.[35]

The most important radiographic *dif-*

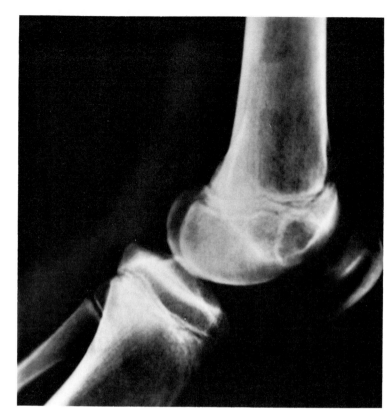

Figure 11–3. Typical chondroblastoma in a 14-year-old boy. The distal femoral epiphysis shows a round radiolucent area surrounded by a sclerotic border. There is no periosteal reaction.

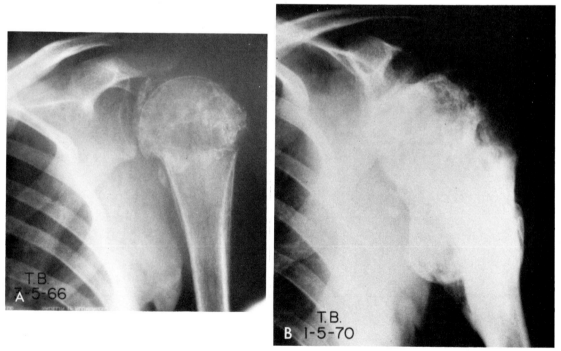

Figure 11–4. Clinically early recurrent chondroblastoma of humerus (A) with a progressive expansion in spite of two curettages with periosteal bone formation (B). Radiopacity developing peripherally (A), then centrally, with fluffy smaller opacities during the 4 year period following the 1966 cryosurgery. The lesion has since remained clinically inactive. (From Huvos, A. G., Marcove, R. C., Erlandson, R. A., et al.: Chondroblastoma of bone. A clinicopathologic and electron microscopy study. Cancer, 29:760–771, 1972.)

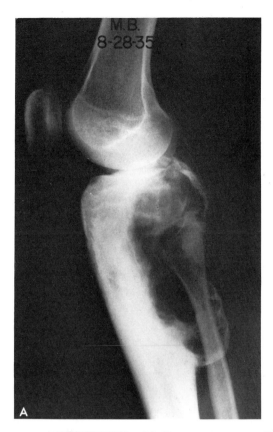

Figure 11–5. Expanding lytic lesion involving epiphysis and metaphysis with early peripheral sclerosis (*A*). Gradual central opacification occurred, followed by progressive peripheral sclerosis involving the entire lesion over a 35 year period (*B* and *C*). (From Huvos, A. G., Marcove, R. C., Erlandson, R. A., et al.: Chondroblastoma of bone. A clinicopathologic and electron microscopy study. Cancer, *29*:760–771, 1972.)

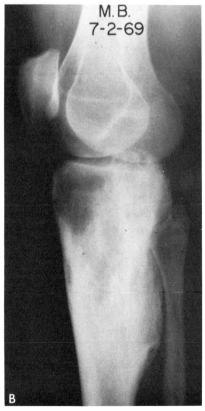

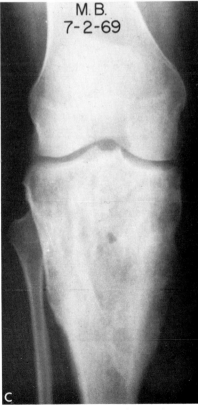

ferential diagnosis is the separation of chondroblastoma from an enchondroma or central chondrosarcoma; all may involve the epiphysis and adjacent metaphysis with thin, sclerotic, bony marginal delimitation. If the intralesional calcific densities are conspicuous, the tumor is more likely than not an enchondroma or a chondrosarcoma. Finely mottled calcifications within a lesion with well-delineated marginal sclerosis leaves the exact classification of the tumor in doubt, and only histologic examination will decide whether one deals with any of the three above-mentioned possibilities. Fibrous dysplasia or nonossifying fibroma rarely affects the epiphysis; they show more intralesional trabeculation and more scalloped borders. Polyostotic involvement has never been reported in chondroblastoma, although it is a prominent feature in fibrous dysplasia. Monostotic fibrous dysplasia appearing in the flat bones of the pelvic girdle and the scapula cannot be separated radiographically from a chondroblastoma. The same applies to nonossifying fibroma. The separation of untreated giant cell tumor of bone from chondroblastoma is usually not too difficult. In giant cell tumors, the fine mottling due to calcification or bone formations is absent, and the sharply defined sclerotic margin is missing. Lack of calcific mottling and the usual nonepiphyseal presentation help keep chondromyxoid fibroma and chondroblastoma roentgenographically distinct. If, however, the chondromyxoid fibroma involves the epiphysis, this distinction becomes illusory and the lesions cannot be distinguished from each other with certainty. On occasion, a chondroblastoma has been seriously considered as a lytic form of osteogenic sarcoma.[83] The spherical or oval configuration, the epiphyseal location, the presence of some cortical thinning and expansion, as well as the relatively distinct borders of the lesion, are all more likely to be displayed by a chondroblastoma. Other helpful features include a fairly small size, an innocuous periosteal buttress-type reaction, an absence of perpendicular shape, and a relatively limited small soft tissue mass, all of which militate against an osteogenic sarcoma.

Inflammatory lesions, especially tuberculosis, may simulate chondroblastoma radiologically. Three of six cases reported by Sundaram were originally diagnosed as tuberculosis.[88] A case of brucellosis involving the proximal epiphysis and adjacent metaphysis of the humerus closely mimicked a chondroblastoma.[72]

Ischemic necrosis of the femoral head may mimic chondroblastoma.[27]

GROSS FINDINGS

On gross examination, the curetted tissue shows soft or friable, mottled, grayish material that appears to be focally gritty. The color varies from gray-yellow to gray-brown and is, on occasion, frankly hemorrhagic. Study of a totally excised intact specimen revealed a central chondroid lesion, within which was a well-delineated cyst (Fig. 11–6). The lesions are usually well-demarcated, present primary epiphyseal involvement, and may destroy adjacent bony cortex as well as medullary cancellous bone. Cystic alterations have been described.[12]

MICROSCOPIC FEATURES

The microscopic examination of the tumor tissue reveals the background to be formed by uniform, polyhedral, closely packed cells, which may sometimes be difficult to distinguish from plasma cells (Figs. 11–7 and 11–8). The cellular elements are separated by scanty interstitial matrix, which may be frankly chondroid in its makeup (Fig. 11–9). The pericellular, lattice-like, fine calcification arranged in the characteristic "chicken wire" or "picket fence" pattern is the hallmark of this lesion. Our experience parallels that of others; chondroblastomas occasionally do occur without these calcifications.[12, 66, 80] Stromal calcific encrustation may be seen, especially in older, long-standing, or recurrent lesions. Controversy exists as to whether this interstitial calcification can exist prior to focal tissue necrosis or is due to necrosis or degeneration. Currently, most observers favor stromal calcification as the primary process, since such calcareous areas can be present in the total absence of tissue necrosis. As calcium deposition builds up, some areas in turn

Text continued on page 180

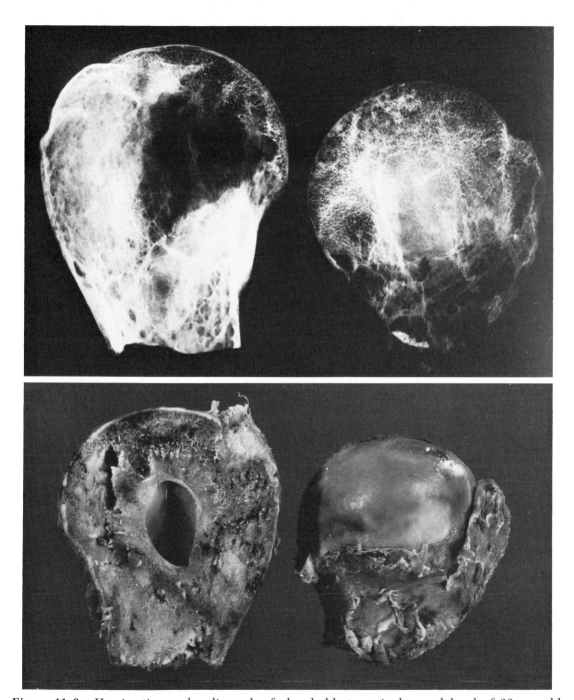

Figure 11–6. Hemisection and radiograph of chondroblastoma in humeral head of 33-year-old woman. Central chondrification and cyst formation are noted. (From Huvos, A. G., Marcove, R. C., Erlandson, R. A., et al.: Chondroblastoma of bone. A clinicopathologic and electron microscopy study. Cancer, 29:760–771, 1972.)

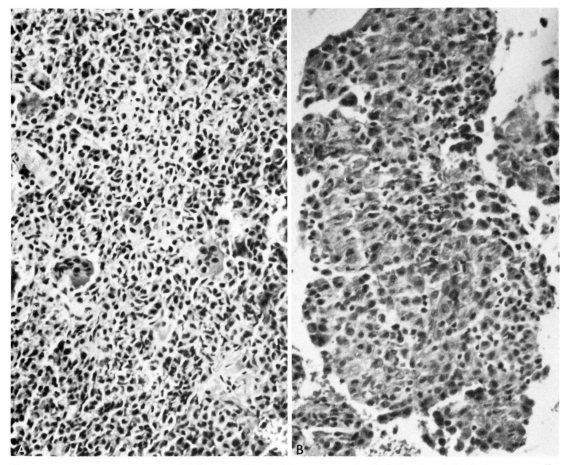

Figure 11–7. Representative fields in a chondroblastoma with ill-defined polyhedral tumor cells interspersed with giant cells. (Hematoxylin-eosin stain. Magnification ×80.)

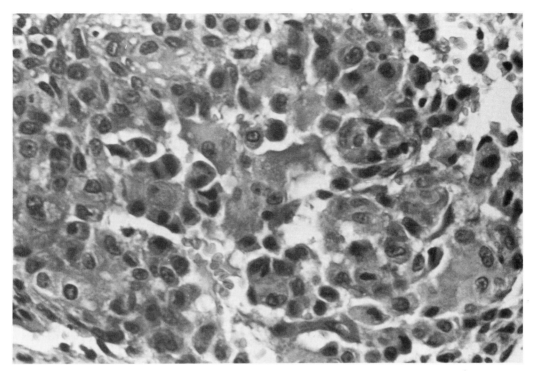

Figure 11–8. Typical chondroblastoma with closely packed cells separated by scanty interstitial matrix. (Hematoxylin-eosin stain. Magnification ×200.) (From Huvos, A. G., and Marcove, R. C.: Chondroblastoma of bone. A critical review. Clin. Orthop., 95:300–312, 1973.)

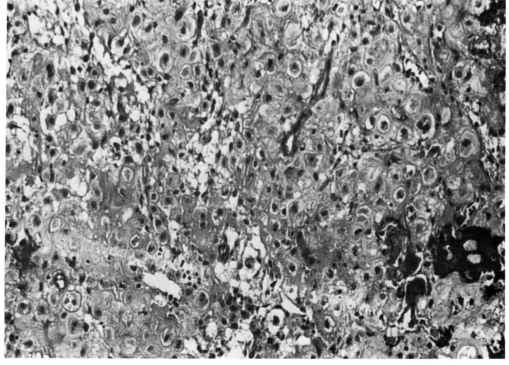

Figure 11–9. Chondroblastoma with typical fully developed calcifications. (Hematoxylin-eosin stain. Magnification ×80.)

become necrotic. It is good to remember that the physiologic maturation process of normal cartilage includes calcium deposition in the matrix. Peripheral areas of the tumor may show fibrosis, while central regions are more apt to reveal hemorrhages and hemosiderin deposition.

The evolutionary progression in chondroblastoma as studied by light microscopy is depicted as follows:

Earliest phase:

Compact round or polyhedral cells of moderate size. Large nuclei. Occasionally more than one nucleus. A sprinkling of multinucleated giant cells.

Intermediate phase:

Focal areas of calcification. The heavier the calcification, the heavier the degeneration and necrosis of tumor cells.

Late phase:

Connective tissue replacement of necrotic tissue. Chondroid or even osseous matrix formation.

Small foci of osteoid and bone are present in many cases. Occasionally, they meld gradually with islands of chondroid material, indicating transformation of cartilage into osteoid and bone.[29] Sometimes, ossification is of such magnitude that classification of the tumor as an osteoblastoma is seriously considered. One such case was reported as an "osteochondroblastoma."[102]

The presence of numerous multinucleated giant cells within a chondroblastoma as an integral part of this lesion raises the question as to whether these cells are secondary to hemorrhage or necrosis due to spontaneous or operative trauma or whether they are indeed tumor cells. In many instances, the clustering of giant cells is more confined to hemorrhages and necrosis than conventional giant cell tumors, which would favor the giant cells to be of the reactive type. On the other hand, ultramicroscopic study in some cases shows the nuclei of both giant cells and stromal tumor cells in chondroblastoma to be similar, if not identical.

Often, prominent dilated vascular channels may be seen in the center as well as at the periphery of the tumor (Fig. 11–10). In approximately 20 to 25 per cent of the cases, such aneurysmally dilated blood vessels can be seen, signaling an in-

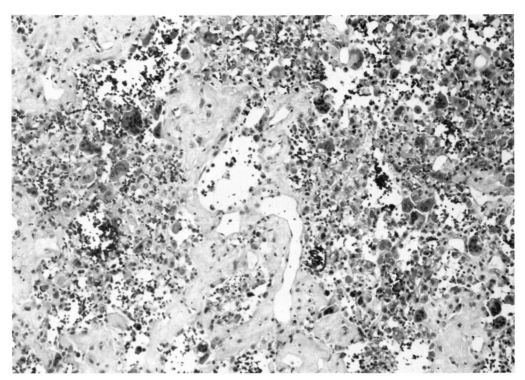

Figure 11–10. Chondroblastoma with associated secondary aneurysmal bone cyst formation. (Hematoxylin-eosin stain. Magnification ×100.)

creased propensity for clinical recurrence.[4, 52] Such lesions, which display the microscopic features of an aneurysmal bone cyst engrafted on a chondroblastoma, clinically manifest heavy bleeding at the time of surgical intervention and are sometimes referred to as "cystic chondroblastoma."[17, 81]

It has been emphasized by Jaffe[40] and by Kunkel and his coworkers[47] that the microscopic features of chondroblastoma may mimic those of chondromyxoid fibroma because of the cartilaginous, myxocartilaginous, or myxoid appearance of areas of both tumors. As a rule of thumb, the decision about classifying such a lesion should be based on its predominant characteristics. In our experience at Memorial Hospital with approximately 40 chondroblastomas, no overlapping microscopic fields with chondromyxoid fibroma were recognized.

Soft tissue extension or implantation of chondroblastoma nodules is usually surrounded, but also traversed, by metaplastic new bone formation, a not uncommon occurrence when cartilaginous cells grow within extraosseous soft tissues or even in cases of pulmonary "metastasis." This bone is composed of well-formed lamellae lined by regular, uniform osteoblasts and does not indicate osteoid or bone production by the tumor or a change to osteogenic sarcoma.[43]

ULSTRASTRUCTURAL FINDINGS

Several studies deal with the ultrastructural aspects of chondroblastoma.[39, 51, 98, 99] Electron microscope examination reveals spherical to oblong, closely packed cells with the nuclei having a multilobulated appearance (Fig. 11–11).

The characteristic dense nuclear band originally described by Welsh and Meyer,[99] and later by Wellmann,[98] closely resembles the fibrous lamina of the nuclei in certain invertebrates and vertebrates, including humans. This fibrous lamina is closely adherent to the inner aspect of the nuclear envelope.[21, 39, 58] The chondromucoprotein intercellular matrix in chondroblastomas is scanty and is composed of a finely fibrillar material containing occasional collagen fibers. The cell membrane of the tumor cells exhibits numerous microvilli. The Golgi region shows multiple electron-lucent mitochondria and irregularly distributed segments of rough endoplasmic reticulum with rare cystic dilatations. Glycogen particles and scattered lipid droplets, as well as small fascicles of cytoplasmic filaments, characterize the cytoplasm of the tumor cells. Distinct prominent cytoplasmic indentations, each usually containing a small nucleolus, can be seen (Fig. 11–12). The multinucleated giant cells in two cases studied at Memorial Hospital showed definite ultrastructural similarities to the single chondroblastic tumor cells.[39] Comparison of chondroblasts and chondrocytes establishes the former as being larger and more spherical with an increased nucleocytoplasmic ratio. Under normal circumstances, chondrocytes exhibit lipid droplets, large stores of glycogen, and pools of mucoprotein in the cytoplasm. They also tend to show degenerative changes within the cartilage lacunae. These features strongly suggest that chondroblasts closely resemble chondrocytes and fail to support the idea that they are of reticulohistiocytic origin.

AGGRESSIVE BEHAVIOR AND METASTASIS

As experience with the management of chondroblastomas was broadened, more precise follow-up information became available and an understanding of the natural history expanded. As a result, one can now better appreciate their capricious nature, i.e., increased local recurrence rate, aggressive clinical behavior, and even rare metastases.[13, 17, 24, 36, 37, 43, 60, 76, 81, 85] Curettage with intraoperative implantation often results in clinical soft tissue recurrence or tumor invasion of adjacent bones.[84, 95] Synovial membrane and articular recurrences follow transarticular curettage, thereby emphasizing the importance of avoiding entering the adjacent joints.[13, 59, 64] Longstanding, neglected lesions may extend spontaneously into adjacent joints, articular surfaces, and soft tissues, necessitating major ablation.[88, 98] All these lesions, al-

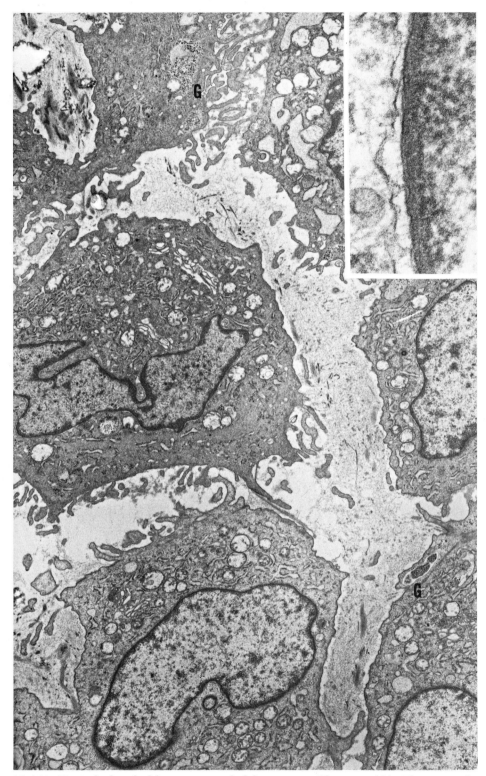

Figure 11–11. Typical chondroblasts surrounded by matrix. Glycogen (G). The inset shows the fibrous lamina at high magnification. (Magnification ×8000; inset magnification ×90,000.) (From Huvos, A. G., Marcove, R. C., Erlandson, R. A., et al.: Chondroblastoma of bone. A clinicopathologic and electron microscopy study. Cancer, 29:760–771, 1972.)

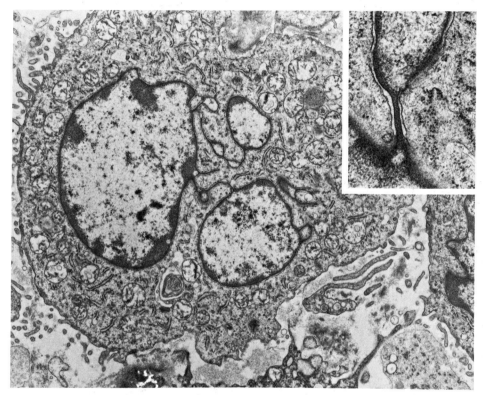

Figure 11–12. A chondroblast containing a multilobulated nucleus. The opposed fibrous laminae have fused in the thin stalk connecting the two lobes (*inset*). (Magnification ×8000; *inset*, magnification ×24,000.) (From Huvos, A. G., Marcove, R. C., Erlandson, R. A., et al.: Chondroblastoma of bone. A clinicopathologic and electron microscopy study. Cancer, *29*:760–771, 1972.)

though histologically benign, did indeed exhibit aggressive but self-limited clinical behavior.[37]

Histologically, well-documented une-quivocal "benign" chondroblastoma may exhibit pulmonary metastases following vigorous curettage (Figs. 11–13 and 11–14).[17, 30, 37, 76, 89] In spite of these pulmo-

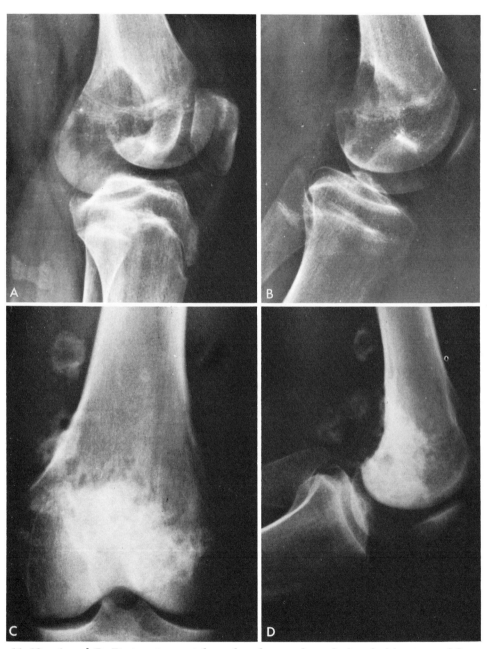

Figure 11–13. A and B, Destructive epiphyseal and metaphyseal chondroblastoma of femur with mottled opacities and slight sclerotic borders in a 14-year-old boy. C and D, Soft tissue opacifications along the medial longitudinal border of the femur. This represents soft tissue chondroblastoma implants from the first operative intervention. Curettage of the bone revealed no tumor. (From Huvos, A. G., Higinbotham, N. L., Marcove, R. C., et al.: Aggressive chondroblastoma. Review of the literature on aggressive behavior and metastases with a report of one new case. Clin. Orthop., *126*:266–272, 1977.)

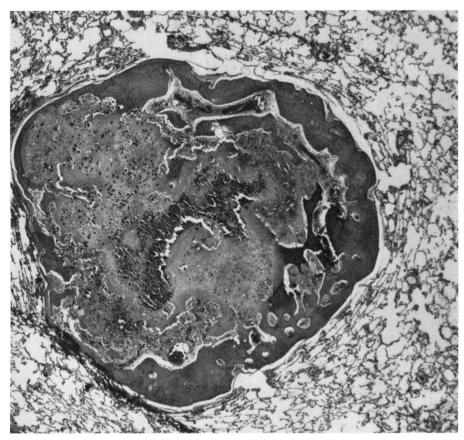

Figure 11–14. Pulmonary metastatic nodule with a rim of heavy ossification, chondroblastic core, and calcification. (Hematoxylin-eosin stain. Magnification ×50.) (From Huvos, A. G., Higinbotham, N. L., Marcove, R. C., et al.: Aggressive chondroblastoma. Review of the literature on aggressive behavior and metastases with a report of one new case. Clin. Orthop., *126*:266–272, 1977.)

nary "metastases," treatment should be based upon the concept that chondroblastoma is basically a benign neoplasm and that the lung "metastases" represent purely transport phenomena secondary to surgical intervention. Study of the pulmonary "metastases" in such cases makes one realize that, in most instances, they will be self-limiting in their growth potential.

Primary malignant chondroblastomas, although rare, do indeed exist.[24] Other examples may represent either a radiation-induced transformation of a benign chondroblastoma into a chondrosarcoma or a spontaneous sarcomatous change to an anaplastic spindle-cell sarcoma.[32, 64, 81, 85] Occasionally, one may also encounter a case of chondrosarcoma that was originally mistaken for a chondroblastoma. Still more data are needed to establish whether unequivocal chondroblastoma metastases are

biologically malignant some of the time, all of the time, or not at all.

TREATMENT AND PROGNOSIS

The various modalities of treatment affect the recurrence rates; they also bear a close relationship to the rates of recurrence for patients with chondroblastoma alone and those with aneurysmal bone cyst associated with chondroblastoma.[4, 5, 39, 52, 82] The overall recurrence rates at Memorial Hospital, first recurrence if there were several, for patients with or without aneurysmal bone cysts and for those with aneurysmal bone cysts unassociated with other bone lesions are depicted in Figure 11–15. It is shown that pure chondroblastoma, without associated aneurysmal bone cyst, yields a 20 per cent,

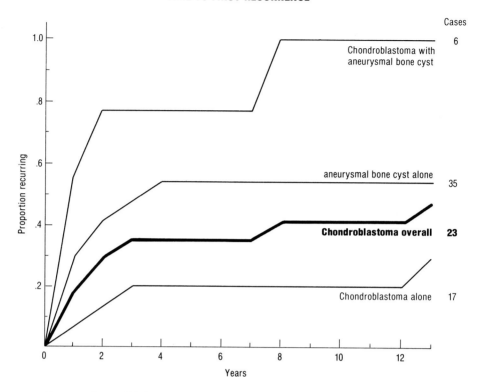

Figure 11–15. Three year recurrence rates for patients with or without associated aneurysmal bone cyst. (From Huvos, A. G., and Marcove, R. C.: Chondroblastoma of bone. A critical review. Clin. Orthop., 95:300–312, 1973.)

three year postoperative recurrence rate. In those patients in whom the chondroblastoma is accompanied by an aneurysmal bone cyst, a 100 per cent recurrence is expected (P < 0.01). This recurrence rate is also higher than that reported for aneurysmal bone cyst without associated lesions, although this difference is not statistically significant.[4, 38, 39] The overall recurrence rate in the 25 cases studied at Memorial Hospital was 38 per cent. Other series claim lower recurrence rates.[17, 81]

Among the various modalities of therapy, curettage with bone chip grafting yields the lowest recurrence rates (25 per cent), which is significantly different from the rate of recurrence after curettage only (60 per cent). This suggests that bone packing increases the cure rate. The recurrence rate for patients treated by cryosurgery at Memorial Hospital is also lower

than that for those who underwent curettage only. In cases in which there have been several recurrences or the chondroblastoma is associated with aneurysmal bone cyst, curettage coupled with cryosurgery yields consistently good results, with a high cure rate when the entire tumor can be adequately frozen with liquid nitrogen. Lesions located in the pelvic bones are best treated by *en bloc* resection.[17]

Approximately six months after unsuccessful curettage and packing with bone chips of a conventional chondroblastoma, there is a fairly rapid dissolution of these chips. The bone destruction then extends further into the involved portion and the adjacent bony cortex becomes less distinct. Extending through the cortex, breached by a previous operation, a large soft tissue mass may be seen with calcific deposits, giving the radiologic picture of a malignant tumor. Radiographic evaluation of a suspected recurrence treated by curettage and packing with bone chips is hampered by the fact that areas of smudgy increased densities may be the result of remnants of bone chips or may represent the calcific cartilaginous matrix of a recurrent chondroblastoma.

Chondroblastomas are radiosensitive tumors, but this therapeutic modality should not be used for uncomplicated cases because of the increased potential hazard incurred with irradiation-induced malignant transformation and the generally favorable results with conservative surgical measures.[8, 82]

REFERENCES

1. Aronsohn, R. S., Hart, W. R., and Martel, W.: Metaphyseal chondroblastoma of bone. Am. J. Roentgenol. Radium Ther. Nucl. Med., 127:686–688, 1976.
2. Assor, D.: Chondroblastoma of the rib. Report of a case. J. Bone Joint Surg. [Am.], 55:208–210, 1973.
3. Benedetti, G. B.: Il condroblastoma benigno dell'osso (revisione critica della letteratura e rilievi istologici e istochimici). Arch. Putti Chir. Organi Mov., 16:21–49, 1962.
4. Biesecker, J. L., Marcove, R. C., Huvos, A. G., et al.: Aneurysmal bone cysts: a clinicopathologic study of 66 cases. Cancer, 26:615–625, 1970.
5. Bonakdarpour, A., Levy, W. M., and Aegerter, E.: Primary and secondary aneurysmal bone cyst: a radiological study of 75 cases. Radiology, 126:75–83, 1978.
6. Breck, L. W., and Emmett, J. E.: Chondroblastoma of the talus; a case report. Clin. Orthop., 7:132–135, 1956.
7. Buraczewski, J., Lisakowska, J., and Rudowski, W.: Chondroblastoma (Codman's tumor) of the thoracic spine. J. Bone Joint Surg. [Br.], 39:705–710, 1957.
8. Capuano, G., Boulet, R., and Morin, A.: Le chondroblastome bénin. Lyon Med., 227:721–727, 1972.
9. Cares, H. L., and Terplan, K.: Chondroblastoma of the skull. Case report. J. Neurosurg., 35:614–618, 1971.
10. Case records of the Massachusetts General Hospital. Case 33–1964. N. Engl. J. Med., 271:94–100, 1964.
11. Codman, E. A.: Epiphyseal chondromatous giant cell tumors of the upper end of the humerus. Surg. Gynecol. Obstet., 52:543–548, 1931.
12. Cohen, J., and Cahen, I.: Benign chondroblastoma of the patella: a case report. J. Bone Joint Surg. [Am.], 45:824–826, 1963.
13. Coleman, S. S.: Benign chondroblastoma with recurrent soft-tissue and intra-articular lesions.

14. Coley, B. L., and Santoro, A. J.: Benign central cartilaginous tumors of bone. Surgery, 22:411–423, 1947.
15. Copeland, M. M., and Geschickter, C. F.: Chondroblastic tumors of bone. Benign and malignant. Ann. Surg., 129:724–735, 1949.
16. Dahlin, D. C.: Chondromyxoid fibroma of bone with emphasis on its morphological relationship to benign chondroblastoma. Cancer, 9:195–203, 1956.
17. Dahlin, D. C., and Ivins, J. C.: Benign chondroblastoma. A study of 125 cases. Cancer, 30:401–413, 1972.
18. Denko, J. V., and Krauel, L. H.: Benign chondroblastoma of bone. (An unusual localization in temporal bone.) Arch. Pathol., 59:710–711, 1955.
19. Dominok, G. W., and Knoch, H. G.: Das benigne Chondroblastom. Beitr. Orthop. Traumatol., 17:453–458, 1970.
20. Ewing, J.: Neoplastic Diseases. A Treatise on Tumors. 3rd ed. Philadelphia, W. B. Saunders Co., 1928, p. 293.
21. Fawcett, D. W.: On the occurrence of a fibrous lamina on the inner aspect of the nuclear envelope in certain cells of vertebrates. Am. J. Anat., 119:129–145, 1966.
22. Fechner, R. E., and Wilde, H. D.: Chondroblastoma in the metaphysis of the femoral neck. A case report and review of the literature. J. Bone Joint Surg. [Am.], 56:413–415, 1974.
23. Fontaine, R., Muller, J. N., and Le Gal, Y.: Un cas de chondroblastome épiphysair bénin. Presse Méd., 68:154–156, 1960.
24. Gawlik, Z., and Witwicki, T.: Chondroblastoma malignum primarium. Patol. Pol., 15(2):181–189, 1965.
25. Genovesi, A., and Barbareschi, A.: Sul condroblastoma epifisario (studio di 2 casi). Biol. Lat., 15:279–305, 1962.
26. Geschickter, C. F., and Copeland, M. M.: Chondroblastic tumors of bone: benign and malignant. Ann. Surg., 129:724–735, 1949.
27. Gohel, V. K., Dalinka, M. K., and Edeiken, J.: Ischemic necrosis of the femoral head simulating chondroblastoma. Radiology, 107:545–546, 1973.
28. Goodsell, J. O., and Hubinger, H. L.: Benign chondroblastoma of mandibular condyle: report of case. J. Oral Surg., 22:355–363, 1964.
29. Gravanis, M. B., and Giansanti, J. S.: Benign chondroblastoma: report of 4 cases with a discussion of the presence of ossification. Am. J. Clin. Pathol., 55:624–631, 1971.
30. Green, P., and Whittaker, R. P.: Benign chondroblastoma. Case report with pulmonary metastasis. J. Bone Joint Surg. [Am.], 57:418–420, 1975.
31. Hadders, H. N., Donner, R., and Van Rijssel, T. G.: Chondroblastoma benignum. Ned. Tijdschr. Geneeskd., 100:2648–2652, 1956.
32. Hatcher, C. H., and Campbell, J. C.: Benign chondroblastoma of bone. Its histologic variations and a report of late sarcoma in the site of one. Bull. Hosp. Joint Dis., 12:411–430, 1951.
33. Hellner, H.: Semimaligne Geschwülste. Arch. Geschwulstforsch., 18:107–119, 1961.

Report of a case. J. Bone Joint Surg. [Am.], 48:1554–1560, 1966.

34. Hiertonn, T., and Salen, E.: Cystic lesions of bone resembling giant cell tumours. Acta Orthop. Scand., 32:281–289, 1962.

35. Hirth, R., Städtler, F., and Piepgras, U.: An intracranial chondroblastoma. Arch. Psychiatr. Nervenkr., 216:359–369, 1972.

36. Hull, M. T., Gonzalez-Crussi, F., DeRosa, G. P., et al.: Aggressive chondroblastoma. Report of a case with multiple bone and soft tissue involvement. Clin. Orthop., 126:261–265, 1977.

37. Huvos, A. G., Higinbotham, N. L., Marcove, R. C., et al.: Aggressive chondroblastoma. Review of the literature on aggressive behavior and metastases with a report of one new case. Clin. Orthop., 126:266–272, 1977.

38. Huvos, A. G., and Marcove, R. C.: Chondroblastoma of bone. A critical review. Clin. Orthop., 95:300–312, 1973.

39. Huvos, A. G., Marcove, R. C., Erlandson, R. A., et al.: Chondroblastoma of bone. A clinicopathologic and electron microscopy study. Cancer, 29:760–771, 1972.

40. Jaffe, H. L.: Tumors and Tumorous Conditions of the Bones and Joints. Philadelphia, Lea & Febiger, 1958, p. 44.

41. Jaffe, H. L., and Lichtenstein, L.: Benign chondroblastoma of bone. A reinterpretation of the so-called calcifying or chondromatous giant cell tumor. Am. J. Pathol., 18:969–983, 1942.

42. Kadell, B. M., Coulson, W. F., Desilets, D. T., et al.: Congenital atypical benign chondroblastoma of a rib. J. Pediatr. Surg., 5:46–52, 1970.

43. Kahn, L. B., Wood, F. M., and Ackerman, L. V.: Malignant chondroblastoma. Report of 2 cases and review of the literature. Arch. Pathol., 88:371–376, 1969.

44. Kingsley, T. C., and Markel, S. F.: Extraskeletal chondroblastoma. A report of the first recorded case. Cancer, 27:203–206, 1971.

45. Kolodny, A.: Bone sarcoma. The primary malignant tumors of bone and the giant-cell tumor. Surg. Gynecol. Obstet., 44 (Supplement 1):1–214, 1927.

46. Kuhlman, R. E., and McNamee, M. J.: Quantitative microchemical studies of chondroblastoma, giant-cell tumor, chondromyxoid fibroma and desmoplastic fibroma. Clin. Orthop., 69:264–270, 1970.

47. Kunkel, M. G., Dahlin, D. C., and Young, H. H.: Benign chondroblastoma. J. Bone Joint Surg. [Am.], 38:817–826, 1956.

48. Lagrot, F., and Tordjeman, G.: Un cas de chondroblastome du fémur. Pediatrie, 16:708–716, 1961.

49. Le Gal, Y., and Keiling, R.: Un cas de chondroblastome épiphysaire bénin. Ann. Anat. Pathol. (Paris), 4:476–482, 1959.

50. Le Sec, G., Forest, M., Abelanet, R., et al.: La distribution squelettique des chondroblastomes. Les rapports avec les territoires d'ossification. J. Radiol. Electrol. Med. Nucl., 57:623–625, 1976.

51. Levine, G. D., and Bensch, K. G.: Chondroblastoma—the nature of the basic cell. A study by means of histochemistry, tissue culture, electron microscopy, and autoradiography. Cancer, 29:1546–1562, 1972.

52. Levy, W. M., Miller, A. S., Bonakdarpour, A., et al.: Aneurysmal bone cyst secondary to other osseous lesions. Report of 57 cases. Am. J. Clin. Pathol., 63:1–8, 1975.

53. Lichtenstein, L., and Bernstein, D.: Unusual benign and malignant chondroid tumors of bone. Cancer, 12:1142–1157, 1959.

54. Lichtenstein, L., and Kaplan, L.: Benign chondroblastoma of bone. Unusual localization in femoral capital epiphysis. Cancer, 2:793–798, 1949.

55. Litsios, B. I., and Papacharalampous, N. X.: Die benignen Chondroblastome. Zentralbl. Allg. Pathol., 114:344–349, 1971.

56. Maestre Herrero, J.: Chondroblastoma epifisario benigno tibial. Contribucion al diagnostico diferencial de un infrecuente proceso osteoarticular, tumoral, de rodilla. Acta Ortop. Traumatol. Ibér., 3:319–334, 1955.

57. Mangini, U.: Benign chondroblastoma localized in the capitate bone: a case report. Bull. Hosp. Joint Dis., 25:50–56, 1964.

58. Mazanec, K.: Présence de la "zonula nucleum limitans" dans-quelques cellules humaines. J. Microscopie, 6:1027–1032, 1967.

59. McBryde, A., Jr., and Goldner, J. L.: Chondroblastoma of bone. Am. Surg., 36:94–108, 1970.

60. McLaughlin, R. E., Sweet, D. E., Webster, T., et al.: Chondroblastoma of the pelvis suggestive of malignancy. Report of an unusual case treated by wide pelvic excision. J. Bone Joint Surg. [Am.], 57:549–551, 1975.

61. McLeod, R. A., and Beabout, J. W.: The roentgenographic features of chondroblastoma. Am. J. Roentgenol. Radium Ther. Nucl. Med., 118:464–471, 1973.

62. Milazzo, F.: On an unusual case of chondroblastoma of the mandible. Arch. Ital. Otol. Rinol. Laringol., 78:61–72, 1967.

63. Moore, T. M., Roe, J. B., and Harvey, J. P., Jr.: Chondroblastoma of the talus. A case report. J. Bone Joint Surg. [Am.], 59:830–831, 1977.

64. Netherlands Committee on Bone Tumours: Radiological Atlas of Bone Tumours. Vol. 2. Baltimore, Williams & Wilkins, 1973, p. 313.

65. Neviaser, R. J., and Wilson, J. N.: Benign chondroblastoma in the finger. J. Bone Joint Surg. [Am.], 54:389–392, 1972.

66. Nézelof, C., Mazabraud, A., and Jobard, P.: Bénin chondroblastome des os. À propos de 4 cas. Arch. Anat. Pathol., 10:111–117, 1962.

67. Nolan, D. J., and Middlemiss, H.: Chondroblastoma of bone. Clin. Radiol., 26:343–350, 1975.

68. Onuigbo, W. I. B.: A definition problem in cancer metastasis. Neoplasma, 22:547–550, 1975.

69. Oppenheim, J. M., and Boal, R. W.: Benign chondroblastoma (Codman's tumor). Case report and review of literature. U.S. Armed Forces Med. J., 6:279–282, 1955.

70. Paunier, J. P., Candardjis, G., and Wettstein, P.: Le chondroblastome. Description de 3 nouveaux cas. Radiol. Clin. Biol., 36:237–242, 1967.

71. Pizzoferrato, A., Piccaluga, A., and Giunti, A.: Il condroblastoma epifisario benigno. Arch. Ital. Anat. Istol. Patol., 41:165–288, 1967.

72. Plum, G. E., and Pugh, D. G.: Roentgenologic aspects of benign chondroblastoma of bone.

Am. J. Roentgenol. Radium Ther. Nucl. Med., 79:584–591, 1958.

73. Popp, D. D., and MacCarthy, J. D.: Chondroblastoma of the cuboid. Case report. Northwest Med., 59:916–918, 1960.

74. Ravault, P. P., Vignon, G., Lejeune, E., et al.: Benign chondroblastoma of bone. (Report of 6 clinical anatomical observations.) Rev. Rhum. Mal. Osteoartic, 36:215–224, 1969.

75. Renfer, H. R.: Chondroblastoma (a rare primary tumor of bones). Radiol. Clin. (Basel), 29:288–297, 1960.

76. Riddell, R. J., Louis, C. J., and Bromberger, N. A.: Pulmonary metastases from chondroblastoma of the tibia. Report of a case. J. Bone Joint Surg. [Br.], 55:848–853, 1973.

77. Ross, J. A., and Dawson, E. K.: Benign chondroblastoma of bone. Report of a case. J. Bone Joint Surg. [Br.], 57:78–81, 1975.

78. Ruziczka, O., and Haslhofer, L.: Zur Klinik und Pathologie des Chondroblastoma "benignum". Monatsschr. Kinderheilkd., 110:201–202, 1962.

79. Salzer, M., Salzer-Kuntschik, M., and Kretschmer, G.: Das benigne Chondroblastom. Arch. Orthop. Unfallchir., 64:229–244, 1968.

80. Salzer-Kuntschik, M.: Atypical chondroblastic tumour. Beitr. Pathol. Anat. Allg. Pathol., 138:337–341, 1969.

81. Schajowicz, F., and Gallardo, H.: Epiphysial chondroblastoma of bone. A clinicopathological study of 69 cases. J. Bone Joint Surg. [Br.], 52:205–226, 1970.

82. Schauwecker, F., Weller, S., Klumper, A., et al.: Therapeutische Möglichkeiten beim benignen Chondroblastom. Bruns' Beitr. Klin. Chir., 217:155–159, 1969.

83. Sherman, R. S., and Uzel, A. R.: Benign chondroblastoma of bone. Its roentgen diagnosis. Am. J. Roentgenol. Radium Ther Nucl. Med., 76:1132–1140, 1956.

84. Shoji, H., and Miller, T. R.: Benign chondroblastoma with soft-tissue recurrence. N.Y. State J. Med., 71:2786–2789, 1971.

85. Sirsat, M. V., and Doctor, V. M.: Benign chondroblastoma of bone: report of a case of malignant transformation. J. Bone Joint Surg. [Br.], 52:741–745, 1970.

86. Smith, D. A., Graham, W. C., and Smith, F. R.: Benign chondroblastoma of bone. Report of an unusual case. J. Bone Joint Surg. [Am.], 44:571–577, 1962.

87. Steiner, G. C.: Postradiation sarcoma of bone. Cancer, 18:603–612, 1965.

88. Sundaram, T. K. S.: Benign chondroblastoma. J. Bone Joint Surg. [Br.], 48:92–104, 1966.

89. Sweetnam, R., and Ross, K.: Surgical treatment of pulmonary metastases from primary tumours of bone. J. Bone Joint Surg. [Br.], 49:74–79, 1967.

90. Trapeznikov, N. N., and Plotnikov, V. I.: Unusual site for bone chondroblastoma. Vopr. Onkol., 11:97–99, 1965.

91. Treasure, E. R.: Benign chondroblastoma of bone. Report of a case. J. Bone Joint Surg. [Br.], 37:462–465, 1955.

92. Uehlinger, E.: Die pathologische Anatomie der Knochengeschwülste. Helv. Chir. Acta, 26:597–620, 1959.

93. Uehlinger, E.: Pathologische Anatomie der Knochengeschwülste. Helv. Chir. Acta, 40:5–27, 1973.

94. Valls, J., Ottolenghi, C. E., and Schajowicz, F. Epiphyseal chondroblastoma of bone. J. Bone Joint Surg. [Am.], 33:997–1009, 1951.

95. Varma, B. P., and Gupta, I. M.: Atypical chondroblastoma of tibia. Report of a recurrent lesion. Clin. Orthop., 89:241–245, 1972.

96. Vinogradova, T. P., and Golubev, N. A.: Chondroblastoma. Arkh. Patol., 22(7):20–25, 1960.

97. Weickert, H., and Dominok, G. W.: Benign chondroblastoma in the knee joint. Zentralbl. Allg. Pathol., 118:321–327, 1974.

98. Wellmann, K. F.: Chondroblastoma of the scapula. A case report with ultrastructural observations. Cancer, 24:408–416, 1969.

99. Welsh, R. A., and Meyer, A. T.: A histogenetic study of chondroblastoma. Cancer, 17:578–589, 1964.

100. Werthammer, S., and MacCracken, W. B.: The so-called Codman tumor. Clin. Orthop., 5:193–199, 1955.

101. Wright, J. L., and Sherman, M. S.: An unusual chondroblastoma. J. Bone Joint Surg. [Am.], 46:597–600, 1964.

102. Zabski, Z. A., Cutler, S. S., and Yermakov, V.: Unclassified benign tumor of the rib. Osteochondroblastoma. Cancer, 36:1009–1015, 1975.

12

CHONDROMYXOID FIBROMA.
MYXOMA OF THE FACIAL SKELETON.
MYXOMA AND FIBROMYXOMA OF EXTRAGNATHIC BONES.

CHONDROMYXOID FIBROMA

DEFINITION

Chondromyxoid fibroma is a benign tumor of bone characterized by chondroid and myxoid differentiation of its basic tissue growing in a lobular pattern.

AGE AND SEX DISTRIBUTION

The detailed frequency of age occurrence in 358 patients, as reported in the literature, is summarized in Figure 12–1. The youngest patient is 4 years old and the oldest is 79 years old. In a single case, a congenital occurrence was noted.[34] The lesion is most common in the second decade of life, and about 60 per cent of the patients are less than 30 years old. Increasing age does not appear to affect the skeletal locations. Of these 358 patients, 52 per cent were male and 37 per cent female; in 11 per cent of the cases, no sex was recorded.

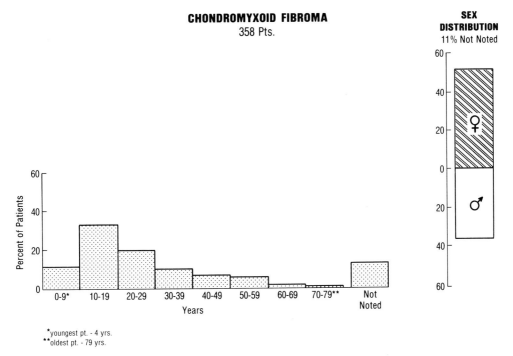

CHONDROMYXOID FIBROMA
358 Pts.

SEX DISTRIBUTION
11% Not Noted

*youngest pt. - 4 yrs.
**oldest pt. - 79 yrs.

Figure 12–1. Age and sex distribution of 358 patients with chondromyxoid fibroma of bone. Data collected from the published literature. In 11 per cent of the reported cases the sex was not recorded.

SYMPTOMS

There is usually a history of slowly and gradually evolving clinical symptoms, often resulting in a delay of months, or years, before the initial examination is performed. Some maintain that the majority of lesions discovered in late adulthood actually arose when the patients were still young.[111] The cardinal symptoms relate to pain, swelling, and restriction of movement and are of approximately two years duration, although the history may vary from as short a time as two weeks to over 10 years.[101] The pain may be spontaneous or elicited by activity of the corresponding bone and is often described by the patient as "rheumatoid" joint pain.[25] Swelling in the absence of pain is rarely encountered and averages less than one year in duration. Occasional cases are entirely asymptomatic and the lesions are only discovered on routine roentgenograms prepared for apparently unrelated reasons. Location at the base of the skull may result in long-standing pain in the back of the head.[38] Spinal cord compression by a lesion in the twelfth rib with spread into the epidural space of the spinal canal has been reported.[103]

LOCATION

It is difficult to tally the exact skeletal locations in the cases collected from the literature, since many of the reports do not specify which end of the long bone was affected. All studies agree, however, that the tibia is involved in about one third of the cases, with proximal tibial metaphysis being by far the most frequent (Fig. 12–2). There is a definite predilection for bones of the lower extremity — the femur (distal metaphysis), fibula, and small bones of the foot. It should be noted that practically no skeletal site is immune to the occurrence of chondromyxoid fibroma and, except for the clavicle, all bones have been reported to be involved.[11] In a most unusual presentation, the histologically proved lesion affected the two distal phalanges of the great toe and crossed the interphalangeal joint.[12] The rare tumor at the base of the skull may extend intracranially through the foramen magnum with infiltration of

CHONDROMYXOID FIBROMA
Location in 340 cases

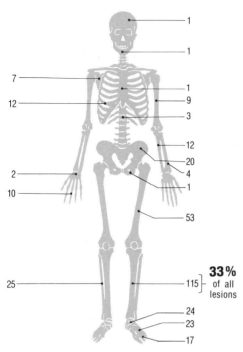

Figure 12–2. Skeletal location in 340 cases of chondromyxoid fibroma reported in the literature.

the spinal canal.[1, 38] A primarily multicentric, histologically proved case of chondromyxoid fibroma of the lower extremity has been encountered in a 26-year-old woman. During the seven year follow-up period, a spontaneous subcutaneous extraskeletal involvement became apparent; i.e., it was not in an area of prior surgery.[92]

RADIOGRAPHIC FINDINGS

The roentgenographic features of a chondromyxoid fibroma are consistently those of a benign bone tumor and therefore provide an important safeguard against histologically overdiagnosing the lesion as a chondrosarcoma. The typical presentation shows an eccentric, oval, or round lesion in the metaphyseal area of a major long bone, especially the tibia (Fig. 12–3). The longitudinal axis of an oval lesion corresponds to that of the bone, and the size ranges from approximately 1 to 10

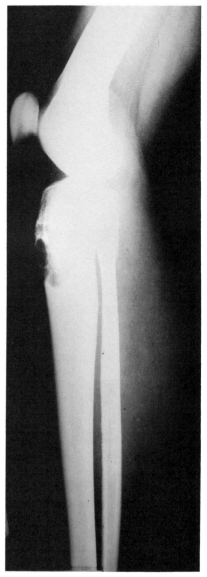

Figure 12–3. Chondromyxoid fibroma of proximal end of tibia in a 31-year-old woman. Curettage with cautery and tibial graft provided long-term cure. Original pathologic diagnosis was low-grade chondromyxosarcoma.

cm, with an average of 3 cm. The scalloped borders are well circumscribed by a distended shell of surrounding sclerotic bone (Fig. 12–4). In places, this external shell may be difficult to appreciate if no subperiosteal reactive bone has been formed.[112] This reactive bone sclerosis may be so accentuated as to mimic osteomyelitis.[142] In the absence of intralesional calcification, the tumor is wholly radiolucent

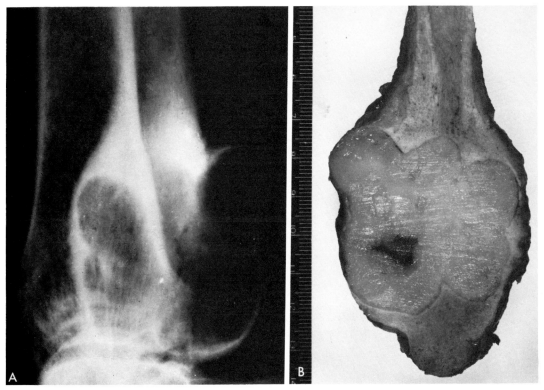

Figure 12–4. Chondromyxoid fibroma in distal end of fibula. *A,* Eccentric radiolucent lesion with sclerotic borders. The soft tissue extension is partially surrounded by irregular periosteal bone. *B,* Gross specimen shows a well-demarcated, homogeneous, rubbery firm tumor with an area of necrosis.

with a trabecular appearance. These trabeculations do not exemplify true bony septa formation but are due to ridges and grooves with scalloping at the border of the lesion. They are referred to as "pseudotrabeculations" by Feldman and associates.[40] Small lesions appear as evenly outlined cystic defects without cortical expansion.[102] Large eccentric lesions demonstrate a distended, attenuated, overlying cortex that may, on occasion, be frankly eroded. Bulging into adjacent soft tissues by a bulky lesion with cortical erosion, which suggests a malignant process, is infrequently seen (Fig. 12–5).[62]

In three of eight cases reported by Lanzi and Conti,[76] large cortical interruption with limited periosteal reaction was noted, thereby making the interpretation difficult. The epiphyseal cartilaginous growth plate is only occasionally involved, practically never when an unfused epiphysis exists, and only a few cases show exclusively diaphyseal presentation. Exceptionally, marked periosteal reaction may be elicited, or it may be limited to a Codman type of triangle.[111] In a few predominantly diaphyseal small tumors, enhanced periosteal bone formation was noted. Intralesional calcifications are rarely demonstrated by the radiographs but are seen in approximately one fourth of the cases on microscopic evaluation.[101] Pathologic fracture is rarely a problem.[3, 40, 58, 122]

In the small bones of the hands and feet, the lesions are usually centrally situated, filling up the entire width of the corresponding bone and resulting in pronounced cortical expansion. The lesions affecting the flat bones appear to be, on the average, quite large, irregularly outlined, and loculated. The general appearance of the lesions in other than the long tubular bones is not characteristic. For instance, lesions may extend throughout the entire width of the involved bone, expand-

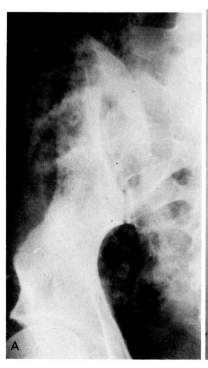 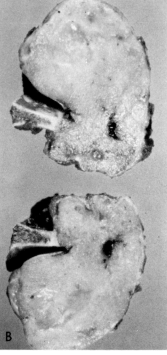

Figure 12–5. Chondromyxoid fibroma of the right iliac wing. *A*, Radiograph reveals an oval, lobular, trabeculated, radiolucent lesion with well-marginated and scalloped borders. *B*, Grossly, this is a large (13 by 9 by 8 cm), encapsulated, yellow, rubbery, slightly granular tumor demonstrating cortical destruction.

ing both surfaces and making the differentiation from fibrous dysplasia or enchondroma difficult.

RADIOGRAPHIC DIFFERENTIAL DIAGNOSIS

It is important to remember that chondromyxoid fibroma characteristically presents the roentgenographic appearance of a benign bone tumor, and the alternatives from other entities are only benign lesions.

Giant cell tumor of bone may be seriously considered in the radiologic differential diagnosis. It is most often located in the end of a long bone, usually around the knee joint after epiphyseal-diaphyseal fusion. Whereas chondromyxoid fibroma has well-defined outlines, the endosteal border of a giant cell tumor is frequently ill-defined, hazy, and not well-demarcated; the entire width of the bone is involved.[93, 136]

Unicameral bone cysts may occasionally cause diagnostic uncertainty. They occur most frequently in children and adolescents, with only extremely rare appearances after the second decade of life.

Their central metaphyseal location with the resultant fusiform swelling of the shaft and pathologic fracture, as a clinical presentation, may be of help in distinguishing them from chondromyxoid fibroma.

The mottled calcification and predilection for the short tubular bones of the hands and the propensity for polyostotic involvement in *enchondromas* are useful features of distinction. *Nonossifying fibroma* presents as a small radiolucent diaphyseal lesion with a markedly sclerotic rim and bony expansion, both of which are more subdued in chondromyxoid fibroma.

Chondroblastomas are epiphyseal lesions and only rarely touch the metaphysis. Intralesional calcification and periosteal reaction are common in chondroblastoma but are quite rare in chondromyxoid fibromas.

GROSS EXAMINATION

On gross examination, the lesion resembles fibrocartilage, but without a bluish opalescence and a smooth flat circumscribed surface; it is usually glistening, homogeneously white, and firm when the chondroid component predominates or gray-white and soft when the myxoid component prevails (Fig. 12–4*B*). As a rule, the lesion is a well-circumscribed, ovoid, lobulated mass (Fig. 12–5*B*). The overlying cortical bone is commonly eroded, occasionally bulging, with some scalloping on the inner aspect. Bony streaks and trabeculations are not seen within the lesional tissue.

MICROSCOPIC APPEARANCE

By studying a relatively large number of cases, one is impressed by the great variability in the microscopic make-up from lesion to lesion, or even in various regions of the same tumor (Figs. 12–6 and 12–7). In some, the myxomatous fields predominate and one has to search for chondroid zones of differentiation (Fig. 12–8). Such tumors feature various degrees of collagenization, providing a definite fibrous appearance and character. The chondroid aspects vary from minute microscopic fields of ill-formed cartilage to overwhelming amounts, simulating a chondroma or even

a chondrosarcoma. In such instances, the histologic growth pattern, especially the presence of large pleomorphic tumor cells, in chondromyxoid fibroma may easily have the appearance of a myxoid type of chondrosarcoma. It is good to remember that the concentration of these strikingly large pleomorphic cells with hyperchromatic nuclei always appears at the periphery of the well-delineated lobules, providing an important feature of recognition. This sharply demarcated lobular arrangement of the lesional tissue, separated from the surrounding uninvolved bone, in addition to branching tumor cells in a myxoid background is quite characteristic, presenting the histologic hallmark of chondromyxoidfibroma.

Silver reticulin stains reveal delicate argyrophilic fibrils coursing about these cells. Giant cells of the osteoclastic variety are frequent in some cases and rare in others. They show a strong acid phosphatase activity and some PAS-positive diastase-resistant material in the cytoplasm.

The apparently biphasic histologic pat-

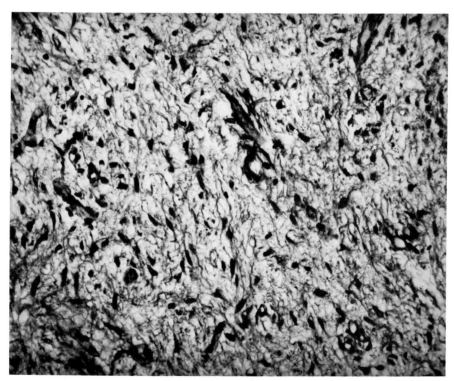

Figure 12–6. Loosely dispersed spindle-shaped and stellate cells in a myxoid background. (Hematoxylin-eosin stain. Magnification × 180.)

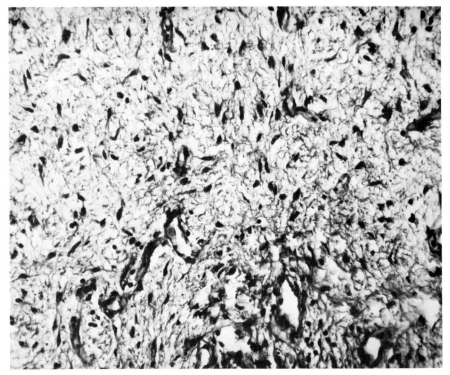

Figure 12–7. The abundant myxoid intercellular material is separated by scanty stellate tumor cells. (Hematoxylin-eosin stain. Magnification × 180.)

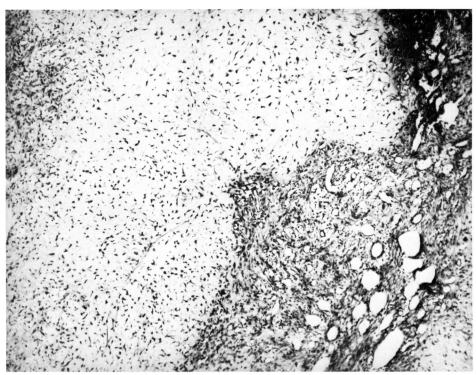

Figure 12–8. The myxoid intercellular material here changes into chondroid. The periphery of this lobular chondroid area is markedly vascular and contains somewhat pleomorphic spindle cells. (Hematoxylin-eosin stain. Magnification × 80.)

tern within a lesion is probably due to variation in the tissue maturation, the myxoid areas representing precollagenized, more immature tissue. Increased cellular differentiation may result in collagenization and ultimately, cartilage may be formed. Specific stains for mucin and fat have been negative.[62] Glycogen may be demonstrated in the chondroid components as well as in the stellate cells of the myxoid fields.[113] Both myxoid and chondroid areas demonstrate a positive metachromatic reaction with toluidine and alcian blue stains. Hyaluronidase digestion removes this metachromasia from the myxoid tissue.[10] The intercellular matrix does not give a mucicarminophilic staining reaction.[82]

Electron microscopic study of one lesion revealed two cellular components. One resembled fibroblasts; the other was morphologically similar to chondrocytes.[133] A distinctive feature of both cellular elements appeared to be a uniformly electron-dense zone, 700Å in width, between the inner and outer nuclear membranes.

HISTOGENESIS

The possibility of a close relationship between chondroblastoma and chondromyxoid fibroma was suggested in studies at the Mayo Clinic.[31, 75] In some cases, histologically overlapping patterns are encountered, but it should be emphasized that the histologic diagnosis of any bone tumor should always be based on the dominant tissue pattern. No such overlap was found in cases studied at Memorial Hospital by this author. Aegerter and Kirkpatrick[2] also link these two tumors and postulate that both arise from the epiphyseal growth plate. While chondromyxoid fibroma subsequently moves towards the diaphysis, chondroblastoma moves towards the epiphysis. Taking previous suggestions, Lipkin[83] distinguishes two variants: the typical or classic and the mixed pattern, i.e., lesions with both chondromyxoid and chondroblastoma growth traits.

Many cases reported in the literature under the diagnosis of "myxoma" or "central myxoma" involving extragnathic bones are probably misinterpreted instances of chondromyxoid fibroma, chondrosarcoma with myxoid traits, fibrosarcoma, enchondroma, or fibrous dysplasia.[13-15, 147] (See discussion on myxoma, p. 200.) This applies especially to cases reported by Bauer and Harell,[8] Chacha and Tan,[24] Herfath,[58] and Scaglietti and Stringa[112] that surely were chondromyxoid fibromas.

CLINICAL BEHAVIOR

In 1948, Jaffe and Lichtenstein[65] pointed out that chondromyxoid fibromas had previously been erroneously diagnosed as chondrosarcomas, even though they are generally benign lesions. It now seems that the pendulum is moving in the opposite direction, for occasional cases appearing in the literature as malignant chondromyxoid fibromas are actually myxoid chondrosarcomas.

Malignant transformation of chondromyxoid fibroma has been noted by several observers.[63, 64, 81, 117, 148] Witwicki and Daniluk reported four cases of malignant chondromyxoid fibroma with metastases within a few months. The two photomicrographs are not entirely convincing, however, and raise the possibility that these cases may, in fact, have been myxoid chondrosarcomas.[148] Such infrequent behavior does not negate the general dictum that this lesion almost always exhibits a benign, nonaggressive clinical course.

TREATMENT

Incomplete removal of a lesion, usually by curettage, with or without packing of the defect with bone graft results in recurrence in approximately 10 to 15 per cent of all tumors. A probable explanation for this may be in the propensity of this neoplasm to grow in a lobular pattern. These lobules, with pseudopod projections extending from the main tumor mass into the spongiosa, may be left behind after simple curettage. An increased tendency to local recurrence has been noted in younger patients.[42, 102, 112] Such clinically recurrent tumors may be adequately treated by recurettage coupled with cauterization or cryosurgery. *En bloc* excision to include a margin of normal bone is preferred by Frank and Rockwood[42] and Schajowicz and Gallardo[113] over conservative treatment.

Curettage followed by 2100 r irradiation to the cervical region showed good results in a lesion that had destroyed the laminal arches and pedicles of the second and third cervical vertebrae, with extension into surrounding soft tissues.[11] The follow-up period in this case, however, was only 15 months.

Although this tumor generally exhibits a benign clinical course, lesions in the hands and feet may require a more aggres-sive surgical approach to adequately re-move all of the tumor. A case in point con-cerns a chondromyxoid fibroma involving the basal phalanx of the fourth finger. The tumor infiltrated adjacent soft tissues and limited the motion of the neighboring fingers. The complete removal of the tumor necessitated amputation of three fingers.[30] A similar case, involving the shaft of the fourth metatarsal, culminated in the total resection of the metatarsal and toe. The extensive involvement of the first metatarsal bone with recurrence led to am-putation of the toe in another case.[102]

MYXOMA OF THE FACIAL SKELETON

DEFINITION

Myxoma, a locally invasive neoplasm of doubtful histogenesis, is formed by small, innocuous, spindle-shaped cells appearing in an abundant mucoid myxoid stroma.

INCIDENCE

In the classic study of 49 myxomas by Stout in 1948, 10 were noted to be in bone, of which 8 were in the mandible and maxilla, one was in the clavicle, and one was in the metatarsal bone.[129] Ten years later, Zimmerman and Dahlin re-ported 26 myxomas of the facial bones.[152] In 1973, Ghosh and associates reported 10 myxomas of the jaws.[47] This relative pau-city of recorded cases from large medical institutions and the uncommon individual case reports attest to the extreme rarity of these tumors in bones.[5, 7, 17, 19, 21, 23, 33, 52, 54, 61, 66, 77, 84, 89, 105, 124, 132, 137, 138, 145]

SIGNS AND SYMPTOMS

Although some patients report pain to be constantly present, in a study of 10 pa-tients by Ghosh and his coworkers this symptom was uniformly absent and the presentation was that of a painless enlarg-ing lump. The rate of growth is inconstant but usually slow. Occasionally, displaced or loose teeth are the initial manifestation. Unerupted or congenitally absent teeth may be associated with this tumor.[47]

LOCATION

The mandible is more commonly affected than the maxilla. Sites of predilection are the posterior and the condylar regions of the jaw and the zygomatic process or the alveo-lar bone in the maxilla.

AGE AND SEX DISTRIBUTION

This tumor most often develops in young adults, but it has been reported to be present at birth and in children and middle-aged persons.[47, 100, 105, 137] In most series of reported cases, there is a slight male predominance.

HISTOGENESIS

Virchow,[141] and later Stout,[129] maintained that these neoplasms were tumors of the primitive mesenchyme, since they greatly resembled embryonal connective tissue. Others, on the other hand, favor the theory that myxomas arising in the mandible or maxilla are derived from odontogenic pri-mordial mesenchyme.[7, 20, 132, 144, 151]

Ultrastructural and histochemical studies

seem to favor fibroblastic derivation.[55, 123, 143, 144] These suggestive features include abundant rough-surfaced endoplasmic reticulum, numerous microfilaments in the cytoplasm, and fibrillar material next to the other cellular membrane. White and associates[144] also demonstrated a finely granular material appearing in the endoplasmic reticulum of the tumor cells, postulating a transfer mechanism whereby this granular substance would be transported into the intercellular matrix and constitute the mucoid component of the neoplasm. Harrison's findings also support this concept of active mucoid secretion.[55] Numerous histochemical investigations of myxomas arising in the jaws proved that these lesions contain large amounts of extracellular mucopolysaccharides, such as hyaluronic acid and chondroitin sulfates.[55, 60, 91, 116] The single myxoma cells contain high alkaline but low acid phosphatase activity. Since osteogenic sarcomas and ossifying fibromas of the jaws concurrently display high alkaline and acid phosphatase secretion, in contrast to fibrosarcomas or fibromas of soft tissues, according to Mori and his coworkers,[91] myxoma may be derived from odontogenic or osteogenic tissues.

Many of the reported tumors have been designated as myxoma, fibromyxoma, or myxofibroma.[16, 20, 57, 143, 151] This indicates that a prominent fibrous component may be an integral part of this neoplasm or, as Fu and Perzin suggest,[43] may represent pre-existing fibrous tissue supporting the bone that has not yet been overwhelmed by the advancing myxoma.

Ultrastructural investigation by White and associates reveals fibrils of collagen in the distended cisternae of the endoplasmic reticulum, a finding that may point to an interruption of and interference with the progress of collagen secretion.[144] Based on the results of electron microscopic and histochemical studies, Westwood and his colleagues believe the basic neoplastic cell to be a fibroblast with the ability to synthesize the abundant mucopolysaccharide incurring the myxoid appearance.[143]

RADIOGRAPHIC FEATURES

On radiographic examination, the lesion in the facial skeleton shows a uni- or multiloculated radiolucent area of varying size divided by straight or curvilinear osseous trabeculations, giving it a "soap bubble" or "honeycomb" appearance. A well-delineated sclerotic margin is often present between the teeth. Various degrees of resorptive changes in the roots of teeth may be observed. Early cortical changes are characterized by thinning and expansion, but later destruction of the thinned cortex is noted. The lesion may be without well-defined margin extending into adjacent soft tissues. Often, the radiographic features of a myxoma are indistinguishable from those of an ameloblastoma.

PATHOLOGIC FEATURES

On gross examination, the mandible shows a tapering expansion covered by a bony shell of variable thickness. Maxillary tumors may fill the entire antrum. On cut section, the lesional tissue is gray-white and gelatinous with a typical slimy, slippery character. The lesion peels off from the surrounding bone with ease if a capsule has been formed, but often this is lacking and an infiltrative growth is demonstrated that may extend through bone into soft tissues.

Microscopically, the lesional tissue is quite acellular with a large amount of myxoid or mucoid intercellular substance. The triangular or stellate cells show long cytoplasmic processes. The nuclei are small and bland with the cytoplasm having a faintly basophilic staining reaction. Occasionally, a variable amount of bandlike intralesional collagenization is featured, prompting the designation of fibromyxoma or myxofibroma. Scattered foci of odontogenic epithelium may be enrobed by abundant myxomatous tissue in some tumors, suggesting that the lesion arises from dental anlage. In such instances, an "odontogenic myxoma" diagnosis may be in order.[26, 55, 56, 68, 95, 100, 114, 123, 144]

PROGNOSIS AND TREATMENT

Myxomas are aggressive, locally infiltrating lesions that will recur in an appreciable number of cases (up to 25 per cent) if treated by less than complete curettage or a shelling-out procedure.[7, 43, 47, 125, 152] The incomplete surgical excision is often the result of the surgeon's mistaken belief that the lesion is encapsulated and amenable to enucleation.

Inadequate excision may result in a larger recurrent tumor that is more difficult to resect.[43] A 35 year follow-up study of a patient with mandibular myxoma revealed numerous recurrences following attempts at excision.[23] Adequate, sufficiently radical surgery at the very onset will avoid subsequent, more major, surgical procedures. Small mandibular lesions are best handled by conservative excision with tumor-free lines of resection.[66] Larger mandibular tumors or recurrent lesions are optimally treated by segmental resection of the involved mandible with immediate prosthetic bridging of the defect.[21, 27, 47, 89] In the maxilla, partial maxillectomy is the usual treatment of choice to adequately encompass the entire lesion.[21, 47] Mere irradiation is of no demonstrated value in the treatment of these tumors,[152] although Attie and associates[6] used this method of treatment as a preoperative measure to facilitate maxillary resection.

MYXOMA AND FIBROMYXOMA OF EXTRAGNATHIC BONES

The dearth of reported cases of myxoma arising in long bones seems to support the opinion of many observers that such an entity is nonexistent in extragnathic osseous sites.[64, 82] This contention is further corroborated by the finding of many of the previously reported myxomas to be, in fact, chondromyxoid fibromas or myxoid chondrosarcomas.[8, 13–15, 24, 29, 112, 127] The proximal tibial lesion reported as a myxoma by Soren is most probably a bursal ganglionic cyst secondarily producing a cystic defect in the bone.[126] The problem is compounded even more: despite the fact that pure myxoma of long bone may be extraordinarily rare, myxomatous areas are not uncommon as a component of many bone tumors, both benign and malignant, especially in those of cartilaginous and fibrous derivation. Some suspect that pure myxoma may have commenced as an enchondroma and subsequently underwent complete myxomatous degeneration.[28]

In spite of this well-grounded skepticism toward the existence of pure myxomas affecting the appendicular skeleton, McClure and Dahlin, in 1977, reported three indubitable cases occurring in the femur in women aged 60, 67, and 74 years respectively. Grossly and microscopically, the lesions were entirely typical of myxomas seen in other sites. Radiographs suggested aggressively expansile rarefied tumors, but conservative surgical management yielded a recurrence-free clinical course.[88] Another acceptable case of pure myxoma arising in an anomalous toe with congenital absence of the middle phalanx occurred in a 72-year-old woman.[97] An additional case arose in the distal phalanx of the fifth toe.[59]

This author's experience is restricted to only one such myxoma affecting the proximal end of the tibia in an adult female (Fig. 12–9). Its appearance and location suggest an early conventional giant cell tumor with a totally lytic presentation in the absence of marginal reactive bone formation. Curettage produced a 15 year disease-free survival.

Four cases of *fibromyxoma* of long bones, a benign tumor having both fibrous and myxoid traits, have been reported: one by Lehmann in 1943[79] and three by Marcove and associates in 1964.[86] These slowly growing, painful lesions appeared in males over the age of 48 years, with involvement of the tibia, the iliac bone, ischiopubic ramus, and the upper end of the ulna. The purely lytic lesions were well-demarcated and on gross examination showed a rubbery firm, light-gray tumor. Microscopic evaluation revealed a fibrous and myxomatous tumor of benign morphologic appearance lacking the characteristic lobular growth pattern or cartilage formation of a chondromyxoid fibroma. Colla-

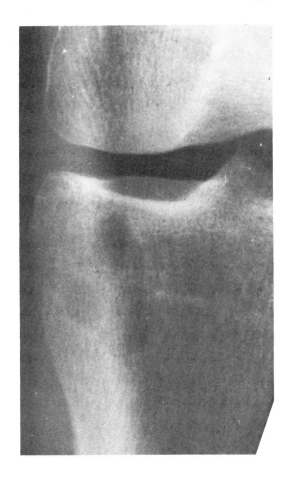

Figure 12-9. Pure myxoma of tibia. This is an entirely osteolytic lesion without marginal reactive bone formation, suggesting an incipient giant cell tumor.

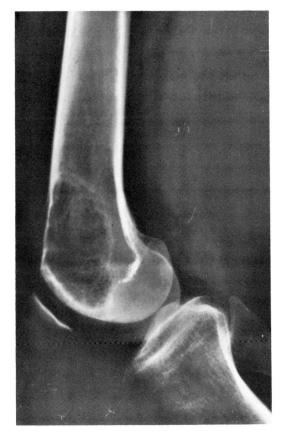

Figure 12-10. Well-delineated, lytic defect in the distal femur in a 34-year-old man. Diagnosis: Fibromyxoma.

genization and focal calcifications were noted. Follow-up information of up to seven years revealed no recurrence following conservative surgical management.[79, 86]

This author has seen and studied other similar examples, one of which occurred in a 34-year-old man with a lytic lesion in the distal end of the femur (Fig. 12–10). As already stated, chondromyxoid fibromas characteristically occur in younger persons, and microscopically, the lesions demonstrate cartilage formation and lobulation.

REFERENCES

1. Acquaviva, R., Tamic, P. M., Thevenot, C., et al.: Los condromas intracraneales. Revisión de la literatura a propósito de dos casos. Rev. Esp. Otoneurooftalmol. Neurocir., 24:15–34, 1965.

2. Aegerter, E., and Kirkpatrick, J. A., Jr.: Orthopedic Diseases. 4th ed. Philadelphia, W. B. Saunders Co., 1975.

3. Andreev, I., Georgiev, V., Krăstin, A., et al.: Bone chondromyxoid fibroma. Vestn. Rentgenol. Radiol., 15(2):110–115, 1976.

4. Antonov, A., Filipović, M., and Nedeljković, J.: Chondromyxoid fibroma of bone. Libri Oncol., 4:53–56, 1975.

5. Attar, S.: Myxoma, a clinicopathologic study. Am. J. Surg., 91:755–760, 1958.

6. Attie, J. N., Catania, A., and Brenner, S.: Myxoma of the maxilla; preoperative irradiation to facilitate resection. Am. J. Roentgenol. Radium Ther. Nucl. Med., 96:19–24, 1966.

7. Barros, R. E., Dominguez, F. V., and Cabrini, R. L.: Myxoma of the jaws. Oral Surg., 27:225–236, 1969.

8. Bauer, W. H., and Harell, A.: Myxoma of bone. J. Bone Joint Surg. [Am.], 36:263–266, 1954.

9. Benedetti, G. B., Canepa, G., and Garcia, M.: Il fibroma condromixoide dell'osso. Arch. Putti Chir. Organi Mov., 17:44–72, 1962.

10. Benedetti, G. B., and Garcia, M.: Il fibroma condromixoide dell'osso. Minerva Ortop., 11:693–698, 1960.

11. Benson, W. R., and Bass, S., Jr.: Chondromyxoid fibroma. First report of occurrence of this tumor in vertebral column. Am. J. Clin. Pathol., 25:1290–1292, 1955.

12. Betts, W. E., Jr., Hitrys, A., Pulich, J. J., et al.: Unusual presentation of chondromyxoid fibroma of bone: report of case. J. Am. Osteopath. Assoc., 74:206–208, 1974.

13. Bloodgood, J. C.: Bone tumors. Myxoma, central and periosteal. Their recurrence after exploratory excision and piecemeal removal. Ann. Surg., 72:713–724, 1920.

14. Bloodgood, J. C.: Bone tumors. Metastasis to lungs from a pure myxoma. Ann. Surg., 77:106–107, 1923.

15. Bloodgood, J. C.: Bone tumors. Myxoma. Second paper with report of three new cases. Ann. Surg., 80:817–833, 1924.

16. Bochetto, J., Minkowitz, F., Minkowitz, S., et al.: Antral fibromyxoma presenting as a giant nasal polyp. Oral Surg., 23:201–206, 1967.

17. Brewer, A. C., and Johnson, J. H.: Myxoma of the mandible. Br. J. Surg., 43:325–326, 1955.

18. Browne, R. M., and Rivas, P. H.: Chondromyxoid fibroma of the mandible: a case report. Br. J. Oral Surg., 15:19–25, 1977.

19. Bruce, K. W., and Royer, R. Q.: Central fibromyxoma of the maxilla. Oral Surg., 5:1277–1281,1952.

20. Buchner, A., and Ramon, Y.: Fibromyxoma of the maxilla. J. Oral Surg., 23:145–148, 1965.

21. Canalis, R. F., Smith, G. A., and Konrad, H. R.: Myxomas of the head and neck. Arch. Otolaryngol., 102:300–305, 1976.

22. Carsin, M., Daverne, A., Denizet, D., et al.: Aspects radiologiques des fibromes chondromyxoides. J. Radiol. Electrol. Med. Nucl., 55:901–902, 1973.

23. Cawson, R. A.: Myxoma of the mandible with a 35 year follow-up. Br. J. Oral Surg., 10:59–63, 1972.

24. Chacha, P. B., and Tan, K. K.: Periosteal myxoma of the femur: a case report. J. Bone Joint Surg. [Am.], 54:1091–1094, 1972.

25. Christ, B.: Über das chondromyxoide Fibrom des Knochens. Dissertation. Faculty of Medicine, University of Basel, 1957, pp. 3–12.

26. Cohen, P. B., and Gamble, J. W.: Maxillary resection for odontogenic myxoma: report of case. J. Oral Surg., 35:573–577, 1977.

27. Colburn, J. F., and Epker, B. N.: Myxoma of the mandibular condyle — surgical excision with immediate reconstruction. J. Oral Surg., 33:351–355, 1975.

28. Coley, B. L., and Higinbotham, N. L.: Tumors of Bone: A Roentgenographic Atlas. New York, Paul B. Hoeber, Inc., 1953.

29. Copello, O.: Mixoma del metatarsiano. Bol. Trab. Cir. Buenos Aires 19:1151–1154, 1935.

30. Dabska, M., Rudowski, W., and Loth, F.: Fibroma chondromyxoides. A new oncological entity of the skeletal system. Nowotwory, 9:275–285, 1959.

31. Dahlin, D. C.: Chondromyxoid fibroma of bone, with emphasis on its morphological relationship to benign chondroblastoma. Cancer, 9:195–203, 1956.

32. Dahlin, D. C., Wells, A. H., and Henderson, E. D.: Chondromyxoid fibroma of bone. Report of 2 cases. J. Bone Joint Surg. [Am.], 35:831–834, 1953.

33. Daniels, D. W.: A case of pure myxoma of the lower jaw. Lancet, 2:1747, 1908.

34. Dihlmann, W., and Müller, G.: Konnatales Chondromyxoidfibrom des Radius. Fortschr. Geb. Roentgenstr. Nuklearmed., 110:759–761, 1969.

35. Dutt, A. K., Dhillon, D. S., and bin Din, O.: Chondromyxoid fibroma of the ilium: report of a case. Med. J. Malaysia, 24:71–73, 1977.

36. Dutz, W., and Stout, A. P.: The myxoma in childhood. Cancer, 14:629–635, 1961.

37. Edmunds, L. H., and Jones, H.: Chondromyxoid fibroma of bone. Bull. Mason Clin., 10:1–9, 1956.

38. Everke, H.: Ein Myxochondrom — Chondro-

myxoid-Fibrom — der Schädelbasis mit Ausdehnung in den Canalis spinalis. Acta Neurochir., *15*:150–158, 1966.

39. Farman, A. G., Nortjé, C. J., Grotepass, F. W., et al.: Myxofibroma of the jaws. Br. J. Oral Surg., *15*:3–18, 1977.

40. Feldman, F., Hecht, H. L., and Johnston, A. D.: Chondromyxoid fibroma of bone. Radiology, *44*:249–260, 1970.

41. Fleischmann, L.: Osteomyxom der Siebbeinzellen. Monatsschr. Ohrenheilkd. Laryngorhinol., *81*:349–352, 1947.

42. Frank, W. E., and Rockwood, C. A.: Chondromyxoidfibroma: review of the literature and report of 4 cases. South. Med. J., *62*:1248–1253, 1969.

43. Fu, Y.-S., and Perzin, K. H.: Non-epithelial tumors of the nasal cavity, paranasal sinuses and nasopharynx: A clinicopathologic study. VII. Myxomas. Cancer, *39*:195–203, 1977.

44. Gacyk, W., Pikiel, L., Bilczuk, B., et al.: Chondro-myxoid fibroma of the calcaneus. Chir. Narzadow Ruchu Ortop. Pol., *36*:127–132, 1971.

45. Gandin, J., and Mollaret, L.: Un cas de fibrome chondromyxoïde d'une phalange traité par evidement-bourrage. Mem. Acad. Chir., *87*:381–386, 1961.

46. Gérard-Marchant, M. P.: Un cas de fibrome chondro-myxoïde. Mem. Acad. Chir., *84*:126–127, 1958.

47. Ghosh, B. C., Huvos, A. G., Gerold, F. P., et al.: Myxoma of the jaw bones. Cancer, *31*:237–240, 1973.

48. Giambelli, G., and Mincione, A.: Fibroma condromixoide del calcagno. Minerva Ortop., *15*:20–23, 1964.

49. Goorwitch, J.: Chondromyxoid fibroma of rib. Report of an unusual benign primary tumor. Dis. Chest, *20*:186–193, 1951.

50. Grumillier, H., Gaussin, D., Parache, R., et al.: Fibrome chondro-myxoïde de l'os iliaque. Ann. Med. (Nancy), *13*:411–418, 1974.

51. Hadders, H. N., and Oterdoom, H. J.: Chondromyxoid fibroma of the bone. Ned. Tijdschr. Geneeskd., *48*:555–559, 1954.

52. Harbert, F., Gerry, R. G., and Dimette, R. M.: Myxoma of the mandible. Oral Surg., *2*:1414–1421, 1949.

53. Harnes, D., Finstervosh, A., and Fuchs, T.: Chondro-myxoid fibroma. Harefuah, *80*:382–384, 1971.

54. Harris, R. J., Garrow, E., and Spinnato, G.: Myxoma of the maxilla. Report of case. J. Oral Surg., *35*:70–73, 1977.

55. Harrison, J. D.: Odontogenic myxoma: ultrastructural and histochemical studies. J. Clin. Pathol., *26*:570–582, 1973.

56. Harrison, J. D., and Eggleston, D. J.: Odontogenic myxoma of the maxilla; a case report and some interesting histological findings. Br. J. Oral Surg., *11*:13 17, 1973.

57. Hayward, J. R.: Odontogenic myxofibroma of the mandible: report of a case. J. Oral Surg., *13*:149–155, 1955.

58. Herfath, H.: Ein zentrales Myxom der Tibia. Arch. Klin. Chir., *170*:283–286, 1932.

59. Hill, J. A., Victor, T. A., Dawson, W. J., et al.: Myxoma of the toe. A case report. J. Bone Joint Surg. [Am.], *60*:128–130, 1978.

60. Hodson, J. J., and Prout, R. E. S.: Chemical and histochemical characterization of mucopolysaccharides in a jaw myxoma. J. Clin. Pathol., *21*:582–589, 1968.

61. Hovnanian, A. P.: Myxoma of the maxilla. Report of two cases. Oral Surg., *6*:927–936. 1953.

62. Hutchison, J., and Park, W. W.: Chondromyxoid fibroma of bone. Report of a case. J. Bone Joint Surg. [Br.], *42*:542–548, 1960.

63. Iwata, S., and Coley, B. L.: Report of 6 cases of chondromyxoid fibroma of bone. Surg. Gynecol. Obstet., *107*:571–576, 1958.

64. Jaffe, H. L.: Tumors and Tumorous Conditions of the Bones and Joints. Philadelphia, Lea & Febiger, 1958.

65. Jaffe, H. L., and Lichtenstein, L.: Chondromyxoid fibroma of bone. A distinctive benign tumor likely to be mistaken especially for chondrosarcoma. Arch. Pathol., *45*:541–551, 1948.

66. Kangur, T. T., Dahlin, D. C., and Turlington, E. G.: Myxomatous tumors of the jaws. J. Oral Surg., *33*:523–528, 1975.

67. Knysh, I. T.: Diagnosis and treatment of chondromyxoid fibroma of bones. Vestn. Khir., *117*(12):59–63, 1976.

68. Koblin, I.: Klinik, Beurteilung und Behandlung der odontogenen Myxome (Fibromyxome). Dtsch. Zahnaerztl. Z, *32*:788–293, 1977.

69. Komitowski, D.: On histogenesis and differential diagnosis of chondromyxoid fibroma. Chir. Narzadow Ruchu Ortop. Pol., *34*:673–678, 1969.

70. Korolev, V. Í., Goldshmidt, B. Ya., and Trushkevich, L. Í.: A rare localization of chondromyxoid fibroma. Vopr. Onkol., *22*(8):89–91, 1976.

71. Kothare, S. N., Morris, S. E., and Joshi, B. B.: Chondromyxoid fibroma of bone. A report of two cases. Indian J. Radiol., *19*:208–213, 1965.

72. Krauspe, C.: Über einen chondroblastischen Riesenzelltumor (Chondromyxoidfibrom). Zentralbl. Allg. Pathol., *97*:16–24, 1957–58.

73. Kreikenbaum, D., Foth, K., and Ringk, H.: Chondromyxoidfibrom der Fibula. Dtsch. Gesundh.-Wes., *26*:1451–1453, 1971.

74. Kuhlman, R. E., and McNamee, M. J.: Quantitative microchemical studies of chondroblastoma, giant-cell tumor, chondromyxoid fibroma and desmoplastic fibroma. Clin. Orthop., *69*:264–270, 1970.

75. Kunkel, M. G., Dahlin, D. C., and Young, H. H.: Benign chondroblastoma. J. Bone Joint Surg. [Am.], *38*:817–826, 1956.

76. Lanzi, F., and Conti, R.: Concerning chondromyxoid fibroma. Arch. Ortop., *78*:345–363, 1965.

77. Large, N. D., Niebel, H. H., and Fredericks, W. H.: Myxoma of the jaws. Report of two cases. Oral Surg., *13*:1462–1468, 1960.

78. Lehmann, O.: "Myxofibroma" of bone: report of case involving tibia. Bull. Hosp. Joint Dis., *4*:12–15, 1943.

79. Lehmann, P.: Fibrome chondro-myxoïde de l'aile iliaque chez un enfant de dix ans. Ann. Chir. Infant., *10*:209–212, 1969.

80. Lelaidier, B. L. C.: Contribution à l'étude du fibrome chondromyxoide des os. Thesis. Faculté de Médecine de Paris, 1957.

81. Levy, W. M., Aegerter, E. E., and Kirkpatrick, J.

A., Jr.; The nature of cartilaginous tumors. Radiol. Clin. North. Am., 2:327–336, 1964.

82. Lichtenstein, L.: Bone Tumors. 4th ed. St. Louis, C. V. Mosby Co., 1972.

83. Lipkin, S. E.: Chondromyxoid fibroma (concerning the variants and microscopic diagnosis). Arkh. Pathol., 33(8):25–31, 1971.

84. Lund, B. A., and Waite, D. B.: Mandibular myxoma: report of case. J. Oral Surg., 24:454–459, 1966.

85. Manfrini, M.: Considerazioni sul fibroma condromixoide dell'osso. Atti Soc. Emiliana Romagnola Triveneta Ortop. Traum., 9:109–122, 1964.

86. Marcove, R. C., Kambolis, C., Bullough, P. G., et al.: Fibromyxoma of bone: a report of 3 cases. Cancer, 17:1209–1213, 1964.

87. Mauck, R. H., and Carpenter, E. B.: Chondromyxoid fibroma of bone. Report of case. Va. Med. Mon., 86:210–212, 1959.

88. McClure, D. K., and Dahlin, D. C.: Myxoma of bone. Report of 3 cases. Mayo Clin. Proc., 52:249–253, 1977.

89. Miglani, D. C., and Ballantyne, A. J.: Myxoma of the mandible, followed by resection and prosthetic repair. Report of a case. Oral Surg., 12:1032–1039, 1959.

90. Mikulowski, P., and Ostberg, G.: Recurrent chondromyxoid fibroma. Acta Orthop. Scand., 42:385–390, 1971.

91. Mori, M., Murakami, M., Hirose, I., et al.: Histochemical studies of myxoma of the jaws. J. Oral Surg., 33:529–536, 1975.

92. Münzenberg, K. J., and Cremer, H.: Multicentric chondro-myxoid-fibroma of bone with extraskeletal foci. Z. Orthop., 115:355–362, 1977.

93. Murphy, N. B., and Price, C. H. G.: The radiological aspects of chondromyxoid fibroma of bone. Clin. Radiol., 22:261–269, 1971.

94. Orso, C. A.: Considerazioni sul fibroma condromixoide. Minerva Ortop., 18:42–47, 1967.

95. Papp, P., and Toth, K.: Odontogenic myxoma of the mandible. Report of a case. Oral Surg., 20:82–84, 1965.

96. Parrini, L., and Spina, G. M.: Considerazioni sui mixomi dell'osso. Minerva Ortop., 13:253–259, 1962.

97. Perou, M. L., Kolis, J. A., Zaeske, E. V., et al.: Myxoma of the toe: case report. Cancer, 20:1030–1034, 1967.

98. Pisar, D. E.: Chondromyxoid fibroma of the ilium with postresection subluxation of the hemipelvis. Tex. Med., 65:52–55, 1969.

99. Prichard, R. W., Stoy, R. P., and Barwick, J. T. F.: Chondromyxoid fibroma of the scapula. Report of a case. J. Bone Joint Surg. [Am.], 46:1759–1760, 1964.

100. Radden, B. G., and Reade, P. C.: Odontogenic myxoma of the jaw. Oral Surg., 15:355–361, 1962.

101. Rahimi, A., Beabout, J. W., Ivins, J. C., et al.: Chondromyxoid fibroma: a clinicopathologic study of 76 cases. Cancer, 30:726–736, 1972.

102. Ralph, L. L.: Chondromyxoid fibroma of bone. J. Bone Joint Surg. [Br.], 44:7–24, 1962.

103. Ramani, P. S.: Chondromyxoid fibroma: a rare cause of spinal cord compression. Case report. J. Neurosurg., 40:107–109, 1974.

104. Randelli, M.: Sul fibroma condromixoide osseo. Arch. Ortop., 74:857–864, 1961.

105. Rao, T. V., and Rao, K. S.: Central myxoma of the mandible in a child: report of case. J. Oral Surg., 32:617–619, 1974.

106. Riachi, E.: Chondromyxoid fibroma du calcanéum. Rev. Med. Moy. Or., 19:615–617, 1962.

107 Rossi, P., and Marinosci, M.: Il fibroma condromixoide. Rass. Fisiopatol. Clin. Ter., 33:52–61, 1961.

108. Roy, B., and Jobard, P.: Un cas de fibrome chondro-myxoïde du tibia. Mem. Acad. Chir., 85:536–540, 1959.

109. Royer, M.: Fibrome chondromyxoïde de la hanche. Laval Méd., 29:467–470, 1960.

110. Saigal, R. K., Khanna, S. D., and Singh, H.: Chondromyxoid fibroma of bone. A clinicopathological study of 9 cases and review of literature. Indian J. Cancer, 11:102–107, 1974.

111. Salzer, M., and Salzer-Kuntschik, M.: Das Chondromyxoidfibrom. Langenbecks Arch. Chir., 312:216–231, 1965.

112. Scaglietti, O., and Stringa, G.: Myxoma of bone in childhood. J. Bone Joint Surg. [Am.], 43:67–80, 1961.

113. Schajowicz, F., and Gallardo, H.: Chondromyxoid fibroma (fibromyxoid chondroma) of bone. A clinico-pathological study of 32 cases. J. Bone Joint Surg. [Br.] 53:198–216, 1971.

114. Schultz, L. W., and Vazirani, S. J.: Central odontogenic fibromyxoma of the mandible. Report of a case. Oral Surg., 10:690–695, 1957.

115. Schutt, P. G., and Frost, H. M.: Chondromyxoid fibroma. Clin. Orthop., 78:323–329, 1971.

116. Sedano, H. O., and Gorlin, R. J.: Odontogenic myxoma: some histochemical considerations. Arch. Oral Biol., 10:727–729, 1965.

117. Sehayik, S., and Rosman, M. A.: Malignant degeneration of a chondromyxoid fibroma in a child. Can. J. Surg., 18:354–360, 1975.

118. Seror, J., Mussini-Montpellier, Mme., Azoulay, Cl., et al.: Fibrome chondromyxoïde du tibia. Afr. Franc. Chir., 18:172–173, 1960.

119. Seth, H. N., and Rao, B. D. P.: Chondromyxoid fibroma of bone. Report on 3 cases. Indian J. Pathol. Bacteriol., 7:112–117, 1964.

120. Shafranski, L. L., Kushinkov, I. U. A., and Isakova, E. V.: Spectroscopic study of an extract of a chondromyxoid fibroma. Vopr. Onkol., 17(5):96–99, 1971.

121. Shrikhande, S. S., and Sirsat, M. V.: Chondromyxoid fibroma bone. (Observations on 5 cases.) Indian J. Radiol., 19:8–11, 1965.

122. Sideman, S., Sarrafian, S., and Topouzian, L. K.: Chondromyxoid fibroma of bone. Review of the literature. Report of a case with pathological fracture. Q. Bull. Northw. Univ. Med. Sch., 35:346–351, 1961.

123. Simes, R. J., Barros, R. E., Klein-Szanto, A. J. P., et al.: Ultrastructure of an odontogenic myxoma. Oral Surg., 39:640–646, 1975.

124. Sirsat, M. V.: Central myxoma of the jaw. Report of a case. Indian J. Med. Sci., 8:639, 1954.

125. Sonesson, A.: Odontogenic cysts and cystic tumours of the jaws; roentgen-diagnostic and patho-anatomic study. Acta Radiol., 81(Supplement):1–159, 1950.

126. Soren, A.: Myxoma in bone. Clin. Orthop., 37:145–149, 1964.

127. Soubeyran, P.: Le myxome pur des os. Rev. Chir., 29:239–252, 588–601, 1904.

128. Spina. G. M.: Fibroma condromixoide della scapola. Chir. Organi Mov., 50:418–426, 1961.

129. Stout, A. P.: Myxoma, the tumor of primitive mesenchyme. Ann. Surg., 127:706–719, 1948.

130. Stradford, H. T.: Chondromyxoid fibroma of bone. Bull. Charlotte Mem. Hosp., 3:7–11, 1948.

131. Teitelbaum, S. L., and Bessone, L.: Resection of a large chondromyxoid fibroma of the sternum. Report of the first case and review of the literature. J. Thorac. Cardiovasc. Surg., 57:333–340, 1969.

132. Thoma, K. H., and Goldman, H. M.: Central myxoma of the jaw. Am. J. Orthod., 33:532–540, 1947.

133. Tornberg, D. N., Rice, R. W., and Johnston, A. D.: The ultrastructure of chondromyxoid fibroma. Its biologic and diagnostic implications. Clin. Orthop., 95:295–299, 1973.

134. Trifaud, A., and Bureau, H.: Fibrome chondromyxoide de l'extrémité inférieure du péroné. Mem. Acad. Chir., 87:386–390, 1961.

135. Trifaud, A., and Bureau, H.: Diagnostic radiologique des fibromes chondromyxoïdes. Ann. Chir. Infant., 5:223–229, 1964.

136. Turcotte, B., Pugh, D. G., and Dahlin, D. C.: The roentgenologic aspects of chondromyxoid fibroma of bone. Am. J. Roentgenol. Radium Ther. Nucl. Med., 87:1085–1095, 1962.

137. Uthman, A. A., and Perriman, A. O.: Myxoma of the mandible. Br. J. Oral Surg., 9:151–153, 1971.

138. Villalobos de Montiel, A., Sánchez, H. A., and Plumacher, A.: Histologic variant of juxta-articular myxoma. Rev. Fac. Med. (Maracaibo), 6:232–236, 1973.

139. Vinogradova, T. P., and Berman, A. M.: Chondromyxoid fibroma of bone. Khirurgiia (Mosk), 36(6):128–131, 1960.

140. Vinogradova, T. P., and Lipkin, S. I.: Chondromyxoid fibroma. Arkh. Patol., 36(4):83–84, 1974.

141. Virchow, R.: Die Cellularpathologie in ihrer Begründung auf physiologische und pathologische Gewebelehre. Berlin, August Hirschwald, 1871, p. 563.

142. Vix, V. A., and Fahmy, A.: Unusual appearance of a chondromyxoid fibroma. Radiology, 92:365–366, 1969.

143. Westwood, R. M., Alexander, R. W., and Bennett, D. E.: Giant odontogenic myxofibroma. Report of a case with histochemical and ultrastructural studies and a review of the literature. Oral Surg., 37:83–92, 1974.

144. White, D. K., Chin, S. Y., Mohnac, A. M., et al.: Odontogenic myxoma. A clinical and ultrastructural study. Oral Surg., 39:901–917, 1975.

145. Whitman, R. A., Stewart, S., Stopack, J. G., et al.: Myxoma of the mandible: Report of a case. J. Oral Surg., 28:63–70, 1971.

146. Wiart, P., Saout, J., Bizard, J., et al.: Fibrome chondromyxoïde costal. J. Sci. Méd. Lille, 88:673–676, 1970.

147. Wirth, W. A., Leavitt, D., and Enzinger, F. M.: Multiple intramuscular myxomas: another extraskeletal manifestation of fibrous dysplasia. Cancer, 27:1167–1173, 1971.

148. Witwicki, T., and Daniluk, A.: Three cases of malignant chondro-myxo-fibroma of bone. Chir. Narzadow Ruchu Ortop. Pol., 36:653–659, 1971.

149. Witwicki, T., and Dziak, A.: Malignant and benign chondromyxoid fibroma. Wiad. Lek., 20(24):2211–2213, 1967.

150. Wrenn, R. N., and Smith, A. G.: Chondromyxoid fibroma. South. Med. J., 47:848–854, 1954.

151. Young, W. G., and Ball, A. T.: Central myxofibroma of the jaws. J. Oral Surg., 26:408–410, 1968.

152. Zimmerman, D. C., and Dahlin, D. C.: Myxomatous tumors of the jaws. Oral Surg., 11:1069–1080, 1958.

Cartilage-forming Tumors — Malignant Chapters 13 and 14

13

CHONDROSARCOMA AND MESENCHYMAL CHONDROSARCOMA

CHONDROSARCOMA

DEFINITION

Chondrosarcoma is a malignant tumor in which the basic neoplastic tissue is fully developed cartilage without tumor osteoid being directly formed by a sarcomatous stroma. Myxoid changes, calcification, or ossification may be present.

INCIDENCE

Excluding multiple myeloma, chondrosarcoma is second to osteogenic sarcoma in frequency as a malignant tumor of bone. It makes up approximately 17 to 22 per cent of all primary bone tumors.

TYPES OF CHONDROSARCOMA — NOMENCLATURE

Primary chondrosarcoma arises *de novo* in a previously normal bone; i.e., the tumor shows its sarcomatous properties from the very onset. *Secondary chondrosarcoma* develops from a pre-existent benign cartilage tumor. Usually, this is an enchondroma, the cartilage cap of an osteocartilaginous exostosis, or, quite uncommonly, a juxtacortical chondroma. Repeated surgical excisions following recurrences often precede malignant transformation. In advanced lesions, it is sometimes difficult to ascertain whether the chondrosarcoma is of primary or of secondary origin, and it is almost impossible to estimate the relative frequency of primary and secondary chondrosarcomas (Fig. 13–1). Protracted clinical history or densely calcified lesions suggest, but do not definitely prove, that a chondrosarcoma is derived from a pre-existent benign condition. The only truly acceptable evidence is the histologic confirmation of a preceding tumor. In the case of a malignant transformation of an osteochondroma, the histologic identification of the still-remaining unchanged base or ped-

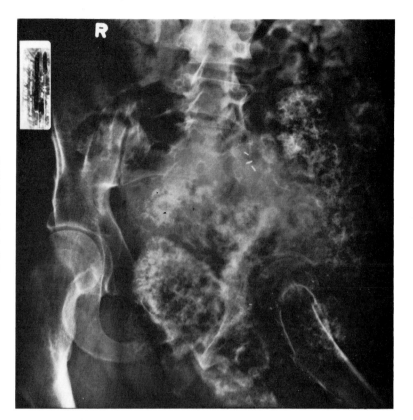

Figure 13–1. Inoperable chondrosarcoma involving the left femur and pelvic bones in a 24-year-old man who had multiple osteochondromatosis from the age of seven. Sudden increase in the size of the pelvic lesion occurred three years ago.

icle is of importance. The problem in proving that chondrosarcomas arise in enchondroma is due to the difficulty in identifying remnants of a benign cartilaginous lesion. In most cases of presumed preexistent enchondroma, one will find that the unequivocal histologic evidence is lacking and that the majority of such lesions are low-grade chondrosarcoma from the very onset.

Chondrosarcoma may be designated as *peripheral* or *central* depending on the location in the involved bone. Rarely, malignant cartilage lesions may also arise in relation to the cortex in periosteal structures and are referred to as *juxtacortical chondrosarcomas.*[24, 70, 145, 175]

On occasion, the problem arises as to whether the lesion represents a juxtacortical or extraskeletal chondrosarcoma. If the lesion is not connected to bone (including *periosteum*) or cartilage (including perichondrium), the tumor is an extraosseous chondrosarcoma, unless previous radiographic or pathologic examination clearly shows the lesion to be secondarily involving bone or cartilage.

It is a relatively easy matter to classify chondrosarcomas in their early stages of evolution, whether they are central or peripheral, especially if they arise in a long tubular bone. In large lesions, or in those involving flat bones with massive osseous destruction, it is frequently futile to attempt to designate the exact position of origin. For instance, O'Neal and Ackerman studied 40 chondrosarcomas, but in 5, they were unable to determine the exact site of origin.[119] Lindbom and associates failed to establish whether the lesions were central or peripheral in 6 of 39 chondrosarcomas studied.[90] The examination of a slice of the whole specimen, however, in some instances indicates whether the origin is central or peripheral.

Chondrosarcomas may be induced by irradiation. Among the 168 cases of radiation-induced bone sarcomas culled from the literature approximately 9 per cent were chondrosarcomas.[43]

Among 68 chondrosarcomas reported by Thomson and Turner-Warwick, 6 arose in association with Paget's disease.[162] Chondrosarcomas may be associated with fibrous dysplasia,[42, 68] unicameral bone cyst,[58] or Maffucci's syndrome[87] (see Chapter 10).

Many instances of chondrosarcomas have been described as superimposed on enchondromatosis (Ollier's disease),[26, 66] multiple hereditary exostosis,[77] chondromyxoid fibroma, and chondroblastoma. Some patients with multiple enchondromatosis or hereditary exostoses may develop more than one chondrosarcoma, either synchronously or metachronously.[10, 19]

SIGNS AND SYMPTOMS

In spite of the wide publicity, pain and tenderness are not reliable and consistent features of primary or secondary chondrosarcoma since only approximately one third of the patients with chondrosarcomas arising in ribs manifested this discomfort initially. When present, these symptoms are rarely severe but provide a valuable diagnostic aid, since benign cartilage lesions are not tender or painful. Peripheral chondrosarcomas especially are often symptomless, usually presenting with only a minor discomfort and palpable swelling (Fig. 13–2). In several reports, a painless tumor mass of long standing appears to be the presenting symptom in many cases.[100, 160] Pelvic tumors, however large, remain hidden for a very long time in the pelvic cavity until the lesions grow sufficiently large to be palpable through the abdominal musculature or nerve compression with radiating pain of sciatic, femoral, or obturator distribution is evidenced. This extremely slow growth of an asymptomatic tumor delays the discovery and treatment of pelvic chondrosarcoma. In cases in which the tumor involves the inner aspect of the innominate bone, its growth is complicated by disturbances in intestinal and vesical function and by lymphatic obstruction with severe lymphedema.[49] Occasionally, a disk syndrome may be the presenting sign and unnecessary myelograms are performed in the search for the source of the pain. Persistent and unrelenting pain in a supposed enchondroma involving the long bones or the pelvic and shoulder girdles is suspicious for chondrosarcoma until proved otherwise!

Rapidly expanding high-grade central chondrosarcomas may cause excruciating pain that is usually commensurate with their rate of cortical destruction.[119] The duration of symptoms, as reported by pa-

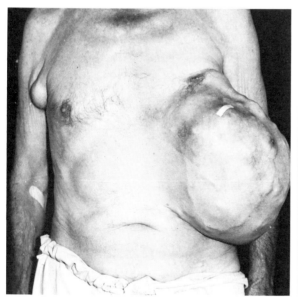
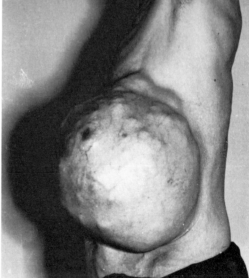

Figure 13–2. Huge chondrosarcoma of rib slowly progressing for over 15 years. Patient arrested several times on suspicion of shoplifting.

tients, varies considerably; it was less than two years for 75 per cent of the patients and less than five years for the rest.[100]

ALTERED CARBOHYDRATE METABOLISM

An altered carbohydrate metabolism has been reported in various neoplastic conditions.[170] The proliferating neoplastic cells utilize greater amounts of glucose,[64] and an increased glycolysis is noted in tumor tissue.[75] Similar to the findings by Marks and Bishop[103] in patients with malignant disease, Marcove[101] observed decreased intravenous glucose tolerance test results in a series of 75 chondrosarcoma patients. Often, normal blood glucose levels are found in the face of a diabetic glucose tolerance curve. In an autopsy study of 15 chondrosarcoma patients, there was definite hypertrophy and hyperplasia of the islets of Langerhans as compared to normal controls.[50] The patients with chondrosarcoma had a greater number of cells per islet in the pancreas, with increase in the number of alpha and beta cells.

AGE AND SEX DISTRIBUTION

Among 264 patients with chondrosarcomas studied at Memorial Hospital from 1949 to 1973, 149 were male and 115 were female (Fig. 13–3). Their ages ranged from 7 to 73 years. The average age was 40 years among the male patients and 43 years among female patients. A considerable number of cases occurred in the first two decades of life, thereby pointing out the common misconception that chondrosarcomas do not occur in this age group.

LOCATION

Chondrosarcoma may develop in any bone preformed in cartilage (Fig. 13–4). The most frequent locations are in the pelvis (31 per cent), the femur (21 per cent), especially the proximal femoral diaphysis, the ribs (9 per cent), the craniofacial bones (9.4 per cent), and the shoulder girdle (13 per cent). The least common sites of involvement are the forearm, or hand, the

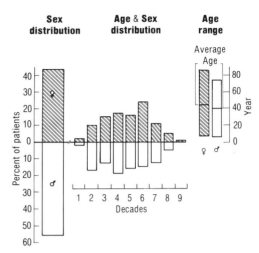

Figure 13–3. Age and sex distribution of 264 patients (149 men and 115 women) treated at Memorial Hospital from 1949 to 1973 (inclusive).

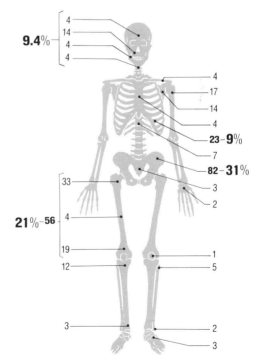

Figure 13–4. Skeletal location of 264 cases of chondrosarcoma treated at Memorial Hospital from 1949 to 1973 (inclusive).

spine, and the bones of the foot.[9, 10, 35, 57] Chondrosarcoma is the most common malignant tumor of the scapula[151] and the sternum.[104] There have been only 21 reported cases of chondrosarcoma in the bones of the hand and in only 4 of these was there evidence of a pre-existing enchondroma.

RADIOGRAPHIC FINDINGS

Central chondrosarcomas demonstrate large, thick-walled areas of radiolucency with trabeculation and central areas of multilocular medullary bone destruction (Fig. 13–5). Foci of irregularly scattered spotty or blotchy calcification represented by densities throughout the lesion are noted. These calcifications have also been described as appearing as "fluffy," "cotton wool," "popcorn," or "breadcrumb" configuration. Cortical destruction occurs late in the course of the disease, and periosteal bone formation is usually limited (Fig. 13–

6). On its endosteal surface, the cortex is scalloped by the lobular outlines of the tumor. The diagnosis of chondrosarcoma is quite difficult when there is only a solitary lytic defect without calcification.[134] Some lesions may show thinning and bulging expansion of the cortex, or a cystic radiolucent appearance may even be presented. In such cases, the evidence for a truly malignant tumor may be lacking (Fig. 13–8).[21] The Netherlands Bone Tumour Registry reported several cases in which the lesion extended over almost the entire length of the long bone with heavy layering of coarse periosteal bone formation. This presentation may mimic Paget's disease of the bone.[115] The rapidly evolving central tumors may show no evidence of radiolucency at all, but periosteal bone formation adjacent to the lesion may be evident. Late in the development of the disease process, the soft tissues adjacent to the osseous site of the lesion may be massively infiltrated by chondrosarcoma, but radiopa-

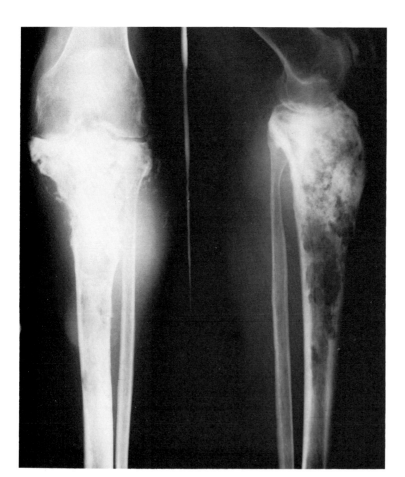

Figure 13–5. Low-grade central chondrosarcoma of upper end of left tibia in a 48-year-old man. The roentgenograph shows a highly calcified, central, irregularly radiolucent lesion occupying large portion of the shaft with cortical destruction.

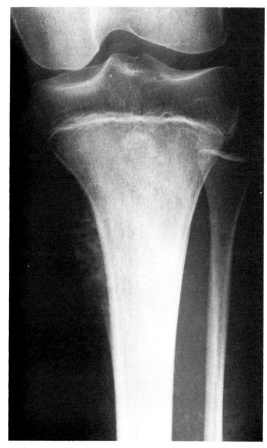

Figure 13–6. Low-grade chondrosarcoma of upper end of tibia in an 11-year-old girl. Centrally located, irregularly dense radiolucency with periosteal lipping and bone formation.

are characteristic of chondrosarcoma, reach the length of 2.5 cm or more, while those in osteogenic sarcoma usually measure less than 1.5 to 2 cm in length. The flattened outer surface of the spicules distinguishes chondrosarcoma from osteogenic sarcoma.[126] It is probably caused by molding of the outermost ends of the spicules on the overlying muscles.

In the early peripheral chondrosarcoma, the radiographs may show a faintly radiopaque wedge-shaped shadow between the cortex and the elevated periosteum. This elevation is commonly referred to as "lipping" or the so-called "Codman's triangle" and is a useful diagnostic feature of this lesion. Periosteal stripping at the level of tumor involvement, and adjacent to it, is seen with some radiating calcified spicules and ossification. Cortical or medullary involvement is slight in the early cases.

Secondary Chondrosarcoma

Radiographically, in early central chondrosarcomas arising in enchondromas, there may be evidence of the original benign primary lesion, but more often than not the pre-existent condition is not demonstrable. The superimposed malignant change is characterized by a fuzzy infiltrating periosteal density. Once the tumor is in an advanced stage, the entire lesion becomes irregularly and coarsely granular, and infiltration with scattered foci of ossifications is noted. The adjacent soft tissues show evidence of stippled calcification, another time-honored diagnostic feature.[25, 129] Frequently, it is very difficult to establish radiographically the pre-existence of an osteocartilaginous exostosis in secondary peripheral chondrosarcomas (Fig. 13–7). The progressive gradual erasure of the smooth outlines of a cartilaginous cap from the periphery inward toward the cortex and a soft tissue mass with foci of irregular calcific speckles represent fairly good evidence that malignant transformation has taken place.[88]

The evaluation of cortical destruction at the base of the tumor is made difficult by the large mass hiding it. The lesions present with lobulated contours with an intermixture of radiolucent and radiopaque areas. Radiopacity is due to calcification and ossification, but there is a great varia-

city, a sign of calcification, may be missing entirely. At the site of cortical invasion by a central chondrosarcoma, the cortical shadow is fuzzy. Pathologic fracture through the lesion results in rapid tumor penetration into the soft tissues with concurrent calcific densities of the extraosseous mass.

The *peripheral chondrosarcoma* reveals a faintly visible, sparsely calcified shadow in the soft tissues next to the lesion, with radiating spicules or large speckles arranged at right angles to the cortex. The adjacent periosteum is elevated but no medullary involvement is demonstrated, and the cortex is rarely affected. The soft tissue shadow cast by the lesion is usually so faint that its presence may be entirely missed. The perpendicular radiating spicules with flattened outer surface, which

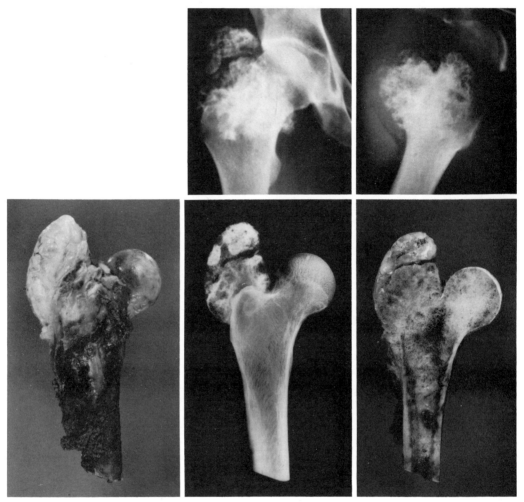

Figure 13–7. Low-grade chondrosarcoma arising in osteochondroma of femur. A 10 by 7 by 6 cm, lobulated cartilaginous mass involves the greater trochanter. A central core of bone and peripheral hyaline cartilage cap are present. The mass overlies and compresses, but does not involve, the femoral neck. *En bloc* resection of proximal femur with total hip replacement. (Courtesy of Dr. R. C. Marcove.)

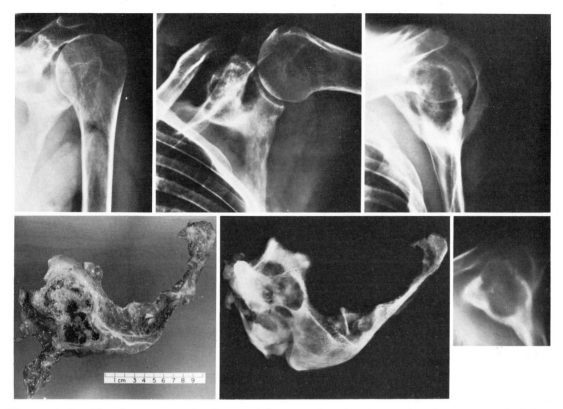

Figure 13–8. Chondrosarcoma, Grade II, of the scapula. This 5 cm, sharply circumscribed lytic lesion of the coracoid process shows a central area of sclerosis with extension into the anterior surface of the glenoid cavity. The lateral tomograms, using trispiral motion, show an irregular destructive lesion with superior expansion and multiple calcifications. The superior cortex is thin with questionable break-through in several areas. (Courtesy of Dr. R. Booher.)

bility in the amount and extent of the radiopaque lesional density in the various tumors. The spectrum varies from massive calcification to stippled flecks of calcium in a largely radiolucent lesion (Fig. 13–8). There may be variation in the extent of calcification within the different areas of the same tumor. Peripheral areas are usually more radiolucent than the center, and more than occasionally, the most peripheral portion of the tumor is totally radiolucent and lacks confining borders, thereby remaining undetectable on radiologic examination. Accordingly, the exact size of the tumor is, more often than not, grossly underestimated by the radiologist. Contrast radiography of adjacent structures and organs, e.g., intravenous pyelogram and so on, may be used to establish the exact dimensions of the cartilaginous mass.

In the roentgenologic evaluation of sternal chondrosarcomas, not only posteroanterior and lateral views are useful but also oblique and cross-table lateral positions make the diagnosis less difficult.[104] Chondrosarcomas of the sternum show coarse, mottled, intralesional calcifications (Fig. 13–9). The roentgenographic distinction between benign and malignant cartilage tumors at this location is quite tenuous, unless cortical destruction and soft tissue involvement are demonstrable.[104]

RADIOGRAPHIC DIFFERENTIAL DIAGNOSIS

1. Chondromas are generally more radiopaque.
2. Radiolucent lesion with stippled and blotchy calcification is more likely to be a chondrosarcoma; however, heavy calcification may indeed occur in chondrosarcoma.
3. Bone destruction may occur in both

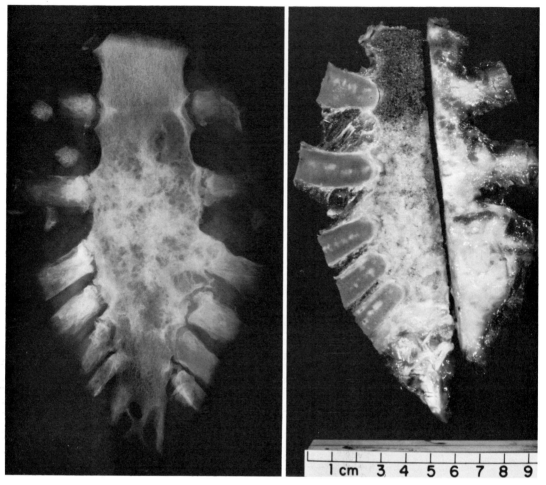

Figure 13–9. Chondrosarcoma of sternum in a 55-year-old man. Specimen radiograph shows a mottled, calcific lesion. The gross specimen reveals a total replacement of the sternum by a cartilaginous tumor. (Case 2 from Martini, N., Huvos, A. G., Smith, J., et al.: Primary malignant tumors of the sternum. Surg. Gynecol. Obstet., *138*:391–395, 1974.)

benign and malignant cartilaginous tumors.

4. Features favoring a benign cartilage lesion include slow growth, increasing intralesional calcifications, and sclerotic perilesional boundaries. On the other hand, rapid enlargement, decreasing intralesional calcifications, and lytic perilesional borders favor chondrosarcomas.

Occasionally, bone infarct may demonstrate a radiographic presentation similar to a central chondrosarcoma. A typical infarct in bone shows interspersed irregular calcifications and ossification with areas of medullary radiolucencies. The pattern of ossification may produce a castlike structure engulfing the surrounding cortex. The irregular areas of ossification within the infarct are segregated from the overlying normal cortical bone by a radiolucent zone.

PROGNOSTIC ASPECTS

The location of the cartilage tumor within a bone, its radiographic features, and the findings at the time of biopsy are of significance in assessing prognosis. A moderately well-delineated diaphyseal lesion, for instance, that is surrounded by an intact cortex, as shown on the roentgenograms and on surgical exploration, will have a more optimistic prognosis, a lower grade of malignancy. On the other hand, a lesion involving the same bone as well as the same location but showing cortical expansion, feathery, poorly defined, translucent outlines will have a worse prognosis. This clinical prospect becomes even more dismal if cortical invasion by tumor is demonstrated at the time of biopsy.

Considerable sclerosis of bone about the area destroyed by tumor represents an encouraging finding. The slow growth of the lesion elicits an osseous confining defense reaction; i.e., well-defined scalloped borders are seen, thereby signifying a relatively lower grade of malignancy.

Angiographic findings in chondrosarcomas reveal a close correlation between the vascularity and the degree of malignancy.[82] In general, the more abundant the vascularity is, the more malignant the tumors are on microscopic examination. The consistent separation of low-grade chondrosarcomas from various chondromas demonstrating poor vascularity is not feasible. In such instances, angiography may be useful in selecting the part of the tumor showing the most marked vascularity.

GROSS FINDINGS

Central chondrosarcomas are characterized by a bluish-white, pearly, translucent tissue that is faceted and lobulated, with the adjacent endosteal cortical surface showing scalloping. Areas of calcification and ossification within the lesions are represented by yellow or white areas of speckling. A mucoid, slimy character is occasionally seen in degenerating or myxoid types of tumors, since the tumor often insinuates itself between the marrow spaces without actual osseous trabecular destruction; the extent and the exact boundaries of the lesion are hardly identifiable either on gross examination or even on radiologic study.[54] The adjacent cortex may show slight swelling and increase in volume due to reactive ossification.[119, 128, 129] Slowly expanding low-grade lesions elicit more reactive new bone formation, while the rapidly progressive high-grade chondrosarcomas exhibit less.[51] Instead of new bone formation, rapid cortical bone destruction with invasion through the cortex into surrounding soft tissues is the rule in fast-growing chondrosarcomas.

In peripheral chondrosarcomas, a pre-existent base or a pedicle may be identifiable, but in most instances, no such structures are retained and the lesion is entirely cartilaginous (Fig. 13–7). Depending on the location, cartilaginous, peripherally situated chondrosarcomas may be huge, especially those arising in the pelvis, the shoulder girdle, or the chest wall. They range in size from 1 cm to gargantuan proportions (Fig. 13–1). The advancing edge of the tumor invading soft tissues is bosselated and may show a pseudocapsule. These pseudopod-like, small, nodular extensions appear to be well demarcated. This appearance may encourage the surgeon to attempt to shell out the lesion without adequate surgical margins, resulting in prompt recurrence.

Frequently, when a huge chondrosarcoma is first examined by the pathologist, it is difficult to determine whether the tumor arose centrally or peripherally. Study of a slice of the whole pathologic specimen, however, in some cases, will indicate whether the origin was central or peripheral.[100]

The median size (greatest diameter) of chondrosarcomas, at the time of initial treatment, was 11 cm in the femur, ranging from 1 to 36 cm, and 13 cm in the pelvis, ranging from 2 to 32 cm.[100] Most of the chondrosarcomas of the scapula are larger than 6 cm in diameter.[151] The size of the rib lesion at the time of initial presentation was found to be of great diagnostic help.[98] Cartilage tumors arising in ribs and measuring more than 4 cm in greatest diameter are chondrosarcomas in most instances.

HISTOLOGIC APPEARANCE AND GRADING

Any pathologist who tries to render a histologic evaluation of a cartilaginous lesion without examining the pertinent radiographs will be wrong more often than right when arriving at the diagnosis. The examination of the radiographs will provide a fair estimate of the size — lesions over 6 to 10 cm in diameter are chondrosarcomas until proved otherwise. The radiographs will also indicate aggressiveness manifested by bony destruction and, in addition, the stippled or blotchy calcifications will steer one away from underdiagnosing the lesion. In assessing the histologic appearance of cartilage lesions, age must be a major consideration. Chondrosarcomas are very uncommon in patients less than 20 years old. In childhood and adolescence, especially during puberty, more cellular atypia may be permitted. The benign cartilage lesions in multiple enchondromatosis (Ollier's disease) are much more cellular than those in the solitary form without signifying a chondrosarcomatous change.

The over-reliance on the histologic appearance as the sole guide to diagnosis, treatment, and prognosis can lead to an unmitigated disaster. Two cartilage tumors with identical histologic features can behave in entirely different ways. For instance, a metacarpal cartilaginous lesion in a growing child may be totally benign, while a tumor of identical appearance in the femur or humerus of an adult may behave in a sinister fashion. Biologic behavior and histologic appearance do not always match. It is to be emphasized that the study of the pathologic material in cartilage lesions requires the closest cooperation between the pathologist, radiologist, and surgeon to properly evaluate the biologic parameters of a given lesion. The ideal multidisciplinary approach in the diagnosis and treatment of cancer reaches its fullest expression in cartilage tumors.

The histological criteria used for the modern diagnosis of chondrosarcoma were developed and outlined in 1943 by Lichtenstein and Jaffe.[88] These criteria include an increased number of cartilage cells with plump nuclei, more than occasional binucleate cells, and mononuclear or multinucleated giant cartilage cells. Many clinicopathologic studies in which the degree of malignancy was graded have clearly indicated that useful and reproducible assessments of the biologic behavior of cartilage neoplasms can be made.[19, 30, 63, 98, 100, 119, 136, 162] In the cytologic grading of cartilage lesions, nuclear pleomorphism and hyperchromatism, as well as increased numbers of multinucleated tumor cells, are important features in establishing the exact grade of a given lesion. Two or more cells within a cartilage lacuna in more than occasional microscopic fields characterize a Grade I chondrosarcoma (Figs. 13–10, 13–11, and 13–12). A careful search for these binucleate or multinucleated cells will help in arriving at the proper diagnosis in those locally aggressive, large, pelvic chondrosarcomas that pose considerable difficulty in the microscopic evaluation. The periphery of the cartilage lobules presents increased cellularity, and careful examination of these regions facilitates appraisal.

The presence of myxomatous change and cystic degeneration correlates well with the low and medium grades of chondrosarcoma, whereas the microscopic absence of cartilage lobules and the presence of fibrosarcomatous areas ("dedifferentiation") are characteristic of the high-grade variants. In these tumors, groups of chondromatous cells lose their usual lobulation and begin to spindle out (Figs. 13–13 through 13–16).[29, 71, 107, 110] The lesion is designated a myxoid chondrosarcoma when a basophilic intercellular substance separates the tumor cells without definite lacunar formation (Fig. 13–17). Ossification of the cartilage matrix may cause confusion with osteogenic sarcoma but is the result of either metaplasia or endochondral ossification in low-grade chondrosarcoma.[128, 129] In the presence of endochondral ossification, cartilaginous cores are, at times, still evident within some of the bony spicules, and rings of ossification can be seen surrounding cartilage lobules (Fig. 13–18). On occasion, marrow elements may be seen within the bone.

Of 152 chondrosarcomas arising in the pelvic bones, 56 were Grade I, 53 were Grade II, and 43 were Grade III.[100] In this group of neoplasms, changes of grade in the recurrent lesions were noted only infrequently. In two cases, the lesion changed from Grade I to II, and in three cases it changed from Grade II to III.

CLEAR CELL TYPE OF CHONDROSARCOMA

A newly recognized clear cell type of chondrosarcoma has been described by Unni and his colleagues.[165] In the 16 cases

Text continued on page 221

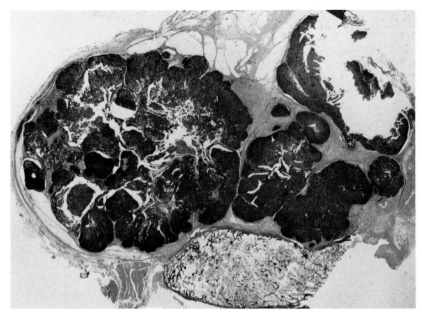

Figure 13–10. Cross section of the entire peripheral chondrosarcoma of pelvis demonstrating lack of encapsulation and nodular growth pattern with pseudopod-like projections. (Hematoxylin-eosin stain. Reduction × 2.)

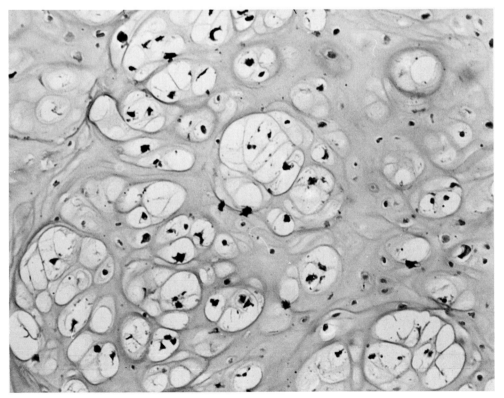

Figure 13–11. Chondrosarcoma, Grade I. Some variation in size and shape of the cartilage cells with binucleate forms. Slight increase in the number of cells. (Hematoxylin-eosin stain. Magnification × 250.)

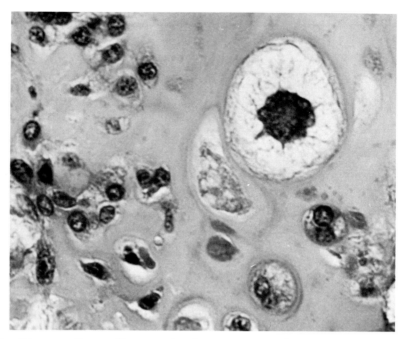

Figure 13–12. Giant cartilage cells in a chondrosarcoma, Grade I. This cell mimicks a physaliphorous cell of a chordoma. (Hematoxylin-eosin stain. Magnification × 430.)

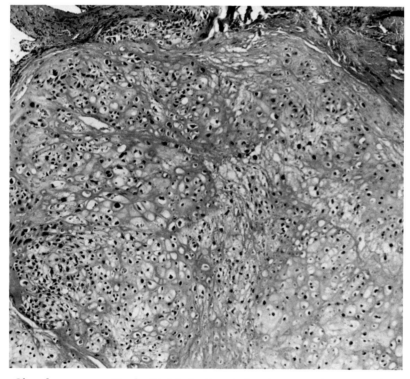

Figure 13–13. Chondrosarcoma, Grade II. Marked variation in size and increased numbers of cartilage cells, some of them with bizarre shapes. (Hematoxylin-eosin stain. Magnification × 100.)

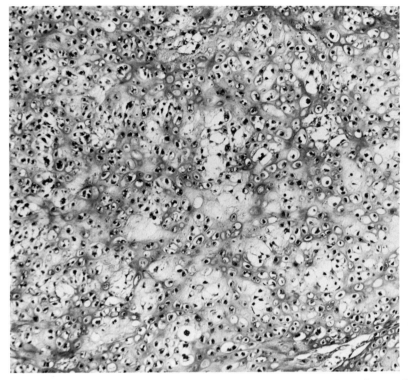

Figure 13-14. Chondrosarcoma, Grade II. Markedly increased number of cartilage cells with pleomorphism of the nuclei. (Hematoxylin-eosin stain. Magnification × 100.)

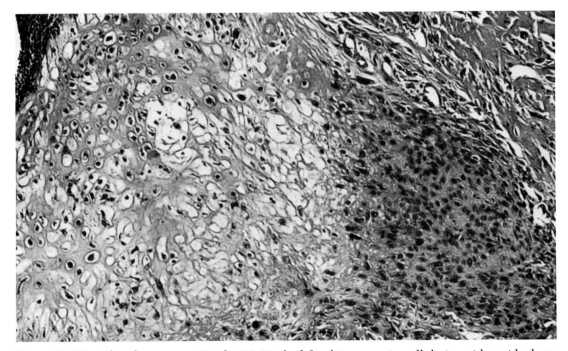

Figure 13-15. Chondrosarcoma, Grade III. Marked focal increase in cellularity with residual cartilage matrix still present. (Hematoxylin-eosin stain. Magnification × 100.)

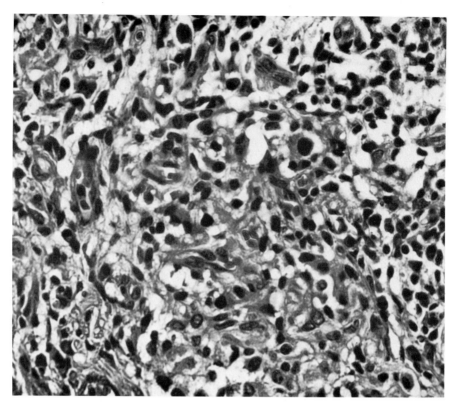

Figure 13–16. Chondrosarcoma, Grade III. Some spindling and increased cellularity of the tumor. (Hematoxylin-eosin stain. Magnification × 250.)

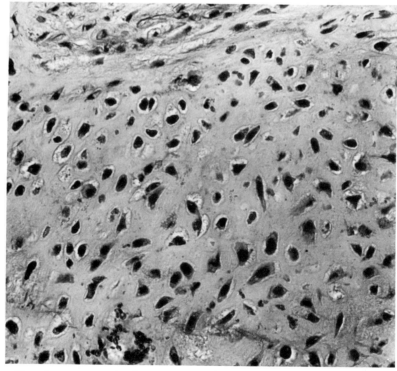

Figure 13–17. Chondrosarcoma, Grade II. Increased number of moderately pleomorphic cells with early myxomatous change. (Hematoxylin-eosin stain. Magnification × 250.)

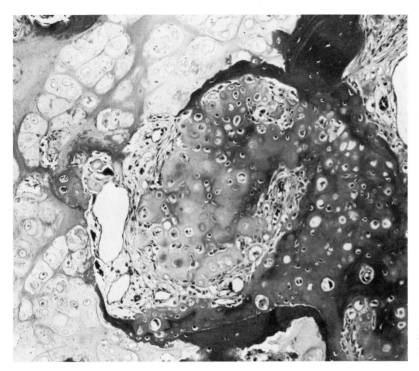

Figure 13–18. Chondrosarcoma with endochondral bone formation at the periphery of the cartilage growth. (Hematoxylin-eosin stain. Magnification × 100.)

reported, males were predilected over females two to one, and all patients were adults. There was a striking preference for the lesions to involve secondary centers of ossification in the epiphyses and abutting metaphyses of long tubular bones, most commonly in the femoral head and greater trochanter as well as in the head of the humerus. Similarities in the location and microscopic features make one postulate a close relationship to chondroblastoma, especially to "malignant" chondroblastoma. Histologically, the lesions show numerous giant cells, osteoid, and mature bone formation, as well as the rounded neoplastic clear cell component. The clinical course is distinguished by local recurrences and eventual metastases.

ELECTRON MICROSCOPIC FINDINGS

Electron microscopic observations show similarities between cells of chondrosarcoma and immature cartilage cells.[38, 48, 61, 69, 147, 167] Consequently, one would have difficulties pointing out the consistent differ-

ences between normal chondrocytes and neoplastic cartilage cells present in low-grade chondrosarcoma, while higher grade chondrosarcomas are easier to identify on electron microscopic examination.

HISTOLOGIC GRADE AND ITS RELATIONSHIP TO PROGNOSIS

Malignant cartilage tumors, especially those in the pelvis, are probably the largest lesions encounterd in oncologic pathology (Fig. 13–1). A small biopsy specimen may not be representative of the entire neoplasm and, accordingly, the path to exact microscopic grading is fraught with the possibility of error. On histologic examination of the biopsy specimen, it is not uncommon for an extremely well-differentiated chondrosarcoma to display relatively normal-appearing cartilage cells while the patient may have a huge tumor that may necessitate major amputation or, even worse, be inoperable. Examination of multiple sections is mandatory for proper interpretation in order to avoid, or at least minimize, errors since only limited portions of the tumor may show the features of a higher grade chondrosarcoma. This diagnostic problem in grading will only occur in differentiating Grade I and Grade II lesions. High-grade lesions, especially the spindle cell fibrosarcomatous variants, may contain microscopic foci of residual Grade I chondrosarcoma, but these extremely limited areas, in practice, do not cause diagnostic confusion. Since mesenchymal chondrosarcoma displays spindly sarcomatous areas, an occasional pitfall in the diagnosis may be encountered, such as mistaking it for a high-grade fibrosarcomatous chondrosarcoma of the "dedifferentiated" variety.[29, 71, 107, 110] If proper attention is paid to the spindle cell sarcomatous component in mesenchymal chondrosarcoma, a hemangiopericytomatoid, vascular growth pattern becomes evident. This is entirely missing in the high-grade (Grade III) fibrosarcomatous chondrosarcomas.

Histologic grading of malignant cartilage lesions shows interesting correlations with prognosis. Despite the fact that the prognosis did not show any significant difference between Grades I and II chondrosarcomas of the pelvis, these two grades were significantly different from Grade III lesions.[100] In another study of chondrosarcoma arising in ribs, Grade II and III tumors were found to have a similar prognosis, whereas the Grade I lesions carried a much better prognosis (Figs. 13–19 and 13–20).[98] From these data, and from others, it seems that the natural history of chondrosarcoma may be related to the specific location of the tumor as well as to the tumor grade.

The histologic grade of the tumor seems to determine the rate of metastasis. None of the Grade I lesions metastasized, while 71 per cent of the Grade III chondrosarcomas metastasized in the series reported

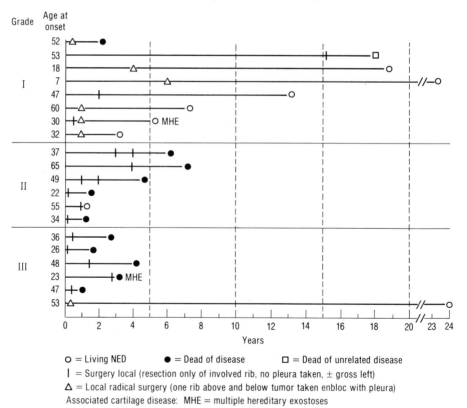

Figure 13–19. Rib chondrosarcomas that did not change grade while under clinical observation. From Marcove, R. C., and Huvos, A. G.: Cartilaginous tumors of the ribs. Cancer, *27*:794–801, 1971.)

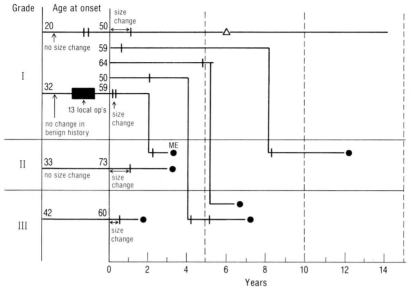

RIB CHONDROSARCOMAS WHICH CHANGED GRADE OR GROWTH RATE PATTERN WHILE UNDER CLINICAL OBSERVATION

O = Living NED   ● = Dead of disease
I = Surgery local (resection only of involved rib, no pleura taken, ± gross left)
△ = Local radical surgery (one rib above and below tumor taken enbloc with pleura)
Associated cartilage disease: ME = multiple enchondromatoses

Figure 13–20. Rib chondrosarcomas that changed grade or growth rate pattern while under clinical observation. (From Marcove, R. C., and Huvos, A. G.: Cartilaginous tumors of the ribs. Cancer, 27:794–801, 1971.)

from the M. D. Anderson Hospital.[41] Other studies, however, found a definite but low metastatic potential for Grade I lesions.[30, 90] Most of the metastases in all grades occurred in less than five years. Also, most local recurrences become evident within five years.

Patients with low-grade, well-differentiated chondrosarcomas at all sites have a significantly longer survival rate and longer interval between treatment and recurrence than those with higher grade tumors. The disease-free interval between surgery and recurrence for patients with low-grade chondrosarcomas of the pelvic girdle was over 40 per cent at five years, compared with only 15 per cent for those with less-differentiated (Grade III) tumors (Fig. 13–21). The combination of pain and higher grade of tumor appeared to impart a cumulatively worse prognosis of the patients. About three fourths of the painless tumors are of the low-grade variety, while

only about one third of patients presenting with pain will have low-grade chondrosarcomas on histologic examination.[73]

Chondrosarcomas with a low or intermediate degree of malignancy (Grades I and II) tend to grow slowly, may recur locally, and metastasize late in their clinical course. The five year recurrence or metastatic rate in this group of patients is about 63 per cent, including even those cases in which the primary treatment was deemed inadequate.

Grade III chondrosarcomas behave in a highly malignant fashion and metastasize early. Early radical ablative surgery is indicated for their treatment, but even then the results are quite disappointing.[159] The local recurrence or metastatic rate in these high-grade lesions is about 85 per cent at five years even after radical ablative surgery.

The importance of mitotic activity and cellularity as prognostic indicators was

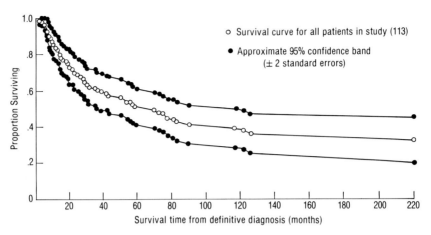

Figure 13–21. Survival curve for patients with chondrosarcoma of the pelvis and upper end of the femur. (From Marcove, R. C., Miké, V., Hutter, R. V. P., et al.: Chondrosarcoma of the pelvis and upper end of the femur. An analysis of factors influencing survival time in 113 cases. J. Bone Joint Surg. [Am.], *54*:561–572, 1972.)

emphasized by Evans and associates,[41] although every other study stressed the value of nuclear hyperchromatism, pleomorphism, and cellularity in order to reliably grade chondrosarcomas and predict behavior.[30, 63, 90, 98, 100, 119, 127] In all of the larger reported series except two,[41, 90] it was found that recurrent chondrosarcomas may show a higher grade of malignancy than the original lesion (Figs. 13–19 and 13–20).[19, 30, 98, 100, 119]

The secondary chondrosarcomas arising in patients having either multiple hereditary exostoses or multiple enchondromatoses are most often of the low-grade variety. The chondrosarcomas associated with Maffucci's disease (soft tissue hemangiomas) are usually of higher grade malignancy (Grade II or III chondrosarcomas).

HISTOLOGIC DIFFERENTIAL DIAGNOSIS

The separation of chondrosarcoma from osteogenic sarcoma was not always clear-cut. In the past, some considered chondrosarcoma to be a sarcoma that did not produce bone at all.[74] Others, like Phemister,[129] designated those tumors that contained largely cartilage as chondrosarcoma and those exhibiting tumor bone with cartilage either absent or present in small quantities in the region of ossification as osteogenic sarcoma. In 1943, Lich-

tenstein and Jaffe clearly separated these two entities.[88] In their opinion, chondrosarcomas arose from fully developed cartilage, even though they may show endochondral or metaplastic ossification or myxomatous changes. In contrast to osteogenic sarcoma, they maintained, malignant cartilaginous tumors should not show direct osteoid or bone production by the sarcomatous stroma. The unambiguous separation of osteogenic sarcoma with prominent cartilage component, also designated as chondroblastic osteogenic sarcoma, from chondrosarcoma with calcification and ossification is of paramount importance since the prognosis and the treatment is entirely different in these two entities. Occasionally, this poses a practical problem in microscopically examining a limited piece of bulky tumor in a child or an adult that only reveals malignant cartilaginous differentiation. In such cases, a mistaken diagnosis of chondrosarcoma, instead of the correct one of osteogenic sarcoma, is rendered. As a practical guide, it should be borne in mind that primary chondrosarcomas in children and adolescents are extremely rare.[8] In this age group, with only negligible exceptions, the carefully sampled tumor tissue will reveal neoplastic osteoid or bone directly formed by the sarcomatous stroma, thereby establishing the true diagnosis of osteogenic sarcoma. Before a final conclusion of a chondrosarcoma is reached in an adult, the tumor tissue should be meticulously searched for unequivocal tumor bone formation, since the prognosis and probably the treatment is dependent on the exact diagnosis.

A chondromyxoid fibroma occasionally may be mistaken for a chondrosarcoma that has prominent myxoid characteristics. In addition to the clinical features and the radiologic appearance, the microscopic characteristics are of help in keeping these two entities apart. On histologic examination, a chondromyxoid fibroma exhibits a pseudolobular growth pattern in which the crowding and condensation of tumor cells at the periphery imitates that of cartilage lobules. In contradistinction, chondrosarcomas, even in a relatively limited biopsy specimen, will exhibit true cartilage lobules with a hyaline intercellular substance separated by collagen strands. Well-developed lacunae with binucleated or multinucleated chondrocytes are features of low-grade chondrosarcoma in more than occasional microscopic fields.

TREATMENT AND PROGNOSIS

A chondromatous tumor that starts to grow in an adult is potentially malignant and must be removed. Clinical evidence of renewed growth may be characterized by the onset of pain, pathologic fracture, extension of the lesion as demonstrated by serial radiographs, or the disappearance of previously visible calcification. Cartilage tumors arising in the axial skeleton, or involving the long bones of the appendicular skeleton close to the torso, are usually malignant while those in more distal locations, especially the hands and feet, are ordinarily benign.

The "borderline" group of cartilage lesions causes most of the problems in diagnosis and treatment. The subtle but significant histologic changes remove these tumors from the clearly benign category. Our experience has shown that those "atypical" or "borderline" cartilage lesions, for which the pathologist is hesitant to make a definite diagnosis, will almost certainly turn out to be and behave like a low-grade chondrosarcoma. These lesions are the most frequently underdiagnosed and underestimated tumors in the patholo-

gy of bones. Closer attention to the supporting clinical data, such as age, location, size, radiographic appearance, and so forth, in addition to histologic features, will clearly point away from a benign cartilage tumor designation. There is no good excuse for equivocation or temporizing in these slowly evolving low-grade chondrosarcomas, since prompt and proper therapy results in a high percentage of cures. In general, secondary chondrosarcomas have a lower growth potential and progress slowly in contrast to primary chondrosarcomas, which may grow rapidly and progressively with a more malignant clinical course.

Cartilaginous tumors, especially chondrosarcomas, may be implanted with ease in soft tissues. The lack of mechanical containment by bone with abundant vascular supply in soft tissues results in a remarkably accelerated growth potential and increased invasiveness. The biopsy, therefore, should be performed through an incision that can be completely excised at the time of definitive surgery.

The recommended treatment, when feasible, is total removal of the entire tumor mass with an adequate margin of surrounding uninvolved tissue so that the lesion is not cut into or seen.

Radical surgical excision of tumors is quite successful in secondary chondrosarcomas, in low-grade central or peripheral chondrosarcomas, and in those central chondrosarcomas that do not perforate the cortical bone. The excision of humeral and femoral lesions may be coupled with functional restoration by endoprosthetic devices[18] or with massive amounts of fresh autogenous cancellous bone surrounding the autoclaved segment of resected bone.[152]

In the assessment of therapeutic approaches for the excision of bulky cartilaginous lesions involving the shoulder girdle, an upper limb–saving modification may be attempted instead of the traditional Berger type of interscapulothoracic amputation.[84] Serious consideration should be given to the Tikhoff-Linberg procedure.[89, 99, 121] This was originally devised by Tikhoff in 1922 and described by Linberg in 1928 as an interscapulothoracic resection instead of amputation.[89] In this operation, the entire pectoral girdle is re-

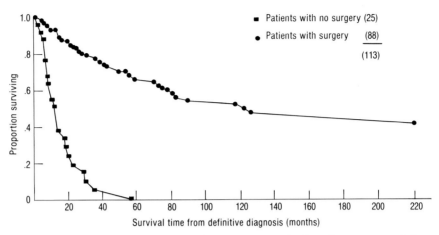

Figure 13–22. Comparison of survival curves for patients with chondrosarcoma of the pelvis and upper end of the femur who had only biopsy with those who had some form of definitive surgical treatment. (From Marcove, R. C., Miké, V., Hutter, R. V. P., et al.: Chondrosarcoma of the pelvis and upper end of the femur. An analysis of factors influencing survival time in 113 cases. J. Bone Joint Surg. [Am.], 54:561–572, 1972.)

moved *en bloc* with the upper portion of the humerus, the rest of the extremity, and the distal part of the arm, forearm, and hand remaining intact. Naturally, this procedure is feasible only if the vessel and nerve bundles are not involved by tumor, since the subclavian vessels may not be ligated.[99, 121]

Simple local excision with stripping away of an involved rib from the adjacent pleura without adequate margins may be curative for cartilage tumors of ribs measuring 4 cm or less.[98] This type of surgical intervention is considered to be insufficient for lesions measuring more than 4 cm in diameter. In such instances, the successful eradication of disease, notwithstanding the pathologist's inability to confirm the diagnosis of chondrosarcoma, requires radical surgical excision with removal of adjacent uninvolved ribs and the pleura *en bloc* with the lesion.[98] Less than this radical intervention seems to yield at least a local recurrence, if not eventual death from disease.

Five year survival rates for those patients with pelvic chondrosarcomas who had "curative" surgery were 47 per cent, 38 per cent, and 15 per cent in Grade I, II, and III lesions respectively (Fig. 13–21).[100]

The adequacy of surgical therapy bears an important relationship to the survival of patients with chondrosarcomas. In those patients for whom only a biopsy was per-

formed as treatment, the average survival time is approximately 1.8 years, with a five year survival rate of approximately 6 per cent (Fig. 13–22).[73] The five year overall survival rate for all grades of chondrosarcoma at all sites ranges between 42 per cent and 69 per cent for those patients who had operations with attempt at cure and 32 per cent for those who only underwent local resections without attempt at curative surgical excisions.

The survival curve for patients with chondrosarcoma of the pelvic girdle reveals an estimated five year survival rate of 52 per cent (Fig. 13–21). It is also suggested that it is more meaningful to employ a 10 or 15 year survival rate as an indicator of cure since about 15 per cent of the patients die of their disease more than five years after initial diagnosis. The 10 and 15 year survival rates in this study were 40 per cent and 37 per cent respectively.[100]

Is there any difference in prognosis between central and peripheral chondrosarcomas? Tumors of the femur were classified as central (32 patients) or peripheral (11 patients).[100] The distribution of the histologic grades and of the types of surgery in these two groups was quite similar. The survival curves for central or peripheral chondrosarcomas of the femur were also nearly identical.

If one compares the survival rates of osteogenic sarcoma and chondrosarcoma in patients less than 21 years of age, interesting findings emerge.[100] The median survival time from definitive diagnosis was 13.5 months for patients with osteogenic sarcoma as compared to 27 months for those with chondrosarcoma. The two year survival rates were 26 per cent for osteogenic sarcoma patients and 54 per cent for chondrosarcoma patients. The five year survival rates were 18 per cent and 37 per cent respectively.

Careful analysis of data in 121 patients treated for chondrosarcoma of the pelvis and of the proximal end of the femur reveals that the best overall cure rate may be attained if there is a wide margin of normal tissue between the tumor and the surgical line of resection. If this conclusion is correct, the optimal surgical treatment for these lesions should be hemipelvectomy.[60] Some attempts at devising limb-saving radical resections of chondrosarcoma of the pelvis have been reported.[37]

Marcove pioneered cryosurgery coupled with curettage as an effective method in the treatment of low- and medium-grade chondrosarcoma, and the preliminary results are encouraging.[99]

In the search for newer and more successful methods in the treatment of chondrosarcoma, radioactive sulphur (^{35}S) has been introduced.[11, 12, 55, 56, 92, 93] On the basis of experimental studies, ^{35}S is incorporated into the chondrocytes and inhibits the tumor growth by interfering with the biosynthesis of the sulfated glycosaminoglycan matrix. It is possible, but not yet proved, that the amount of irradiation directly destroys the chondrocytes since, in the experience at Memorial Hospital, these cells show considerable degeneration and necrosis.[99, 105] Although about 80 per cent of the radioactive sulphur is excreted through the kidney in 24 hours, profound hematologic changes were noted, characterized not only by a marked reduction in the number of granulocytes and thrombocytes but also by a leukemoid marrow reaction in some cases.[105]

The role of radiotherapy is a limited one. It should be reserved for those cases in which regional tumor excision removes the visible lesion and radiotherapy is used as an adjuvant to control microscopic foci of residual disease. Similarly, chemotherapy may be employed in an adjuvant therapy regimen, and adriamycin, in the experience at the Roswell Park Memorial Institute, may bring about remissions.[73]

METASTATIC PATTERN

Following inadequate excisions, local recurrences are the rule, and distant metastases to lungs and so on may occur many years later. In rare cases, however, tumors may disseminate within a short while, as soon as a few months after the diagnosis has been established. Intravascular hematogenous spread via venous channels reaching the right atrium and lung were noted by Virchow in 1855,[168] Weber in 1866,[172] Biesiadecki in 1868,[7] Ernst in 1900,[39] and Kósa in 1929.[80] A rare example of chondrosarcoma of the femur metastatic to the lung with direct extension via the pulmonary veins to the left atrium has been reported.[142] Regional lymph node metastases are rare occurrences.[20]

REFERENCES

1. Ahmed, H.: A case of chondrosarcoma of rib involving the right upper lobe. Br. J. Surg., 51:390–391, 1964.
2. Arnold, P. G., and Pairolero, P. C.: Chondrosarcoma of the manubrium. Resection and reconstruction with pectoralis major muscle. Mayo Clin. Proc., 53:54–57, 1978.
3. Avdiunichev, V. I.: Successful operation of shoulder-girdle excision in osteochondrosarcoma. Khirurgiia (Mosk.), 10:58–59, 1954.
4. Barnes, R., and Catto, M.: Chondrosarcoma of bone. J. Bone Joint Surg. [Br.], 48:729–764, 1966.
5. Bessler, W.: Das Beckenchondrom und Chondrosarkom. Virchows Arch., 323:72–92, 1953.
6. Bessler, W.: Die malignen Potenzen der Skelettchondrome. Schweiz. Med. Wochenschr., 96:461–466, 1966.
7. Biesiadecki, A.: Zottenchondrom des Darmbeines, enchondromatöse Thromben der Beckenvenen und Pulmonalarterien. S.-B. Akad. Math. Naturw., 57:793–808, 1868.
8. Bizer, V. A.: Clinical aspects and treatment of chondrosarcoma in children and adolescents. Vestn. Khir., 118(2):93–97, 1977.
9. Blaylock. R. L., and Kempe, L. G.: Chondrosarcoma of the cervical spine. Case report. J. Neurosurg., 44:500–503, 1976.
10. Block, R. S., and Burton, R. I.: Multiple chondrosarcomas in a hand: a case report. J. Hand Surg., 2:310–313, 1977.

11. Boström, H., Edgren, B., Friberg, U., et al.: Case of chondrosarcoma with pulmonary and skeletal metastases after hemipelvectomy, successfully treated with ^{35}S-sulfate. Acta Orthop. Scand., 39:549–564, 1968.

12. Boström, H., Friberg, U., Larsson, K. S., et al.: *In vitro* incorporation of S^{35}-sulfate in chondrosarcomatous tissue. Acta Orthop. Scand., 39:58–72, 1968.

13. Boström, H., Friberg, U., Larsson, K. S., et al.: Biochemical and autoradiographic studies in a case of fulminant, metastatic chondrosarcoma unsuccessfully treated with 35S-sulfate. Acta Orthop. Scand., 41:57–73, 1970.

14. Brodey, R. S., Misdorp, W., Riser, W. H., et al.: Canine skeletal chondrosarcoma: a clinicopathologic study of 35 cases. J. Am. Vet. Med. Assoc., 165:68–78, 1974.

15. Brozmanová, E., and Škrovina, B.: Serum alkaline phosphatase in malignant bone tumours (osteosarcoma, chondrosarcoma, fibrosarcoma, Ewing's sarcoma). Neoplasma, 20:419–425, 1973.

16. Brozmanová, E., and Škrovina, B.: Biochemical and haematological findings in malignant bone tumours. Neoplasma, 21:75–82, 1974.

17. Brozmanová, E., and Škrovina, B.: Biochemical and hematologic findings in chondrosarcomas. Bratisl. Lek. List, 62:424–429, 1974.

18. Burrows, H. J., Wilson, J. N., and Scales, J. T.: Excision of tumours of humerus and femur, with restoration by internal prostheses. J. Bone Joint Surg. [Br.], 57:148–159, 1975.

19. Campanacci, M., Guernelli, N., Leonessa, C., et al.: Chondrosarcoma. A study of 133 cases, 80 with long term follow-up. Ital. J. Orthop. Traum., 1:387–414, 1975.

20. Castrén, H.: Zur Kenntnis der metastasenbildenden Chondrome. Acta Soc. Med. Fenn. B15:3–18, 1931.

21. Chavanne, G., Calle, R., and Schlienger, P.: Bone chondrosarcomas (a radioclinical study of 44 cases). J. Radiol. Electrol. Med. Nucl., 52:425–438, 1971.

22. Coley, B. L., and Higinbotham, N. L.: Secondary chondrosarcoma. Ann. Surg., 139:547–559, 1954.

23. Cooper, A.: Exostosis. *In*, Cooper, A., and Travers, B. (eds.): Surgical Essays. 3rd ed. London, Cox and Son, 1818, pp. 169–226.

24. Cooper, R. R.: Juxtacortical chondrosarcoma. A case report. J. Bone Joint Surg. [Am.], 47:524–528, 1965.

25. Copeland, M. M.: Tumors of cartilaginous origin. Clin. Orthop., 7:9–26, 1956.

26. Cowan, W. K.: Malignant change and multiple metastases in Ollier's disease. J. Clin. Pathol., 18:650–653, 1965.

27. Culver, J. E., Jr., Sweet, D. E., and McCue, F. C.: Chondrosarcoma of the hand arising from a pre-existent benign solitary enchondroma. Clin. Orthop., 113:128–131, 1975.

28. Dahlin, D. C.: Chondrosarcoma and its "variants." In Ackerman, L. V., Spjut, H. J., and Abell, M. R. (eds.): Bones and Joints. Baltimore, Williams & Wilkins, 1976, pp. 300–311.

29. Dahlin, D. C., and Beabout, J. W.: Dedifferen-

30. Dahlin, D. C., and Henderson, E. D.: Chondrosarcoma, a surgical and pathological problem. Review of 212 cases. J. Bone Joint Surg. [Am.], 38:1025–1038, 1956.

31. Dahlin, D. C., and Salvador, A. H.: Chondrosarcomas of bones of the hands and feet — a study of 30 cases. Cancer, 34:755–760, 1974.

32. Daniels, A. C., Conner, G. H., and Straus, F. H.: Primary chondrosarcoma of the tracheobronchial tree. Report of a unique case and brief review. Arch. Pathol., 84:615–624, 1967.

33. del Castillo, J. J., Gianfrancesco, H., and Mannix, E. P.: Pulmonic stenosis due to compression by sternal chondrosarcoma. J. Thorac. Cardiovasc. Surg., 52:255–260, 1960.

34. Dorner, R. A., and Marcy, D. S.: Primary rib tumors. Survey of literature and a report of seven additional cases. J. Thorac. Cardiovasc. Surg., 17:690–704, 1948.

35. Durbin, F. C., and Smith, G. S.: A chondromatous tumour of the calcaneum. J. Bone Joint Surg. [Br.], 37:584–590, 1955.

36. Eisenbarth, G. S., Wellman, D. K., and Lebovitz, H. E.: Prostaglandin A_1 inhibition of chondrosarcoma growth. Biochem. Biophys. Res. Commun., 60:1302–1308, 1974.

37. Erickson, U., and Hjelmstedt, A.: Limb-saving radical resection of chondrosarcoma of the pelvis. Case report. J. Bone Joint Surg. [Am.], 58:568–570, 1976.

38. Erlandson, R. A., and Huvos, A. G.: Chondrosarcoma: a light and electron microscopic study. Cancer, 34:1642–1652, 1974.

39. Ernst, P.: Ungewöhnliche Verbreitung einer Knorpelgeschwulst in der Blutbahn. Beitr. Pathol. Anat. Allg. Pathol., 28:255–295, 1900.

40. Ernst, P.: Über den feineren Bau der Knorpelgeschwülste. Beitr. Pathol. Anat. Allg. Pathol., 38:67–100, 1905.

41. Evans, H. L., Ayala, A. G., and Romsdahl, M. M.: Prognostic factors in chondrosarcoma of bone. A clinicopathologic analysis with emphasis on histologic grading. Cancer, 40:818–831, 1977.

42. Feintuch, T. A.: Chondrosarcoma arising in a cartilaginous area of previously irradiated fibrous dysplasia. Cancer, 31:877–881, 1973.

43. Fitzwater, J. E., Cabaud, H. E., and Farr, G. H.: Irradiation-induced chondrosarcoma. A case report. J. Bone Joint Surg. [Am.], 58:1037–1039, 1976.

44. Flörcken, H.: Ein selten grosses Chondrom der Lendengegend und seine Behandlung. Z. Krebsforsch., 35:354–359, 1932.

45. Fodden, J. H.: The central malignant chondroma of bone. Can. Med. Assoc. J., 63:362–364, 1950.

46. Franke, D., and Hennig, K.: Totalersatz des Humerus einschliesslich Schulter- und Ellenbogengelenk. Chirurg., 47:531–533, 1976.

47. Froimson, A. I.: Metastatic chondrosarcoma of the hand. Clin. Orthop., 53:155–160, 1967.

48. Fu, Y.-S., and Kay, S.: A comparative ultrastructural study of mesenchymal chondrosarcoma and myxoid chondrosarcoma. Cancer, 33:1531–1542, 1974.

tiation of low-grade chondrosarcomas. Cancer, 28:461–466, 1971.

49. Ghormley, R. K.: Chondromas and chondrosarcomas of the scapula and the innominate bone. Arch. Surg., 36:48–52, 1951.

50. Ghosh, L., Huvos, A. G., and Miké, V.: The pancreatic islets in chondrosarcoma. A qualitative and quantitative study in humans. Am. J. Pathol., 71:23–32, 1973.

51. Gilmer, W. S., Jr., Kilgore, W., and Smith, H.: Central cartilage tumors of bone. Clin. Orthop., 26:81–103, 1963.

52. Gilula, L. A., and Staple, T. W.: Central chondrosarcoma. Orthop. Rev., 3:43–45, 1974.

53. Godman, G. C., and Porter, K. R.: Chondrogenesis studied with the electron microscope. J. Biophys. Biochem. Cytol., 8:719–760, 1960.

54. Goldenberg, R. R.: Chondrosarcoma. Bull. Hosp. Joint Dis., 25:30–49, 1964.

55. Gottschalk, R. G., Alpert, L. K., and Albert, R. E.: The use of large amounts of radioactive sulfur in patients with advanced chondrosarcomas. I. Clinical and hematologic observations. Cancer Res., 19:1070–1077, 1959.

56. Gottschalk, R. G., Alpert, L. K., and Miller, P. O.: The use of large amounts of radioactive sulfur in patients with advanced chondrosarcomas. II. Distribution and tissue irradiation. Cancer Res., 19:1078–1085, 1959.

57. Gottschalk, R. G., and Smith, R. T.: Chondrosarcoma of the hand. Report of a case with radioactive sulphur studies and review of literature. J. Bone Joint Surg. [Am.], 45:141–150, 1963.

58. Grabias, S., and Mankin, H. J.: Chondrosarcoma arising in histologically proved unicameral bone cyst. A case report. J. Bone Joint Surg. [Am.], 56:1501–1509, 1974.

59. Greer, J. A., Jr., Devine, K. D., and Dahlin, D. C.: Gardner's syndrome and chondrosarcoma of the hyoid bone. Arch. Otolaryngol., 103:425–427, 1977.

60. Grigorova, T. M.: Immediate and late results secondary to the treatment of pelvic bones chondrosarcoma. Sov. Med., 38(3):101–105, 1975.

61. Halliwell, W. H., and Kinden, D. A.: Chondrosarcoma: a light and electron microscopic study of a case in a dog. Am. J. Vet. Res., 38:1647–1652, 1977.

62. Harrington, S. W.: Surgical treatment of intrathoracic tumors and tumors of the chest wall. Arch. Surg., 14:406–431, 1927.

63. Henderson, E. D., and Dahlin, D. C.: Chondrosarcoma of bone — a study of 288 cases. J. Bone Joint Surg. [Am.], 45:1450–1458, 1963.

64. Henderson, F. J., and LePage, G. A.: The nutrition of tumors: a review. Cancer Res., 19:887–902, 1959.

65. Higgins, G. M., Levy, B. M., and Yollick, B. L.: A transplantable beryllium-induced chondrosarcoma of rabbits. J. Bone Joint Surg. [Am.], 46:789–796, 1964.

66. Hochheim, W.: Malignant evolution of osteochondromatosis type Ollier. Acta Chir. Orthop. Traumatol. Cech., 33:161–163, 1966.

67. Holz, U., and Weller, S.: Hemipelvectomy after malignant degeneration of a chondroblastoma. Aktuel. Traum., 4:197–203, 1974.

68. Huvos, A. G., Higinbotham, N. L., and Miller, T. R.: Bone sarcomas arising in fibrous dysplasia. J. Bone Joint Surg. [Am.], 54:1047–1056, 1972.

69. Imura, S.-I., Tanaka, S., and Takase, B.: Intracytoplasmic segment long spacing fibrils in chondrosarcoma. J. Electron Microsc. (Tokyo), 24:87–95, 1975.

70. Jokl, P., Albright, J. A., and Goodman, A. H.: Juxtacortical chondrosarcoma of the hand. J. Bone Joint Surg. [Am.], 53:1370–1376, 1971.

71. Kahn, L. B.: Chondrosarcoma with dedifferentiated foci. A comparative and ultrastructural study. Cancer, 37:1365–1375, 1976.

72. Kaufman, J. H., Cedermark, B. J., Parthasarathy, K. L., et al.: The value of ⁶⁷Ga Scintigraphy in soft-tissue sarcoma and chondrosarcoma. Radiology, 123:131–134, 1977.

73. Kaufman, J. H., Douglass, H. O., Jr., Blake, W., et al.: The importance of initial presentation and treatment upon the survival of patients with chondrosarcoma. Surg. Gynecol. Obstet., 145:357–363, 1977.

74. Keiller, V. H.: Cartilaginous tumors of bone. Surg. Gynecol. Obstet., 40:510–521, 1925.

75. Kit, S., and Griffin, A. C.: Cellular metabolism and cancer: a review. Cancer Res., 28:621–656, 1958.

76. Kitagawa, T.: Chondroma and chondrosarcoma (case report). Kumamoto Med. J., 27:55–65, 1974.

77. Knight, J. D. S.: Sarcomatous change in three brothers with diaphysial aclasis. Br. Med. J., 1:1013–1015, 1960.

78. Knowles, H. C., Jr.: Evaluation of a positive urinary sugar test. J.A.M.A., 234:961–963, 1975.

79. Koepke, J. A., and Brower, T. W.: Chondrosarcoma mimicking pseudotumor of hemophilia. Arch. Pathol., 80:655–659, 1965.

80. Kósa, M.: Chondroblastom in der venösen Blutbahn. Virchows Arch. [Pathol. Anat.], 272:166–204, 1929.

81. Kraft, J. R.: Detection of diabetes mellitus *in situ* (occult diabetes). Lab. Med., 6:10–22, 1975.

82. Lagergren, C., Lindbom, A., and Söderberg, G.: The blood vessels of chondrosarcomas. Acta Radiol., 55:321–328, 1961.

83. Laroye, G. J.: Cancer caused by an inherited selective defect in immunological surveillance. Lancet, 1:641–643, 1973.

84. Levinthal, D. H., and Grossman, A.: Interscapulo-thoracic amputation for malignant tumors of the shoulder region. Surg. Gynecol. Obstet., 69:234–239, 1939.

85. Levy, W. M., Aegerter, E. E., and Kirkpatrick, J. A., Jr.: The nature of cartilaginous tumors. Radiol. Clin. North Am., 2:327–336, 1964.

86. Lewis, M. M., Marcove, R. C., and Bullough, P. G.: Chondrosarcoma of the foot. A case report and review of the literature. Cancer, 36:586–589, 1975.

87. Lewis, R. J., and Ketcham, A. S.: Maffucci's syndrome: functional and neoplastic significance. Case report and review of the literature. J. Bone Joint Surg. [Am.], 55:1465–1479, 1973.

88. Lichtenstein, L., and Jaffe, H. L.: Chondrosarcoma of bone. Am. J. Pathol., 19:553–573, 1943.

89. Linberg, B. E.: Interscapulo-thoracic resection for malignant tumors of the shoulder joint region. J. Bone Joint Surg., 10:344–349, 1928.

90. Lindbom, A., Söderberg, G., and Spjut, H. J.: Primary chondrosarcoma of bone. Acta Radiol., 55:81–96, 1961.

91. Ling, G. V., Morgan, J. P., and Pool, R. R.: Primary bone tumors in the dog: a combined clinical, radiographic, and histologic approach to early diagnosis. J. Am. Vet. Med. Assoc., 165:55–67, 1974.

92. Löbe, J.: On ^{35}S therapy of chondrosarcoma. Radiobiol. Radiother., 16:207–213, 1975.

93. Löbe, J., and Wohlgemuth, B.: Autoradiographische und hämatologische Befunde bei der hochdosierten ^{35}S-Therapie des Chondrosarkoms. Strahlentherapie, 74:481–486, 1975.

94. Luck, J. V.: A correlation of roentgenogram and pathological changes in ossifying and chondrifying primary osteogenic neoplasms. Radiology, 40:253–276, 1943.

95. Mack, G. R., Robey, D. B., and Kurman, R. J.: Chondrosarcoma secreting chorionic gonadotropin. Report of a case. J. Bone Joint Surg. [Am.], 59:1107–1111, 1977.

96. Makrycostas, K.: Zur Histologie des bösartigen embryonalen Enchondroms. Virchows Arch., 282:737–760, 1931.

97. Marcove, R. C.: Chondrosarcoma: diagnosis and treatment. Orthop. Clin. North Am., 8:811–820, 1977.

98. Marcove, R. C., and Huvos, A. G.: Cartilaginous tumors of the ribs. Cancer, 27:794–801, 1971.

99. Marcove, R. C., Lewis, M. M., and Huvos, A. G.: En bloc upper humeral interscapulo-thoracic resection. The Tikhoff-Linberg procedure. Clin. Orthop., 124:219–228, 1977.

100. Marcove, R. C., Miké, V., Hutter, R. V. P., et al.: Chondrosarcoma of the pelvis and upper end of the femur. An analysis of factors influencing survival time in 113 cases. J. Bone Joint Surg. [Am.], 54:561–572, 1972.

101. Marcove, R. C., Shoji, H., and Arlen, M.: Altered carbohydrate metabolism in cartilaginous tumors. Contemp. Surg., 5:53–54, 1974.

102. Marcove, R. C., Stovell, P. B., Huvos, A. G., et al.: The use of cryosurgery in the treatment of low and medium grade chondrosarcoma. A preliminary report. Clin. Orthop., 122:147–156, 1977.

103. Marks, P. A., and Bishop, J. S.: The glucose metabolism of patients with malignant disease and of normal subjects as studied by means of an intravenous glucose tolerance test. J. Clin. Invest., 36:245–264, 1957.

104. Martini, N., Huvos, A. G., Smith, J., et al.: Primary malignant tumors of the sternum. Surg. Gynecol. Obstet., 138:391–395, 1974.

105. Mayer, K., Pentlow, K. S., Marcove, R. C., et al.: Sulfur-35 therapy of chondrosarcoma and chordoma. In Spencer, R. P. (ed.): Therapy in Nuclear Medicine. New York, Grune & Stratton, 1978, pp. 185–192.

106. Mayer, L.: Chondro-sarcoma of the rib. Five year cure after resection. J. Mt. Sinai Hosp., 7:467–470, 1941.

107. McFarland, G. B., Jr., McKinley, L. M., and Reed, R. J.: Dedifferentiation of low grade chondrosarcomas. Clin. Orthop., 122:157–164, 1977.

108. Menanteau, B. P., and Dilenge, D.: Angiographic findings in chondrosarcomas. J. Can. Assoc. Radiol., 28:193–198, 1977.

109. Merle d'Aubigné, R., Meary, R., Gauthier-Villars, P., et al.: A propos du diagnostic de malignité dans les tumeurs cartilagineuses des os. Mem. Acad. Chir., 84:83–92, 1958.

110. Mirra, J. M., and Marcove, R. C.: Fibrosarcomatous dedifferentiation of primary and secondary chondrosarcoma. Review of 5 cases. J. Bone Joint Surg. [Am.], 56:285–296, 1974.

111. Monro, R. S., and Golding, J. S. R.: Chondrosarcoma of the ilium complicating hereditary multiple exostoses. Br. J. Surg., 39:73–75, 1951.

112. Morgan, A. D., and Salama, F. D.: Primary chondrosarcoma of the lung. Case report and review of the literature. J. Thorac. Cardiovasc. Surg., 64:460–466, 1972.

113. Morton, J. J., and Mider, G. B.: Chondrosarcoma. Ann. Surg., 126:895–931, 1947.

114. Nardo, C.: Contributo alla conoscenza radiologica dei condrosarcomi. Tumori, 39:308–326, 1953.

115. Netherlands Committee on Bone Tumours: Radiological Atlas of Bone Tumours. Vol. 1. Baltimore, Williams & Wilkins, 1966, p. 76.

116. Neumann, H. W., and Fleissner, H. K.: Behandlungsergebnisse bei Osteosarkomen, Chondrosarkomen und Fibrosarkomen. Beitr. Orthop. Traumatol., 21:559–568, 1974.

117. Odom, J. A., Jr., DeMuth, W. E., Jr., and Blakemore, W. S.: Chest wall chondrosarcoma in youth. J. Thorac. Cardiovasc. Surg., 50:550–554, 1965.

118. O'Neal, L. W., and Ackerman, L. V.: Cartilaginous tumors of ribs and sternum. J. Thorac. Surg., 21:71–108, 1951.

119. O'Neal, L. W., and Ackerman, L. V.: Chondrosarcoma of bone. Cancer, 5:551–577, 1952.

120. Pachter, M. R., and Alpert, M.: Chondrosarcoma of the foot skeleton. J. Bone Joint Surg. [Am.], 46:601–607, 1064.

121. Pack. G. T.: On the management of giant cartilaginous tumors of the pelvic and shoulder girdles. Surgery, 62:405–406, 1967.

122. Parrish, F. F.: Allograft replacement of all or part of the end of a long bone following excision of a tumor. Report of 21 cases. J. Bone Joint Surg. [Am.], 55:1–22, 1973.

123. Parrish, F. F.: Total and partial half joint resection followed by allograft replacement in neoplasms involving ends of long bones. Transplant. Proc. 8(Supplement 1):77–81, 1976.

124. Patel, M. R., Pearlman, H. S., Engler, J., et al.: Chondrosarcoma of the proximal phalanx of the finger. Review of the literature and report of a case. J. Bone Joint Surg. [Am.], 59:401–403, 1977.

125. Peabody, C. N.: Chondrosarcoma of sternum. Report of a six-year survival. J. Thorac. Cardiovasc. Surg., 61:636–640, 1971.

126. Pendergrass, E. P., Lafferty, J. O., and Horn, R. C.: Osteogenic sarcoma and chondrosarcoma; with special reference to the roentgen diagnosis. Am. J. Roentgenol. Radium Ther. Nucl. Med., 54:234–256, 1945.

127. Phelan, J. T., and Cabrera, A.: Chondrosarcoma of bone. Surg. Gynecol. Obstet., 119:42–46, 1964.

128. Phemister, D. B.: A study of the ossification in bone sarcoma. Radiology, 7:17–23, 1926.

129. Phemister, D. B.: Chondrosarcoma of bone. Surg. Gynecol. Obstet., 50:216–233, 1930.

130. Potdar, G. G.: Chondrosarcoma. Indian J. Cancer, 7:280–287, 1970.

131. Potdar, G. G., and Srikhande, S. S.: Chondrogenic tumors of the jaws. Oral Surg., 30:649–658, 1970.

132. Rabinovich, Yu.Ya.: Chondrosarcomas and osteochondrosarcomas of the bones. Khirurgiia (Mosk.), 35(11):78–86, 1959.

133. Reimann, H., and Kienböck, R.: Über Gelenks-Osteochondromatose mit Sarkombildung. Roentgenpraxis, 3:942–944, 1931.

134. Reiter, F. B., Ackerman, L. V., and Staple, T. W.: Central chondrosarcoma of the appendicular skeleton. Radiology, 105:525–530, 1972.

135. Relkin, R.: Hypocalcemia resulting from calcium accretion by a chondrosarcoma. Cancer, 34:1834–1837, 1974.

136. Roberg, O. T., Jr.: Chondrosarcoma. The relation of structure and location to the clinical course. Surg. Gynecol. Obstet., 61:68–82, 1935.

137. Roberts, P. H., and Price, C. H. G.: Chondrosarcoma of the bones of the hand. J. Bone Joint Surg. [Br.], 59:213–221, 1977.

138. Roger, A., and Meary, R.: Les chondrosarcomes. Rev. Prat., 19:2415–2422, 1969.

139. Šafář, J.: Chondrosarcoma of the chest wall in a three-month-old infant with prolonged survival. Cesk. Pediatr., 19(5):422–424, 1964.

140. Salib, P. I.: Chondrosarcoma. A study of the cases treated at the Massachusetts General Hospital in 27 years (1937–1963). Am. J. Orthop., 9:240–242, 1967.

141. Salmon, M.: Chondrosarcome de l'extrémité supérieure du fémur: radiothérapie, résection de l'épiphyse, prothèse en acrylic, resultat tardif (6 ans). Rev. Chir. Orthop., 42:621–629, 1956.

142. Samii, M., and Faupel, G.: Chondrosarcoma with intraspinal, intra- and extrathoracal extension. Acta Neurochir., 39:71–80, 1977.

143. Sanchez, J. E., and Herrera, N. E.: Chondrosarcoma of the sternum. A case report. Conn. Med., 38:589–592, 1974.

144. Schabel, S. I., and Burgener, F. A.: Osteitis pubis in renal failure simulating chondrosarcoma. Br. J. Radiol., 48:1027–1028, 1975.

145. Schajowicz, F.: Juxtacortical chondrosarcoma. J. Bone Joint Surg. [Br.], 59:473–480, 1977.

146. Schajowicz, F., and Bessone, J. E.: Chondrosarcoma in three brothers. A pathological and genetic study. J. Bone Joint Surg. [Am.], 49:129–141, 1967.

147. Schajowicz, F., Cabrini, R. L., Simes, R. J., et al.: Ultrastructure of chondrosarcoma. Clin. Orthop., 100:378–386, 1974.

148. Sharma, O. P., Pinto, J. M., and Hingorani, C. B.: Chondrosarcoma — a roentgenographic and follow-up study. Indian J. Cancer, 11:326–335, 1974.

149. Sinkovics, J. G., Shirato, E., Martin, R. G., et al.: Chondrosarcoma. I. A brief review of 83 patients. J. Med., 1:15–25, 1970.

150. Sinkovics, J. G., Shirato, E., Martin, R. G., et al.: Chondrosarcoma. Immune reactions of a patient to autologous tumor. Cancer, 27:782–793, 1971.

151. Smith, J., McLachlan, D. L., Huvos, A. G., et al.: Primary tumors of the clavicle and scapula. Am. J. Roentgenol. Radium Ther. Nucl. Med., 124:113–123, 1975.

152. Smith, W. S., and Simon, M. A.: Segmental resection for chondrosarcoma. J. Bone Joint Surg. [Am.], 57:1097–1103, 1975.

153. Sobolev, A.: Osteoid chondroma. Dissertation. Moscow, 1873.

154. Solomon, L.: Chondrosarcoma in hereditary multiple exostosis. S. Afr. Med. J., 48:671–676, 1974.

155. Spjut, H. J.: Cartilagenous malignant tumors arising in the skeleton. In: Proceedings Seventh National Cancer Conference. Philadelphia, J. B. Lippincott Co., 1973, pp. 921–924.

156. Spuler, R.: Ueber den feineren Bau der Chondrome. Beitr. Pathol. Anat. Allg. Pathol., 32:253–265, 1902.

157. Sugarbaker, E. D., and Ackerman, L. V.: Disarticulation of the innominate bone for malignant tumors of the pelvic parietes and upper thigh. Surg. Gynecol. Obstet., 81:36–52, 1945.

158. Sweet, M. B. E., Thonar, E. J., and Immelman, A. R.: Glycosaminoglycans and proteoglycans of human chondrosarcoma. Biochim. Biophys. Acta, 437:71–86, 1976.

159. Taylor, G. W., and Rogers, W. P., Jr.: Hindquarter amputation. Experience with eighteen cases. N. Engl. J. Med., 249:963–969, 1953.

160. Thomine, J. M.: Cartilaginous tumours of the pelvic girdle. In Price, C. H. G., and Ross, F. G. M. (eds.) Bone — Certain Aspects of Neoplasia. Philadelphia, F. A. Davis Co. (Butterworths), 1973, pp. 451–459.

161. Thompson, V. P., and Steggall, C. T.: Chondrosarcoma of the proximal portion of the femur treated by resection and bone replacement. A six-year result. J. Bone Joint Surg. [Am.], 38:357–367, 1956.

162. Thomson, A. D., and Turner-Warwick, R. T.: Skeletal sarcomata and giant-cell tumour. J. Bone Joint Surg. [Br.], 37:266–303, 1955.

163. Ujiki, G. T., Method, H. L., Putong, P. B., et al.: Primary chondrosarcoma of the diaphragm. Am. J. Surg., 122:132–134, 1971.

164. Ungar, F.: Revisione clinico-statistica di 187 condromi a di 94 condrosarcomi osservati nel Centro Tumori degli Organi di Movimento di Firenze. Arch. Putti Chir. Organi Mov., 25:257–278, 1970.

165. Unni, K. K., Dahlin, D. C., Beabout, J. W., et al.: Chondrosarcoma: clear-cell variant. A report of sixteen cases. J. Bone Joint Surg. [Am.], 58:676–683, 1976.

166. Uno, Y., Kasumi, H., Takemoto, T., et al.: Poorly differentiated so called collagenochondrosarcoma. Jap. J. Cancer Clin., 21:51–55, 1975.

167. Vernick, S. H., Kay, S., Escobar, M., et al.: Intracisternal tubules in myxoid chondrosarcoma. Letter to the editor. Arch. Pathol. Lab. Med., 101:556, 1977.

168. Virchow, R.: Ueber Perlgeschwülste. Arch. Pathol. Anat., 8:371–418, 1855.

169. Volkmann, R.: Acutes, schmerzhaftes Enchondrom des Metacarpus; Enchondrome der Lunge. Dtsch. Klin., 7:577–578, 1855.

170. Warburg, O.: The metabolism of carcinoma cells. J. Cancer Res., 9:148–163, 1925.

171. Warren, S.: Chondrosarcoma with intravascular growth and tumor emboli to lungs. Am. J. Pathol., 7:161–167, 1931.

172. Weber, O.: Zur Geschichte des Enchondroms namentlich in Bezug auf dessen hereditäres Vorkommen und secundäre Verbreitung in inneren Organen durch Embolie. Arch. Pathol. Anat., 35:501–524, 1866.

173. Weisel, W., Watson, R. R., and O'Connor, T. M.: Sternal resection for chondrosarcoma. Wis. Med. J., 73:97–100, 1974.

174. Wolfe, H. J., and Vickery, A. L., Jr.: The use of

175. Wu, K. K., and Kelly, A. P.: Periosteal (juxtacortical) chondrosarcoma: report of a case occurring in the hand. J. Hand Surg., 2:314–315, 1977.

176. Yaghmai, I., and Ghahremani, G. G.: Chondrosarcoma of the esophagus. Am. J. Roentgenol. Radium Ther. Nucl. Med., 126:1175–1177, 1976.

177. Zanoli, R., and Domeniconi, S.: Il condrosarcoma dello scheletro. Chir. Organi Mov., 42:243–290, 1955.

S^{35}-labeled sulfate in studies on human normal and neoplastic cartilage tissues. Lab. Invest., 13:743–751, 1964.

MESENCHYMAL CHONDROSARCOMA (POORLY DIFFERENTIATED CHONDROSARCOMA)

A relatively recently described, rare variety of chondrosarcoma is mesenchymal chondrosarcoma. Originally, 2 examples were described by Lichtenstein and Bernstein among 25 unusual benign and malignant cartilaginous tumors of bone.[15] This type of tumor is a distinct clinicopathologic entity differing from the usual chondrosarcoma by its generally unfavorable clinical outcome, predilection for unusual osseous sites, and frequent origin in extraskeletal tissues. The designation "mesenchymal" is a rather unfortunate one; it is a tautology in that all sarcomas, including chondrosarcomas, except malignant schwannomas are mesenchymal. Azar has suggested a more apt descriptive term: poorly differentiated chondrosarcoma.[1] These tumors were referred to in previous publications as "chondroblastoma with peculiar histologic character,"[2] "primitive multipotential primary sarcoma of bone,"[11] "hemangiopericytoma with cartilaginous differentiation,"[25] or "polyhistioma."[12]

The tally of the literature reveals about 70 reported cases. The most common skeletal locations, in descending order of frequency, include ribs, mandible, maxilla, skull, pelvis, and vertebral column. Only infrequently are the long tubular bones involved (Fig. 13–23). About one third of the cases arise in extraskeletal sites, such as various skeletal muscles, orbit, meninges, and brain (Fig. 13–24). More than half of the patients are in the second and third decades of life, with an age range from 5 to 70 years.[27] A slight (64 per cent) female predilection is noted. The clinical course is quite variable but is generally characterized by local recurrences and eventual metastases. The recommended treatment favors radical surgical removal with postoperative chemotherapy since the available data so far suggest that these tumors are practically radioresistant.[17] Late metastases, even in the face of complete resection, may occur in other bones, the lungs, lymph nodes, and brain.

Histologically, the tumor is defined by a bimorphic or biphasic growth pattern with sheets of undifferentiated small round cells similar to those of Ewing's sarcoma and lobules of cartilage showing the characteristics of a low-grade chondrosarcoma (Fig. 13–25). In some areas, instead of, or adjacent to, the sheets of round small tumor cells, the pattern of the tumor indicates a hemangiopericytoma (Figs. 13–26 and 13–27). The cartilage component contains ample matrix and may show areas of calcifications or ossification. Several articles describe the ultrastructural features of this neoplasm.[7, 31]

Text continued on page 237

Figure 13–23. Mesenchymal chondrosarcoma of distal end of femur in a 37-year-old man. The mottled, trabeculated, largely lytic metaphyseal lesion destroys the medullary bone and extends through cortex into surrounding soft tissue. The radiographic diagnosis here includes aggressive giant cell tumor. Note hemorrhagic character of lesion. (Courtesy of Dr. R. C. Marcove.)

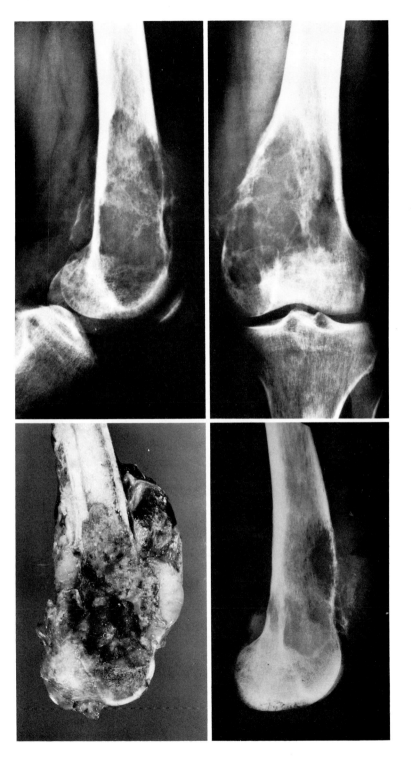

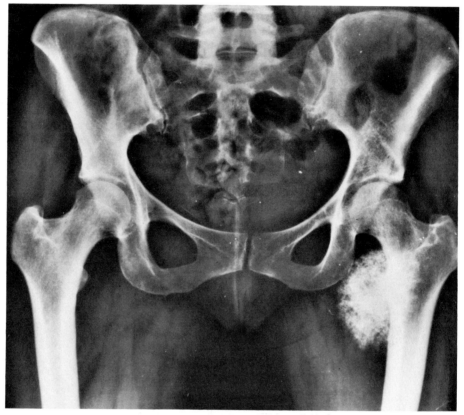

Figure 13–24. Extraosseous mesenchymal chondrosarcoma of thigh with heavy calcification in a 39-year-old woman. Other radiographic views clearly showed the lesion not to be arising in bone. (Courtesy of Dr. R. C. Marcove.)

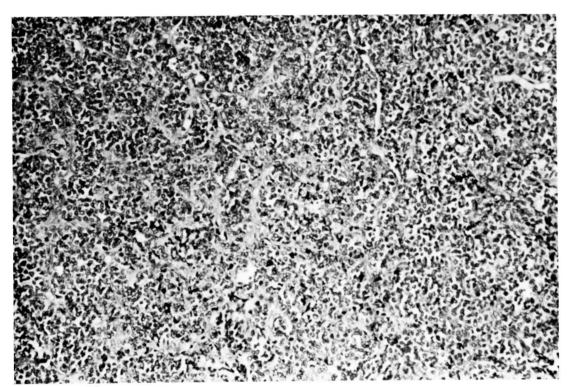

Figure 13–25.   Microscopic field from a mesenchymal chondrosarcoma exhibiting an undifferentiated small cell sarcoma pattern similar to Ewing's sarcoma. (Hematoxylin-eosin stain. Magnification × 100.)

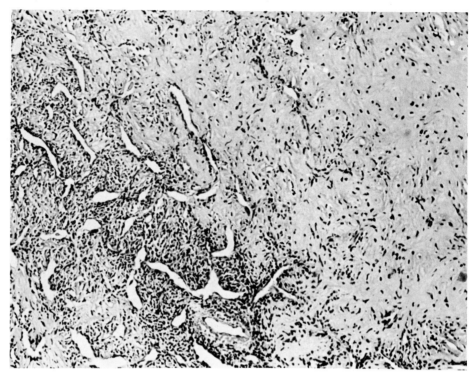

Figure 13–26. Mesenchymal chondrosarcoma. A hemangiopericytomatoid growth pattern is seen (left lower corner) melding imperceptibly into a cartilaginous tumor. (Hematoxylin-eosin stain. Magnification × 100.)

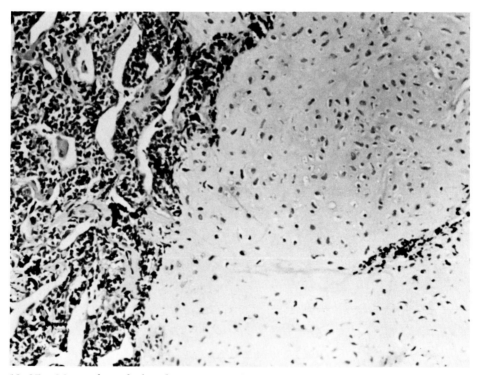

Figure 13–27. Mesenchymal chondrosarcoma. The hemangiopericytoma-like area is more characteristic here and the cartilage growth traits are also well shown. (Hematoxylin-eosin stain. Magnification × 180.)

REFERENCES

1. Azar, H. A.: Discussion. Cancer Seminar, *1*:39, 1976.
2. Benedetti, G. B.: Tumore condroblastico della mandibola a caratteri istologici peculiari. Chir. Organi Mov., *50*:135–144, 1951.
3. Cárdenas-Ramírez, L., Albores-Saavedra, J., and de Buen, S.: Mesenchymal chondrosarcoma of the orbit. Report of the first case in orbital location. Arch. Ophthalmol., *86*:410–413, 1971.
4. Chaves, E.: Condrosarcoma mesenquimal. Hospital (Rio de J.), *68*:1217–1225, 1965.
5. Dahlin, D. C., and Henderson, E. D.: Mesenchymal chondrosarcoma: further observations on a new entity. Cancer, *15*:410–417, 1962.
6. Dowling, E. A.: Mesenchymal chondrosarcoma. J. Bone Joint Surg. [Am.], *46*:747–754, 1964.
7. Fu, Y.-S., and Kay, S.: A comparative ultrastructural study of mesenchymal chondrosarcoma and myxoid chondrosarcoma. Cancer, *33*:1531–1542, 1974.
8. Gawlik, Z.: Chondrosarcoma mesenchymale. Patol. Pol., *19*:289–297, 1968.
9. Goldman, R. L.: "Mesenchymal" chondrosarcoma, a rare malignant chondroid tumor usually primary in bone. Report of a case arising in extraskeletal soft tissue. Cancer, *20*:1494–1498, 1967.
10. Guccion, J. G., Font, R. L., Enzinger, F. M., et al.: Extraskeletal mesenchymal chondrosarcoma. Arch. Pathol., *95*:336–340, 1973.
11. Hutter, R. V. P., Foote, F. W., Francis, K. C., et al.: Primitive multipotential primary sarcoma of bone. Cancer, *19*:1–25, 1966.
12. Jacobson, S. A.: Polyhistioma. A malignant tumor of bone and extraskeletal tissues. Cancer, *40*:2116–2130, 1977.
13. Klein, H., and Spinelli, M.: Mesenchymal chondrosarcoma. Report of two extraskeletal cases. Zentralbl. Allg. Pathol., *120*:51–55, 1976.
14. Koselnik-Glugla, B., and Ejsmont, K.: Mesenchymal chondrosarcoma of maxilla. Otolaryngol. Pol., *27*:671–673, 1973.
15. Lichtenstein, L., and Bernstein, D.: Unusual benign and malignant chondroid tumors of bone. Cancer, *12*:1142–1157, 1959.
16. Mandalenakis, N.: Mesenchymatous chondrosarcoma. Histological and ultrastructural study. Ann. Anat. Pathol., *19*:175–188, 1974.
17. Mazabraud, A.: Mesenchymal chondrosarcoma. Six cases. Rev. Chir. Orthop., *60*:197–203, 1974.
18. Muir, C. S., and Seah, C. S.: Primary chondrosarcomatous mesenchymoma of the mitral valve. Thorax, *21*:254–262, 1966.
19. Nezelof, C., Mazabraud, A., and Meary, R.: Le chondrosarcome mésenchymateux. A propos d'un cas de localisation pararachidienne. Arch. Anat. Pathol., *13*:26–28, 1965.
20. Pavon, S. J., Bullough, P. G., and Marcove, R. C.: Mesenchymal chondrosarcoma. Medullary lesion of humerus. N. Y. State J. Med., *71*:1662–1664, 1971.
21. Pepe, A. J., Kuhlmann, R. F., and Miller, D. B.: Mesenchymal chondrosarcoma. A case report. J. Bone Joint Surg. [Am.], *59*:256–258, 1977.
22. Pirschel, J.: Ein mesenchymales Chondrosarkom des Sternum. Fortschr. Geb. Roentgenstr. Nuklearmed., *124*:91–93, 1976.
23. Pittman, M. R., and Keller, E. E.: Mesenchymal chondrosarcoma: report of case. J. Oral Surg., *32*:443–447, 1974.
24. Raskind, R., and Grant, S.: Primary mesenchymal chondrosarcoma of the cerebrum. Report of a case. J. Neurosurg., *24*:676–678, 1966.
25. Reeh, M. J.: Hemangiopericytoma with cartilaginous differentiation involving orbit. Arch. Ophthalmol., *75*:82–83, 1966.
26. Rengachary, S. S., and Kepes, J. J.: Spinal epidural metastatic "mesenchymal" chondrosarcoma. Case report. J. Neurosurg., *30*:71–73, 1969.
27. Salvador, A. H., Beabout, J. W., and Dahlin, D. C.: Mesenchymal chondrosarcoma — observations on 30 new cases. Cancer, *28*:605–615, 1971.
28. Sears, W. P., Tefft, M., and Cohen, J.: Postirradiation mesenchymal chondrosarcoma. Pediatrics, *40*:254–258, 1967.
29. Sengupta, P., and Sarcar, S. K.: Mesenchymal chondrosarcoma — report of 4 cases. Indian J. Cancer, *12*:84–90, 1975.
30. Sevel, D.: Mesenchymal chondrosarcoma of the orbit. Br. J. Ophthalmol., *58*:882–887, 1974.
31. Steiner, G. C., Mirra, J. M., and Bullough, P. G.: Mesenchymal chondrosarcoma. A study of the ultrastructure. Cancer, *32*:926–939, 1973.
32. Trzcinska-Dabrowska, Z., Witwicki, T., and Zielinska, K.: Primary "mesenchymal" chondrosarcoma of the orbit (chondrosarcoma mesenchymale primitivum orbitae) treated by biological resection. Ophthalmologica, *157*:24–35, 1969.
33. Wu, W. Q., and Lapi, A.: Primary non-skeletal intracranial cartilaginous neoplasms: report of a chondroma and a mesenchymal chondrosarcoma. J. Neurol. Neurosurg. Psychiatry, *33*:469–475, 1970.

14

CHONDROSARCOMA OF THE CRANIOFACIAL BONES

INCIDENCE

Just under 10 per cent of chondrosarcomas in adults develop in the craniofacial osseous system, an incidence roughly comparable to that of osteogenic sarcomas of the same region (see Fig. 13–4). Approximately 20 per cent of the rare chondrosarcomas arising in children involve the head and neck.

SIGNS AND SYMPTOMS

The majority of the symptoms relate to the site of origin and the size of the tumor. An enlarging, usually painless mass is the most frequent symptom noted. Loosening of the teeth or poorly fitting dentures are initial features. Nasal obstruction, epistaxis, headaches, proptosis, and visual disturbances are present with nasal septal lesions. Pain is not a consistent and early symptom, and only about one third of the patients manifest it initially. Since the development of the tumor is usually slow and gradually progressive, the overall period from onset of symptoms to diagnosis ranges from three months to one year. Occasional patients, however, report

symptoms for longer than five years before definitive diagnosis is established. Chondrosarcomas of the mandibular condyle may manifest the typical symptoms of the temporomandibular joint dysfunction syndrome and can reach a considerable size without producing clinically demonstrable swelling.[44]

AGE AND SEX DISTRIBUTION

The average age of patients with chondrosarcomas of all sites is approximately 40 years; the average age of those with tumors arising in the craniofacial bones is 32 years (Fig. 13–3). One third of the patients are under 20 years of age, and two thirds are under 40. The youngest patient reported was a 16-month-old baby boy.[23] The oldest patient at Memorial Hospital was 72 years.[2] About two thirds of the patients are male.

LOCATION

The maxilla, preferentially in its anterior alveolar region, is involved most frequently (approximately 60 per cent).[5, 53, 54] The mandible is the second most common site of occurrence with a predilection for the coronoid process, the condyles, the premolars or molars, and the symphyseal regions (approximately 30 per cent).[58] The rest of the cases involve the cranial vault.[3] In comparison, osteogenic sarcomas of the head and neck grow more frequently in the mandible. The calvarium, the nasal bones,[17, 36, 55] the upper alveolar ridge, and the cervical spine may, on occasion, give rise to chondrosarcomas. Malignant cartilage tumors of the skull associated with Maffucci's syndrome have been reported.[16] The temporomandibular joint may be a rare site of chondrosarcoma.[34, 48] Primary malignant cartilaginous laryngeal or tracheobronchial tree tumors have been reported.[24, 33]

EMBRYOLOGIC CONSIDERATIONS

As was already pointed out in the discussion of osteogenic sarcomas of craniofacial bones, the maxilla and mandible are formed in membrane bone and are not preformed in cartilage. Cartilage, however, is intimately associated with the embryonic development of these bones since, for instance, Meckel's cartilage is noted in the mandibular arch prior to the appearance of bone. The process of ossification in this region usually eliminates the foci of cartilage, but it is conceivable that some may persist. The fibrocartilage arising from the mandibular symphysis may develop secondarily from midline connective tissues and therefore does not evolve from the embryonic chondrocranium. The mandibular condyle and the coronoid process also develop from fibrocartilage. Miles has convincingly demonstrated the relation of the maxilla to the chondrocranium, thereby postulating how cartilage remnants may be encountered in this region.[42] The nasal capsule and the paranasal septum may provide foci of residual cartilage from which chondroid tumors may arise. It is well known that under normal circumstances cartilage may be recognized in the palate in adults. Those who do not completely agree with these explanations suggest that some of the chondrosarcomas so reported are in fact chondroblastic osteogenic sarcomas.[32]

RADIOGRAPHIC FEATURES

Radiographic examination, especially tomograms, are of great help in pointing to a diagnosis and defining the extent of the lesion. The newly developed technique of computerized axial tomographic scan clearly outlines the dimensions of tumor involvement, thereby establishing operability. This method of C.T. scanning, coupled with contrast enhancement, not only establishes the extent of bone destruction but also reveals the often considerable displacement of the surrounding soft tissues and the distortion of the ventricular system of the brain. Carotid angiography may also help to clearly outline the lesion. Roentgen examination reveals osteolytic, radiopaque, or mixed type of lesion. On occasion, a large tumor of minor salivary gland origin arising in the sinuses may simulate a chondrosarcoma. Frequently, a localized, uniform widening of the periodontal membrane space is seen in chondrosarcomas arising in the jaws similarly to osteogenic sarcomas.[1] This finding is especially valuable, since some of these lesions lack calcific intralesional densities, especially in more advanced cases in which lytic changes are prominent. Sinus opacification[13, 32] or a densely calcified mass may also be encountered.

HISTOLOGIC FEATURES

The key to a proper diagnosis is an adequate sample of tissue, preferably obtained from various areas of the lesion. One should be wary of the diagnosis of a "chondroma" arising in craniofacial bones, since chondrosarcomas outnumber benign cartilage lesions in this region at least two to one.[14] This is especially so in large cartilage tumors.

Lesions histologically considered to be benign, upon recurrence, are found to be more cellular and often frankly malignant. In general, the microscopic features of chondrosarcomas arising in the jaws are those of malignant cartilage tumors of other sites. It should be noted that mesenchymal chondrosarcoma has a special preference for the jaws.[6, 47]

Since about half of the osteogenic sarcomas arising in the jaws have a prominent cartilage component (chondroblastic osteogenic sarcoma), the most important differential diagnostic consideration is to separate this entity. Endochondral ossification or metaplastic bone formation are features of chondrosarcoma, and direct osteoid production by the neoplastic stromal cells identify osteogenic sarcoma. Large, locally aggressive, benign mixed tumors of minor salivary gland origin with a prominent cartilage component may cause diagnostic difficulty, especially if only a small biopsy specimen is available for microscopic examination. The cartilage component in a benign mixed tumor closely resembles well-differentiated hyaline cartilage with foci of myxochondroid growth traits. There is, of course, no microscopic evidence for a chondrosarcoma in such salivary gland tumors. Chordomas of the spheno-occipital region and chondrosarcomas arising at the skull base may be distinguished, on occasion, with considerable difficulty histologically, clinically, and radiographically.[28]

TREATMENT AND PROGNOSIS

Patients with chondrosarcomas arising in the craniofacial osseous structures present an interesting group that challenges the inventiveness of the head and neck surgeon when devising sufficiently extensive but curative procedures that are restricted by the very nature of the anatomic location. Freedom from recurrence depends so much on the complete eradication of the growth. It was generally found that radical surgery, with the lines of surgical excision carried well into uninvolved normal tissues, provides the most effective treatment.

The treatment of chondrosarcoma of the craniofacial bones includes radical and local surgery, supervoltage radiotherapy,[40, 45] chemotherapy, and various combinations thereof but results are, in general, unsatisfactory.

Mandibular resection is employed to remove lesions of the lower jaw. The classic commando type of resection or radical neck dissection has not been employed as part of this procedure.[2] Partial maxillectomy is used to encompass small lesions in the upper alveolar region. Orbital exenteration, in addition to the maxillary resection, may be necessary for large tumors.

The surgical resection should go well beyond the margin of the lesion as demonstrated by radiography. A radiograph of the specimen prepared immediately following the resection is of help in determining the adequacy of the surgical procedure. In order to establish the surgical lines of resection intraoperatively, they may be examined, if feasible, by frozen section. Resection margins of the mandible, for instance, may be scraped by a sharp instrument and the tissue smeared on a glass slide and stained by hematoxylin and eosin.

Ballantyne summarizes his view of mandibular resections, the disability following such major surgery, and the various prosthetic replacement methods.[4] The surgeon and the maxillofacial prosthodontist should plan every phase of the postoperative reconstruction preoperatively.[57]

When the primary radical excision is incomplete or the tumor has invaded the floor of the orbit, recurrence is prompt and death ensues within one to two years.[2] The local recurrence rate for all therapeutic modalities is quite high, and the cure rate (44 per cent at five years) is directly related to the ability for successful local control. Survival is best in cases initially treated by radical surgery, and a precipitous drop in cure rate is evidenced in patients with local recurrence or with persistent lesions. Most of the patients who die succumb to uncontrolled local disease, and only a few will show distant metastatic spread.[19] The major factor leading to death is extension of chondrosarcoma into the brain. Sites of metastases include the lungs and the other bones. Lymph nodes are rarely involved.[48] A rare patient will survive free of disease for more than five years after secondary resection for recurrent disease. In summarizing the results of treatment, Fu and Perzin outlined three important factors influencing prognosis.[21]

1. *The location and extent of the tumor.* Nasopharyngeal, posterior nasal, and sphenoid sinus tumors have a guarded prognosis since they are large when detected and consequently cannot be removed in their entirety.

2. *The adequacy of the primary surgical removal.*

3. *The grade of malignancy of the chondrosarcoma* correlates with prognosis. This factor seems to be logical but is difficult to prove with only relatively few cases available for such evaluation.

Although chondrosarcomas of the jaws in general are slowly progressive neoplasms characterized by multiple recurrences prior to hematogenous metastases, Fronstin and associates[20] found that two thirds of the patients died within 5 years owing to their disease, either from locally destructive tumor or from widespread metastases. Chondrosarcomas are usually not considered to be radiosensitive lesions, but an occasional case like that reported by Paddison and Hanks in 1971 seems to regress following irradiation.

REFERENCES

1. Anderson, J. A., and Cornyn, J.: Radiographic and pathologic diagnosis of tumors of the jaws. J. Natl. Med. Assoc., 67:277–282, 1975.
2. Arlen, M., Tollefsen, H. R., Huvos, A. G., et al.: Chondrosarcoma of the head and neck. Am. J. Surg., 120:456–460, 1970.
3. Bahr, A. L., and Gayler, B. W.: Cranial chondrosarcomas. Report of four cases and review of the literature. Radiology, 124:151–156, 1977.
4. Ballantyne, A. J.: A surgeon's view of mandibular resection and replacement. J. Prosthet. Dent., 38:42–51, 1977.
5. Batsakis, J. G., and Dito, W. R.: Chondrosarcoma of the maxilla. Arch. Otolaryngol., 75:55–61, 1962.
6. Benedetti, G. B.: Tumore condroblastico della mandibola a caratteri istologici peculiari. Chir. Organi Mov., 50:135–144, 1951.
7. Berkmen, Y. M., and Blatt, E. S.: Cranial and intracranial cartilaginous tumours. Clin. Radiol., 19:327–333, 1968.
8. Bhatt, A. P., Dholakia, H. M., and Bhoweer, A. L.: Chondrosarcoma of maxilla (report of a case). J. Oral Med., 32:51–54, 1977.
9. Blum, T.: Cartilage tumors of the jaws: report of three cases. Oral Surg., 7:1320–1334, 1954.
10. Boskov, H.: Chondrosarcoma maxillae. God. Zb. Med. Fak. Skopje, 20:405–414, 1974.
11. Brocheriou, C., and Payen, J.: Cartilaginous tumors of the jaws. Ann. Anat. Pathol., 20:23–34, 1975.
12. Cendelin, E.: Chondromatous tumours in the maxillofacial region. Dtsch. Stomat., 19:746–753, 1969.
13. Cernéa, P., Payen, J., and Brocheriou, C.: Sarcomes osseux des maxillaires: Etude statistique de 41 observations. Bull. Cancer, 61:151–160, 1974.
14. Chaudhry, A. P., Robinovitch, M. R., Mitchell, D. F., et al.: Chondrogenic tumors of the jaws. Am. J. Surg., 102:403–411, 1961.
15. Cohen, B., and Smith, C. J.: Chondrosarcoma of the mandible. Ann. R. Coll. Surg. Engl., 32:303–313, 1963.
16. Cook, P. L., and Evans, P. G.: Chondrosarcoma of the skull in Maffucci's syndrome. Br. J. Radiol., 50:833–836, 1977.
17. Coyas, A. J.: Chondrosarcoma of the nose. J. Laryngol. Otol., 79:69–72, 1965.
18. Curphey, J. E.: Chondrosarcoma of the maxilla: report of case. J. Oral Surg., 29:285–290, 1971.
19. El-Gindi, S., Abd-El-Hafeez, M., and Salama, M.: Extracranial skeletal metastases from an intracranial meningeal chondrosarcoma. Case report. J. Neurosurg., 40:651–653, 1974.
20. Fronstin, M. H., Hutcheson, J. B., and Sanders, H. L.: Chondrosarcoma of the mandibular symphysis. Oral Surg., 25:665–669, 1968.
21. Fu, Y.-S., and Perzin, K. H.: Non-epithelial tumors of the nasal cavity, paranasal sinuses, and nasopharynx: a clinicopathologic study. III. Cartilaginous tumors (chondroma, chondrosarcoma). Cancer, 34:453–463, 1974.
22. Gabrielsen, T. O., and Kingman, A. F., Jr.: Osteocartilaginous tumors of the base of the skull. Report of a unique case and review of the literature. Am. J. Roentgenol. Radium Ther. Nucl. Med., 91:1016–1023, 1964.
23. Gallagher, T. M., and Strome, M.: Chondrosarcomas of the facial region. Laryngoscope, 82:978–984, 1972.
24. Goethals, P. L., Dahlin, D. C., and Devine, K. D.: Cartilaginous tumors of the larynx. Surg. Gynecol. Obstet., 117:77–82, 1963.
25. Goldstein, I. H., and Goldstein, M. C.: Jaw metastases in chondroblastic osteogenic sarcoma. Am. J. Orthod., 29:57–59, 1943.
26. Greer, J. A., Jr., Devine, K. D., and Dahlin, D. C.: Gardner's syndrome and chondrosarcoma of the hyoid bone. Arch. Otolaryngol., 103:425–427, 1977.
27. Harris, M.: The enigmatic chondrosarcoma of the maxilla. Oral Surg., 34:13–20, 1972.
28. Heffelfinger, M. J., Dahlin, D. C., MacCarty, C. S., et al.: Chordomas and cartilaginous tumors at the skull base. Cancer, 32:410–420, 1973.
29. Hofmann, L.: Contribution à l'étude histologique et clinique des ostéo et chondrosarcomes du maxillaire supérieur. Ann. Mal. Oreil. Larynx, 45:433–457, 1926.
30. Kemper, J. W., and Bloom, H. J.: Metastatic osteochondroma of maxilla from primary tumor of tibia. Report of case. Am. J. Orthod., 30:704–708, 1944.
31. Krantz, S., and Gay, B. B., Jr.: Primary chondrosarcoma of the occipital bone. Am. J. Roentgenol. Radium Ther. Nucl. Med., 69:598–604, 1953.
32. Kragh, L. V., Dahlin, D. C., and Erich, J. B.: Cartilaginous tumors of the jaws and facial regions. Am. J. Surg., 99:852–856, 1960.
33. Kurtz, D. M.: Primary cartilaginous laryngeal neoplasm. N. Y. State J. Med., 75:85–86, 1975.
34. Lanier, V. C., Jr., Rosenfeld, L., and Wilkinson, H. A.: Chondrosarcoma of the mandible. South. Med. J., 64:711–714, 1971.
35. Lapidot, A., Ramm, C., and Fani, K.: Chondrosarcoma of maxilla (case report). J. Laryngol. Otol., 80:743–747, 1966.
36. Lawson, L. J.: Intranasal chondrosarcoma. Report of a case. Arch. Otolaryngol., 55:559–565, 1952.

37. Leedham, P. W., and Swash, M.: Chondrosarcoma with subarachnoid dissemination. J. Pathol., *107*:59–61, 1972.

38. Link, J. F.: Chondrosarcoma of maxilla. Oral Surg., 7:140–144, 1954.

39. Looser, K. G., and Kuehn, P. G.: Primary tumors of the mandible. A study of 49 cases. Am. J. Surg., *132*:608–614, 1976.

40. Lott, S., and Bordley, J. E.: A radiosensitive chondrosarcoma of the sphenoid sinus and base of the skull. Report of a case. Laryngoscope, *82*:57–60, 1972.

41. Lynch, P. G., and Uriburu, E.: An intracranial cartilage-containing meningeal tumor. Case report. J. Neurosurg., *39*:261–264, 1973.

42. Miles, A. E. W.: Chondrosarcoma of the maxilla. Br. Dent. J., *88*:257–269, 1950.

43. Minagi, H., and Newton, T. H.: Cartilaginous tumors of the base of skull. Am. J. Roentgenol. Radium Ther. Nucl. Med., *105*:308–313, 1969.

44. Nortjé, C. J., Farman, A. G., Grotepass, F. W., et al.: Chondrosarcoma of the mandibular condyle. Report of a case with special reference to radiographic features. Br. J. Oral Surg., *14*:101–111, 1976.

45. Paddison, G. M., and Hanks, G. E.: Chondrosarcoma of the maxilla. Report of a case responding to supervoltage irradiation and review of the literature. Cancer, *28*:616–619, 1971.

46. Paterson, W.: Chondrosarcoma of the maxilla. J. Laryngol. Otol., *69*:132–139, 1955.

47. Potdar, G. G., and Srikhande, S. S.: Chondrogenic tumors of the jaws. Oral Surg., *30*:649–658, 1970.

48. Richter, K. J., Freeman, N. S., and Quick, C. A.: Chondrosarcoma of the temporomandibular joint: report of case. J. Oral Surg., *32*:777–781, 1974.

49. Robinson, H. B. G.: Metastasis of chondromyxosarcoma to the jaw and tooth. Am. J. Orthod., *33*:558–566, 1947.

50. Roper-Hall, H. T. and Adcock, A. H.: Cartilaginous tumours of the palate. Dent. Gaz., *5*:417–425, 1939.

51. Roukkula, M.: Roentgenologic findings in chondromas of the pontine angle. Acta Radiol. [Diagn.] (Stockh.), *2*:120–128, 1964.

52. Sandler, H. C.: Chondrosarcoma of the maxilla; report of a case. Oral Surg., *10*:97–104, 1957.

53. Sato, K., Nukaga, H., and Horikoshi, T.: Chondrosarcoma of the jaws and facial skeleton: a review of the Japanese literature. J. Oral Surg., *35*:892–897, 1977.

54. Smatt, V.: Chondrosarcoma of maxillary bone, report of a case. Rev. Stomatol.. Chir. Maxillofac., *78*:45–51, 1977.

55. Soboroff, B. J., and Lederer, F. L.: Chondrosarcoma of the nasal cavity. Ann. Otol. Rhinol. Laryngol., *64*:718–727, 1955.

56. Swerdlow, R. S., Som, M. L., and Biller, H. F.: Cartilaginous tumors of the larynx. Arch. Otolaryngol., *100*:269–272, 1974.

57. Terezhalmy, G. T., and Bottomley, W. K.: Maxillary chondrogenic sarcoma: management of a case. Oral Surg., *44*:539–546, 1977.

58. Tullio, G., and D'Errico, P.: Il condrosarcoma della mandibola. Considerazioni cliniche ed istologiche. Ann. Stomatol., *23*:191–206, 1974.

59. Wakumoto, F., and Ishikawa, G.: An autopsy case of chondrosarcoma of the cranial basis and upper jaw. Gann, *44*:248–250, 1953.

Tumors of Fibrous Connective Tissue Origin Chapters 15 and 16

15

DESMOPLASTIC FIBROMA AND PERIOSTEAL "DESMOID"

DEFINITION

Desmoplastic fibroma is a rare benign tumor of fibrous connective tissue derivation characterized by abundant collagen formation. The lesional tissue is sparsely cellular with ovoid or fusiform nuclei. The absence of both cellularity and pleomorphism and decreased mitotic activity separate this tumor from fibrosarcoma.

INCIDENCE

This tumor is extremely infrequent and only about 50 cases have been reported in the literature.[32]

AGE AND SEX DISTRIBUTION

The age incidence varies widely and ranges from 20 months to 71 years. A soli-

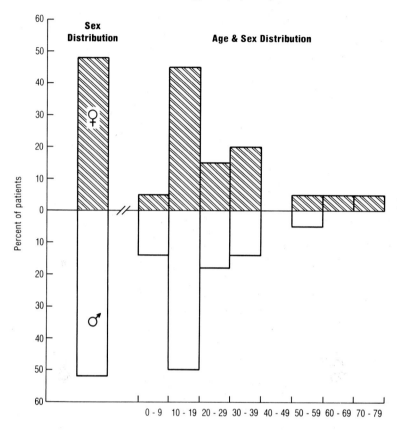

DESMOPLASTIC FIBROMA
42 Pts. (♂ = 22, ♀ = 20)

Figure 15–1. Age and sex distribution in 42 patients with desmoplastic fibroma as reported in the literature.

Average age males : 20   youngest: 20 mos. ; oldest: 56 yrs.
Average age females: 26   youngest: 8 yrs. ; oldest: 71 yrs.

tary congenital case has been recorded.[21] Most of the patients are in their second decade of life; i.e., they are adolescents and young adults. The average age in male patients is 20 years, and it is 6 years more in female patients (Fig. 15–1). The sexes are affected equally.

LOCATION

A wide distribution in the osseous sites of involvement is noted (Fig. 15–2). The most common regions affected are the ilium and the jaws (10 cases each). About half of the lesions arose in the long bones. When the lesion involves long bones, it preferentially affects the metaphyseal ends or both ends of the diaphysis. Epiphyseal extension has also been reported.[37] Only

one of the ten cases reported in the head and neck region involved the maxilla. The rest were in the mandible.

SIGNS AND SYMPTOMS

Most of the lesions fail to produce early symptoms and when discovered are of considerable size. This indicates a slow progressive course. About one case in ten manifests with pathologic fracture.[32] Pain presenting late in the already fully developed tumor is a common finding and swelling follows even later in the course. Location near a joint may present as an effusion.

The concept of desmoplastic fibroma of bone was conceived by Jaffe in 1958 to delineate an extremely rare group of fi-

DESMOPLASTIC FIBROMA
Location in 47 Cases

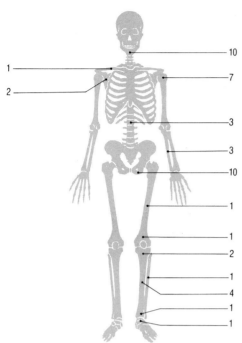

Figure 15–2. Skeletal location in 47 cases of desmoplastic fibroma as reported in the literature.

brous tissue lesions distinct from fibrosarcoma on one end of the spectrum and from various other benign lesions, like nonossifying fibroma or chondromyxoid fibroma, on the other.[14] Since nonossifying fibroma is now considered by many to be a tumor of fibrous histiocytic derivation, the delineation of these two entities is made somewhat easier. In 1935, Cappel described an intramedullary central fibular lesion, which he designated as endosteal fibroma, and this seems now to be the first case of desmoplastic fibroma in the literature.[3]

Periosteal "desmoids," also known as fibromatosis of periosteal location, have been recognized since 1951.[15] This lesion is histologically identical with that of desmoplastic fibroma, and only the location distinguishes the two entities. Central fibromas of the jaws are variants of desmoplastic fibroma in this region and they are histologically indistinguishable.[11, 17] Tumors of fibrous derivation (so-called fibromatoses) may secondarily extend into, or invade, adjacent bones. The clinical and roentgen findings help to separate primary and secondary osseous involvement since

microscopic features are identical.[9, 25] Because of its location, parosteal fasciitis and periosteal desmoid may be confused.[13, 18] Parosteal fasciitis, the analog of the pseudosarcomatous nodular fasciitis of soft tissues, may histologically simulate an aggressive neoplasm, yet it behaves in an innocuous way. Periosteal desmoid, on the other hand, histologically is entirely benign, but it is a clinically aggressive lesion prone to recurrence and requiring numerous re-excisions. Many of the cases reported as "fibroma" of bone are, in fact, examples of ossifying fibroma or fibrous dysplasia, especially those instances that arose in the jaws, and only a few cases of pure fibromas have been reported.[36] Desmoplastic fibromas occurring in the jaws are occasionally referred to as nonodontogenic fibroma.[16] The lack of associated dental abnormalities and the abundantly desmoplastic, collagen-forming properties separate this lesion from an odontogenic fibroma, which is often accompanied by unerupted teeth and noncollagenized fibrous tissue.

RADIOGRAPHIC FEATURES

Radiographically, the lesion is purely osteolytic and well-demarcated and arises centrally from the bone (Fig. 15–3). It presents as medullary, expanded radiolucency with thinned overlying cortex but without any periosteal reaction and usually is located in the metaphyseal end of a long bone. On occasion, diaphyseal or epiphyseal locations have been reported.[37] The borders of the lesion are often irregular and slightly sclerotic, exhibiting a trabeculated appearance. Marked bony destruction may lead to the erroneous impression of a malignant bone tumor.

Radiographic differential diagnosis includes nonossifying fibroma, giant cell tumor, chondromyxoid fibroma, monostotic fibrous dysplasia, and medullary fibrosarcoma. The cortical expansion and lesional trabeculation may also imitate solitary unicameral bone cyst, hemangioma, aneurysmal bone cyst, and eosinophilic granuloma. The mimicry of an osteolytic osteogenic sarcoma[20] or a metastatic renal or thyroid carcinoma is also a serious distinguishing consideration.[37] Maxillary or mandibular lesions may present as a hon-

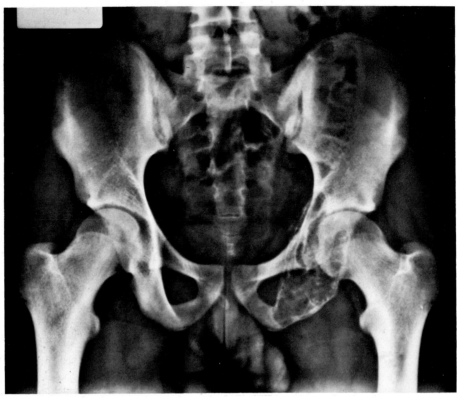

Figure 15–3. Desmoplastic fibroma of ischium presenting as a fine trabeculated soap bubble radiolucency in a 15-year-old boy.

eycombed lytic area and are suspicious of an ameloblastoma.

PATHOLOGIC FEATURES

Grossly, the tumor is whitish gray, rubbery firm, without ossification or calcifications. Delicate trabeculations may be seen on the cut surface. Overall, there is a striking resemblance to the fibromatoses involving soft tissues. Larger lesions show cystic degeneration with clear fluid appearing in the cavities. A pseudocapsule creates the impression of true encapsulation, encouraging the surgeon to make an inadequate excision.

Histologically, the lesions closely resemble the various fibromatoses of soft tissues. The lesional tissue may vary in the different areas of the tumor. On the one hand, there are regions with only a few cells exhibiting heavy wavy bands of collagen fibers (Fig. 15–4). In other areas, the collagen bundles are loosely deposited, with more fibrous cellular forms being present (Fig. 15–5). The individual cells

are uniform throughout with slender spindly nuclei without any atypia. Mitotic figures are virtually nonexistent. Metaplastic ossification or cartilage formation is not demonstrable except at the periphery, where pre-existent nontumorous bony trabeculae may be incorporated into the lesion. The innocuous histologic appearance does not change, even upon recurrence; i.e., the tumor shows no increased cellular anaplasia. The most important microscopic differential diagnosis concerns the separation of desmoplastic fibroma from low-grade medullary fibrosarcoma. Whereas in the former, thick wavy collagen bundles accompany the sparsely cellular uniform fibroblasts with practically no mitotic figures, in the latter, the fibroblastic tumor cells are enlarged and long, the nuclei are plump and hyperchromatic, and the mitoses are easier to recognize. These sometimes elusive distinctions may make the separation of these two entities extremely difficult. It is good to remember that the presence of occasional mitoses does not necessarily signify a malignant tumor nor can one always identify mitotic figures in

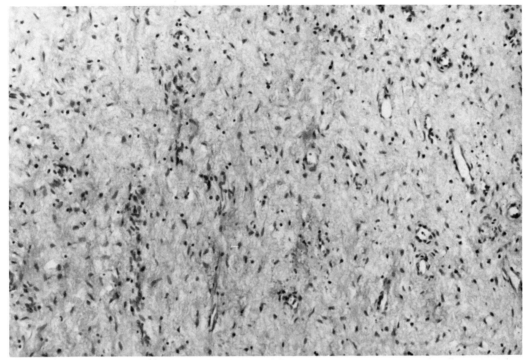

Figure 15–4. Desmoplastic fibroma, with pale-staining fusiform cells and collagenized intercellular matrix. No mitotic figures or cellular atypia. (Hematoxylin-eosin stain. Magnification ×80.)

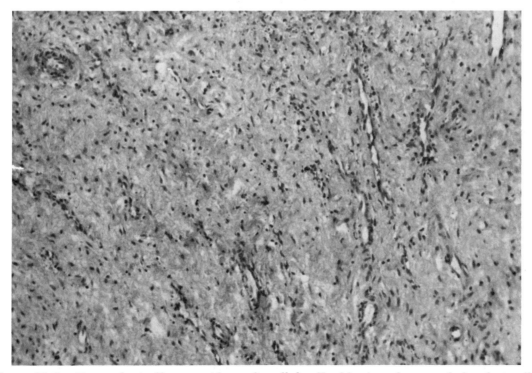

Figure 15–5. Desmoplastic fibroma with poorly cellular fibroblastic make-up and abundant collagen formation. (Hematoxylin-eosin stain. Magnification ×80.)

low-grade fibrosarcomas with ease. Careful long-term follow-up may help to decide the exact nature of the tumor in question.

TREATMENT

Wide resection and thorough curettage, coupled with bone grafting, are the most commonly employed treatment methods. Painstaking curettage followed by cryosurgery is a treatment of great promise. Curettage often fails to eradicate disease and results in persistent tumor growth. Irradiation or amputation are contraindicated and are probably not acceptable as proper management. In about 20 per cent of the reported cases, local recurrence of the tumor was noted, most often attributable to incomplete tumor removal. The false impression of pseudocapsule formation at the tumor margin encourages the surgeon to underestimate the true boundaries, thereby leaving viable tumor behind.

REFERENCES

1. Agazzi, C., and Belloni, L.: Non-osteogenic fibroma of the jaw. Ann. Otol. Rhinol. Laryngol., 60:365–369, 1951.
2. Browne, W. G.: Central fibroma of the mandible. Br. J. Oral Surg., 7:127–130, 1969.
3. Cappell, D. F.: Endosteal fibroma of the fibula. Br. J. Surg., 22:891–895, 1935.
4. Cohen, P., and Goldenberg, R. R.: Desmoplastic fibroma of bone. Report of 2 cases. J. Bone Joint Surg. [Am.], 47:1620–1625, 1965.
5. Cunningham, C. D., Smith, R. O., Enriquez, P., et al.: Desmoplastic fibroma of the mandible. A case report. Ann. Otol. Rhinol. Laryngol., 84:125–129, 1975.
6. Dahlin, D. C., and Hoover, N. W.: Desmoplastic fibroma of bone. Report of 2 cases. J.A.M.A., 188:685–687, 1964.
7. Godinho, F. S., Chiconelli, J. R., and Lemos, C.: Desmoplastic fibroma of bone. Report of a case. J. Bone Joint Surg. [Br.], 49:560–561, 1967.
8. Griffith, J. G., and Irby, W. B.: Desmoplastic fibroma. Report of a rare tumor of oral structures. Oral Surg., 20:269–275, 1965.
9. Hardy, R., and Lehrer, H.: Desmoplastic fibroma vs. desmoid tumor of bone. Two cases illustrating a problem in differential diagnosis and classification. Radiology, 88:899–901, 1967.
10. Heiple, K. G., Perrin, E., and Aikawa, M.: Congenital generalized fibromatosis. A case limited to osseous lesions. J. Bone Joint Surg. [Am.], 54:663–669, 1972.
11. Hinds, E. C., Kent, J. N., and Fechner, R. E.: Desmoplastic fibroma of the mandible: report of case. J. Oral Surg., 27:271–274, 1969.
12. Hovinga, J., and Ingenhoes, R.: A desmoplastic fibroma in the mandible. Int. J. Oral Surg., 3:41–44, 1974.
13. Hutter, R. V. P., Foote, F. W., Jr., Francis, K. C., et al.: Parosteal fasciitis. A self-limited benign process that simulates a malignant neoplasm. Am. J. Surg., 104:800–807, 1962.
14. Jaffe, H. L.: Tumors and Tumorous Conditions of the Bones and Joints. Philadelphia, Lea & Febiger, 1958.
15. Kimmelstiel, P., and Rapp, I. H.: Cortical defect due to periosteal desmoids. Bull. Hosp. Joint Dis., 12:286–297, 1951.
16. Lucas, R. B.: Pathology of Tumours of the Oral Tissues. 3rd ed. Edinburgh, Churchill Livingstone, 1976, p. 171.
17. Martis, C., and Karakasis, D.: Central fibroma of the mandible: report of case. J. Oral Surg., 30:758–760, 1972.
18. McCarthy, E. F., Ireland, D. C., Sprague, B. L., et al.: Parosteal (nodular) fasciitis of the hand. A case report. J. Bone Joint Surg. [Am.], 58:714–716, 1976.
19. Melanotte, P. L.: Il desmoide paraostale. Clin. Ortop., 12:436–444, 1960.
20. Nilsonne, U., and Göthlin, G.: Desmoplastic fibroma of bone. Acta Orthop. Scand., 40:205–215, 1969.
21. Nissan, S., Aviad, I., and Levy, E.: Congenital central fibroma of the mandible. J. Dent. Child., 38:236–238, 1971.
22. Nussbaum, G. B., Terz, J. J., and Joy, E. D., Jr.: Desmoplastic fibroma of the mandible in a 3-year-old child. J. Oral Surg., 34:1117–1121, 1976.
23. Pranzo-Zaccaria, C. L.: Neoplasm of the femur with the histological and radiographic characteristics of a desmoplastic fibroma, but following a malignant clinical course. Scalpello, 2:179–184, 1973.
24. Rabhan, W. N., and Rosai, J.: Desmoplastic fibroma. Report of 10 cases and review of the literature. J. Bone Joint Surg. [Am.], 50:487–502, 1968.
25. Randelli, G.: Desmoid tumours of bone. Arch. Ortop., 77:523–527, 1964.
26. Scheer, G. E., and Kuhlman, R. E.: Vertebral involvement by desmoplastic fibroma. J.A.M.A., 185:669–670, 1963.
27. Schenkar, D. L., and Kleinert, H. E.: Desmoplastic fibroma of the hand. Case report. Plast. Reconstr. Surg., 59:128–133, 1977.
28. Scudese, V. A.: Desmoplastic fibroma of the radius. Report of a case with segmental resection. Clin. Orthop., 79:141–144, 1971.
29. Specchiulli, F., and Florio, U.: Desmoplastic fibroma of bone (a study of three cases). Ital. J. Orthop. Traum., 2:141–150, 1976.
30. Stadler, H. E., and Williams, H. L.: Benign lytic tumor of the ilium (desmoplastic fibroma) — a case report. J. Indiana Med. Assoc., 70:642–643, 1977.
31. Streit, W., and Kirsch, W.: Multiple fibroplastische Proliferationsherde bei einem Neugeborenen. Helv. Paediatr. Acta, 22:271–277, 1967.
32. Sugiura, I.: Desmoplastic fibroma. Case report and review of the literature. J. Bone Joint Surg. [Am.], 58:126–130, 1976.

33. Triantafyllou, N. M., Triantafyllou, D. N., and Antonados, D. N.: Desmoid tumors of the bone. Int. Surg., 57:793–797, 1972.

34. Wagner, J. E., Lorandi, C. S., and Ebling, H.: Desmoplastic fibroma of bone. A case in the mandible. Oral Surg., 43:108–111, 1977.

35. Walker, D. G.: Benign nonodontogenic tumors of the jaws. J. Oral Surg., 28:39–57, 1970.

36. Wesley, R. K., Wysocki, G. P., and Mintz, S. M.: The central odontogenic fibroma. Clinical and morphologic studies. Oral Surg., 40:235–245, 1975.

37. Whitesides, T. E., Jr., and Ackerman, L. V.: Desmoplastic fibroma. A report of 3 cases. J. Bone Joint Surg. [Am.], 42:1143–1150, 1960.

16

FIBROSARCOMA OF BONE

DEFINITION

Fibrosarcoma of bone is a malignant fibroblastic tumor characterized by varying amounts of collagen production and lacking any tendency to form tumor bone, osteoid, or cartilage, either in its primary site or in its metastases.

These sarcomas may occur in intramedullary or periosteal locations. They may arise as "primary" lesions without any associated pre-existent osseous conditions, or they may be "secondary" to such benign bone lesions as fibrous dysplasia, Paget's disease, bone infarct or cyst, and osteomyelitis. (Fig. 16–1.[2, 21, 27, 41, 46] Fibrosarcomas can also occur spontaneously or be induced by irradiation, as a secondary malignant conversion of a giant cell tumor of bone, or they may follow irradiation in the absence of any pre-existent bone lesion. About 30 per cent of the fibrosarcomas in the Mayo Clinic series were secondary to other pre-existent bone lesions or followed prior radiation.[19, 67] An interesting study of a family revealed that three of six siblings were developing medullary fibrosarcomas associated with bone infarcts inherited as an autosomal dominant trait.[3]

Fibrosarcoma is one of the two least common primary malignant tumors of bone, representing less than 5 per cent of all such lesions, the other being primary non-Hodgkin's lymphoma.[5, 74] Fibrosarcoma of bone is the most "maligned" malignant bone tumor. Some deny its existence in bone while contending that such lesions are poorly differentiated osteogenic sarcomas or chondrosarcomas.[53, 79] Others doubt the actual occurrence of the medullary type, since they feel these represent periosteal or soft tissue fibrosarcomas secondarily extending into the medullary cavity.[25, 28, 79] Some studies, on the other hand, exclude the periosteal variety, considering most of them soft tissue fibrosarcomas merely abutting on bone.[17, 19] The 158 cases of fibrosarcomas arising in bones, studied at the Mayo Clinic, include 17 examples of malignant fibrous histiocytoma.[67]

The separation of fibroblastic osteogenic sarcoma and fibrosarcoma is considered by some as purely "didactic" and "artificial" since they "are very closely related as to histology and as to prognosis."[18, 59] These "bones of contention" should be settled by now in favor of accepting the existence of medullary and periosteal fibrosarcomas (Fig. 16–2).[15, 31, 34, 42, 43, 64] It should be realized, however, that in advanced cases the periosteal variant may be difficult to distinguish from a soft part sarcoma, and a

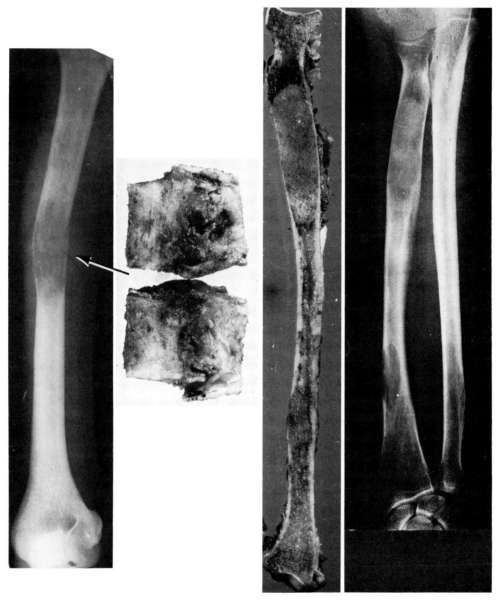

Figure 16–1. Medullary fibrosarcoma arising in the midhumerus of a 20-year-old woman with polyostotic fibrous dysplasia, at least since age 9. Bulbous cortical expansion with medullary destruction of humerus. Shoulder disarticulation specimen reveals a pathologic fracture and a sarcoma of the humerus. The radius shows two areas typical of fibrous dysplasia. (Case #3 from Huvos, A. G., Higinbotham, N. L., and Miller, T. R.: Bone sarcomas arising in fibrous dysplasia. J. Bone Joint Surg. [Am.], *54*:1047–1056, 1972.)

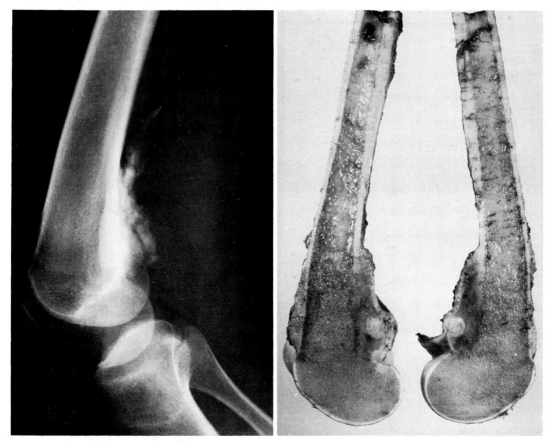

Figure 16–2. Periosteal fibrosarcoma of distal end of femur in a 19-year-old girl. Periosteal reaction due to sarcoma is noted.

fibroblastic osteogenic sarcoma may show only very limited areas of definite osteoid formation.[4]

SIGNS AND SYMPTOMS

The most often encountered symptom with medullary lesions is pain, and in periosteal tumor presentations it is mass with or without pain or tenderness. The average duration of symptoms is about two years — 24 months in medullary lesions and 20 months in periosteal lesions. Not unexpectedly, a recent history of injury is volunteered by patients, especially if the tumor arose in the knee region, giving credence to Ewing's idea of "traumatic determinism"; i.e., trauma draws attention to sites of tumor and not vice versa. About one third of the tumors present with pathologic fracture.[49]

Mandibular and maxillary presentations manifest with pain, swelling, and loosening of teeth.

AGE AND SEX DISTRIBUTION

The age distribution is similar in both medullary and periosteal fibrosarcomas and ranges from 4 to 83 years, with an average of 38 years (Fig. 16–3). Figure 16–4 details the relative age incidence in both groups while pinpointing two distinct age peaks in the third and fifth decades of life. Among the 130 patients studied at Memorial Hospital, there were 11 children and adolescents below the age of 15 years, 8 with medullary lesions and 3 with periosteal lesions.[40] The sex distribution is nearly equal, 71 male patients and 59 female patients with only a slight male predominance (50 male patients to 39 female patients with the medullary variety) (Fig. 16–3).

PRIMARY FIBROSARCOMA OF BONE

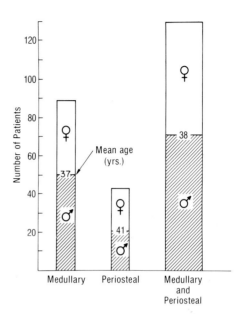

AGE & SEX DISTRIBUTION OF PATIENTS

Figure 16–3. Age and sex distribution of 130 patients with primary fibrosarcoma of bone. (From Huvos, A. G., and Higinbotham, N. L.: Primary fibrosarcoma of bone. A clinicopathologic study of 130 patients. Cancer, 35:837–847, 1975.)

PRIMARY FIBROSARCOMA OF BONE

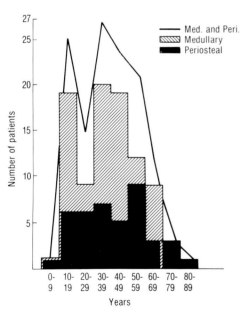

Figure 16–4. Age distribution in 130 patients with primary fibrosarcoma of bone (89 medullary and 41 periosteal). (From Huvos, A. G., and Higinbotham, N. L.: Primary fibrosarcoma of bone. A clinicopathologic study of 130 patients. Cancer, 35:837–847, 1975.)

Fibrosarcomas arising in bone are quite rare in children and adolescents. Dodge reported several such examples, however, occurring in the bones of Uganda African children, six of eight cases manifesting at 13 years of age or younger. He noted, "There seems to be a definite difference in the rate of normal bone growth between African and European children, the rate being substantially greater in the African until the age of 3, when bone retardation occurs."[20] Congenital generalized fibromatosis, limited to osseous lesions, has been reported.[36, 63, 65, 66, 76, 80]

LOCATION

Of the 130 lesions studied at Memorial Hospital, 89 were medullary in location and 41 were periosteal — a ratio of 2:1. The tumors show a strong predilection for long bones, with the most common sites being the femur (43 cases), the humerus (16 cases), and the tibia (12 cases) (Fig. 16–5). The classic locations within the bones are the condyles of the femur or the epicondyles of the humerus. Numerous ex-

LOCATION OF
MEDULLARY AND PERIOSTEAL
FIBROSARCOMA

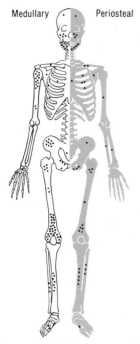

Medullary   Periosteal

Figure 16–5. Skeletal locations of 130 cases of primary medullary and periosteal fibrosarcoma of bone. (From Huvos, A. G., and Higinbotham, N. L.: Primary fibrosarcoma of bone. A clinicopathologic study of 130 patients. Cancer, 35:837–847, 1975.)

amples may occur in the midshaft as well, however (Fig. 16–1).[1] At Memorial Hospital, the craniofacial bones were the primary locations in 19 instances. Fibrosarcoma in this region occurs more commonly in the mandible,[6, 30, 35, 47, 54, 70, 81, 86, 89] but single cases have been reported in the maxilla as well.[14, 24, 38, 71, 82, 87, 88] Fibrosarcoma is a rare occurrence in the skull.[56] A largely equal incidence of both medullary and periosteal lesions occurs in the head and neck region as well as in the upper end of the femur. On the other hand, the upper end of the humerus, the pelvic bones, the lower end of the femur, and other bones below the knee are more frequently affected by medullary fibrosarcomas.

Multifocal bone involvement has been reported in a few instances.[37, 61, 78] Before

accepting such a presentation, metastases from a spindle cell variant of a renal carcinoma should be ruled out.[52] In two of the three cases reported, a complete postmortem examination revealed tumor involvement of the kidneys, leaving one with some uncertainty as to a possible renal primary site. A discontinuous medullary spread within the same bone may simulate multifocal deposits.

RADIOGRAPHIC FEATURES

The typical appearance of a medullary fibrosarcoma is that of a lytic lesion in the bone, with thinning and widening of the overlying cortex (Fig. 16–6).[84, 85] The radiolucent areas indicating bone destruction are often eccentrically located and totally lack radiopacity since the lesions contain no calcification or bone production (Fig. 16–7). A unique case of a humeral fibrosarcoma revealed a fusiform midshaft lesion with very fine spiculations, almost corallike in appearance, cloaking the area of bone destruction.[77] Only minimal periosteal reaction was noted (Fig. 16–8). In some cases, a peripheral ring of bony condensation is noted, and only rarely can one appreciate periosteal new bone formation or a Codman's triangle. There seems to be a straight relationship between the radiographic appearance and the progressive rate of tumor growth. In the relatively slow-growing lesions, the radiolucent areas are well-defined, suggesting a diagnosis of unicameral bone cyst or giant cell tumor. The more aggressive, rapidly progressing lesions demonstrate fuzzy indistinct contours, with scanty or no periosteal bone formation.[12] Osteolytic osteogenic sarcoma shows a similar, if not identical, picture; however, the periosteal reaction is less in fibrosarcoma. Both lesions may present with a deceptively small size. The underestimation of the lesional size is due to the tumor's propensity to involve and permeate cancellous bony trabeculae before totally destroying them. Cortical destruction provides good evidence of aggressive behavior. This cortical permeation is frequently accompanied by a periosteal reaction. Other entities that should be considered in the differential diagnosis include malignant giant cell tumor or an os-

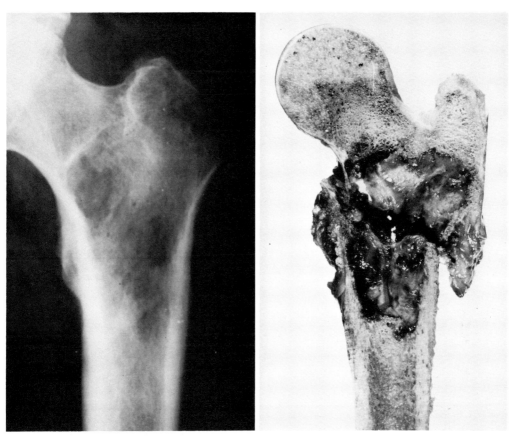

Figure 16–6.   High-grade medullary fibrosarcoma of proximal end of femur with pathologic fracture in a 55-year-old man.

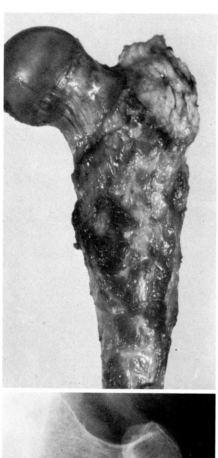
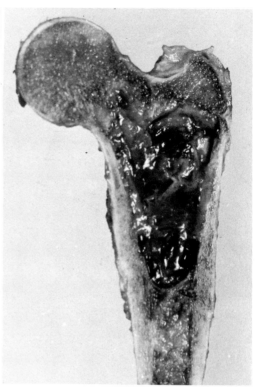
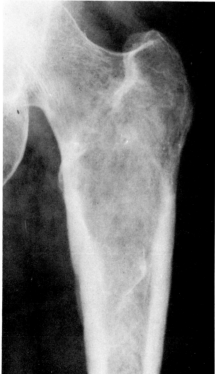

Figure 16–7. Medullary fibrosarcoma of proximal end of femur with osteolytic medullary bone destruction and marked circumferential cortical thickening in a 60-year-old woman. Grossly, the lesion is wholly intramedullary with areas of hemorrhage and necrosis. (From Huvos, A. G., and Higinbotham, N. L.: Primary fibrosarcoma of bone. A clinicopathologic study of 130 patients. Cancer, 35:837–847, 1975.)

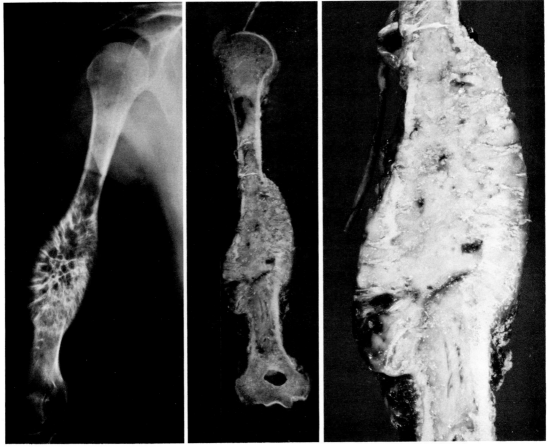

Figure 16–8. Unusual medullary fibrosarcoma of humerus showing a fusiform expanding lesion with delicate spiculation cloaking the area of destruction. Cut sections reveal a fleshy tumor of the medullary cavity with cortical penetration and peripheral, slender, hard-pointed prickle formation. (From Smith, J., and Huvos, A. G.: A spectacular fibrosarcoma of bone. Clin. Bull., 6:24–27, 1976.)

teolytic metastasis from an unknown primary cancer. Occasionally, a solitary plasmacytoma diagnosis is also entertained. Fibrosarcoma may also imitate a pseudotumor of hemophilia.[51] One should be reminded of Lichtenstein's rule of thumb: "If a lesion suggests a primary malignant bone tumor, but not any one in particular, then think of fibrosarcoma as a possibility, especially if the lesion is in the femur or tibia of an adult."[50] The angiographic features of fibrosarcomas of bone have been described.[48, 90]

PATHOLOGIC FEATURES

On *gross examination*, fibrosarcomas most frequently arise toward the ends of long bones in metaphyseal location; how-

ever, several examples have been noted in the midshaft as well (Figs. 16–1 and 16–8). The tumor tissue is grayish white and rubbery firm. The larger the lesion, the more tendency there is for hemorrhagic necrotic areas, usually in the center of the tumor (Figs. 16–6 and 16–7). The rapidly proliferating and aggressive high-grade fibrosarcomas are of soft consistency and are white with hemorrhagic and necrotic areas.[83]

On *histologic examination*, fibrosarcomas of bones have features identical with those arising in soft tissues.[13, 16, 55, 68, 79] The low-grade, well-differentiated tumor exhibits ample intercellular collagen deposition and a distinctive herring bone pattern.[7, 13] (Fig. 16–9 and 16–10). In the secondary fibrosarcomas complicating Paget's disease, focally abundant collagen

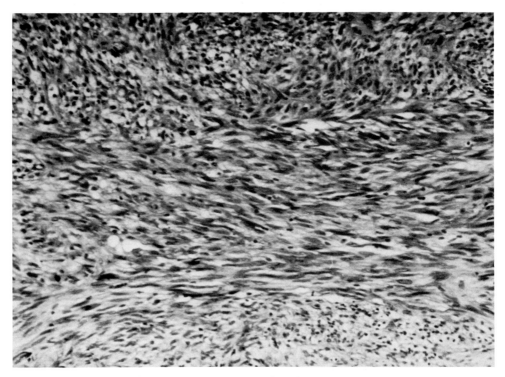

Figure 16–9. Low-grade fibrosarcoma of bone with typical herringbone pattern. (Hematoxylin-eosin stain. Magnification × 80.) (Figure from Huvos, A. G., and Higinbotham, N. L.: Primary fibrosarcoma of bone. A clinicopathologic study of 130 patients. Cancer, 35:837–847, 1975.)

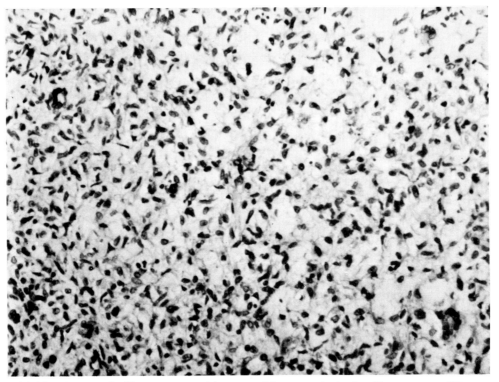

Figure 16–10. Low-grade fibrosarcoma with a myxoid pattern imitating liposarcoma. (Hematoxylin-eosin stain. Magnification × 80.) (From Huvos, A. G., and Higinbotham, N. L.: Primary fibrosarcoma of bone. A clinicopathologic study of 130 patients. Cancer, 35:837–847, 1975.)

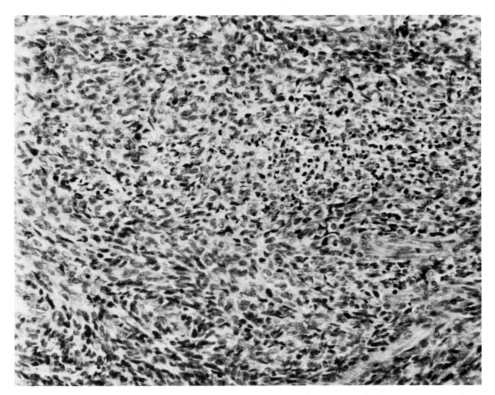

Figure 16–11. High-grade fibrosarcoma demonstrating cellular pleomorphism, mitotic figures, and increased numbers of tumor cells. (Hemotoxylin-eosin stain. Magnification × 80.) (From Huvos, A. G., and Higinbotham, N. L.: Primary fibrosarcoma of bone. A clinicopathologic study of 130 patients. Cancer, 35:837–847, 1975.)

production in the absence of increased cellularity may be demonstrated.[26] In these tumors, the fascicles of fusiform tumor cells appear in direct angles to each other with minimal variation in size and shape. Mitoses appear only occasionally. The more anaplastic, high-grade lesions reveal a disruption of this characteristic growth pattern with interspersed tumor giant cells and increased numbers of abnormal mitoses (Fig. 16–11). The spindly tumor cells here exhibit marked pleomorphism. The presence of tumor giant cells and cellular pleomorphism raises the possibility of a malignant fibrous histiocytoma; the lack of a pinwheel, and a matted or storiform growth pattern, so characteristic of the fibrous histiocytic lesions, helps to rule out a fibrosarcoma diagnosis.[39] On occasion, periosteal or endosteal reactive bone formation may be encountered, causing diagnostic difficulties.[83] Silver impregnation techniques, both Wilder's and Laidlaw's, demonstrate a close relationship between the individual tumor cells and the fine reticulum fibers or fibrils.[26] In heavily collagen-producing lesions, the presence of a fibroblastic osteogenic sarcoma masquerading as a fibrosarcoma is a real consideration. In such diagnostic dilemmas, the unfixed tumor tissue may be examined for the presence of phosphatase values. Histochemical examination shows no alkaline phosphatase activity by the tumor cells in fibrosarcoma but registers increased values in osteogenic sarcomas.[8, 9, 44] For increased accuracy, samples of both the intramedullary and soft tissue extension should be examined, since they may vary significantly in their alkaline phosphatase content. Cortical invasion by the medullary lesions may elicit reactive bone formation or a pathologic fracture will result in callus formation (Fig. 16–2). The most important differential diagnostic considerations include desmoplastic fibroma, fibrous dysplasia, and a metastasis of a spindle cell variant of a renal carcinoma[52] (see Chapter 15). The diagnostic pitfall most often encountered concerns separation of desmoplastic fibroma and well-differentiated fibrosarcoma. The presence of small fibroblasts forming ample thick strands and bundles of collagen, the lack of a herringbone growth pattern, and the absence of nuclear pleomorphism or mitotic figures clearly separate desmoplastic fibroma from fibrosarcoma (see Chapter 15). Periosteal fibrosarcoma may be mimicked by periosteal fasciitis, periosteal desmoids, the various fibromatoses secondarily involving bone, or, very rarely, an unusually cellular fibrous cortical defect (see Chapter 15).

TREATMENT AND PROGNOSIS

The uniformly practiced treatment of fibrosarcomas, whether periosteal or medullary, is amputation.[62] More than three fourths of these sarcomas arising in the extremities are treated by major ablative procedures, either hip or shoulder joint disarticulations or forequarter or hindquarter amputations. Major amputation is usually performed in all medullary lesions irrespective of the histologic grade of malignancy. The recently introduced surgical techniques of total femur and total knee replacement with metallic prosthesis in association with intensive chemotherapy seem to provide a realistic limb-saving alternative to radical amputation.[58] Tumors involving the shoulder girdle, upper end of humerus, clavicle, or scapula may also be resected without performing a major amputation by considering an *en bloc* upper humeral interscapulothoracic resection, the so-called Tikhoff-Linberg procedure.[57] The role of preoperative or adjuvant multidrug multicycle chemotherapy has not been well established and results are not yet available. At this time, it seems that patients with high-grade fibrosarcomas, either medullary or periosteal, may benefit from preoperative and adjuvant chemotherapy. Low-grade tumors may be treated, if feasible, by surgical means alone, i.e., a radical *en bloc* resection instead of amputation.

The presence of pulmonary metastases on admission is not an absolute contraindication for *en bloc* resection since pulmonary resection, coupled with chemotherapy, may provide long-term disease-free survival or even cure. In 59 of the 130 patients studied at Memorial Hospital, metastases complicated the clinical course of the disease.[40] The most frequent sites of metas-

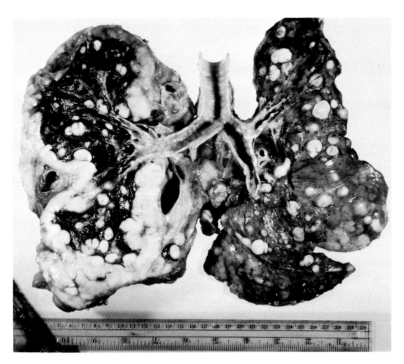

Figure 16–12. Fibrosarcoma of bone with massive pulmonary metastases at autopsy. Note tumor encasing the left lung. (From Huvos, A. G., and Higinbotham, N. L.: Primary fibrosarcoma of bone. A clinicopathologic study of 130 patients. Cancer, 35:837–847, 1975.)

tases were the lungs, in 48 instances, and other bones, in 20 (Fig. 16–12). Regional lymph node involvement occurred in only two cases. The pattern of dissemination is comparable with that of osteogenic sarcoma.[45] The overall survival for all patients with primary fibrosarcoma of bone studied at Memorial Hospital was 34 per cent, 28 per cent, 27 per cent, and 25 per cent at 5, 10, 15, and 20 years respectively (Fig. 16–3). The survival curve suggests that for fibrosarcoma it is more meaningful to use 10 or 15 year survival rates as a fair indication for cure.[75] In separately analyzing curves for the medullary and periosteal lesions, one finds instructive and significant differences. Patients with medullary lesions had a uniformly worse prognosis, with survival rates of 27 per cent, 20 per cent, 17 per cent, and 17 per cent at 5, 10, 15, and 20 year intervals respectively (Fig. 16–13). Patients with periosteal lesions, however, had a relatively more favorable prognosis in all of these time intervals: at 5 years (52 per cent), 10 years (48 per cent), 15 years (48 per cent), and 20 years (40 per cent).[15] The periosteal location consistently provided the patient with lesions in the craniofacial bones with a more favorable outcome, since the 5 through 20 year survival rates were uniformly at the

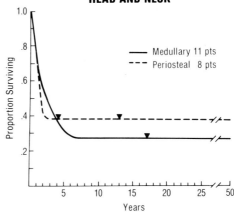

Figure 16–14. Rate of survival of patients at Memorial Hospital with primary fibrosarcoma of craniofacial bones from time of diagnosis to death or last follow-up. (From Huvos, A. G., and Higinbotham, N. L.: Primary fibrosarcoma of bone. A clinicopathologic study of 130 patients. Cancer, 35:837–847, 1975.)

38 per cent level (Fig. 16–14). If the patient with a fibrosarcoma in this region survived the first two and one-half years following the initial diagnosis and definitive treatment, the survival rate remained

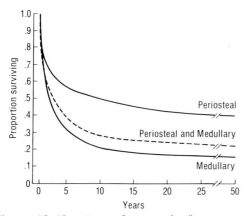

Figure 16–13. Rate of survival of patients at Memorial Hospital with primary fibrosarcoma of bone from time of diagnosis to death or last follow-up. (From Huvos, A. G., and Higinbotham, N. L.: Primary fibrosarcoma of bone. A clinicopathologic study of 130 patients. Cancer, 35:837–847, 1975.)

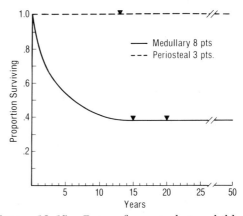

Figure 16–15. Rate of survival in children under the age of 15 at Memorial Hospital with primary fibrosarcoma of bone from time of diagnosis to death or last follow-up. (From Huvos, A. G., and Higinbotham, N. L.: Primary fibrosarcoma of bone. A clinicopathologic study of 130 patients. Cancer, 35:837–847, 1975.)

uniform throughout. Patients with a medullary lesion in the jaws had a relatively less favorable prognosis compared to the periosteal tumors, since their 5, 10, 15, and 20 year estimated survival rates remained at the 27 per cent level throughout the observation period (Fig. 16–14). In contrast to all other reports, 24 patients with medullary fibrosarcomas, recorded in the Swedish Cancer Registry, had a five year survival rate of only 4.2 per cent.[49]

There were 11 children below the age of 15 years in the Memorial Hospital study.[40] Local excision of the periosteal lesions provided these children and adolescents with perfect cure (Fig. 16–15). The medullary tumors, however, proved to be more aggressive and only a 50 per cent five year survival rate was reached (Fig. 16–15). Subsequent to this time period, the survival leveled off at the 38 per cent level.

REFERENCES

1. Aegerter, E., and Kirkpatrick, J. A., Jr.: Orthopedic Diseases. 3rd ed. Philadelphia, W. B. Saunders Co., 1968, pp. 670–678.
2. Akbarnia, B. A., Wirth, C. R., and Colman, N.: Fibrosarcoma arising from chronic osteomyelitis. Case report and review of the literature. J. Bone Joint Surg. [Am.], 58:123–125, 1976.
3. Arnold, W. H.: Hereditary bone dysplasia with sarcomatous degeneration. Study of a family. Ann. Intern. Med., 78:902–906, 1973.
4. Batts, M., Jr.: Periosteal fibrosarcoma. Arch. Surg., 42:566–576, 1941.
5. Boyd, J. T., Doll, R., Hill, G. B., et al.: Mortality from primary tumours of bone in England and Wales 1961–63, Br. J. Prev. Soc. Med., 23:12–22, 1969.
6. Breslin, W. W.: Fibrosarcoma of the mandible. J. Can. Dent. Assoc., 22:151–153, 1956.
7. Broders, A. C., Hargrave, R., and Meyerding, H. W.: Pathological features of soft tissue fibrosarcoma. With special reference to the grading of its malignancy. Surg. Gynecol. Obstet., 69:267–280, 1939.
8. Brozmanová, E., and Škrovina, B.: Biochemical and haematological findings in malignant bone tumours. Neoplasma, 21:75–82, 1974.
9. Brozmanová, E., and Škrovina, B.: Osseous fibrosarcoma — laboratory and clinical evaluation. Acta Chir. Orthop. Traumatol. Cech., 42:454–458, 1975.
10. Burns, W. A., Kanhouwa, S., Tillman, L., et al.: Fibrosarcoma occurring at the site of a plastic vascular graft. Cancer, 29:66–72, 1972.
11. Burton, M. E.: Well-differentiated fibrosarcoma of the scapula. A case report. Bull. Hosp. Joint Dis., 15:85–89, 1954.
12. Chen, V., and Lennartz, K. J.: A case of sarcoma of the talus giving the radiographic appearance of a "cyst." Z. Orthop., 113:1027–1031, 1975.
13. Conley, J., Stout, A. P., and Healey, W. V.: Clinicopathologic analysis of 84 patients with an original diagnosis of fibrosarcoma of the head and neck. Am. J. Surg., 114:564–569, 1967.
14. Cronin, J.: Fibrosarcoma of the paranasal air sinuses. J. Laryngol. Otol., 87:667–674, 1973.
15. Cunningham, M. P., and Arlen, M.: Medullary fibrosarcoma of bone. Cancer, 21:31–37, 1968.
16. Dahl, I., Save-Soderbergh, J., and Angervall, L.: Fibrosarcoma in early infancy. Pathol. Eur., 8:193–209, 1973.
17. Dahlin, D. C.: Bone tumors. 2nd ed. Springfield, Illinois, Charles C Thomas, 1967, p. 212.
18. Dahlin, D. C.: Discussion. Cancer Seminar, 1:25, 1976.
19. Dahlin, D. C., and Ivins, J. C.: Fibrosarcoma of bone. A study of 114 cases. Cancer, 23:35–41, 1969.
20. Dodge, O. G.: Bone tumours in Uganda Africans. Br. J. Cancer, 18:627–633, 1964.
21. Dorfman, H. D., Norman, A., and Wolff, H.: Fibrosarcoma complicating bone infarction in a caisson worker. A case report. J. Bone Joint Surg. [Am.], 48:528–532, 1966.
22. Edeiken, J., Farrell, C., Ackerman, L. V., et al.: Parosteal sarcoma. Am. J. Roentgenol. Radium Ther. Nucl. Med., 111:579–583, 1971.
23. Edeiken, J., and Hodes, P. J.: Roentgen Diagnosis of Diseases of Bone. 2nd ed. Vol. 2. Baltimore, Williams & Wilkins, 1973, pp. 983–998.
24. Eversole, L. R., Schwartz, W. D., and Sabes, W. R.: Central and peripheral fibrogenic and neurogenic sarcoma of the oral region. Oral Surg., 36:49–62, 1973.
25. Ewing, J.: Neoplastic Diseases. A Treatise of Tumors. Philadelphia, W. B. Saunders Co., 1934, p. 296.
26. Eyre-Brook, A. L., and Price, C. H. G.: Fibrosarcoma of bone. Review of fifty consecutive cases from the Bristol Bone Tumour Registry. J. Bone Joint Surg. [Br.], 51:20–37, 1969.
27. Furey, J. G., Ferrer-Torells, M., and Reagan, J. W.: Fibrosarcoma arising at the site of bone infarcts. A report of two cases. J. Bone Joint Surg. [Am.], 42:802—810, 1960.
28. Geschickter, C. I.: So-called fibrosarcoma of bone: bone involvement by sarcoma of neighboring soft parts. Arch. Surg., 24:231–291, 1932.
29. Gilmer, W. S., Jr., and MacEwen, G. D.: Central (medullary) fibrosarcoma of bone. J. Bone Joint Surg. [Am.], 40:121–141, 1958.
30. Gingrass, R. P., and Hinz, L. E.: Fibrosarcoma of the mandible. J. Oral Surg., 19:241–244, 1961.
31. Goidanich, I. F., and Venturi, R. I.: I fibrosarcomi primitivi dello scheletro. Chir. Organi Mov., 46:1–90, 1958.
32. Goldenberg, R. R.: Well differentiated fibrosarcoma of the calcaneus. Report of a case treated by resection. J. Bone Joint Surg. [Am.], 42:1151–1155, 1960.
33. Grubb, R. L., Jr., and Dehner, L. P.: Congenital fibrosarcoma of the thoracolumbar region. J. Pediatr. Surg., 9:785–786, 1974.
34. Hadders, H. N.: Fibrosarcoma centrale seu medullare ossium. Jaarboek van Kankeronderzoek en Kankerbestrijding, 10:219–229, 1960.
35. Hamilton, I.: Fibro-sarcoma of the lower jaw. Aust. N. Z. J. Surg., 15:54–57, 1945.
36. Heiple, K. G., Perrin, E., and Aikawa, M.: Congenital generalized fibromatosis. A case limited

to osseous lesions. J. Bone Joint Surg. [Am.], 54:663–669, 1972.

37. Hernandez, F. J., and Fernandez, B. B.: Multiple diffuse fibrosarcoma of bone. Cancer, 37:939–945, 1976.

38. Hoggins, G. S., and Brady, C. L.: Fibrosarcoma of maxilla. Report of a case. Oral Surg., 15:34–38, 1962.

39. Huvos, A. G.: Primary malignant fibrous histiocytoma of bone. Clinicopathologic study of 18 patients. N.Y. State J. Med., 76:552–559, 1976.

40. Huvos, A. G., and Higinbotham, N. L.: Primary fibrosarcoma of bone. A clinicopathologic study of 130 patients. Cancer, 35:837–847, 1975.

41. Huvos, A. G., Higinbotham, N. L., and Miller, T. R.: Bone sarcomas arising in fibrous dysplasia. J. Bone Joint Surg. [Am.], 54:1047–1056, 1972.

42. Jaffe, H. L.: Tumors of the skeletal system: pathological aspects. Bull. N.Y. Acad. Med., 23:497–511, 1947.

43. Jaffe, H. L.: Tumors and Tumorous Conditions of the Bones and Joints. Philadelphia, Lea & Febiger, 1958, pp. 298–313.

44. Jeffree, G. M.: Enzymes in fibroblastic lesions. J. Bone Joint Surg. [Br.], 54:535–546, 1972.

45. Jeffree, G. M., and Price, C. H. G.: Metastatic spread of fibrosarcoma of bone. A report on forty-nine cases, and a comparison with osteosarcoma. J. Bone Joint Surg. [Br.], 58:418–425, 1976.

46. Johnson, L. C., Vetter, H., and Putschar, W. G. J.: Sarcomas arising in bone cysts. Virchows Arch. [Pathol. Anat.], 335:428–451, 1962.

47. Kangur, T. T., Dahlin, D. C., and Turlington, E. G.: Myxomatous tumours of the jaws. J. Oral Surg., 33:523–528, 1975.

48. Lagergren, C., Lindbom, A., and Söderberg, G.: Vascularization of fibromatous and fibrosarcomatous tumors. Histopathologic, microangiographic and angiographic studies. Acta Radiol., 53:1–16, 1960.

49. Larsson, S. E., Lorentzon, R., and Boquist, L.: Fibrosarcoma of bone. A demographic, clinical and histopathological study of all cases recorded in the Swedish Cancer Registry from 1958 to 1968. J. Bone Joint Surg. [Br.], 58:412–417, 1976.

50. Lichtenstein, L.: Bone Tumors. 4th ed. St. Louis, C. V. Mosby Co., 1972, pp. 244–255, 377.

51. Lieberg, O. U., Penner, J. A., and Bailey, R. W.: Fibrosarcoma presenting as a pseudotumor of hemophilia. Report of an unusual case. J. Bone Joint Surg. [Am.], 57:422–424, 1975.

52. LiVolsi, V. A.: Fibrosarcoma metastatic to the brain. Letter to the editor. Arch. Pathol., 97:126, 1974.

53. MacDonald, I., and Budd, J. W.: Osteogenic sarcoma. I. A modified nomenclature and a review of 118 five year cures. Surg. Gynecol. Obstet., 77:413–421, 1943.

54. MacFarlane, W. I.: Fibrosarcoma of the mandible with pulmonary metastases: a case report. Br. J. Oral Surg., 10:168–174, 1972.

55. Mackenzie, D. H.: The Differential Diagnosis of Fibroblastic Disorders. Philadelphia, F. A. Davis (Blackwell), 1970, pp. 132–137.

56. Mansfield, J. B.: Primary fibrosarcoma of the skull. Case report. J. Neurosurg., 47:785–787, 1977.

57. Marcove, R. C., Lewis, M. M., and Huvos, A. G.: En bloc upper humeral interscapulo-thoracic resection. The Tikhoff-Linberg procedure. Clin. Orthop., 124:219–228, 1977.

58. Marcove, R. C., Lewis, M. M., Rosen, G., et al.: Total femur and total knee replacement. Clin. Orthop., 126:147–152, 1977.

59. McLeod, J. J., Dahlin, D. C., and Ivins, J. C.: Fibrosarcoma of bone. Am. J. Surg., 94:431–437, 1957.

60. Moritani, M.: DMBA-induced fibrosarcoma in bone. Histochemical and electron microscopical studies on new transplantable bone tumor of 7,12-dimethylbenz (α) anthracene-induced fibrosarcoma in rats. Neoplasma, 24:165–176, 1977.

61. Nielsen, A. R., and Poulsen, H.: Multiple diffuse fibrosarcomata of the bones. Acta Pathol. Microbiol. Scand., 55:265–272, 1962.

62. Nilsonne, U., and Mazabraud, A.: Fibrosarcoma of bone. Rev. Chir. Orthop., 60:109–122, 1974.

63. Peede, L. F., Jr., and Epker, B. N.: Aggressive juvenile fibromatosis involving the mandible: surgical excision with immediate reconstruction. Oral. Surg., 43:651–657, 1977.

64. Phemister, D. B.: Cancer of the bone and joint. J.A.M.A., 136:545–552, 1948.

65. Pingitore, R., and Bachechi, P.: Congenital fibrosarcoma. Tumori, 61:351–356, 1975.

66. Ponzone, A.: Un caso di fibrosarcoma congenito. Minerva Pediatr., 18:221–224, 1966.

67. Pritchard, D. J., Sim, F. H., Ivins, J. C., et al.: Fibrosarcoma of bone and soft tissues of the trunk and extremities. Orthop. Clin. North Am., 8:869–881, 1977.

68. Pritchard, D. J., Soule, E. H., Taylor, W. F., et al.: Fibrosarcoma — a clinicopathologic and statistical study of 199 tumors of the soft tissues of the extremities and trunk. Cancer, 33:888–897, 1974.

69. Rabhan, W. N., and Rosai, J.: Desmoplastic fibroma. Report of ten cases and review of the literature. J. Bone Joint Surg. [Am.], 50:487–502, 1968.

70. Reade, P. C., and Radden, B. G.: Oral fibrosarcoma. Oral Surg., 22:217–225, 1966.

71. Richardson, J. F., Fine, M. A., and Goldman, H. M.: Fibrosarcoma of the mandible: a clinicopathologic controversy: report of case. J. Oral Surg., 30:664–668, 1972.

72. Scarff, R. W.: Discussion on malignant tumours of bone. Proc. R. Soc. Med., 30:796–804, 1937.

73. Scarff, R. W.: Symposium on primary malignant tumours of bone. Br. J. Radiol., 20:19–30, 1947.

74. Sissons, H. A.: Malignant tumors of bone and cartilage. In Raven, R. W. (ed.): Cancer. Vol. 2. Philadelphia, F. A. Davis (Butterworths), 1958.

75. Sissons, H. A., and Duthie, R. B.: A survey of the biological properties of tumours of bone. In Carling, E. Rock, and Ross, J. P. (eds.): British Surgical Progress. Philadelphia, F. A. Davis 1959, pp. 157–175.

76. Slavens, J. J.: Congenital fibromyxosarcoma of os calcis. Pediatrics, 11:617–621, 1953.

77. Smith, J., and Huvos, A. G.: A spectacular fibrosarcoma of bone. Clin. Bull., 6:24–27, 1976.

78. Steiner, P. E.: Multiple diffuse fibrosarcoma of bone. Am. J. Pathol., 20:877–893, 1944.

79. Stout, A. P.: Fibrosarcoma: the malignant tumor of fibroblasts. Cancer, 1:30–63, 1948.

80. Streit, W., and Kirsch, W.: Multiple fibroplas-

tische Proliferationsherde bei einem Neugeborenen. Helv. Paediatr. Acta, 22:271–277,
1967.

81. Stuteville, O. H.: Fibrosarcoma of the mandible.
Report of a case. Q. Bull. Northw. Univ. Med.
Sch., 29:400–402, 1955.

82. Swain, R. E., Sessions, D. G., and Ogura, J. H.:
Fibrosarcoma of the head and neck: a clinical
analysis of 40 cases. Ann. Otol. Rhinol. Laryngol., 83:439–444, 1974.

83. Tarasov, B. P.: Diagnosis of fibrosarcoma of the
bone. Arkh. Patol., 32:23–28, 1969.

84. Tseshkovsky, M. S., and Soloviev, Yu.N.: Primary
central fibrosarcoma of the bone (roentgeno-
morphological characteristics). Vestn. Rentgenol. Radiol., 51(3):6–14, 1976.

85. Uehlinger, E.: Zentrales osteolytisches Fibrosar-
kom des Femurschaftes. Arch. Orthop. Unfallchir., 87:357–359, 1977.

86. Van Blarcom, C. W., Masson, J. K., and Dahlin,
D. C.: Fibrosarcoma of the mandible. A clinicopathologic study. Oral Surg., 32:428–439,
1971.

87. Van Wyk, C. W., and Jonck, L. M.: A peripheral
fibrosarcoma of the upper jaw and a central fibrosarcomatous tumour of the lower jaw. J.
Dent. Assoc. S. Afr., 19:18–22, 1964.

88. Vazirani, S. J., and Bolden, T. E.: Oral fibromyxosarcoma of the maxilla. Report of a case. Oral
Surg., 11:227–234, 1958.

89. Wright, J. A., and Kuehn, P. G.: Fibrosarcoma of
the mandible. Report of a case. Oral Surg.,
36:16–20, 1973.

90. Yaghmai, I.: Angiographic features of fibromas
and fibrosarcomas. Radiology, 125:57–64, 1977.

Tumors of Histiocytic or Fibrohistiocytic Origin
Chapters 17 through 20

17

GIANT CELL TUMOR OF BONE

DEFINITION

Giant cell tumor of bone is an aggressive lesion characterized by well-vascularized tissue made up of plump, spindly, or ovoid cells in addition to numerous multinucleated giant cells uniformly dispersed throughout the tumor tissue. This lesion represents about 5 per cent of all primary bone tumors.

HISTORICAL ASPECTS

In 1818, Sir Astley Cooper seems to have been the first to describe giant cell tumor of bone, emphasizing its essentially benign nature.[25] Others during the 19th century referred to it as a "myeloid sarcoma," realizing that these lesions were not as lethal as other primary bone sarcomas.[7] In 1853, Paget lectured on this entity, calling it a "brown or myeloid tumor," and gave its classic description.[117] The noted French surgeon Nélaton outlined the multifaceted clinical and histologic features well, pointing out that this tumor is only locally aggressive (Fig. 17–1).[113] He named this entity a "tumor of myeloplaxes," myeloplaxes being osteoclastic giant cells according to the then prevalent terminology. Virchow insisted that these tumors may not only recur but also eventually turn into a fully malignant cancer.[170] Samuel W.

D'UNE

NOUVELLE ESPÈCE

DE TUMEURS BÉNIGNES DES OS,

OU

TUMEURS A MYELOPLAXES.

PAR

le Docteur Eugène NÉLATON,

Prosecteur à la Faculté de Médecine de Paris,
ancien Interne des Hôpitaux de Paris,
Membre de la Société Anatomique.

Mémoire orné de 3 Planches soigneusement coloriees.

PARIS.

ADRIEN DELAHAYE, LIBRAIRE-ÉDITEUR,

place de l'École-de-Médecine, 23.

1860

Figure 17–1. Title page and figure from Nélaton's classic book on giant cell tumors, *D'Une Nouvelle Espèce de Tumeurs Bénignes des Os, ou Tumeurs à Myéloplaxes.*

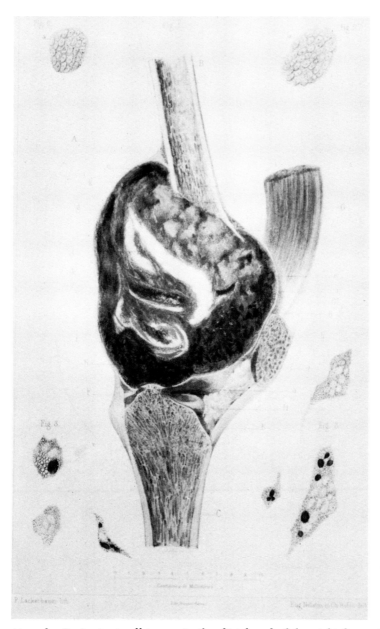

Figure 17–1. Continued. B, A giant cell tumor in the distal end of the right femur in a 21-year-old woman.

Gross of Philadelphia, after studying 70 cases, maintained the tumor's essential benignity while conceding that there were problems in separating it from an aneurysmal variety of medullary sarcoma.[55] During the preroentgen era, most of these tumors were treated by radical amputations, but more precise clinical criteria employing roentgenographic studies permitted a more accurate recognition and less radical treatment, independently championed by Bloodgood[9] and by W. B. Coley.[24] In 1910, Bloodgood even proposed to change the original designation of giant cell sarcoma to "benign giant cell tumor."[8] Stewart, in 1922, introduced the term "osteoclastoma" into the British orthopedic literature, where it received instant adoption and, until very recently, wide use.[155] Following the Soviet pathologist Rusakov's suggestion in 1939, the Russian literature still refers to giant cell tumors as "osteoblastoclastoma."[30, 173] As recently as 1975, Aegerter and Kirkpatrick, after ignoring this tumor for many years, reluctantly listed it under the heading of osteoclastoma while still doubting its authenticity.[2]

SIGNS AND SYMPTOMS

Suggestive physical findings relate to the involved bone and are manifested by often intermittent aching pain, local swelling, tenderness, and limited motion. Neither physical signs nor symptoms are distinctly characteristic of this particular lesion, but they are helpful in drawing prompt attention to the affected site. It is recommended that radiographs include adjacent bones to evaluate joint space involvement. Small lesions do not form an appreciable mass and cause only slight pain, thereby misleading the examiner to suspect arthritis or poorly documented trauma. When palpable swelling is produced, the diagnosis is rapidly forthcoming, since roentgen examination is promptly ordered. Tumors located in the spine and sacrum often present with neurological disturbances.[90]

A case of Goltz syndrome with multiple giant cell tumor–like bone lesions has been reported.[142] A unique instance of three histologically proved distinct bone lesions — a metacarpal giant cell tumor, a sternal osteoblastoma, and a pubic osteogenic sarcoma — has been described in the same patient.[132] An unusual association of a tibial aggressive giant cell tumor in a 17-year-old woman with congenital adrenal virilism (adrenogenital syndrome) has been reported.[15]

AGE AND SEX DISTRIBUTION

There is considerable variation in the age incidence, ranging from 5 to 73 years. More than 80 per cent of the giant cell tumors of bone occur in patients older than 20 years of age, however, i.e., in individuals who are skeletally mature. If a patient under the age of 15 years is diagnosed as having a giant cell tumor, it should be seriously questioned and further investigations are in order. The average age is 33 years; the median age is 30 and the mode is 23 years. These tumors are most common in the third (35 per cent) and fourth (21 per cent) decades and are distinctly rare (12 per cent) above the age of 50 years. Although it is true that 17 per cent of patients at Memorial Hospital were under the age of 20 years, all but three were in the latter half of the second decade of life and the majority of these almost reached the upper limit. The average age of patients with malignant giant cell tumors is slightly higher than that of those with benign ones.

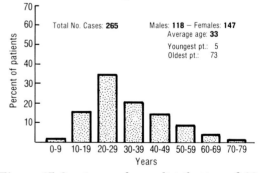

Figure 17–2. Age and sex distribution of 265 patients with giant cell tumors treated at Memorial Hospital. Percentage of age distribution is according to decades.

There are slightly more women than men affected, the ratio being 3:2 (Fig. 17–2). Among the 265 patients in the Memorial Hospital Registry, 55.5 per cent were female and 44.5 per cent were male. As was already reported, the benign tumors predominate in female patients in a proportion of 3:2; the malignant variants predilect male patients in a ratio of 3:1.[66]

LOCATION

More than 75 per cent of giant cell tumors are situated at or near the articular end of a long tubular bone. The distal femur, proximal tibia, and fibula were predilected by half of the tumors (Fig. 17–3). The distal radius, proximal femur, sacrum, and humerus were also relatively frequent sites of involvement. In 10 cases, the vertebrae above the sacrum were the primary sites, and three lesions involved the craniofacial bones. The latter cases were associated with well-documented Paget's disease of bones.[65] (See Chapter 8.) The vertebral column, including sacrum, was involved in 8 per cent of cases. In the spine, giant cell tumor may be located in the vertebral body, the spinous process, or the transverse process. Infrequent sites are the os calcis,[120, 144] patella,[81, 183] innominate bone, rib,[98] and carpal bones.[41, 86 135, 150] The bones of the hands and feet were affected in 6 per cent of the cases. In eight instances the lesions were multifocal (Fig. 17–3). Multifocal giant cell tumors in the proved absence of hyperparathyroidism have been reported.[23, 68, 80, 146, 160, 169]

RADIOGRAPHIC APPEARANCE

Small lesions, and those arising in long tubular bones, have a characteristic presentation.[39, 68, 100] They are slightly eccentric to the long axis of a tubular bone, showing an expanding central area of radiolucency appearing in the epiphyseal end with a slight suggestion of fine trabeculation. The presence or absence of trabeculae is related to the rapidity of tumor growth. The center of the lesion is more lucent, with gradually increasing density toward the periphery (Fig. 17–4). As long as the tumor is actively growing, there is essentially no peripheral zone of new bone formation. Large tumors may extend secondarily into the metaphysis or, even more rarely, into the diaphysis; crossing adjacent joints is an uncommon occurrence.[179] Some controversy exists as to whether all giant cell tumors arise in the epiphysis or the metaphysis.[10, 17, 18, 123, 143] Most experts favor an exclusive epiphyseal origin, but it is difficult to settle this question with great certainty because instances in which this tumor is discovered before the closure of the epiphyseal plate are quite infrequent (Fig. 17–5).[49] Larger lesions expand the overlying cortex with a thin well-developed sclerotic outline. This is due to either the corrugations of the residual expanded inner cortical surface or the periosteal reactive bone formation.

When cortical erosion is present, radiolucent areas of varying size are seen representing interruptions of the cortex. The occurrence of infraction complicates this evaluation. The extraosseous extension by

SKELETAL LOCATION IN 265 CASES OF GIANT CELL TUMOR OF BONE

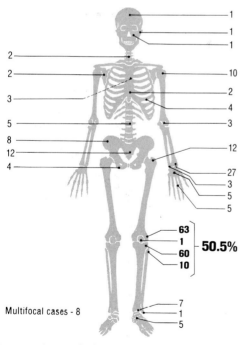

Multifocal cases - 8

Figure 17–3. Skeletal location in 265 cases of giant cell tumor of bone treated at Memorial Hospital.

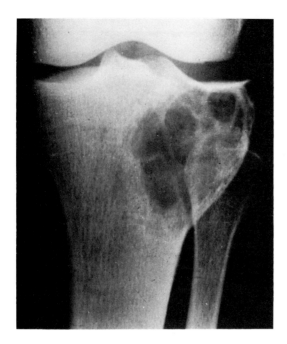

Figure 17–4. Typical epiphyseal giant cell tumor involving the lateral tuberosity of the proximal tibia. This circumscribed purely lytic lesion with soap bubble-like trabeculations encroaches on the articular cartilage but does not expand the thin overlying cortex.

Figure 17–5. Large distal metaphyseal giant cell tumor of the femur in a 7-year-old girl with a preoperative diagnosis of unicameral bone cyst. Courtesy of Drs. R. C. Marcove and L. Helson.)

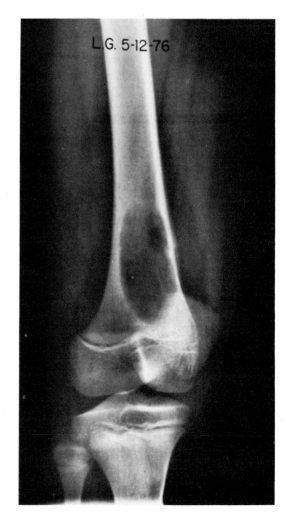

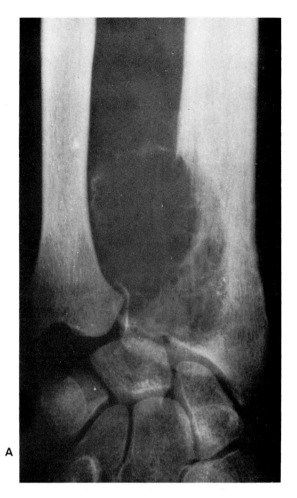

Figure 17–6. Focally malignant giant cell tumor of distal end of left radius in a 44-year-old man with extensive interosseous muscle involvement. Multiple curettages and radiotherapy (TTD 2468 r) followed by total excision and fibula transplant finally resulting in cure.

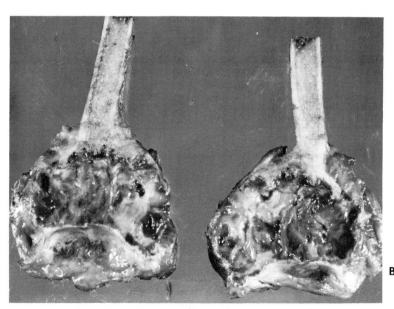

tumor is characterized by limited opacification of soft tissues at the area of infiltration (Fig. 17–6).

On the basis of radiographic appearance,

Erens proposed a grading system of predictive prognostic value.[39] Lesions with intact outer borders and sharp inner margins have a better prognosis. Those with indis-

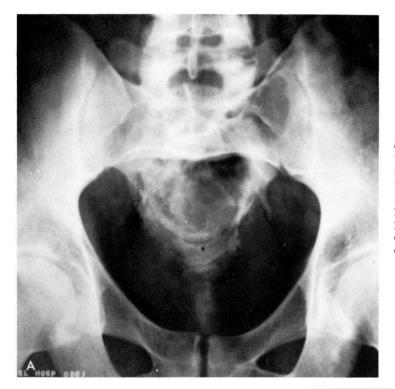

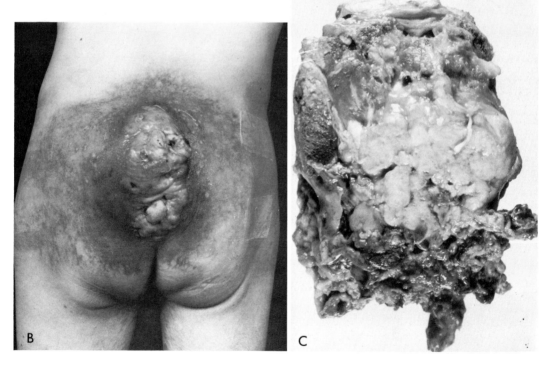

Figure 17–7. Primary fully malignant giant cell tumor of sacrum in a 25-year-old man involving L_5 vertebra. *A* and *B*, Extensive local recurrence five years postresection and four years after irradiation. *C*, Necrotic tumor at autopsy. No distant metastases.

tinct inner margins or outer cortical interruptions or a combination of the two behave in a more aggressive manner.

A "soap bubble" effect of cortical expansion may be the result of a secondary aneurysmal bone cyst component engrafted on the giant cell tumor (Fig. 17–4). In many tumors, on examination after *en bloc* excision, the specimen reveals a totally solid appearance in spite of the "pseudocystic" radiographic features.

Giant cell tumors involving the small bones of the appendicular skeleton or arising in the axial osseous system present as ill-defined lytic areas lacking specific radiographic features, and only a differential diagnosis is feasible.[47, 68] Sacral lesions are especially notorious for lack of consistent recognizability. Even tumors of considerable size may easily be missed. In the

small bones, the lesions are often centrally situated and are not eccentric, especially when they have been presented for a long time.[34]

The radiographic appearance following therapy is quite variable. Radiation therapy results in gradual and progressive ossification, i.e., sclerosis of the lesional area.[71] These changes are most pronounced during the first few years, finally becoming stationary (Fig. 17–7).

Following irradiation, the Herendeen phenomenon, a rare paradoxical reaction, may be observed, characterized by a rapid enlargement of the lesion lasting from a few weeks up to six months.[62] The presence of a growing, rarified, lytic area after curettage is suspicious of recurrence, especially if irregularly and poorly marginated. Considerable areas of cortical erosion also

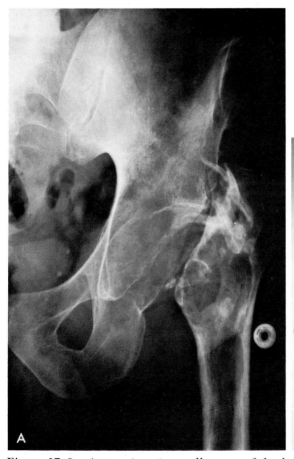
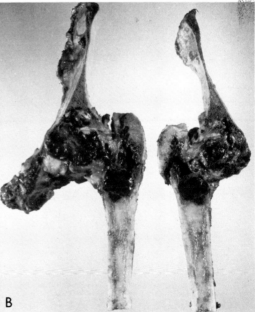

Figure 17–8.   Aggressive giant cell tumor of the left proximal femur in a 35-year-old man who had curettage and bone graft three and one half years previously with diagnosis of benign giant cell tumor. The lesion now extends into ilium. Hemipelvectomy yielded long-term cure.

herald the presence of an active disease process. Clinically, early recurrent lesions are indistinguishable from a secondary malignant giant cell tumor, although such an occurrence in advanced stages may be clearly diagnosable (Fig. 17–8).

Unfortunately, the radiographic features of giant cell tumors frequently are of no aid in distinguishing between benign and malignant forms. Innocuous presentation may culminate in aggressive growth and prompt metastasis; malignant-appearing tumors may never recur. The appearance of a malignant giant cell tumor is that of a medullary fibrosarcoma, an osteolytic osteogenic sarcoma, or even a malignant fibrous histiocytoma.

The *angiographic* assessment of giant

cell tumors reveals marked tumor vascularity with arteriovenous fistula formation.[99] This technique offers additional help in evaluating the size and extent of the lesion, especially the presence of soft tissue involvement. Angiographic distinctions between pure giant cell tumors and aneurysmal bone cysts are elusive and notoriously unreliable.[56]

RADIOGRAPHIC DIFFERENTIAL DIAGNOSIS

The radiographic differential diagnosis includes both benign and malignant bone lesions (Table 17–1).

1. Chondroblastoma   characteristically

TABLE 17–1.   Differential Diagnosis of Giant Cell Lesions of Bone

	Most Common Age Group	Location in Bone	Radiologic Appearance	Gross Features	Microscopic Features	
					Giant Cells	*Stromal Cells*
Giant cell tumor	3rd and 4th decades	Epiphysis	Eccentric expanded radiolucency	Fleshy soft tissue	Abundant number uniformly distributed	Plump and polyhedral with abundant cytoplasm
Non-ossifying fibroma	1st decade	Metaphysis	Eccentric oval defects	Fleshy soft tissue	Focal in distribution, small with few nuclei	Slender and spindly with little cytoplasm
Aneurysmal bone cyst	1st and 2nd decades	Vertebral column or metaphysis of long bone	Eccentric blow-out "soap bubble" appearance	Cavity filled with blood	Focally around vascular channels	Large vascular channels; slender to plump cells with hemosiderin granules
Brown tumor of hyperparathyroidism	Any age	Anywhere in bone	Absent lamina dura of teeth	Fleshy tissue or cystic spaces	Focal around hemosiderin pigment	Fibrous stroma with slender cells
Unicameral bone cyst	1st and 2nd decades	Metaphysis (proximal humerus)	Trabeculations in radiolucency	Cyst filled with clear fluid	Focal around cholesterol clefts	Cyst wall is fibrous tissue
Chondroblastoma	2nd decade	Epiphysis	Radiolucency with spotty opacities	Firm to fleshy tissue	Few and focal	Large, plump, and round cells with pericellular calcifications
Fibrous dysplasia	1st and 2nd decades	Metaphysis (proximal femur)	Ground-glass appearance	Firm and gritty	Few and focal	Woven bone and fibrous tissue
Giant cell reparative granuloma	2nd and 3rd decades	Maxilla and mandible	Radiolucent focus	Soft fleshy tissue	Abundant around hemosiderin pigment	Slender or plump cells
Ossifying fibroma	2nd and 3rd decades	Maxilla and mandible	Radiopaque	Bony hard tissue	Few and focal	Lamellar bony trabeculae in fibrous tissue
Osteogenic sarcoma	2nd and 3rd decades	Metaphysis	Radiolucent	Soft or firm	Focal distribution	Malignant spindle cells with direct osteoid formation
Chondromyxoid fibroma	2nd and 3rd decades	Metaphysis	Eccentric with expanded cortex	Soft to firm	Focal distribution	Chondroid and myxoid components
Osteoblastoma	2nd and 3rd decades	Vertebral column	Radiolucent or dense	Soft to firm	Focal distribution	Abundant osteoblasts between osteoid trabeculae

(Modified from Ghandur-Mnaymneh, L., and Mnaymneh, W. A.: Bone lesions with giant cells: problems in differential diagnosis. J. Med. Liban., 25:91–104, 1972.)

occurs in children and adolescents who have open epiphyses, contrary to giant cell tumor, which afflicts skeletally mature individuals. Solitary or multiple pinpoint calcification characterizes chondroblastoma; giant cell tumor lacks such features.

2. Nonossifying fibroma also occurs in patients with open epiphyses. The lesions here are in the shaft far removed from the epiphysis, have eccentric location within the bone, and have well-delineated, scalloped, sclerotic outlines. The sclerotic margins and diaphyseal location help to distinguish the two lesions in question.

3. On occasion, chondromyxoid fibroma may be confused with a giant cell tumor. The "pseudotrabeculations" so typical of chondromyxoid fibroma are denser and thicker than those occasionally seen in giant cell tumors. Metaphyseal location is the rule in chondromyxoid fibroma and the exception in giant cell tumors.

4. "Brown tumor" of hyperparathyroidism in its localized, destructive form, lacking signs of skeletal demineralization, i.e., loss of lamina dura, subperiosteal bone resorption, or thinned bony cortex, is practically indistinguishable from true giant cell tumor. This difficulty is magnified when the lesion happens to be located in the metaphyseal end of long bones in young adults. Serum calcium determination is the only real help.

5. Slow-growing medullary fibrosarcomas may display prominent cortical expansion. Their frequent diaphyseal location and extensive cortical destruction at a considerable distance from the main tumor mass offer some help in keeping these lesions apart.

6. Osteolytic osteogenic sarcomas may occasionally mimic giant cell tumors, since they preferentially involve the same osseous sites and age groups. Aggressive bony destruction with rapid progression lacking lesional delineation distinctly favors a malignant tumor.

GROSS APPEARANCE

The vast majority of the lesions are eccentrically situated in an epiphyseal location. The lesional tissue is fleshy, grayish-white, within an intermixture of hemor-rhagic or cystic areas and focal fibrous septa formation. Occasionally, when the epiphysis is still open, the lesion may be primarily metaphyseal, or in larger tumors, it may be in that location secondarily. Some are prominently hemorrhagic, soft, and cystic, especially when an aneurysmal bone cyst is engrafted thereon. At the area of cortical destruction, the bony contour is expanded, but the tumor is usually contained by a shell of new bone. The distended, thin cortex in larger lesions, which is associated with periosteal reactive bone formation only, incompletely delimits the tumor, thereby providing an ineffective barrier for soft tissue invasion. Direct penetration of the articular cartilage is quite rare, and joint space involvement usually occurs through lateral cortical erosion.

MICROSCOPIC APPEARANCE

The histologic appearance of giant cell tumor of bone is not distinctively characteristic, since the mere presence of giant cells, even in large numbers, is not sufficient to establish the diagnosis.[70, 174] Several other benign lesions may simulate it by containing giant cells (Table 17–1).[29] Aneurysmal or unicameral bone cysts, nonossifying fibroma, chondroblastoma, reparative granuloma, or "brown tumor" of hyperparathyroidism primarily come to mind. This tumor should be diagnosed only after a complete appraisal of the clinical, radiographic, operative, and pathologic data.[7, 105] The diagnosis of giant cell tumor is only tenable when *all* considerations, both major and minor, including age, anatomic site, signs, and symptoms, are satisfied.

In the conventional giant cell tumor, large numbers of multinucleated giant cells dominate the picture (Fig. 17–9). These are separated by inconspicuous mononuclear stromal cells with indistinct cellular outlines and scanty intercellular substance. The nuclei of the stromal and the giant cells have an identical appearance on both light microscopic and ultramicroscopic examination.[152] The loosely arranged stromal cells focally may become spindly and elongated, and focal collagenization may be featured (Fig. 17–10). These focal areas of collagen production

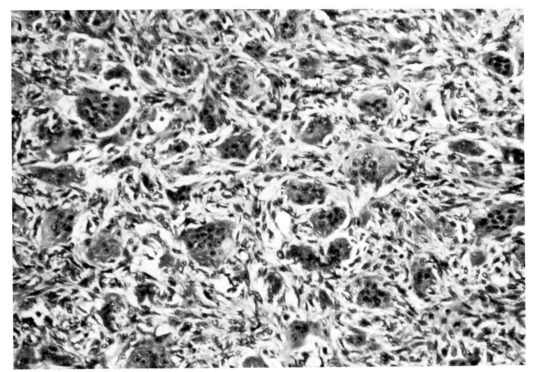

Figure 17–9. Giant cell tumor of conventional appearance. Note the abundance of multinucleated giant cells and sparse stromal component (Grade I). (Hematoxylin-eosin stain. Magnification × 80.)

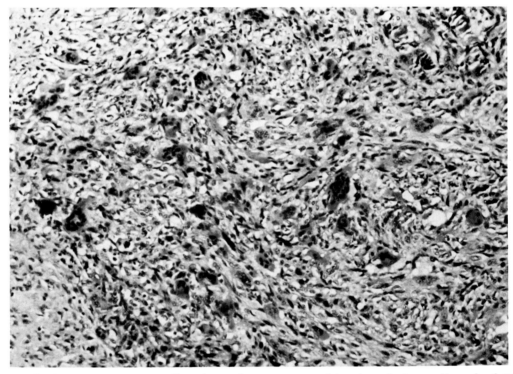

Figure 17–10. Recurrent giant cell tumor with numerous multinucleated giant cells and relatively increased stromal component. (Hematoxylin-eosin stain. Magnification × 50.)

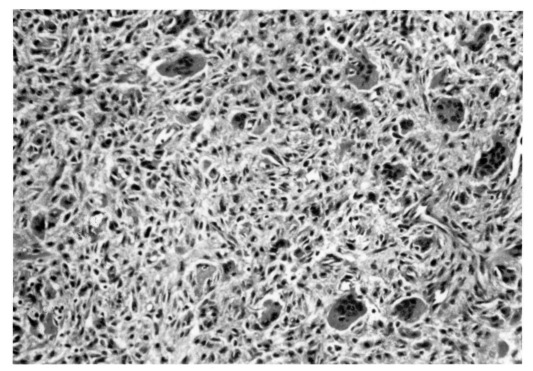

Figure 17–11. Focally atypical giant cell tumor with loosely dispersed giant cells but irregular spindle cell stroma with variation in size and shape of the cells as well as mitotic figures (Grade II). (Hematoxylin-eosin stain. Magnification × 80.)

correspond to the fibrous septa formation as seen on gross examination. When the stromal component becomes more prominent, i.e., the relative number of the giant cells decreases, the proliferative capacity, the growth of the lesion, is augmented. The frequency of giant cells is directly related to the amount of stroma. In instances in which the stroma features prominent spindle cell forms, variation of nuclear and cytoplasmic staining intensity, large nucleoli, increased nucleocytoplasmic ratio, as well as moderate numbers of mitotic figures are seen (Fig. 17–11). It should be emphasized that an occasional stromal cell may be quite atypical in almost every lesion but such an isolated finding has no adverse effect on the prognosis. Small clusters of spindle cells in the stroma also do not alter an otherwise benign designation. Large fields of dense collagenous scarring within the lesion are, in general, suspicious for a malignant transformation, but previously incompletely removed lesions, or those treated by bone grafts and irradiation, may show such areas without

necessarily signifying such a sinister behavioral alteration. In several microscopic foci, osteoid production and ossification may be noted (in about 30 per cent of our cases at Memorial Hospital), but these areas never become conspicuous, thereby avoiding the possibility of considering the lesion an osteoblastoma or even an osteogenic sarcoma. The tumor may also show osteoid and a reactive type of bone formation after fracture. On rare occasions, especially when the lesion involves atypical osseous sites, such as the small bones of the hands or feet, the patella, and so on, microscopic foci of poorly formed cartilage may be identified. Such instances are referred to as "enchondromatous giant cell tumor" and may lead to a misdiagnosis of chondroblastoma. Areas of hemorrhages with hemosiderin pigment deposition and a display of xanthomatous features with lipid-laden histiocytes may be present and usually represent involutional alterations or effects of previous treatment. Vacuolar degeneration and phagocytic properties of the multinucleated giant cells may be

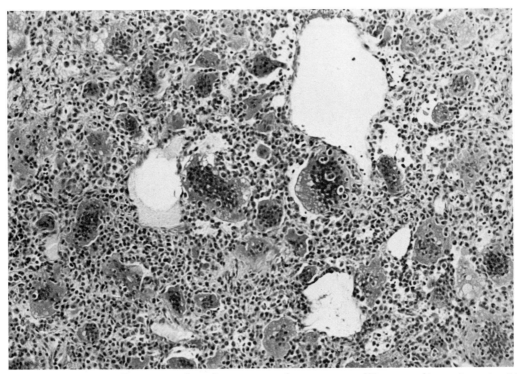

Figure 17–12.   Giant cell tumor with early aneurysmal component. (Hematoxylin-eosin stain. Magnification × 80.)

noted. These degenerating giant cells may appear in the peripheral sinusoid of the regional lymph nodes, as pointed out by several investigators, and may not be correctly interpreted as tumor giant cells since they do exhibit vacuolar degeneration and phagocytic activity.[14, 66]

Hutter and associates[66] emphasized in their analysis of the various microscopic patterns that a wide variation does exist under the diagnosis of "benign" giant cell tumor. No consistently predictable microscopic features are available to forecast recurrence or eventual malignant alteration in this "benign" group of lesions. Blood-filled areas may represent a prominent component of a giant cell tumor, raising the possibility of an aneurysmal bone cyst (Fig. 17–12). One should be mindful of the fact that some giant cell tumors may also exhibit such increased vascularity following fracture or treatment. Histologic examination of predominantly osteolytic osteogenic sarcoma may reveal limited but densely cellular areas of giant cells.[48, 164]

The microscopic evaluation of a giant cell tumor may include, in addition to routine histologic study, *cytologic examina-*

tion of material removed at fine needle aspiration biopsy (Fig. 17–13). It must be borne in mind that the mere presence of giant cells in the aspirate is not diagnostic of a giant cell tumor of bone, since such cells may be found in many other osseous lesions, both neoplastic and nontumorous. It is also good to remember that the giant cells in smears are readily separated from the stromal components, thereby making it difficult to obtain clear-cut information concerning the proportion of the various cells in a given bone lesion.[156] If the smears prepared from an aspirate of bone reveal a firm cytoplasmic cohesion between the mononuclear stromal forms and the giant cells, valuable information may be gleaned.[66] In experienced hands, the diagnostic accuracy of this technique is excellent and surgical procedures may be based on it.

GRADING

There are opposing views on the feasibility of grading these lesions and predicting clinical behavior.[57] Some believe that

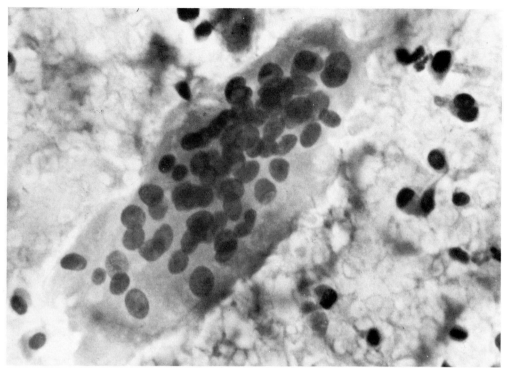

Figure 17-13. Air-dried aspiration smear showing a typical multinucleated giant cell of a conventional giant cell tumor bone. (Hematoxylin-eosin stain. Magnification × 800.)

the histologic features do not reliably and consistently parallel subsequent behavior. Others feel that microscopic features should be coupled with other parameters, such as erosion of cortex and extension to soft tissues, to provide a more predictive gauge for prognostications. Finally, there are those, this author included, who believe that the histologic features reliably mirror subsequent behavior and are of some help in predicting prognosis while providing valuable guidance in treatment.[66] An easily reproducible scheme in grading giant cell tumors provides three histologic grades. In Grade I, or conventional giant cell tumor, the stroma is quite inconspicuous and subservient to the large numbers of giant cells that dominate the histologic picture. The wide variation in the stromal patterns was discussed previously. In Grade II (borderline) lesions the stroma becomes prominent and the giant cells diminish in number in relation to the stromal component. The proliferating stromal cells here are spindly and elongated, and marked cellular atypia is

featured with a moderate number of mitotic figures; however, the cytologic alterations are insufficient to justify a diagnosis of cancer. In the fully malignant, or Grade III, giant cell tumor, the spindle cell sarcomatous stroma entirely overwhelms the giant cells, the latter becoming quite sparse, with microscopic evidence of an overt sarcoma (Figs. 17-14 and 17-15). In general, two distinct but occasionally overlapping histologic patterns may be discerned. In the secondarily "converted" malignant giant cell tumor, the densely collagenized spindle cell sarcoma is accompanied by only a few benign giant cells.[66] In the primary malignant giant cell variant, however, a more vascularized, telangiectatic type of spindle cell, usually fibrosarcoma, is present with large numbers of benign giant cells and scarce collagen fiber deposition (Fig. 17-16). It is quite important to remember, if a successful attempt at grading is contemplated, to evaluate all tissues removed at surgical exploration to be certain that limited areas showing malignant transformation are not

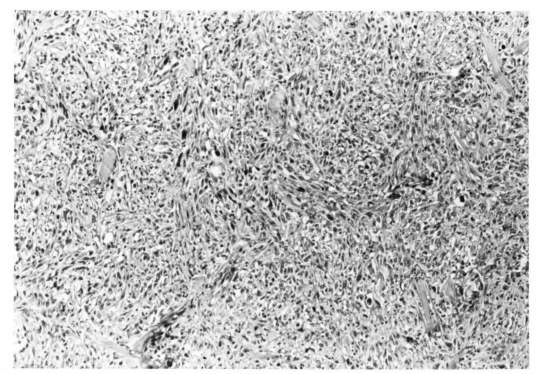

Figure 17–14. Secondary fully malignant giant cell tumor with typical storiform matted growth pattern of the spindly tumor cells. (Hematoxylin-eosin stain. Magnification × 50.)

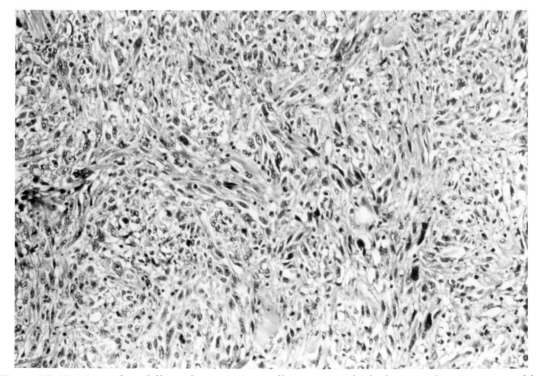

Figure 17–15. Secondary fully malignant giant cell tumor in which the growth pattern resembles that of a malignant fibrous histiocytoma. Other areas showed a conventional giant cell tumor. (Hematoxylin-eosin stain. Magnification × 80.)

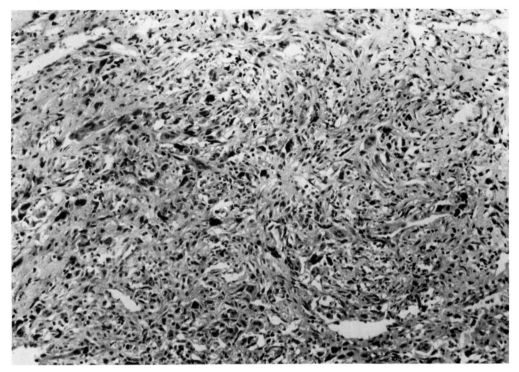

Figure 17–16. Primary fully malignant giant cell tumor with pleomorphic tumor cells, increased vascularity, and only very few benign giant cells. (Hematoxylin-eosin stain. Magnification × 50.)

omitted. The number and size of the multinucleate giant cells have no relation to the benign or malignant nature of the tumor.

ULTRASTRUCTURAL AND HISTOCHEMICAL STUDIES

Ultrastructural findings suggest conversion of stromal cells into multinucleated giant cells.[11, 60, 63, 152] The exact mechanism by which this transformation takes place still remains under discussion, but the favored opinion is that of fusion or conglomeration of the stromal cells,[60, 152] although some prefer amitotic cell division as the likelier explanation.[139]

Mitoses have only been observed in stromal cells, strongly suggesting that these are the proliferating elements and not the giant cells. Various degrees of degenerative changes within the giant cells, visible on light microscopic and ultramicroscopic examination, may suggest an end stage of development resulting in ultimate cell death. The abundance of lysosomes and the large amounts of hydrolytic enzymes, especially acid phosphatase, which is present in the giant cells but absent in the stromal component, may implicate intracellular self-digestion as means of cellular demise.[11, 85, 152]

The derivation of the stromal cells is also a matter of contention, although the majority of the investigators favor the undifferentiated connective tissue cells of the bone marrow as the origin.[70, 95, 139] Additional suggestions are that the stromal component is derived from undifferentiated mesenchymal cells maturing into osteoclasts[181] or that the stromal cells are indeed of endothelial origin.[2, 128]

Ultrastructural comparison of the giant cells and the stromal cells reveals markedly increased numbers of mitochondria in the multinucleated giant cells.[63] This mitochondral abundance is directly related to the succinic dehydrogenase and β-glucuronidase activity.[73, 85]

Until very recently, no definite and consistently demonstrable distinctions between the multinucleated giant cells of giant cell tumors and those of other conditions, both neoplastic and nontumorous, have been found.[52] By employing combined techniques of electron microscopic histochemistry and biochemical measurements, Doty and Schofield demonstrated the multinucleated giant cells in giant cell tumor of bone to be strongly positive for acid phosphatase, phosphamidase, and "neutral" lysosomal reactions. In their experience, osteoclasts, although similar in appearance, do not display "neutral" phosphatase activity, thereby allowing a clearcut distinction.[32]

MALIGNANT TRANSFORMATION OF A PREVIOUSLY HISTOLOGICALLY BENIGN GIANT CELL TUMOR

There is an inherent invasiveness and aggressiveness to these tumors. After multiple or, occasionally, even solitary local recurrence, a previously conventional giant cell tumor may exhibit fully malignant behavior and may show morphologic changes of an overt sarcoma.[109, 126, 138, 139] There is no reliable way of predicting which benign giant cell tumor will convert to a malignant one. A sarcomatous change in a previously benign giant cell tumor may occur without antecedent irradiation but is more common after it. The time required for malignant transformation is less than one year in one third of the patients, between one and five years in one third, and more than five years after the initial diagnosis or treatment in the rest. The overall average is seven years. In those patients treated by surgery alone, the time period of malignant change ranges from 1 to 3 years, and their tumors are mostly well-differentiated, low-grade malignant types. This is in contradistinction to those patients whose primary treatment is solely radiation, where the time period of malignant conversion ranges from 3 to 20 years, and most of the secondary tumors are of the high-grade, anaplastic variants.[66]

These malignant giant cell tumors secondarily evolving from a benign counterpart may be either a fibrosarcoma, usually with a typical herringbone pattern that still retains a benign giant cell component, or an osteogenic sarcoma. Microscopically, the fibrosarcomatous feature is associated with abundant collagen formation, and few retain benign giant cells. An abortive attempt at a storiform, matted, or pinwheel growth pattern is occasionally evident, mimicking that of a fibrous histiocytoma (Figs. 17–14 and 17–15). Marked cellular pleomorphism, increased numbers, and atypical mitoses accompanied by scanty collagen formation characterize the anaplastic variants. The presence of direct osteoid production by the sarcomatous spindle cells, i.e., features of an osteogenic sarcoma, generally follows radiation therapy for an otherwise conventional giant cell tumor.

The pertinent literature is replete with solitary case reports or small series of cases documenting the role of radiotherapy in the induction of sarcomatous change.[13, 165] Seventy per cent of all malignant giant cell tumors were treated by radiation prior to the diagnosis of cancer.[66] It must be emphasized, however, that malignant transformation of giant cell tumors often follows excessive dosages of radiation with old fashioned equipment or conventional small dose fractionations over a protracted length of time.[37, 44, 121] The current use of modern supervoltage radiotherapy and Cobalt[60] teletherapy decreases the intensity of the absorbed dose, thereby greatly reducing the likelihood of future malignant transformation. The therapeutic results of irradiated giant cell tumors employing modern dose and fractionation schedules, in addition to up-to-date equipment, are very encouraging, although no long-term follow-up data are yet available.[35, 88] It is good to remember that several decades may pass before a sarcoma may supervene in a giant cell tumor.

PRIMARY MALIGNANT GIANT CELL TUMOR

Although malignant giant cell tumors make up 30 per cent of all cases at Memorial Hospital, only 8 per cent are malignant from the very onset (Table 17–2).[66] These are considered to be primary malignant giant cell tumors and are often situated in unusual sites.[103] The predominant microscopic pattern in these lesions is that of an anaplastic spindle cell sarcoma with pronounced telangiectatic features and lack of collagenization.[83, 154] (Fig. 17–16.)

TABLE 17-2. Incidence of Malignant Giant Cell Tumor of Bone

Authors	Year Reported	Percentage
1. Hutter et al.	1962	30.0*
2. Dahlin et al.	1970	8.7
3. Goldenberg et al.	1970	6.2
4. McGrath	1972	15.4
5. Larsson et al.	1975	11.3

*The incidence of conversion from a benign to a malignant giant cell tumor is 22 per cent.

No direct osteoid formation by the sarcomatous tumor cells is demonstrated. The most pertinent microscopic differential diagnosis includes a telangiectatic osteogenic sarcoma, but the giant cell tumor lacks "malignant osteoid" production in its entirety. A fair number of benign multinucleated giant cells accompanies the overtly sarcomatous spindle cells. In some foci, a fibrous histiocytoma-like growth pattern may be seen.

METASTASIZING BENIGN GIANT CELL TUMORS

Metastasis may be construed as "the formation of another growth in any site following the transportation of tumor cells from the initial growth."[115] Tumor metastases are usually due to blood vessel or lymphatic invasion. Well-preserved bone and bone marrow particles may be encountered during an autopsy in the pulmonary parenchyma subsequent to forceful cardiac resuscitation resulting in rib fractures. This and other similar examples of essentially transport phenomena represent "benign" metastasis. There are a number of authentic reports of benign giant cell tumors that have metastasized to the lungs.[54, 67, 74, 87, 91, 119, 151, 161] It is conceivable that the pulmonary metastases in a histologically benign giant cell tumor are secondary to iatrogenic "seeding" of blood vessels or lymphatics due to vigorous curettage. This may explain the often observed self-limited growth potential of lung lesions in giant cell tumors of bone not completely excised and the long-term benign clinical course.[161] It is reasonable to suggest that, in histologically equivocal "benign" giant cell tumors, the metastases are biologically benign most of the time, and there should be no hesitation in resecting the pulmonary lesions, with an excellent prospect of total cure. Ossified pulmonary metastases from a benign giant cell tumor of the tibia have been noted.[58]

CLINICAL BEHAVIOR AND TREATMENT

In order to vividly explain the concept of "semimalignant" bone tumors, Professor Uehlinger of Zurich provided the following allegory: On the day of the final judgment of mankind, humans were separated into benign and malignant Christians. It soon became evident, however, that the strict separation into these two groups was not satisfactory, and it was deemed necessary to introduce a third intermediate category reserved for those who, although originally sinners, would have a chance to enter heaven after expiatory purification in purgatory (Fig. 17–17).[167] Experience with classification of tumors according to their biologic behavior is quite similar: in addition to clearly benign and malignant types, Uehlinger, among others, conceived an intermediate group. Giant cell tumor fits this "semimalignant" category and indeed represents the prime example of it.[175]

Approximately 20 per cent of giant cell tumors, even in the total absence of histologic malignancy, invade the cortex and directly extend into adjacent soft tissues.[75] Giant cell tumor may spontaneously involve a neighboring bone through extension into the interosseous muscles or may invade an adjacent vertebra (Figs. 17–6 and 17–7).

The local recurrence rate is approximately 30 per cent within the first two years following curettage, and close to half of the lesions recur within five years (Fig. 17–18). Most of the recurrent disease (about 90 per cent) clinically manifests during this time period, and any evidence of recrudescent tumor activity after this time is highly suspicious of malignant conversion. Only one third of the patients are cured after one attempt at therapy, an additional one third requires a second therapeutic intervention, and about one third must undergo three to five separate efforts to successfully eradicate the disease.[66]

The result of treatment is related to

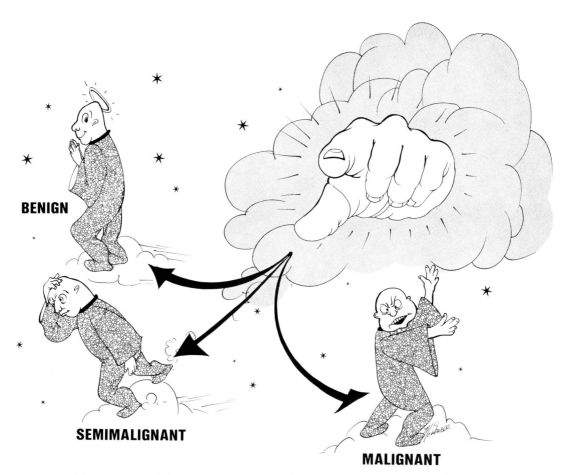

Figure 17–17.   The allegory of "semimalignant" tumors at the time of creation.

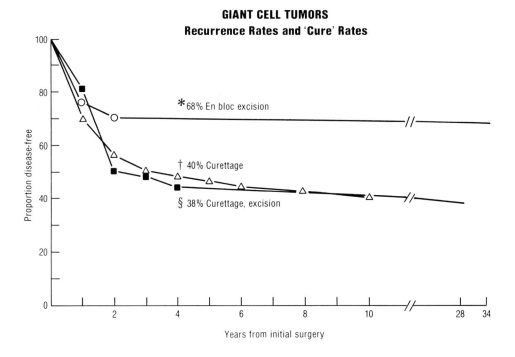

GIANT CELL TUMORS
Recurrence Rates and 'Cure' Rates

*68% En bloc excision

† 40% Curettage

§ 38% Curettage, excision

Proportion disease-free

Years from initial surgery

* Goldenberg, Campbell, Bonfiglio, JBJS, 52A:619, 1970
† Johnson, Dahlin, JBJS, 41A:895, 1959
§ Hutter et al., Cancer, 15:653, 1962

Figure 17–18. Recurrence rates and cure rates of giant cell tumors following various modalities of therapy. (From Marcove, R. C., Weis, L. D., Vaghaiwalla, M. R., et al.: Cryosurgery in the treatment of giant cell tumors of bone. A report of 52 consecutive cases. Cancer, *41*:957–969, 1978.

many factors but especially to the method of tumor removal, the extent and location of the lesion, and adjacent soft tissue involvement.[187] Extensive lesions of the knee region, where about 50 to 60 per cent of the tumors are located, necessitate complete resection of the distal femur or proximal tibia, especially if there is soft tissue involvement, occasionally including the sacrifice of the knee joint (arthrodesis).[188] In smaller lesions of this area, a total excision of the overlying cortex, with unroofing (exteriorizing) of the tumor cavity and thorough curettage followed by iliac or tibial bone graft is employed by most surgeons. It is important to remember that separate preparation and draping techniques should be utilized to avoid the accidental implantation of a giant cell tumor at the donor site of a bone graft.[157] Wound implantation by giant cell tumor is a well-recognized complication resulting in soft tissue recurrences.[131] The chal-

lenge, of course, is to remove all tumor and preserve or restore the function of the knee joint. The wide exposure of the tumorous area gives a better chance for the surgeon to completely remove the tumor. Recurrent large tumors may necessitate a radical *en bloc* resection of the involved bone and adjacent joint, especially if the tumor extends to the articular surface or involves adjacent soft tissues. The Merle d'Aubigné reconstructive technique employs an ingenious method in which a portion of the proximal tibia is divided and shifted upward to traverse the surgical defect.[107, 108] In fully grown individuals of above average height a corresponding portion of bone from the subtrochanteric region of the opposite extremity may be utilized to bridge the created defect. This, of course, makes the patient somewhat shorter, but the lengths of both legs are equal.

Recent improvements in the reconstructive techniques of orthopedic surgery, employing custom-made bone implants and total joint replacement, permit one to safely and successfully restore the functional integrity and physiologic function of a resected bone and joint.

Clinically aggressive giant cell tumors of distal radius have been successfully treated by massive resection and tibial bone graft[20] or by allograft replacement of the involved bone[147] with good functional results. Iliac bone grafts[184, 185] and homograft implants have also been employed with success.[116, 122] In some selected cases, thorough curettage with acrylic cementation, permitting full and early mobility as well as stability, has been successful.[125]

The unacceptably high recurrence rates after curettage and the considerable risk of sarcomatous degeneration in tumors treated by irradiation caused Marcove and associates[102] to seek a newer, more effective method of treatment.[27, 103] This technique, developed at Memorial Hospital, advocates wide incision, thorough curettage, and repetitive exposure of the large curetted bony area to temperatures of $-20°$ C by liquid nitrogen instillation.[102] The use of cryosurgery as a supplement to adequate curettage reliably reduced the incidence of local recurrence to about 12 per cent in 52 consecutive cases of giant cell tumor while usually preserving joint motion and avoiding total arthroplasty, arthrodesis, and amputation. Currently, methyl methacrylate along with corticocancellous onlay graft is used to provide additional structural support until peripheral bone regeneration occurs. This provides increased bone stability and prevents postoperative infraction, especially if coupled with a long-leg, ischial, weight-bearing brace.

Tumors in the sacrum or vertebral bodies are quite difficult to discover early, are less accessible for total removal, necessitating radiation therapy, and have less predictable behavior (Fig. 17–7). Even though sacral lesions may be small and histologically benign when detected, they present a formidable therapeutic challenge. Radiation therapy, or even total sacrectomy, may provide a long-term cure in an otherwise difficult location for treatment. It is generally agreed that the ideal treatment of giant cell tumors of the spine is initial complete removal if possible.[22, 26, 77, 153] This is easier said than done, especially in the face of impending severe neurologic deficit necessitating immediate decompression. A combined early orthopedic and neurological approach should be seriously considered since, if treatment is delayed for more than three months after the onset of nerve root symptoms, irreversible nerve deficits may develop.[90] Surgical treatment by curettage or local excision is preferred.[51] This purely surgical approach should be coupled with radiotherapy for incompletely removed, recurrent, or nonresectable tumors.[35, 40, 88]

REFERENCES

1. Adkins, K. F., Martinez, M. G., and Romaniuk, K.: Ultrastructure of giant-cell lesions. Mononuclear cells in peripheral giant-cell granulomas. Oral Surg., 33:775–786, 1972.
2. Aegerter, E., and Kirkpatrick, J. A., Jr.: Orthopedic Diseases. 4th ed. Philadelphia, W. B. Saunders Co., 1975.
3. Akerman, M., Berg, N. O., and Persson, B. M.: Fine needle aspiration biopsy in the evaluation of tumor-like lesions of bone. Acta Orthop. Scand., 47:129–136, 1976.
4. Alguacil-Garcia, A., Unni, K. K., and Goellner, J. R.: Malignant giant cell tumor of soft parts. An ultrastructural study of four cases. Cancer, 40:244–253, 1977.
5. Alguacil-Garcia, A., Unni, K. K., and Goellner, J. R.: Giant cell tumor of tendon sheath and pigmented villonodular synovitis. An ultrastructural study. Am. J. Clin. Pathol. 69:6–17, 1978.
6. Anthikad, I., and Reddy, G. N.: Giant cell tumour of the bone. J. Indian Med. Assoc., 66:303–304, 1976.
7. Barnes, R.: Giant-cell tumour of bone. J. Bone Joint Surg. [Br.], 54:213–215, 1972.
8. Bloodgood, J. C.: Benign bone cysts, ostitis fibrosa, giant-cell sarcoma and bone aneurism of the long pipe bones: a clinical and pathological study with the conclusion that conservative treatment is justifiable. Ann. Surg., 52:145–185, 1910.
9. Bloodgood, J. C.: Bone tumors. Central (medullary) giant-cell tumor (sarcoma) of lower end of ulna, with evidence that complete destruction of the bony shell or perforation of the bony shell is not a sign of increased malignancy. Ann. Surg., 69:345–359, 1919.
10. Bogumill, G. P., Schultz, M. A., and Johnson, L. C.: Giant-cell tumor — A metaphyseal lesion. Abstract. J. Bone Joint Surg. [Am.], 54:1558, 1972.
11. Boquist, L., Larsson, S. E., and Lorentzon, R.: Genuine giant-cell tumour of bone: a combined cytological, histopathological and ultrastructural study. Pathol. Eur., 11:117–127, 1976.
12. Borsotti, G.: Tumore a mieloplassi ad origine

pluricentrica. Rass. Int. Stomatol. Prat., 16:503–521, 1965.

13. Bradshaw, J. D.: The value of x-ray therapy in the management of osteoclastoma. Clin. Radiol., 15:70–74, 1964.

14. Budzilovich, G. N., Truchly, G., and Wilens, S. L.: Tumor giant cells in regional lymph nodes of a case of recurrent giant cell tumor of bone. Clin. Orthop., 30:182–187, 1963.

15. Burman, M. S., Gardner, R. C., and Lauter, C. B.: Aggressive giant-cell tumor in a young female with congenital adrenal virilism (adrenogenital syndrome). Report of an unusual association of a bone neoplasm with an endocrine disorder. Cancer, 25:1174–1177, 1970.

16. Byers, V. S., Levin, A. S., Johnston, J. O., et al.: Quantitative immunofluorescence studies of the tumor antigen-bearing cell in giant cell tumor of bone and osteogenic sarcoma. Cancer Res., 35:2520–2531, 1975.

17. Campanacci, M., Giunti, A., and Olmi, R.: Giant-cell tumours of bone. Ital. J. Orthop. Traum., 1:249–277, 1975.

18. Campanacci, M., Giunti, A., and Olmi, R.: Metaphyseal and diaphyseal location of the giant cell tumor. Chir. Organi Mov., 62:29–34, 1975.

19. Campbell, C. J.: Place of resection in the management of primary bone tumours. Can. J. Surg., 20:518, 521, 1977.

20. Campbell, C. J., and Akbarnia, B. A.: Giant-cell tumor of the radius treated by massive resection and tibial bone graft. J. Bone Joint Surg. [Am.], 57:982–986, 1975.

21. Chaix, C., and Trifaud, A.: Evolution and treatment of giant cell tumors of bone. Rev. Chir. Orthop., 61:429–432, 1975.

22. Chow, S. P., Leong, J. C. Y., and Yau, A. C. M. C.: Osteoclastoma of the axis. Report of a case. J. Bone Joint Surg. [Am.], 59:550–551, 1977.

23. Coley, B. L., Higinbotham, N. L., and Kogure, T.: Giant cell tumor of bone. Am. J. Surg., 96:479–491, 1958.

24. Coley, W. B.: Prognosis in giant-cell sarcoma of the long bones. Ann. Surg., 79:321–357, 561–595, 1924.

25. Cooper, A., and Travers, B.: Surgical Essays. 3rd ed. London, Cox & Son, 1818.

26. Dahlin, D. C.: Giant-cell tumor of vertebrae above the sacrum. A review of 31 cases. Cancer, 39:1350–1356, 1977.

27. Dahlin, D. C., Cupps, R. E., and Johnson, E. W., Jr.: Giant-cell tumor: a study of 195 cases. Cancer, 25:1061–1070, 1970.

28. d'Alessio, E. S., D'Alessio, C., and Fusco, L.: Osteoclastomas: casistic contribution (33 cases) and clinic and histopathologic considerations. Rass. Int. Clin. Ter., 54:1309–1334, 1974.

29. D'Alonzo, R. T., Pitcock, J. A., and Milford, L. W.: Giant-cell reaction of bone. Report of two cases. J. Bone Joint Surg. [Am.], 54:1267–1271, 1972.

30. Danilov, A. Y.: Juxtaphysary osteoblastoclastomas in children. Ortop. Travmatol. Protez., 34(5):27–30, 1973.

31. DePalma, A. F., Ahmad, I., and Flannery, G.: Treatment of giant cell tumors in bone. Clin. Orthop., 100:232–237, 1974.

32. Doty, S. B., and Schofield, B. H.: Enzyme histochemistry of bone and cartilage cells. Prog. Histochem. Cytochem., 8:1–37, 1976.

33. Duquennoy, A., Decoulx, J., Houche, M., et al.: Evolution of giant cell tumors. Rev. Chir. Orthop., 61:415, 423, 1975.

34. Edeiken, J., and Hodes, P. J.: Giant cell tumors vs. tumors with giant cells. Radiol. Clin. North Am., 1:75–100, 1963.

35. Eilers, H., Habighorst, L. V., Albers, P., et al.: Radiation therapy of an inoperable giant cell tumor. Strahlentherapie, 153:103–105, 1977.

36. Eisenstein, S. M., Levin, C., and Schmaman, A.: Giant cell tumour of the sacrum. A case report. S. Afr. Med. J., 49:1099,–1101, 1975.

37. Ellis, F.: Treatment of osteoclastoma by radiation. J. Bone Joint Surg. [Br.], 31:268–280, 1949.

38. Emley, W. E.: Giant cell tumor of the sphenoid bone. A case report and review of the literature. Arch. Otolaryngol., 94:369–374, 1971.

39. Erens, A. C.: Giant cell tumour of bone. Radiological characteristics. Radiol. Clin. Biol., 42:385–394, 1973.

40. Fitz, G. R., and Carter, H. K.: Giant cell tumor of bone: review and presentation of two unusual cases. J. Am. Osteopath. Assoc., 66:292–302, 1966.

41. FitzPatrick, D. J., and Bullough, P. G.: Giant cell tumor of the lunate bone: a case report. J. Hand Surg., 2:269–270, 1977.

42. Ford, G. H., Empson, R. N., Jr., Plopper, C. G., et al.: Giant cell tumor of soft parts. A report of an equine and feline case. Vet. Pathol., 12:428–433, 1975.

43. Forest, M.: The pathologic appearance of giant cell tumors of bone. Rev. Chir. Orthop., 61:359–375, 1975.

44. Friedman, M., and Pearlman, A. W.: Benign giant-cell tumor of bone: radiation dosage for each type. Radiology, 91:1151–1158, 1968.

45. Gallardo, H., de Lustig, E. S., and Schajowicz, F.: Growth and maintenance of human giant-cell bone tumors (osteoclastomas) in continuous culture. Oncology, 24:146–159, 1970.

46. Garman, R. H., Powell, F. R., and Tompsett, J. W.: Malignant giant cell tumor in a dog. J. Am. Vet. Med. Assoc., 171:546–548, 1977.

47. Gee, V. R., and Pugh, D. G.: Giant-cell tumor of bone. Radiology, 70:33–45, 1958.

48. Ghandur-Mnaymneh, L., and Mnaymneh, W. A.: Bone lesions with giant cells: problems in differential diagnosis. J. Med. Liban., 25:91–104, 1972.

49. Goldenberg, R. R., Campbell, C. J., and Bonfiglio, M.: Giant-cell tumor of bone. An analysis of 218 cases. J. Bone Joint Surg. [Am.], 52:619–664, 1970.

50. Goldring, S. R., Dayer, J. M., Russell, R. G. G., et al.: Cells cultured from human giant cell tumors of bone respond to parathyroid hormone. Calcif. Tissue Res., 22(Supplement):269–274, 1977.

51. Gonem, M. N.: Osteoclastoma of the thoracic spine. Case report. J. Neurosurg., 44:748–752, 1976.

52. Gothlin, G., and Ericsson, J. L. E.: The osteoclast: review of ultrastructure, origin and structure-function relationship. Clin. Orthop., *120*:201–231, 1976.

53. Govallo, V. I., and Shelepina, T. A.: Immunological studies in carcinogenesis. Distribution of the tissue incompatibility antigens (HL-A system) in oncological patients. Vopr. Onkol., *21*(9):13–19, 1975.

54. Gresen, A. A., Dahlin, D. C., Peterson, L. F. A., et al.: "Benign" giant cell tumor of bone metastasizing to lung. Ann. Thorac. Surg., *16*:531–535, 1973.

55. Gross, S. W.: Sarcoma of the long bones: based upon a study of one hundred and sixty-five cases. Am. J. Med. Sci., 78:17–57, 1879.

56. Gunterberg, B., Kindblom, L. G., and Laurin, S.: Giant-cell tumor of bone and aneurysmal bone cyst. A correlated histologic and angiographic study. Skeletal Radiol., 2:65–74, 1977.

57. Hadders, H. N.: Some remarks on the histology of bone tumours. Yearbook Cancer Res. (Amsterdam), 22:7–10, 1973.

58. Hall, F. M., Frank, H. A., Cohen, R. B., et al.: Ossified pulmonary metastases from giant cell tumor of bone. Am. J. Roentgenol. Radium Ther. Nucl. Med., *127*:1046–1047, 1976.

59. Hallowes, R. C., and Chesterman, F. C.: Ultrastructure of giant cells in tumours induced in golden hamsters by murine sarcoma virus-Harvey. Int. J. Cancer, 7:513–525, 1971.

60. Hanaoka, H., Friedman, B., and Mack, R. P.: Ultrastructure and histogenesis of giant-cell tumor of bone. Cancer, 25:1408–1423, 1970.

61. Harwood, A. R., Fornasier, V. L., and Rider, W. D.: Supervoltage irradiation in the management of giant cell tumor of bone. Radiology, *125*:223–226, 1977.

62. Herendeen, R. W.: Results in röntgen-ray therapy of giant-cell tumors of bone. Ann. Surg., 93:398–411, 1931.

63. Horie, A.: An electron microscopic observation of giant cells and stromal cells in the benign giant cell tumor of the bone. Fukuoka Acta Med., 52:817–828, 1961.

64. Howard, E. B., and Kenyon, A. J.: Malignant osteoclastoma (giant cell tumor) in the cat with associated mast-cell response. Cornell Vet., 57:398–409, 1967.

65. Hutter, R. V. P., Foote, F. W., Jr., Frazell, E. L., et al.: Giant cell tumors complicating Paget's disease of bone. Cancer, *16*:1044–1056, 1963.

66. Hutter, R. V. P., Worcester, J. N., Jr., Francis, K. C., et al.: Benign and malignant giant cell tumors of bone. A clinicopathological analysis of the natural history of the disease. Cancer, 15:653–690, 1962.

67. Inoue, H., Ishihara, T., Ikeda, T., et al.: Benign giant cell tumor of femur with bilateral multiple pulmonary metastases. J. Thorac. Cardiovasc. Surg., 74:935–938, 1977.

68. Jacobs, P.: The diagnosis of osteoclastoma (giant-cell tumour): a radiological and pathological correlation. Br. J. Radiol., 45:121–136, 1972.

69. Jaffe, H. L.: Giant-cell tumour (osteoclastoma) of bone: its pathologic delimitation and the inherent clinical implications. Ann. R. Coll. Surg. Engl., *13*:343–355, 1953.

70. Jaffe, H. L., Lichtenstein, L., and Portis, R. B.: Giant cell tumor of bone. Its pathologic appearance, grading, supposed variants and treatment. Arch. Pathol., *30*:993–1031, 1940.

71. Jansson, G.: Roentgen treatment and the course of cure of giant cell tumour in the osseous system. Acta Radiol., 25:569–579, 1944.

72. Jedrzejewska, H.: Remarks on the surgical treatment of giant cell tumor of the proximal end of the humerus. Chir. Narzadow Ruchu Ortop. Pol. 39(5):641–647, 1974.

73. Jeffree, G. M., and Price, C. H. G.: Bone tumours and their enzymes. A study of the phosphatases, non-specific esterase and beta-glucuronidase of osteogenic and cartilaginous tumors, fibroblastic and giant-cell lesions. J. Bone Joint Surg. [Br.], 47:120–136, 1965.

74. Jewell, J. H. and Bush, L. F.: "Benign" giant-cell tumor of bone with a solitary pulmonary metastasis. A case report. J. Bone Joint Surg. [Am.], 46:848–852, 1964.

75. Johnson, E. W., Jr.: Adjacent and distant spread of giant cell tumors. Am. J. Surg., *109*:163–166, 1965.

76. Johnson, E. W., Jr., and Dahlin, D. C.: Treatment of giant-cell tumor of bone. J. Bone Joint Surg. [Am.], *41*:895–904, 1959.

77. Johnson, E. W., Jr., Gee, V. R., and Dahlin, D. C.: Giant-cell tumors of the sacrum. Am. J. Orthop., *4*:302–305, 1962.

78. Johnson, K. A., and Riley, L. H., Jr.: Giant-cell tumor of bone. An evaluation of 24 cases treated at The Johns Hopkins Hospital between 1925 and 1955. Clin. Orthop., *62*:187–191, 1969.

79. Johnston, J.: Giant cell tumor of bone: The role of the giant cell in orthopedic pathology. Orthop. Clin. North Am., 8:751–770, 1977.

80. Kaufman, S. M., and Isaac, P. C.: Multiple giant cell tumors. South. Med. J., 70:105–107, 1977.

81. Kelikian, H., and Clayton, I.: Giant-cell tumor of the patella. J. Bone Joint Surg. [Am.], 39:414–420, 1957.

82. Kikuta, Y., Ishii, S., and Umeda, H.: Electron microscopic studies on the cultured cells from the human benign giant cell tumors and osteosarcomas. J. Jap. Orthop. Assoc. (Nippon Seikeigekagakkai Zasshi), 49:135–143, 1975.

83. Kimball, R. M., and Desanto, D. A.: Malignant giant-cell tumor of the ulna. Report of a case of 18 years' duration. J. Bone Joint Surg. [Am.] , 40:1131–1138, 1958.

84. Knahr, K., Locke, H., Plaue, R., et al.: Hüftendoprothesen bei Tumoren des coxalen Femurendes. Orthop. Prax., *12*:647–.655, 1976.

85. Kraievski, N. A., Raikhlin, N. T., and Soloviev, Yu. N.: Histochemical characteristics of giant cell bone tumours. Folia Histochem. Cytochem. (Krakow),8:3–10, 1970.

86. Kumar, S., and Tuli, S. M.: Giant cell tumor of the middle phalanx of the left fifth finger. Case report. Int. Surg., 55:288–292, 1971.

87. Kutchemeshgi, A. D., Wright, J. R., and Humphrey, R. L.: Pulmonary metastases from a well-differentiated giant cell tumor of bone. Report of a patient with apparent response to cyclophosphamide therapy. Johns Hopkins Med. J., *134*:237–245, 1974.

88. Laddaga, M., Calderazzi, A., Ducci, F., et al.:

Radiotherapy of giant-cell tumour of the vertebral column. Radiol. Med. (Torino), *62*:609–622, 1976.

89. Larsson, S. E., Lorentzon, R., and Boquist, L.: Giant-cell tumor of bone. A demographic, clinical, and histopathological study of all cases recorded in the Swedish Cancer Registry for the years 1958 through 1968. J. Bone Joint Surg. [Am.], *57*:167–173, 1975.

90. Larsson, S. E., Lorentzon, R., and Boquist, L.: Giant-cell tumors of the spine and sacrum causing neurological symptoms. Clin. Orthop., *111*:201–211, 1975.

91. Lasser, E. C., and Tetewsky, H.: Metastasizing giant cell tumor. Report of an unusual case with indolent bone and pulmonary metastases. Am. J. Roentgenol. Radium Ther. Nucl. Med., *78*:804–811, 1957.

92. Le Charpentier, Y., Forest, M., Daudet-Monsac, M., et al.: Ultrastructure of giant cell tumors of bone. Rev. Chir. Orthop., *61*:387–390, 1975.

93. Le Charpentier, Y., Le Charpentier, M., Forest, M., et al.: Intranuclear inclusions in giant cell bone tumor. Demonstration by electron microscopy. Nouv. Presse Méd., *6*:259–262, 1977.

94. Lichtenstein, L.: Giant-cell tumor of bone. Current status of problems in diagnosis and treatment. J. Bone Joint Surg. [Am.], *33*:143–150, 1951.

95. Lichtenstein, L.: Bone Tumors. 4th ed. St. Louis, C. V. Mosby Co., 1972.

96. Liguori, I., Tupputi, M., and Ventura, T.: Su due casi di tumore a cellule giganti benigno del menisco del ginocchio. Chir. Organi Mov., *63*:269–272, 1976.

97. Linder, F., Pieper, M., Ott, G., et al.: Zur Therapie der Knochengeschwülste. Ergebnisse einer Gemeinschaftsstudie an 527 Fällen. Chirurg., *45*:54–62, 1974.

98. Locher, G. W., and Kaiser, G.: Giant-cell tumors and aneurysmal bone cysts of ribs in childhood. J. Pediatr. Surg., *10*:103–108, 1975.

99. Lundström, B., Lorentzon, R., Larsson, S. E., et al.: Angiography in giant-cell tumours of bone. Acta Radiol. (Diagn.), *18*:541–553, 1977.

100. MacIntyre, R. S., Latourette, H. B., and Hodges, F. J.: Radiologic aspects of giant-cell tumor of bone. Clin. Orthop., *7*:82–92, 1956.

101. Mándi, A., and Kiss, I.: Ersatz tumoröser Knochensegmente durch Palacos. Beitr. Orthop. Traumatol., *23*:213–217, 1976.

102. Marcove, R. C., Weis, L. D., Vaghaiwalla, M. R., et al.: Cryosurgery in the treatment of giant cell tumors of bone. A report of 52 consecutive cases. Cancer, *41*:957–969, 1978.

103. McGrath, P. J.: Giant-cell tumour of bone. An analysis of fifty-two cases. J. Bone Joint Surg. [Br.], *54*:216–229, 1972.

104. Méary, R., Merle d'Aubigné, R., Tomeno, B., et al.: Treatment of giant cell tumours. Rev. Chir. Orthop., *61*:391–413, 1975.

105. Meister, P., and Finsterer, H.: Der Riesenzelltumor des Knochens und seine Problematik. Munch. Med. Wochenschr., *114*:55–60, 1972.

106. Menanteau, B. P., and DiLenge, D.: Considérations sémiologiques sur l'aspect angiographique des chondrosarcomes. J. Can. Assoc. Radiol., *28*:193–198, 1977.

107. Merle d'Aubigné, R., and Mazabraud, A.: A propos de 22 observations de "vraies" tumeurs à cellules géantes. Lyon Chir., *58*:389–403, 1962.

108. Merle d'Aubigné, R., Thomine, J. M., Mazabraud, A., et al.: Évolution spontanée et postopératoire des tumeurs à cellules géantes. Indications therapeutiques à propos de 39 cas dont 20 suivis 5 ans ou plus. Rev. Chir. Orthop., *54*:689–714, 1968.

109. Mnaymneh, W. A., Dudley, H.R., and Ghandur-Mnaymneh, L.: Giant-cell tumor of bone. An analysis and follow-up study of the 41 cases observed at the Massachusetts General Hospital between 1925 and 1960. J. Bone Joint Surg. [Am.], *46*:63–75, 1964.

110. Mnaymneh, W. A., and Ghandur-Mnaymneh, L.: Giant-cell tumor of bone. Prog. Clin. Cancer, *3*:245–280, 1967.

111. Motais de Narbonne, J., Thiéry, J. P., Magdelenat, H., et al.: Demonstration of osteoclastic acid phosphatase in the serum of patients with giant cell tumor. Bull. Cancer, *64*:31–36, 1977.

112. Murphy, W. R., and Ackerman, L. V.: Benign and malignant giant-cell tumors of bone. A clinical-pathological evaluation of thirty-one cases. Cancer, *9*:317–339, 1956.

113. Nélaton, E.: D'Une Nouvelle Espèce de Tumeurs Bénignes des Os, ou Tumeurs à Myéloplaxes. Paris, Adrien Delahaye, 1860.

114. Oeseburg, H. B.: Cryochirurgische behandeling van enkele beentumoren. Thesis. University of Groningen, 1977.

115. Onuigbo, W. I. B.: A definition problem in cancer metastasis. Neoplasma, *22*:547–550, 1975.

116. Ottolenghi, C. E.: Massive osteo and osteoarticular bone grafts. Technic and results of 62 cases. Clin. Orthop., *87*:156–164, 1972.

117. Paget, J.: Lectures on Surgical Pathology (delivered at the Royal College of Surgeons of England). London, Longmans, 1853.

118. Pallardy, G., Galmiche, J. M., Chevrot, A., et al.: Tumeurs à cellules géantes. Étude radiologique à propos de 89 observations. J. Radiol. Electrol. Med. Nucl., *57*:637–640, 1976.

119. Pan, P., Dahlin, D. C., Lipscomb, P. R., et al.: "Benign" giant cell tumor of the radius with pulmonary metastasis. Mayo Clin. Proc., *39*:344–349, 1964.

120. Pandey, S.: Giant cell tumor of the talus. A report of two cases. Int. Surg., *55*:179–182, 1971.

121. Papillon, J., Montbarbon, J. F., and Chollat, L.: La roentgenthérapie des tumeurs à myéloplaxes. J. Radiol. Electrol. Med. Nucl., *39*:288–299, 1958.

122. Parrish, F. F.: Treatment of bone tumors by total excision and replacement with massive autologous and homologous grafts. J. Bone Joint Surg. [Am.], *48*:968–990, 1966.

123. Peison, B., and Feigenbaum, J.: Metaphyseal giant-cell tumor in a girl of 14. Radiology, *118*:145–146, 1976.

124. Pepler, W. J.: The histochemistry of giant-cell tumours (osteoclastoma and giant-cell epulis). J. Pathol. Bacteriol., *76*:505–510, 1958.

125. Persson, B. M., and Wouters, H. W.: Curettage and acrylic cementation in surgery of giant cell tumors of bone. Clin. Orthop., *120*:125–133, 1976.

126. Plumacher, A.: Giant cell tumors of the bone

(osteoclastoma). Rev. Fac. Med. (Maracaibo), 6:194–231, 1973.

127. Popp, J. A., and Simpson, C. F.: Feline malignant giant cell tumor of bone associated with C-type virus particles. Cornell Vet., 66:528–535, 1976.

128. Rather, L. J.: A note on the origin of multinucleated giant cells from vascular channels in tumors: tumors arising in thyroid gland, bone and soft tissue. Arch. Pathol., 52:98–103, 1951.

129. Ribári, O., Elemér, G., and Bálint, A.: Laryngeal giant cell tumour. J. Laryngol. Otol., 89:857–861, 1975.

130. Riihim, A. E., Suoranta, H., and Tallroth, K.: Tumor detection in extremities of man with 99MTC-tetracycline. Eur. J. Nucl. Med., 1:123–124, 1976.

131. Riley, L. H., Jr., Hartmann, W. H., and Robinson, R. A.: Soft-tissue recurrence of giant-cell tumor of bone after irradiation and excision. J. Bone Joint Surg. [Am.], 49:365–368, 1967.

132. Roberts, A., Long, J., and Wickstrom, J.: A metacarpal giant cell tumor, a sternal osteoblastoma and a pubic osteogenic sarcoma in the same patient. South. Med. J., 69:660–662, 1976.

133. Robinson, L., Damjenov, I., and Brezina, P.: Multinucleated giant cell neoplasm of pancreas. Light and electron microscopy features. Arch. Pathol. Lab. Med., 101:590–593, 1977.

134. Rockwell, M.A., and Small, C. S.: Giant-cell tumors of bone in South India. J. Bone Joint Surg. [Am.], 43:1035–1040, 1961.

135. Rolle, J., and Liebegott, G.: Osteoclastoma of the 1st metacarpal bone. Handchirurgie, 8:47–48, 1976.

136. Rosai, J.: Carcinoma of pancreas simulating giant cell tumor of bone. Electron-microscopic evidence of its acinar cell origin. Cancer, 22:333–344, 1968.

137. Salm, R., and Sissons, H. A.: Giant-cell tumours of soft tissues. J. Pathol., 107:27–39, 1972.

138. Schajowicz, F.: Sobre la degeneración y la variedad maligna de los tumores a células gigantes. Rev. Ortop. Traum., 10:349–376, 1941.

139. Schajowicz, F.: Giant-cell tumors of bone (osteoclastoma): A pathological and histochemical study. J. Bone Joint Surg. [Am.], 43:1–29, 1961.

140. Schajowicz, F., and Slullitel, I.: Giant-cell tumor associated with Paget's disease of bone. A case report. J. Bone Joint Surg. [Am.], 48:1340–1349, 1966.

141. Sedel, L.: Les tumeurs à cellules géantes des os. A propos d'une série homogene de 74 cas. Thesis. Paris, 1973.

142. Selzer, G., David, R., Revach, M., et al.: Goltz syndrome with multiple giant-cell tumor-like lesions in bones. A case report. Ann. Intern. Med., 80:714–717, 1974.

143. Sherman, N., and Fabricius, R.: Giant cell tumors in the metaphysis in a child. Report of an unusual case. J. Bone Joint Surg. [Am.] 43:1225, 1229, 1961.

144. Sheth, R. D., and Shah, S. N.: Osteoclastoma of the os calcis Int. Surg., 57:748–749, 1972.

145. Shtutin, A. Y., Sazlaj, I. I., and Trifonova, A. D.: Osteoblastoclastoma of the patella. Vopr. Onkol., 20(8):87–89, 1974.

146. Sim, F. H., Dahlin, D. C., and Beabout, J. W.: Multicentric giant-cell tumor of bone. J. Bone Joint Surg. [Am.], 59:1052–1060, 1977.

147. Smith, R. J., and Mankin, H. J.: Allograft replacement of distal radius for giant cell tumor. J. Hand Surg., 2:299—309, 1977.

148. Sokolova, I. N.: Giant celled tumour of bones (osteoblastoclastoma). Arkh. Patol., 35 (12):34–39, 1973.

149. Soman, C. S., and Talvalkar, G. V.: Histopathological study of radiated giant cell tumour of the bone. Indian J. Cancer, 14:241–248, 1977.

150. Srivastava, T. P., Tuli, S. M., Varma, B. P., et al.: Giant cell tumour of metacarpals. Indian J. Cancer., 12:164–169, 1975.

151. Stargardter, F. L., and Cooperman, L. R.: Giant-cell tumour of sacrum with multiple pulmonary metastases and long-term survival. Br. J. Radiol., 44:976–979, 1971.

152. Steiner, G. C., Ghosh, L., and Dorfman, H. D.: Ultrastructure of giant cell tumors of bone. Hum. Pathol., 3:569–586, 1972.

153. Stevens, W. W., and Weaver, E. N.: Giant cell tumors and aneurysmal bone cysts of the spine. Report of 4 cases. South. Med. J., 63:218–221, 1970.

154. Stewart, F. W., Coley, B. L., and Farrow, J. H.: Malignant giant cell tumor of bone. Am. J. Pathol., 14:515–535, 1938.

155. Stewart, M. J.: The histogenesis of myeloid sarcoma. Lancet, 2:1106–1108, 1922.

156. Stormby, N., and Akerman, M.: Cytodiagnosis of bone lesions by means of fine-needle aspiration biopsy. Acta Cytol., 17:166–172, 1973.

157. Tate, R. G.: Giant cell tumour of bone. Can. J. Surg., 7:25–42, 1964.

158. Thommesen, P., and Frederiksen, P.: Fine needle aspiration biopsy of bone lesions: clinical value. Acta Orthop., 47:137–143, 1976.

159. Thurzo, V., Popovic, M., Matoska, J., et al.: Human neoplastic cells in tissue culture: two established cell lines derived from giant cell tumor and fibrosarcoma. Neoplasma, 23(6):577–587, 1976.

160. Tornberg, D. N., Dick, H. M., and Johnston, A. D.: Multicentric giant-cell tumors in the long bones. A case report. J. Bone Joint Surg. [Am.], 57:420–422, 1975.

161. Trifaud, A., and Chaix, C.: Unusual pulmonary metastases complicating giant cell tumors of bone. Rev. Chir. Orthop., 61:439–442, 1975.

162. Trifaud, A., Faysse, R., and Papillon, J.: Les tumeurs à myeloplaxes des os ou tumeurs osseuses à cellules géantes. Rev. Chir. Orthop., 42:413–415, 1956.

163. Troise, G. D., de Lustig, E. S., Schajowicz, F., et al.: Mitosis in tissue cultures of human giant cell tumors of bone. Oncology, 28:193–203, 1973.

164. Troup, J. B., Dahlin, D. C., and Coventry, M. B.: The significance of giant cells in osteogenic sarcoma: do they indicate a relationship between osteogenic sarcoma and giant cell tumor of bone? Mayo Clin. Proc., 35:179–186, 1960.

165. Tudway, R. C.: Giant cell tumour of bone. Br. J. Radiol., 32:315–321, 1959.

166. Tuli, S. M., Gupta, I. M., and Kumar, S.: Giant-cell tumor of the scapula treated by total scap-

ulectomy. J. Bone Joint Surg. [Am.], 56:836–840, 1974.

167. Uehlinger, E.: Primary malignancy, secondary malignancy and semimalignancy of bone tumors. *In* Grundmann, E. (ed.): Malignant Bone Tumors. New York, Springer-Verlag, 1976, pp. 109–119.

168. Veliath, A. J., Sankaran, V., and Aurora, A. L.: Ovarian giant cell tumor with cystadenocarcinoma. Arch. Pathol., 99:488–491, 1975.

169. Verhelst, M. P., Hawkins, R. H., and Mulier, J. C.: Giant-cell tumor of bone. An analysis of twenty cases. Acta Orthop. Belg., 40:308–320, 1974.

170. Virchow, R.: Die Krankhaften Geschwülste. Vol. 2. Berlin, Hirschwald, 1846–1865.

171. Vistnes, L. M., and Vermuelen, W. J.: The natural history of a giant-cell tumor. Case report. J. Bone Joint Surg. [Am.], 57:865–867, 1975.

172. Vohra, V. G., Dholakia, A. N., and Shenoy, S. S.: Giant cell tumour. An analysis of 143 cases seen at the Tata Memorial Hospital, Bombay, during 1941 and 1965. Indian J. Cancer, 8:221–237, 1971.

173. Volkov, M. V.: Childhood Osteology. Bone Tumours and Dysplasias. Moscow, Mir Publishers, 1972.

174. von Albertini, A.: Gutartige Riesenzellgeschwülste. Leipzig, Georg Thieme, 1928.

175. Weber, H. G.: Semimaligne Knochengeschwülste. Tägl. Prax., 11:607–621, 1970.

176. Weidemann, H.: Riesenzelltumor des Sprungbeins. Chirurg., 48:345–347, 1977.

177. Weiland, A. J., Daniel, R. K., and Riley, L. H., Jr.: Application of the free vascularized bone graft in the treatment of malignant or aggressive bone tumors. Johns Hopkins Med. J., 140:85–96, 1977.

178. Welsh, R. A., and Meyer, A. T.: Nuclear fragmentations and associated fibrils in giant cell tumor of bone. Lab. Invest., 22:63–72, 1970.

179. Wilkerson, J. A., and Cracchiolo, A.: Giant-cell tumor of the tibial diaphysis. J. Bone Joint Surg. [Am.], 51:1205–1209, 1969.

180. Williams, R. R., Dahlin, D. C., and Ghormley, R. K.: Giant-cell tumor of bone. Cancer, 7:764–773, 1954.

181. Willis, R. A.: Pathology of Tumours. 4th ed. Philadelphia, F. A. Davis (Butterworths), 1967, pp. 696–701.

182. Willis, R. A.: The Spread of Tumours in the Human Body. 3rd ed. Philadelphia, F. A. Davis (Butterworths), 1973, p. 107.

183. Wilson, J. S., Genant, H. K., Carlsson, A., et al.: Patellar giant cell tumor. Am. J. Roentgenol. Radium Ther. Nucl. Med., 127:856–858, 1976.

184. Wilson, P. D., Jr.: A clinical study of the biomechanical behavior of massive bone transplants used to reconstruct large bone defects. Clin. Orthop., 87:81–109, 1972.

185. Wilson, P. D., and Lance, E. M.: Surgical reconstruction of the skeleton following segmental resection for bone tumors. J. Bone Joint Surg. [Am.], 47:1629–1656, 1965.

186. Windeyer, B. W., and Woodyatt, P. B.: Osteoclastoma. A study of thirty-eight cases. J. Bone Joint Surg. [Br.], 31:252–267, 1949.

187. Witwicki, T., Zacharjasiewicz, I., and Archutowska, M.: Benign and malignant osteoclastoma. Wiad. Lek., 22:1277–1282, 1969.

188. Zenker, H.: Die Kniearthrodese bei En-bloc-Resektion von Riesenzellgeschwülsten. Z. Orthop., 111:438–440, 1973.

18

GIANT CELL TUMOR OF THE CRANIOFACIAL BONES. GIANT CELL "REPARATIVE" GRANULOMA OF JAW BONES

Considerable controversy surrounds the issue of whether true giant cell tumors ever occur in the craniofacial bony structures.[4, 23, 24, 31, 32, 39, 51] This dispute is quite perplexing because of the diagnostic confusion in the past. For instance, a review of more than 800 cases of giant cell tumors prior to 1948 showed that about 11 per cent involved this site.[7] It is certain that many of these cases would be unacceptable by today's standards. Jaffe maintained the extremely rare occurrence of such lesions and considered most of them reparative central giant cell granulomas and not true neoplasms.[36]

In 1953, Waldron reported 28 central giant cell lesions of the jaws with only five cases meeting the strict criteria of a true giant cell tumor.[60] Among 34 intraosseous giant cell lesions assembled at the Mayo Clinic, only two were bona fide giant cell tumors.[5] Many share this opinion while others propose that the incidence of true giant cell tumors in jaw bones, even in the absence of Paget's disease of bone, is more frequent than previously accepted.[9, 12, 29, 35, 46, 54, 56, 61] (see Chapter 8).

Various giant cell lesions in the jaws or calvarium have been considered as true giant cell tumors in the past, since it is undeniable that these entities are microscopically indistinguishable more often than not. Since the reactive, reparative, or traumatic nature is highly unlikely, many refer to it now as simply giant cell granuloma. The lesion chiefly afflicts adolescents and

292

young adults, with approximately one half of the patients being less than 20 years of age. The ages range from 7 to 67 years and three fourths of the patients are younger than 30 years of age.[61] It occurs twice as frequently in female patients as in male patients and involves the mandible more often than the maxilla (Fig. 18–1). The tooth-bearing region of the mandible (horizontal ramus) is most frequently affected, usually anteriorly to the first permanent molars. Extension across the midline is a common finding. Pain and swelling of several weeks duration are the first symptoms, but rapid growth may also be experienced. A simultaneous expansion of opposing vestibular and lingual plates of the mandible may be present. Pronounced expansion of the lesion during pregnancy is a frequent finding.[44] Among the lesions located

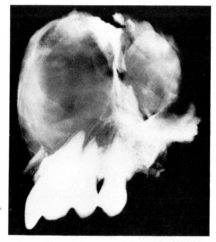

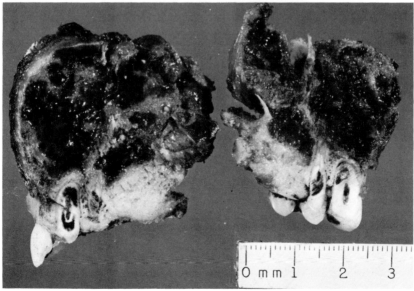

Figure 18–1. Giant cell reparative granuloma of left maxillary antrum. *A*, Radiograph of the partial maxillectomy specimen reveals a bulky tumor mass eroding the anterior and medial walls of the antrum. *B*, A soft, hemorrhagic, and necrotic tumor measuring 3 by 2 by 2 cm replaces the maxilla and maxillary antrum.

in the skull, the sphenoid and the temporal bones are most frequently involved.[38, 50] Only about 15 cases have been encountered in each location.[14, 21, 25, 28, 32, 37, 39, 41, 47, 48, 49, 63] Frontal headaches and diplopia are the most frequent symptoms in sphenoid presentation, with erosion of the dorsum sellae or the floor of the sella, or both, visible on lateral skull radiographs.[24, 26] The temporal lesions may involve different areas of the bone, namely the mastoid, the jugular bulb, the petrous pyramid, and the middle ear.[28] Depending on the exact location within the temporal bone, the symptoms are increasing conductive or sensorineural hearing loss, vertigo, and tinnitus.

RADIOGRAPHIC FEATURES

Radiographically, the lesions are radiolucent and usually well demarcated and may be multiloculated (Fig. 18–1).[55] Slender bony trabeculations may be seen traversing the lesional area, particularly in larger lesions. Pronounced expansion with thinnning of the overlying cortex is the rule. The cortex is usually not eroded, but such an occurrence, even with a soft tissue mass, does not mean the diagnosis is incorrect.[18, 42] Lesions that erode the bony cortex result in a soft tissue swelling of a brownish or bluish hue, rendering the distinction between a peripheral and a central giant cell granuloma quite tenuous.[8, 27] Temporal bone lesions are lytic expansile tumors with poorly defined borders.[40]

HISTOLOGIC FEATURES

Microscopically, the lesions show oval or spindly tumor cells having fibrous properties with collagen production. The multinucleated giant cells are small, moderate in number, and irregularly distributed throughout the lesional tissue. This uneven distribution of the multinucleated giant cells is often related to hemorrhages, iron pigment deposition, and necrosis. Distinct areas of collagenization are present, very unlike that of giant cell tumors occurring in long bones. Osteoid and bone production is demonstrated in about three fourths of the cases.[61] Marked myxomatous

changes occur in patients over 20 years of age.[3] It is alleged that the fibrogenic properties, with appreciable areas of collagen production, uneven distribution of giant cells, in addition to a decreased relative number of giant cells, separates giant cell granuloma from "true" giant cell tumor.[5] "Brown tumor" of hyperparathyroidism is histologically indistinguishable from giant cell granuloma, and the diagnosis must be based on the elevated serum calcium.[6, 11, 15-17] Upon recurrence, giant cell granuloma retains its original microscopic appearance; i.e., no malignant conversion is seen and there is no unequivocal evidence of metastasis in any of the cases. Light microscopic, ultrastructural, as well as histochemical studies of the giant cells in giant cell granuloma and "true" giant cell tumor fail to reveal appreciable differences.[1, 2, 43, 53, 58, 59, 62]

TREATMENT AND PROGNOSIS

The vast majority of the giant cell granulomas are essentially benign lesions with only about 13 per cent showing local recurrence.[3] The treatment is by enucleation or curettage, after which most of the lesions are cured. Occasional lesions, especially in the sphenoid or temporal bones, may require radiation therapy to control recurrent or persistent tumors.

REFERENCES

1. Adkins, K. F., Martinez, M. G., and Hartley, M. W.: Ultrastructure of giant-cell lesions. A peripheral giant-cell reparative granuloma. Oral Surg., 28:713–723, 1969.
2. Adkins, K. F., Martinez, M. G., and Robinson, L. H.: Cellular morphology and relationships in giant-cell lesions of the jaws. Oral Surg., 28:216–222, 1969.
3. Andersen, L., Fejerskov, O., and Philipsen, H. P.: Oral giant cell granulomas. A clinical and histological study of 129 new cases. Acta Pathol. Microbiol. Scand. [A], 81:606–616, 1973.
4. Arseni, C., Horvath, L., Maretsis, M., et al.: Giant cell tumors of the calvaria. J. Neurosurg., 42:535–540, 1975.
5. Austin, L. T., Jr., Dahlin, D. C., and Royer, E. Q.: Giant-cell reparative granuloma and related conditions affecting the jawbones. Oral Surg., 12:1285–1295, 1959.
6. Barlett, N. L., and Cochran, D. Q.: Reparative processes in primary hyperparathyroidism. Radiol. Clin. North Am., 2:261–279, 1964.

7. Bernick, S.: Central giant cell tumors of the jaws. J. Oral Surg., 6:324–330, 1948.

8. Bernier, J. L., and Cahn, L. R.: The peripheral giant cell reparative granuloma. J. Am. Dent. Assoc., 49:141–148, 1954.

9. Bhaskar, S. N., Bernier, J. L., and Godby, F.: Aneurysmal bone cyst and other giant cell lesions of the jaws; report of 104 cases. J. Oral Surg., 17:30–41, 1959.

10. Bonk, U.: Zur Problematik der Riesenzelltumoren und Riesenzellgranulome im Kieferknochen. Fortschr. Kiefer Gesichtschir., 21:161–164, 1976.

11. Bridge, A. J.: Primary hyperparathyroidism presenting as a dental problem. Br. Dent. J., 124:172–176, 1968.

12. Brooke, R. K.: Giant-cell tumor in patients with Paget's disease. Oral Surg., 30:230–241, 1970.

13. Brown, G. N., Darlington, C. G.,and Kupfer, S. R.: A clinicopathologic study of alveolar border epulis with special emphasis on benign giant-cell tumor. Oral Surg., 9:765–775, 888–901, 1956.

14. Cares, H. L., and Bakay, L.: Giant cell lesions of the skull. Acta Neurochir., 25:1–18, 1971.

15. Clark, O. H., and Taylor, S.: Osteoclastoma of the jaw and multiple parathyroid tumors. Surg. Gynecol. Obstet., 135:188–192, 1972.

16. Cohen, B.: A study of bone lesions in a case of hyperparathyroidism. Oral Surg., 12:1347–1356, 1959.

17. Cooke, B. E. D.: The giant-cell epulis: histogenesis and natural history. Br. Dent. J., 93:13–16, 1952.

18. Curtis, M. L., Hatfield, C. G., and Pierce, J. M.: A destructive giant cell lesion of the mandible. J. Oral Surg., 31:705–709, 1973.

19. De Costa, V., Cóser, P. L., and Meller, E. J.: Granuloma reparativo central de celulas gigantes. Rev. Bras. Cir. Cab. Pesc., 2:55–68, 1975.

20. Dechaume, M.: Les tumeurs a myéloplaxes des maxillaires: considérations pathogéniques et thérapeutiques. Rev. Stomatol., 50:670–693, 1940.

21. Dinning, T. A. R.: Osteoclastoma of the petrous temporal bone. Aust. N. Z. J. Surg., 22:253–257, 1953.

22. Doshi, R., Chaudhari, A. B.,and Thomson, G.: Giant cell tumor of the sphenoid bone. Can. J. Neurol. Sci., 4:213–216, 1977.

23. Dziukowa, J.: Giant cell tumors of jaw bones. Nowotwory, 24(3):173–180, 1974.

24. Emley, W. E.: Giant cell tumor of the sphenoid bone. Arch. Otolaryngol., 94:369–374, 1971.

25. Essamma, E.: Osteoclastoma of the temporal bone. J. Laryngol. Otol., 76:229–233, 1962.

26. Geissinger, J. D., Siqueira, E. B., and Ross, E. R.: Giant cell tumors of the sphenoid bone. J. Neurosurg., 32:665–670, 1970.

27. Giansanti, J. S., and Waldron, C. A.: Peripheral giant cell granuloma: review of 720 cases. J. Oral Surg., 27:787–791, 1969.

28. Glasscock, M. E., and Hunt, W. E.: Giant-cell tumor of the sphenoid and temporal bones. Laryngoscope, 84:1181–1187, 1974.

29. Goldstein, B. H., and Laskin, D. M.: Giant cell tumor of the maxilla complicating Paget's disease of bone. J. Oral Surg., 32:209–213, 1974.

30. Greenwood, A. M., and O'Brien, F. V.: The fibrous epulis in the dog. J. Oral Pathol., 4:67–72, 1975.

31. Gupta, I. M., Gupta, O. P., Samant, H. C., et al.: Giant cell tumor of the sphenoid bone. Ann. Otol. Rhinol. Laryngol., 84:359–363, 1975.

32. Hamlin, W. B., and Lund, P. K.: "Giant cell tumors" of the mandible and facial bones. Arch. Otolaryngol., 86:658–665, 1967.

33. Henry, T. C.: A giant cell reparative granuloma? Br. J. Oral Surg., 2:94–99, 1964.

34. Holzer, N. J., Croft, C. B., Walsh, J. B., et al.: Brown tumor of the orbit. J.A.M.A., 238:1758–1759, 1977.

35. Hutter, R. V. P., Foote, F. W., Jr., Frazell, E. L., et al.: Giant cell tumors complicating Paget's disease of bone. Cancer, 16:1044–1056, 1963.

36. Jaffe, H. L.: Giant-cell reparative granuloma, traumatic bone cyst, and fibrous (fibro-osseous) dysplasia of the jawbones. Oral Surg., 6:159–175, 1953.

37. Jamieson, K. G.: Osteoclastoma of the petrous temporal bone. Br. J. Surg., 56:239–241, 1969.

38. Katz, A., and Hirschl, S.: Giant cell reparative granuloma in the temporal bone. Arch. Otolaryngol., 100:380–382, 1974.

39. Lehrer, S., and Roswit, B.: Giant cell tumor of the temporal bone. Letters — Clinical Notes. Arch. Neurol., 33:663, 1976.

40. Livingston, P. A.: Differential diagnosis of radiolucent lesions of the temporal bone. Radiol. Clin. North Am., 12:571–583, 1974.

41. Lord, O. C., and Stewart, M. J.: Osteoclastoma of the temporal bone. J. Laryngol. Otol., 58:263–271, 1943.

42. Marble, H. B., Baker, R. D., Scofield, H. H., et al.: Central giant-cell reparative granuloma with extraosseous manifestations: report of case. J. Oral Surg., 27:215–220, 1969.

43. Matsumura, T., Sugahara, T., Wada, T., et al.: Recurrent giant-cell reparative granuloma: report of case and histochemical patterns. J. Oral Surg., 29:212–216, 1971.

44. McGowan, D. A.: Central giant cell tumour of the mandible occurring in pregnancy. Br. J. Oral Surg., 7:131–135, 1969.

45. Mongini, F., and Mela, F.: Il quadro istopatologico delle neoformazioni delle ossa mascellari con aspetti gigantocellulari. Minerva Stomatol., 15:681–688, 1966.

46. Morton, J. J.: Giant-cell tumor of bone. Cancer, 9:1012–1026, 1956.

47. Moyes, P. D., Bratty, P. J. A., and Dolman, C. L.: Osteoclastoma of the jugular foramen, case report. J. Neurosurg., 32:255–257, 1970.

48. Novaes, V., Pinaud, M., Paranhcs, J. L., et al.: Giant cell tumors of the sphenoid bone. Report of 3 cases and review of the literature. Arq. Neuropsiquiatr., 35:57–67, 1977.

49. Paterson, W.: Giant cell tumor of the middle cranial fossa. J. Laryngol. Otol., 74:581–585, 1960.

50. Pitkethly, D. T., and Kempe, L. G.: Giant cell tumors of the sphenoid. Report of 2 cases. J. Neurosurg., 30:301–304, 1969.

51. Potter, G. D., and McClennan, B. L.: Malignant giant cell tumor of the sphenoid bone and its differential diagnosis. Cancer, 25:167–170, 1970.

52. Schlorf, R. A., and Koop, S. H.: Maxillary giant

cell reparative granuloma. Laryngoscope, 87:10–17, 1977.

53. Schulz, A., Maerker, R., and Delling, G.: Central giant cell granuloma. Histochemical and ultrastructural study on giant cell function. Virchows Arch. [Pathol. Anat.], 371:161–170, 1976.

54. Seldin, H. M., Seldin, S. D., Rakower, W., et al.: Giant cell tumor of the jaws: an analysis of 38 cases. J. Am. Dent. Assoc., 55:210–222, 1957.

55. Selle, G., and Jacobs, H. G.: On the radiological diagnosis of giant cell tumors. Dent. Maxillofac. Radiol., 1:54–57, 1972.

56. Shklar, G., and Meyer, I.: Giant-cell tumors of the mandible and maxilla. Oral Surg., 14:809–827, 1961.

57. Small, G. S., and Rowe, N. H.: A "true giant cell tumor" in the mandible? J. Oral Surg., 33:296–301, 1975.

58. Soskolne, W. A.: Peripheral giant cell granulomas: an ultrastructural study of three lesions. J. Oral Pathol., 1:133–143, 1972.

59. Soskolne, W. A.: Some observations on the pathogenesis and morphology of giant cell granulomas. Proc. R. Soc. Med., 65:1131–1134, 1972.

60. Waldron, C. A.: Giant cell tumors of the jawbones. Oral Surg., 6:1055–1064, 1953.

61. Waldron, C. A., and Shafer, W. G.: The central giant cell reparative granuloma of the jaws. An analysis of 38 cases. Am. J. Clin. Pathol., 45:437–447, 1966.

62. Wertheimer, F. W.: Enzyme histochemistry of giant-cell reparative granulomas. Oral Surg., 23:464–469, 1967.

63. Wolfowitz, B. L., and Schmaman, A.: Giant cell lesions of the temporal bone — with a case report. S. Afr. Med. J., 47:1397–1399, 1973.

19

NONOSSIFYING FIBROMA

DEFINITION

Nonossifying fibroma and metaphyseal fibrous cortical defect appear as well-delineated lytic lesions in the metaphyseal region of long bones, typically in children and adolescents. Histologically, they are characterized by a fibroblastic, dense, cellular proliferation in a mottled, whorled growth pattern admixed with multinucleated giant cells and foamy xanthomatous cells. These structural traits point to a fibrohistiocytic derivation.

SYNONYMS

The synonyms for nonossifying fibroma are as follows: nonosteogenic fibroma, metaphyseal fibrous defect, fibrous cortical defect, giant cell variant of bone cyst or osteitis fibrosa, healing variant of giant cell tumor, xanthic variant of giant cell tumor, and solitary xanthoma or xanthogranuloma of bone.[1, 32, 33, 41, 49, 51]

In general, the fibrous cortical defect is a small, usually asymptomatic, intracortical lesion; nonossifying fibroma is larger and actively growing, involving the medullary cavity of a long tubular bone. Both are referred to as metaphyseal fibrous defect, a term that describes their location and

points out the great likelihood that some of them are not true neoplasms at all.[12]

INCIDENCE

According to periodic radiographic survey data, benign fibrous defects of the cortex occur in 30 to 40 per cent of all normal children past the age of two years.[8] They occur most often between the ages of four and eight years, rarely after puberty. About 90 per cent appear in the distal femur, and 50 per cent of the lesions are bilateral or multiple. A strong familial tendency has also been noted.[54] The earliest example of a tibial, proximal, metaphyseal nonossifying fibroma was found in an approximately 1000-year-old Merovingian grave in Baden, Germany.[2]

SIGNS AND SYMPTOMS

The lesions rarely cause clinical complaints and usually are only discovered when radiographs taken for unrelated reasons reveal their presence. Larger nonossifying fibromas often cause persistent pain and may predispose to pathologic fracture, especially in active adolescents.[16]

In 1945, Hatcher emphasized the association of fibrous cortical defects with Osgood-Schlatter disease, osteochondritis of the patella, osteochondritis dissecans of the medial femoral condyle, and Legg-Calvé-Perthes disease.[27] Von Recklinghausen's neurofibromatosis may, on occasion, show an intraosseous neurofibroma, but the radiolucent lesion may prove to be a nonossifying fibroma.[23]

LOCATION

The lesions, with a few exceptions, arise in the juxtaepiphyseal areas of the metaphyseal regions of long bones of the appendicular skeleton (Fig. 19–1). Distinctly separate foci may appear synchronously in the same metaphysis or in the metaphyses of several long bones, and additional lesions may form after some time.[38] The for-

tuitous coexistence of two nonossifying fibromas and an osteoid osteoma in the same femur has been described.[19] The 48 patients encountered at Memorial Hospital had a more varied distribution of their lesions, probably representing preselection due to a large referral practice (Fig. 19–1). The dorsal and medial aspects of the femur are predilected, although the upper end of the tibia or both ends of the fibula are the most common locations.[22]

AGE AND SEX DISTRIBUTION

In the 48 patients studied at Memorial Hospital between the years 1930 and 1976, about 30 per cent of the lesions occurred in older children and adolescents (Fig. 19–2). The average age was 16 years among male patients and 19 years among female patients, with an age range of 3 to 42 years. Males predominated in this series, as in most others, with a ratio of 2:1.

HISTOGENESIS

The concept of nonossifying fibroma was introduced in 1942 when Jaffe and Lichtenstein used it to describe a benign connective tissue tumor not containing osseous elements, distinctive and separate from the morass of various giant cell lesions.[29] Subsequently, it was recognized that this lesion may be found incidentally, without symptoms, in subcortical or intracortical locations, and the smaller ones may regress spontaneously.

The most plausible etiologic cause of benign fibrous cortical lesions in children and adolescents has been provided by Caffey, who considered these ephemeral growths as patches and segments of focal cortical fibrosis, a fibrous cortical defect.[8] If the progressively growing lesion erodes the cortex and penetrates the medullary cavity, it is referred to as a nonossifying fibroma.[29, 44] Multifocal involvement affecting a single bone or several bones is occasionally encountered.[1, 19, 38, 45, 54] Well-documented spontaneous involution gave rise to the idea that this lesion is not a true neoplasm but a developmental anomaly or metaphyseal fibrous defect.[27] The "cyst

NONOSSIFYING FIBROMA
Location in 48 Patients
Memorial Hospital
1930 - 1976

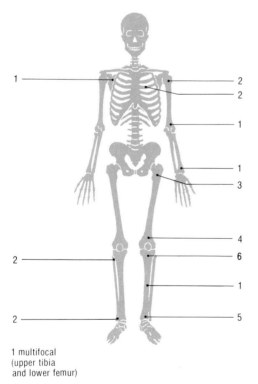

1 multifocal
(upper tibia
and lower femur)

Figure 19–1. Skeletal distribution of 48 nonossifying fibromas of bone seen at Memorial Hospital, 1930–1976.

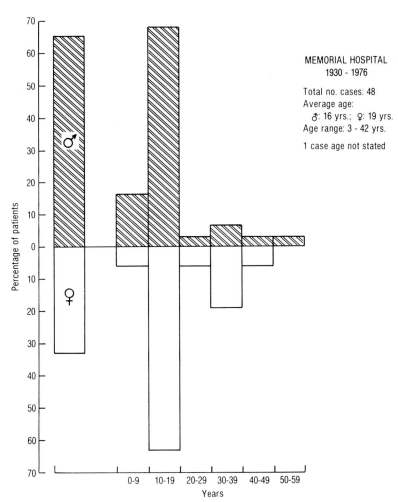

NONOSSIFYING FIBROMA

AGE & SEX DISTRIBUTION

MEMORIAL HOSPITAL
1930 - 1976

Total no. cases: 48
Average age:
♂: 16 yrs.; ♀: 19 yrs.
Age range: 3 - 42 yrs.

1 case age not stated

Figure 19–2. Age and sex distribution in 48 patients with nonossifying fibroma of bone seen at Memorial Hospital, 1930–1976.

like areas" of long bones in children and adolescents, described by Sontag and Pyle in 1941, represent similar if not identical lesions.[56] Lesions complicated by trauma may, on rare occasions, contain a few foci of metaplastic bone formation.[39] This finding, however, does not justify considering nonossifying fibromas to be histologically related to fibrous dysplasia.[1, 38, 39]

Familiarity with a large group of benign soft tissue neoplasms, currently identified as benign fibrous histiocytomas, makes one aware of the fact that fibrous cortical defects and nonossifying fibromas of bones are histologically identical to these soft tis-

sue lesions. Such entities of soft tissue origin include fibrous xanthoma, dermatofibroma, sclerosing hemangioma, and nevoxanthoendothelioma (nevoid histiocytoma).

RADIOGRAPHIC FEATURES

These are fairly characteristic and constant for most lesions, thereby making the correctness of the diagnosis a great certainty.[49] The lesions are situated in the ends of the diaphyses of the long tubular bones, more frequently on the medial

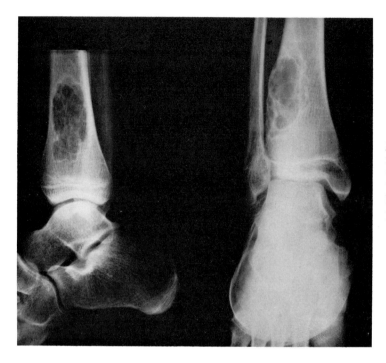

Figure 19–3. Typical nonossifying fibroma of the distal tibia with a characteristic eccentric "bunch of grapes" or "soap bubbles" radiolucent lesion in a 14-year-old girl.

side, in proximity to, but without reaching, the epiphyseal growth plate (Fig. 19–3). Tubulization of the normally maturing bone may bring the lesion next to, or even within, the cortex.[9] They are eccentric and ovoid, with the widest diameter in line with the longitudinal axis of the involved bone. Some of the lesions tend to spread totally across the bone. The extent of loculation within the lesion varies but is always present. A well-delineated thin sclerotic medullary border is usually pres-

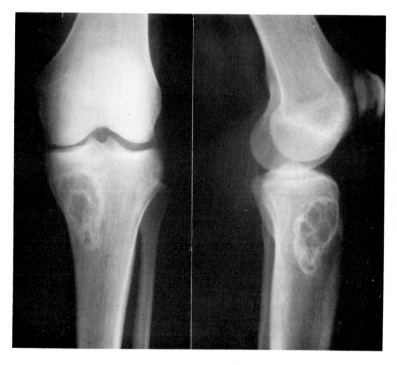

Figure 19–4. Characteristic radiolucent, eccentrically placed tibial lesion with a thin sclerotic rim—a typical nonossifying fibroma. Such obvious lesions can be diagnosed with assurance without biopsy examination.

ent, and the overlying cortex is frequently thinned (Fig. 19–4). Calcified material may be seen outside the line of periosteum.[47] They vary in size from less than 1 cm to about 5 cm, with an average of 3.5 cm. The largest lesion, measuring 15 cm in length, was described by de Moraes and Fialho.[14]

Since the majority of nonossifying fibromas have the characteristic radiographic appearance, most of the lesions do not require histologic examination to confirm their nature. As a rule, biopsy is not indicated unless the lesion occupies more than half the diameter of the tubular bone on anteroposterior and lateral views.[9] Atypical location of the lesion (clavicle, ilium) necessitates biopsy confirmation of the presumptive diagnosis.[24, 35] Angiography may be of help in an occasional case.[30]

PATHOLOGIC FEATURES

On gross examination, the lesions are well-defined and eccentric and vary from soft to firm. On cut surface, they appear yellow to dark brown, the yellow discoloration depending on the extent of xanthomatous areas. The adjacent cortex is intact unless breached by fracture or biopsy (Fig. 19–5).

HISTOLOGIC FEATURES

Histologically, the smaller fibrous cortical defects and the larger nonossifying fibromas display identical appearance. The lesions are composed of spindly fibroblastic cells arranged in matted whorls in a characteristic storiform pattern (Fig. 19–6). (*Storia* or *storea* means rope mat or straw mat in Latin.) These spindle cells are admixed with multinucleated giant cells and larger or smaller aggregates of lipid-laden cells of the xanthoma cell variety (Fig. 19–7).[3, 7, 52, 53] Ingestion of hemosiderin pigment by both the spindly stromal cells and some of the multinucleated giant cells can be seen, but iron deposition is also present and is accompanied by hemorrhage in intercellular areas. Collagen formation is rarely a prominent feature, but a rich feltwork of reticulin fibers is a constant accompaniment (Fig. 19–8).

None of the lesions we examined showed evidence of osteogenesis. However, a thin layer of bone formation occurring along the periphery or at the interface between the tumor and cortex represents reactive bone production provoked in the adjacent tissues.[39]

Are all nonossifying fibromas synonymous with benign fibrous histiocytoma? The majority certainly are. Rarely, we

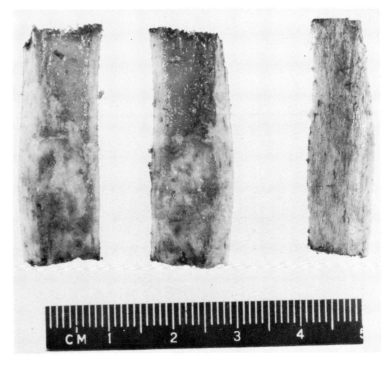

Figure 19–5. A typical nonossifying fibroma of the fibula removed intact in its setting and cut longitudinally. The cut surface shows a mottled, brown-yellow, moderately discrete area having a fibrous consistency and a thin shell of delimiting sclerotic bone.

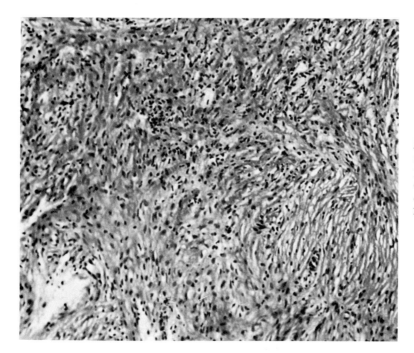

Figure 19–6. Nonossifying fibroma with characteristic pinwheel, matted, spindle cell pattern. (Hematoxylin-eosin stain. Magnification ×50.)

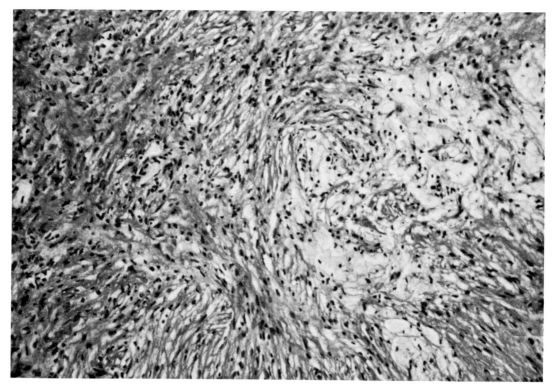

Figure 19–7. Nonossifying fibroma with large areas of xanthoma cells and gradual transition into a more fibrous region. (Hematoxylin-eosin stain. Magnification ×80.)

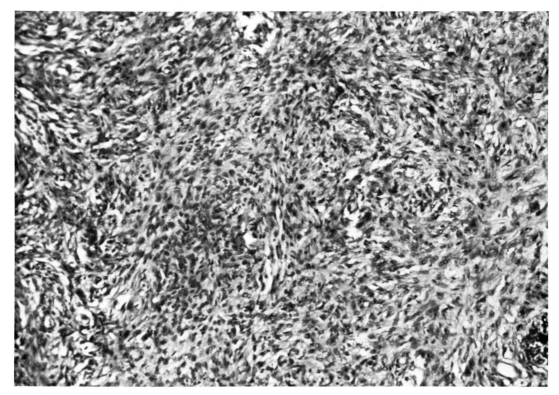

Figure 19–8. The characteristic arrangement of the spindle cells in a nonossifying fibroma without any collagen formation. (Hematoxylin-eosin stain. Magnification ×80.)

have encountered osseous lesions, indistinguishable from fibrous histiocytomas of soft tissue origin, that do not fit the usual age or skeletal location commonly associated with nonossifying fibroma (Figs. 19–1 and 19–2). Such lesions seem to run a more aggressive clinical course.[13]

The most important consideration in the histologic differential diagnosis of a nonossifying fibroma is its confusion with giant cell tumor of bone. Increased collagen production and the typical storiform, whorled, interlacing growth traits of the stroma are often helpful in distinguishing nonossifying fibroma from giant cell tumor.

During the process of healing and resorption, a nonossifying fibroma may show foci of stromal cells that were lipidized and transformed into foam cells. The overemphasis of these focal features can result in the classification of the lesion as a pure xanthoma, xanthogranuloma, or on rare occasion, a healed, lipidized solitary focus of an eosinophilic granuloma.[3, 7, 28, 51–53]

Judging from the pertinent published photomicrographs, the case of a malignant change in a nonossifying fibroma of the upper tibia, diagnosed and treated by curettage 18 months earlier, was most probably a malignant fibrous histiocytoma from the onset.[5] The occurrence of an osteogenic sarcoma in a nonossifying fibroma is a rare phenomenon.[26, 31]

Ultrastructural studies have revealed the basic proliferating cell to be a fibroblast with cytoplasmic fibrils and pinocytotic vesicles reminiscent of connective tissue precursors.[34, 57] Others identified a neoplastic, briskly proliferating, fibroblastic, cellular form with an active protein and lipid synthesis transforming into a xanthomatous foam cell. Histochemically, the basic cells are characterized by elevated alkaline phosphatase activity, ATP-ases, fructose 1,6-diphosphatase, and NADH-NADHPH tetrazolium reductases.[34] The multinucleated giant cells in nonossifying fibromas resemble those seen in giant cell tumors but differ from osteoclasts in that

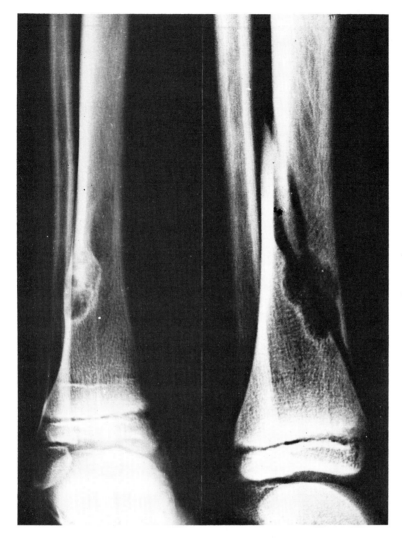

Figure 19–9. Nonossifying fibroma of the distal tibia in a 12-year-old boy before and after pathologic fracture.

ruffled cytoplasmic borders are absent and no osteoclastic bone resorption by these cells can be demonstrated.[57]

TREATMENT

Owing to an increasing awareness of the distinctive features of this lesion by all concerned, the vast majority of asymptomatic patients are not operated upon at all. Progressively enlarging, or already substantial, symptomatic presentation with an incidental pathologic infraction results in orthopedic intervention. Curettage or block excision is recommended for larger, symptomatic lesions in which a pathologic fracture is imminent.

If fracture through the nonossifying fibromas occurs, sliding or iliac bone grafts are the treatment of choice and add stability to the healing process[16] (Fig. 19–9). Internal fixation is seldom called for. In some instances, the lesions are obliterated by the fracture healing process.[12]

REFERENCES

1. Adams, J. P., and Goldner, J. L.: Fibrous lesions of bone. South. Med. J., 46:529–536, 1953.
2. Adler, C. -P., and Klümper, A.: Röntgenologische und pathologische-anatomische Aspekte von Knochentumoren. Radiologe, 17:355–392, 1977.
3. von Bahls, G.: Über ein solitäres Xanthom im Knochen. Zentralbl. Chir., 63:1041–1046, 1936.
4. Berkin, C. R.: Non-ossifying fibroma of bone. Br. J. Radiol., 39:469–471, 1966.

5. Bhagwandeen, S. B.: Malignant transformation of a non-osteogenic fibroma of bone. J. Pathol. Bacteriol., 92:562–364, 1966.

6. Bullough, P. G., and Walley, J.: Fibrous cortical defect and non-ossifying fibroma. Postgrad. Med. J., 41:672–676, 1965.

7. Burman, M. S., and Sinberg, S. E.: Solitary xanthoma (lipoid granulomatosis) of bone. Arch. Surg., 37:1017–1032, 1936.

8. Caffey, J.: On fibrous defects in cortical walls of growing tubular bones: their radiologic appearance, structure, prevalence, natural course, and diagnostic significance. Adv. Pediatr., 7:13–51, 1955.

9. Campbell, C. J., and Harkess, J.: Fibrous metaphyseal defect of bone. Surg. Gynecol. Obstet., 104:329–336, 1957.

10. Cedard, C., Rainaut, J. J., and Aubriot, J.: Non-osteogenic fibroma (Jaffe-Lichtenstein disease). Ann. Chir., 19:1416–1425, 1965.

11. Compere, C. L., and Coleman, S. S.: Nonosteogenic fibroma of bone. Surg. Gynecol. Obstet., 105:588–598, 1957.

12. Cunningham, J. B., and Ackerman, L. V.: Metaphyseal fibrous defects. J. Bone Joint Surg. [Am.], 38:797–808, 1956.

13. Dahlin, D. C., Unni, K. K., and Matsuno, T.: Malignant (fibrous) histiocytoma of bone — fact or fancy? Cancer, 39:1508–1516, 1977.

14. de Moraes, F., and Fialho, F.: Sur un cas de fibrome non ostéogénique du fémur. Rev. Chir. Orthop., 36:35–41, 1950.

15. Devlin, J. A., Bowman, H. E., and Mitchell, C. L.: Non-osteogenic fibroma of bone. A review of the literature with the addition of six cases. J. Bone Joint Surg. [Am.], 37:472–486, 1955.

16. Drennan, D. B., Maylahn, D. J., and Fahey, J. J.: Fractures through large non-ossifying fibromas. Clin. Orthop., 103:82–88, 1974.

17. Duhamel, A., Cohen-Solal, J., and Herrault, A.: Lacunes corticales métaphysaires des os longs. Med. Infant., 72:415–420, 1965.

18. Feldman, F., and Lattes, R.: Primary malignant fibrous histiocytoma (fibrous xanthoma) of bone. Skeletal Radiol., 1:145–160, 1977.

19. Fenton, R. L., and Hoffman, B. P.: Osteoid osteoma and nonossifying fibromas co-existing in one femur: case report. Bull. Hosp. Joint Dis., 14:217–220, 1953.

20. Ferguson, J. W.: Central fibroma of the jaws. Br. J. Oral Surg., 12:205–218, 1974.

21. Gardiner, G. A.: Clavicular nonosteogenic fibroma. An old tumor in a new location. Am. J. Dis. Child., 127:734–735, 1974.

22. Garlipp, M.: Non-osteogenic fibroma of bone. Zentralbl. Chir., 101:1525–1529, 1976.

23. Goodnough, C. P., Kuhlmann, R. P., and Stark, E.: Von Recklinghausen's neurofibromatosis. With nonosteogenic fibroma. N. Y. State J. Med., 75:2407–2409, 1975.

24. Gordon, I. R. S.: Fibrous lesions of bone in childhood. Br. J. Radiol., 37:253–259, 1964.

25. Grepl, J., and Slavik, M.: A contribution to differential diagnosis of ussurative cortical osseous changes, Acta Chir. Orthop. Traumatol. Cech., 40:125–130, 1973.

26. Hastrup, J., and Jensen, T. S.: Osteogenic sarcoma arising in a non-osteogenic fibroma of bone. Acta Pathol. Microbiol. Scand., 63:493–499, 1965.

27. Hatcher, C. H.: The pathogenesis of localized fibrous lesions in the metaphyses of long bones. Ann. Surg., 122:1016–1030, 1945.

28. Jaffe, H. L.: Metabolic, Degenerative, and Inflammatory Diseases of Bones and Joints. Philadelphia, Lea & Febiger, 1972, p. 888.

29. Jaffe, H. L., and Lichtenstein, L.: Non-osteogenic fibroma of bone. Am. J. Pathol., 18:205–221, 1942.

30. Klümper, A.: The differential diagnosis of aneurysmal bone cysts and non-ossifying fibromas. Fortschr. Geb. Roentgenstr. Nuklearmed., 127:261–264, 1977.

31. Koppers, B., Rakow, D., and Schmid, L.: Osteogenic sarcoma combined with non-ossifying fibroma in one bone. Roentgenblaetter, 30:261–266, 1977.

32. Lefebvre, J., and Hassan, M.: Fibromes non ossifiants. Rev. Prat., 19:2133–2141, 1969.

33. Lefebvre, J., Nezelof, C., Fauré, C., et al.: Les lacunes corticales métaphysaires des os longs chez l'enfant et l'adolescent; leurs rapports avec le fibrome non ostéogénique de l'os. A propos de 32 observations. J. Radiol. Electrol. Med. Nucl., 37:300–307, 1956.

34. Llombart-Bosch, A., Pedro-Olaya, A., and Lopez-Fernandez, A.: Non-ossifying fibroma of bone. A histochemical and ultrastructural characterization. Virchows Arch. [Pathol. Anat.], 362:13–21, 1974.

35. Magliato, H. J., and Nastasi, A.: Non-osteogenic fibroma occurring in the ilium. J. Bone Joint Surg. [Am.], 49:384–386, 1967.

36. Marek, F. M.: Fibrous cortical defect (periosteal desmoid). Bull. Hosp. Joint Dis., 16:77–87, 1955.

37. Maudsley, R. H., and Stansfeld, A. G.: Non-osteogenic fibroma of bone (fibrous metaphysial defect). J. Bone Joint Surg. [Br.], 38:714–733, 1956.

38. Meister, P., Konrad, E., and Engert, J.: Polyostische fibröse kortikale Defekte (bzw. nicht ossifizierende Knochenfibrome). Arch. Orthop. Unfallchir., 89:315–318, 1977.

39. Morton, K. S.: Bone production in non-osteogenic fibroma. An attempt to clarify nomenclature in fibrous lesions of bone. J. Bone Joint Surg. [Br.], 46:233–243, 1964.

40. Mubarak, S., Saltzstein, S. L., and Daniel, D. M.: Non-ossifying fibroma. Report of an intact lesion. Am. J. Clin. Pathol., 61:697–701, 1974.

41. Nezelof, C., Fauré, C., Guy, E., et al.: Les lacunes corticales métaphysaires des os longs des enfants et des adolescents (32 observations). Arch. Fr. Pediatr., 12:925–943, 1955.

42. Nissan, S., Aviad, I., and Levy, E.: Congenital central fibroma of the mandible. J. Dent. Child., 38:236–238, 1971.

43. Padovani, P., Rainaut, J. -J., Cédard, C., et al.: Les fibromes non ostéogéniques. Rev. Chir. Orthop., 51:595–603, 1965.

44. Phelan, J. T.: Fibrous cortical defect and nonosseous fibroma of bone. Surg. Gynecol. Obstet., 119:807–810, 1964.

45. Ponseti, I. V., and Friedman, B.: Evolution of metaphyseal fibrous defects. J. Bone Joint Surg. [Am.], *31*:582–585, 1949.

46. Posinković, B.: Non-ossifying fibroma of bone. Libri Oncol., *4*(1):45–48, 1975.

47. Prentice, A. I. D.: Variations on the fibrous cortical defect. Clin. Radiol., *25*:531–533, 1974.

48. Purcell, W. M., and Mulcahy, F.: Non-osteogenic fibroma of bone. Clin. Radiol., *11*:51–59, 1960.

49. Ravelli, A.: Röntgenbild und Deutung bestimmter Knochenherde in den Metaphysen von Tibia und Femur. "Metaphysäres corticales Riesenzellengranulom." Langenbecks Arch. Chir., *280*:205–232, 1955.

50. Rigault, P., and Kliszowski, H.: Non-osteogenic fibroma of the lower tibial extremity in children and teenagers. Rev. Chir. Orthop., *55*:533–541, 1969.

51. Rudy, H. N., and Scheingold, S. S.: Solitary xanthogranuloma of the mandible. Oral Surg., *18*:262–271, 1964.

52. Ruffoni, R.: Solitary bone xanthoma. Panminerva Med., *3*:416–419, 1961.

53. Schröder, F.: Ein zentraler xanthomatöser Riesenzellentumor der Fibula. Gleichzeitig ein Beitrag zur Kenntnis der xanthomatösen Gewebsneubildungen. Arch. Klin. Chir., *168*:118–131, 1931.

54. Selby, S.: Metaphyseal cortical defects in the tubular bones of growing children. J. Bone Joint Surg. [Am.], *43*:395–400, 1961.

55. Skrede, O.: Non-osteogenic fibroma of bone. Acta Orthop. Scand., *41*:369–380, 1970.

56. Sontag, L. W., and Pyle, S. I.: The appearance and nature of cyst-like areas in the distal femoral metaphyses of children. Am. J. Roentgenol. Radium Ther. Nucl. Med., *46*:185–188, 1941.

57. Steiner, G. C.: Fibrous cortical defect and nonossifying fibroma of bone. Arch. Pathol., *97*:205–210, 1974.

58. Vimont, T. R., and Walker, J. H.: Case Note 2. Bull. Mason Clin., *29*:118–119, 1975.

20

MALIGNANT FIBROUS HISTIOCYTOMA OF BONE

DEFINITION

Malignant fibrous histiocytoma is a bone tumor that, similar to lesions of soft tissue origin, is probably of histiocytic derivation. It exhibits both fibrous and histiocytic properties on light microscopic, tissue culture, and ultrastructural examinations.

HISTOGENESIS

Since the early 1960's, many clinicopathologic, tissue culture, and ultramicroscopic studies dealing with a new but distinct tumor entity arising in soft tissues and designated as fibrous histiocytoma, histiocytoma, giant cell tumor, or fibrous xanthoma have appeared in the literature.[10, 18, 29, 30] These soft tissue tumors proved to be aggressive, invasive, and frequently metastasizing.[9, 12, 17, 19, 23, 31, 33, 35, 37, 39, 44, 46, 47, 49] Familiarity with these lesions, especially those involving the deep soft tissues, eventually culminated in their recognition as malignant lesions arising in the skeletal system.[5-7, 14, 28, 41-43, 50] These pleomorphic tumors show a definite "storiform"

histologic pattern of growth with predominantly spindle-shaped cells appearing in a matted, pinwheel, or whorled arrangement. These lesions may be predominantly fibrous, exhibiting exuberant fibrous spindle cell proliferation, with occasional tumor giant cells. The histiocytic components are manifested by the ability of some of the cells to incorporate lipids and ingest hemosiderin and erythrocytes, which are functions not generally attributed to fibrocytes. Tissue culture studies have demonstrated that the tumors arising in soft tissues have a common histiocytic derivation; that is, the cell population that originally seemed to be fibroblastic when explanted to *in vitro* cell cultures assumed histiocytic functional characteristics.[30] Recent ultrastructural studies have further demonstrated that the neoplastic cells in fibrous histiocytomas or fibrous xanthomas can be definitely identified as histiocytes possessing some of the features of fibroblasts.[10] The tissue histiocyte may hide its basic nature and appear to be a fibroblast; i.e., on occasion, it may behave as a "facultative" fibroblast. Electron microscopic examination of these sarcomas may reveal

307

Langerhans cell granules in some of the tumor cells, supporting their identification as histiocytes.[15, 28] There appears to be no doubt that the histologic patterns seen in both benign and malignant soft tissue lesions currently classified as of histiocytic origin are closely duplicated in both primary and secondary bone tumors. Upon reviewing some of the rare variants of malignant primary or secondary osteolytic tumors of the skeleton, which were previously diagnosed as pleomorphic fibrosarcomas, pleomorphic reticulum cell sarcomas, spindle and giant cell sarcomas, osteolytic osteogenic sarcomas, or, occasionally, primary or secondary malignant giant cell tumors, it became clear that many, on histologic examination and on clinical grounds, could now be classified as malignant fibrous histiocytomas.[14]

INCIDENCE

Approximately 100 to 150 cases of primary or secondary malignant fibrous histiocytomas of bone have been reported in the literature.

SIGNS AND SYMPTOMS

A palpable mass and local pain varying from one month to three years' duration represent the most frequent presenting symptoms. A high incidence of pathologic fractures are noted; there were 13 pathologic fractures in 11 of the 23 patients studied by Feldman and Lattes.[6] Serum alkaline phosphatase levels are normal except when the lesion is associated with Paget's disease.

AGE AND SEX DISTRIBUTION

In the reported series of cases, there is a slight male predominance. Of the 18 patients studied at Memorial Hospital, most of the older patients were male; their average age was 36 years, as compared to the average female age of 17 years (Fig. 20–1). The average age of the patients in the reported series is approximately 45 years. The ages range from 6 to 79 years. The average age, therefore, is much higher in

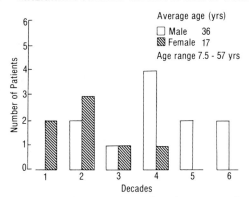

MALIGNANT FIBROUS HISTIOCYTOMA OF BONE

Figure 20–1. Age and sex distribution in 18 patients with primary malignant fibrous histiocytoma of bone studied at Memorial Hospital.

malignant fibrous histiocytomas than in osteogenic sarcomas.

LOCATION

The most common bones involved, in descending order of frequency, are the femur, the tibia, the humerus, the ribs, and the craniofacial bones. The lower portion of the femur is affected slightly more frequently than the upper region.

RADIOLOGIC FINDINGS

On radiologic examination, these highly destructive lesions usually appeared in the metaphyses of long tubular bones, but a secondary extension into the epiphysis was not rare in larger lesions. No favorite sites of involvement were noted in lesions occurring in the spine, since both the vertebral bodies and the posterior elements were equally affected.[6] They presented as permeative, destructive lesions without significant periosteal or endosteal bone production (Figs. 20–2, 20–3, and 20–4). Occasionally, a slight periosteal reaction may be noted, usually associated with previous trauma, fracture, or biopsy (Fig. 20–5). In one case, a periosteal reaction described as an onionskin appearance was noted.[41]

Rarely, areas of mineralization associated with the lesions can be seen.[1] These cases, with a definite blastic response,

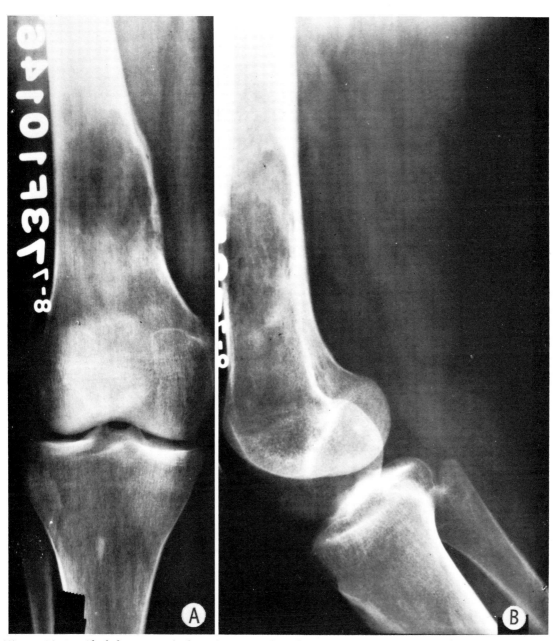

Figure 20-2. Slightly expansile lytic lesion within distal femoral shaft with irregularity, thinning, and, finally, cortical disruption. Periosteal overgrowth is present. (From Huvos, A. G.: Primary malignant fibrous histiocytoma of bone. Clinicopathologic study of 18 patients. N. Y. State J. Med., 76:552–559, 1976.)

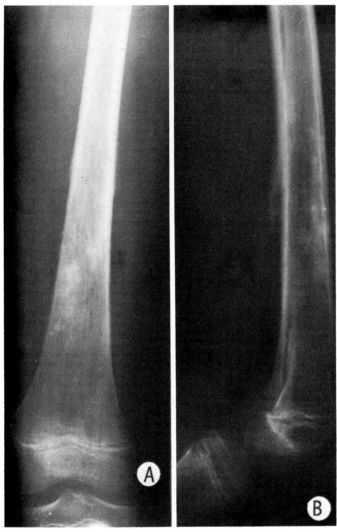

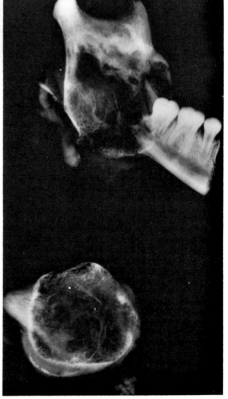

Figure 20–3. Large mottled area of bone destruction of the distal femur with irregular coarsely trabeculated structure in a 7-year-old girl. Periosteal reaction is present. (From Huvos, A. G.: Primary malignant fibrous histiocytoma of bone. Clinicopathologic study of 18 patients. N. Y. State J. Med., 76:552–559, 1976.)

Figure 20–4. Specimen radiograph of a large expansile radiolucent lesion with honeycombed cortical disruption of right mandibular angle in an 11-year-old girl. (Courtesy of Dr. E. W. Strong.) (From Huvos, A. G.: Primary malignant fibrous histiocytoma of bone. Clinicopathologic study of 18 patients. N. Y. State J. Med., 76:552–559, 1976.)

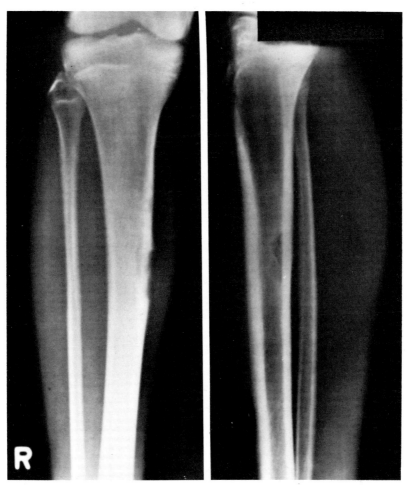

Figure 20–5. Malignant fibrous histiocytoma arising in the medial tibial shaft showing a well-defined lytic lesion with periosteal reaction superiorly and inferiorly. Cortical destruction is well demonstrated. (From Huvos, A. G.: Primary malignant fibrous histiocytoma of bone. Clinicopathologic study of 18 patients. N. Y. State J. Med., 76:552–559, 1976.)

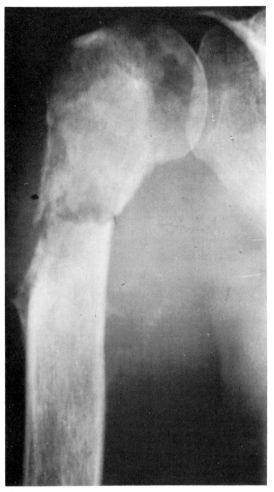

Figure 20–6. Extensive ill-defined area of diffuse destruction of upper humeral shaft with pathologic fracture in a 35-year-old man. (From Huvos, A. G.: Primary malignant fibrous histiocytoma of bone. Clinicopathologic study of 18 patients. N. Y. State J. Med., 76:552–559, 1976.)

show a mottled appearance with ill-defined hazy areas of increased intralesional density (Fig. 20–6). Three of the cases studied at Memorial Hospital and two of those studied at Columbia Presbyterian Medical Center showed irregular calcifications within the area of osteolysis.[6, 14] The permeative destruction of the cortex appears to be without thinning or cortical expansion. Some of the lesions are quite large, reaching up to 10 cm in greatest diameter. Radiologic examination frequently underestimates the size and the extent of the tumor owing to the tumor's propensity for infiltrating the bone marrow without eliciting any secondary response

in the marrow or to the lack of reactive new bone formation. This results in poorly delimited areas of extensive but poorly appreciated bone destruction. Quite often a large soft tissue mass remains hidden at radiologic examination.

Technetium-99 polyphosphate total body scan is of use in determining the extent of the tumor, especially its intraosseous component. The extraosseous portion of the tumor is best demonstrated by selective biplanar angiography.[41]

In some instances, malignant fibrous histiocytoma may be associated with well-developed polyostotic Paget's disease.[5, 41]

Angiographic examination of a malignant fibrous histiocytoma of the talus revealed a highly vascular tumor with beaded, irregularly contoured blood vessels pursuing a haphazard course. Tumor staining and early draining veins were also demonstrated.[32a]

MICROSCOPIC FEATURES

The tumors exhibit densely fibrous, somewhat pleomorphic invasive growth characterized by variable histologic patterns in different areas. The predominantly spindle cell fibrous tumors are arranged in a distinct storiform, matted pattern (Fig. 20–7). Silver reticulum stains reveal many closely placed reticulin and collagen fibers throughout the tumor tissue. In some areas, no such pattern is evident and the vascularization of the lesion is quite prominent. The use of the silver impregnation technique in such areas demonstrates either patchy reticulin fiber production or, on occasion, every tumor cell surrounded by reticulin fibers. The whorls of tumor cells frequently are arranged around blood vessels or in matted aggregates (Fig. 20–8). Densely collagenized fibrous areas, occasionally imitating osteoid, can be seen adjacent to fields of poorly differentiated spindle-shaped fibrogenic cells of moderate to high cellularity. The mitotic activity varies from occasional to numerous mitotic figures. One of the most striking features in these lesions is the presence of many large bizarre cells with hyperchromatic nuclei showing some anaplasia with a few abnormal mitoses and nuclear pyknosis. Some of the cells have several nuclei and many have faintly acidophilic, finely granular cytoplasm with spotty vacuolization. In some areas, xanthomatous histiocytic cells are present, the cytoplasms of which exhibit lipid material (Fig. 20–9). Mucicarmine stains show consistently negative findings. Although in some areas the tumor cells show a distinctly eosinophilic cytoplasm mimicking muscle cells, special stains for intracellular fibers or cross striations are regularly nonrevealing. In the previously treated or recurrent lesions, dense fibrosis and collagenization are evident and most of the tumor giant cells either completely disappear or appear to be an inconspicuous feature. Even if one studies multiple sections of a given tumor, no clear-cut osteoid or tumor bone production or areas of cartilage or chondroid differentiation are seen in any of the lesions. In two instances reported by Spanier, a cartilaginous component was noted, suggesting a pre-existent enchondroma adjacent to the malignant fibrous histiocytoma.[41] Although this may indeed be true, another consideration could be that the lesions in question are low-grade chondrosarcomas showing fibrous dedifferentiation. The subclassification of malignant fibrous histiocytomas of bone into different histologic patterns, namely the fibroxanthoma, the fibrous histiocytoma, and the histiocytoma variants, seems to be arbitrary, and far too few cases have been studied to reliably prognosticate according to such patterns.

Sarcomas arising at the site of a *bone infarct* have attracted wide interest recently.[11] In spite of occurring quite rarely, it has become evident that there is a direct cause and effect relationship between bone infarct and the eventual development of bone sarcoma both in humans and in dogs.[11, 25-27, 34] Most of these cases were originally considered to be fibrosarcoma, but recently it became clear that the majority were of fibrohistiocytic derivation, thereby enabling one to correctly diagnose them as malignant fibrous histiocytomas. Up to the present time, 16 cases of sarcomatous transformation of bone infarcts have been encountered: 13 were male patients, and the lesions developed in the tibia (9 cases), femur (6 cases), and humerus (1 case).[11] The ages of the patients varied from 21 to 80 years, and in all but two the infarctions involved multiple osseous sites. Only four of the patients proved to be caisson workers; the rest had hereditary bone dysplasia (4), sickle cell disease (1), and idiopathic infarcts (8). The prognosis, in spite of radical surgery, proved to be poor, and the majority of the patients succumbed to their disease with widespread metastases within two years following definitive diagnosis. Although one can expect an increasing incidence of bone infarcts to be diagnosed in the general orthopedic practice, the probability for sarcomatous development remains only a remote possibility. The rarity of this occurrence precludes the necessity to treat and excise essentially asymptomatic bone infarcts. If, however, a patient with a demonstrated large medullary bone infarct develops increasing pain, swelling, or tenderness and radiographic alterations are manifested, a malignant transformation should seriously be considered.

DIFFERENTIAL DIAGNOSIS

In the differential diagnosis of malignant fibrous histiocytomas of bone, one should consider osteolytic osteogenic sarcoma, fibrosarcoma of bone, and metastatic carcinoma. *Osteogenic sarcoma* is predominantly an affliction of youth, whereas malignant fibrous histiocytomas usually occur in the mature skeleton. Alkaline phosphatase elevation in osteogenic sarcoma is a regular feature; elevated serum phosphatase levels occur only with fibrous histiocytoma associated with polyostotic Paget's disease of bone. Osteolytic osteogenic sarcomas have minimal or no serum alkaline phosphatase elevation, so this parameter might not be a foolproof method in differentiating these two osteolytic lesions.

Medullary fibrosarcoma is a definite consideration in the differential diagnosis. On clinical grounds, fibrosarcoma cannot be distinguished from malignant fibrous histiocytoma, and histologic examination is necessary to separate these two entities. The presence of homogeneous, predominantly spindle-shaped cells, the distinctive herringbone pattern throughout the tumor tissue, and uniform ground substance usually help to pinpoint fibrosarcomas; fi-

Text continued on page 318

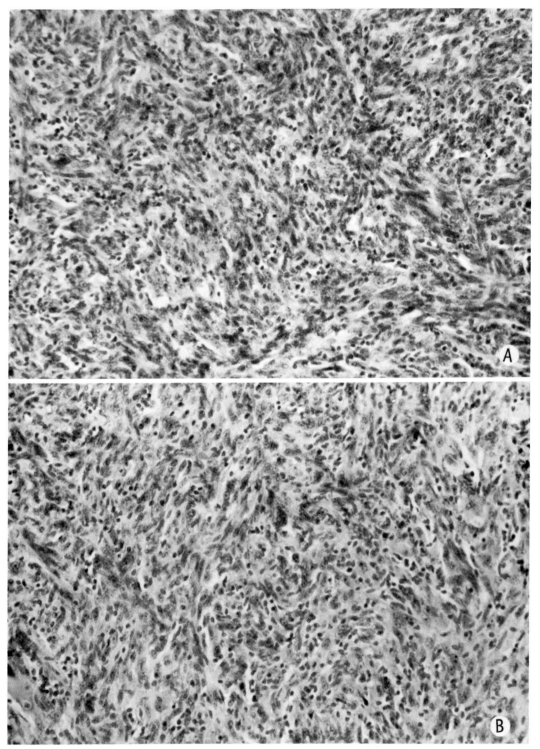

Figure 20–7. A, Malignant fibrous histiocytoma with a typical fibrous pattern and an attempt at pin-wheel, matted arrangement of the spindle-shaped cells. B, Pinwheel arrangement of the fibroblastic cells intermixed with multinucleated giant cells and occasional mitosis.

Illustration continued on opposite page

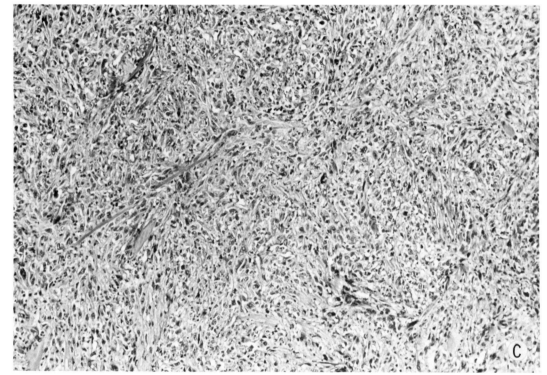

Figure 20–7 Continued. C, Anaplastic fibrous histiocytic pattern with marked cellular anaplasia and tumor giant cells. (From Huvos, A. G.: Primary malignant fibrous histiocytoma of bone. Clinico-pathologic study of 18 patients. N. Y. State J. Med., 76:552–559, 1976.)

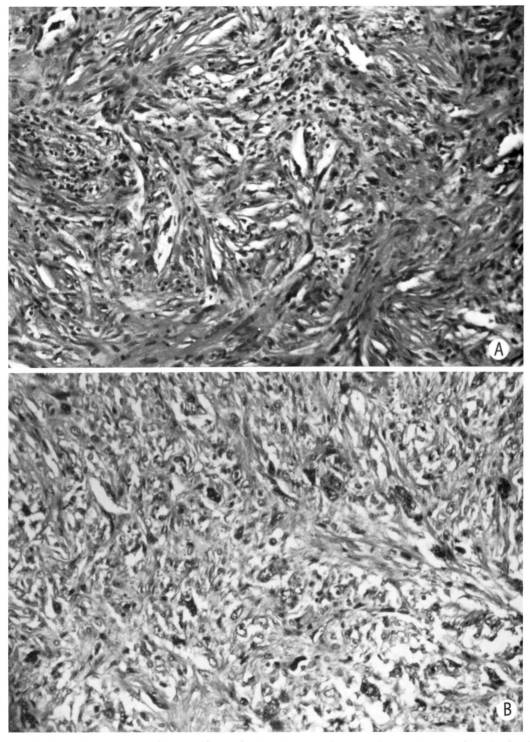

Figure 20–8. *A*, Recurrent malignant fibrous histiocytoma with a storiform pattern and marked collagenization. *B*, Pronounced anaplastic histiocytic pattern with multinucleated tumor giant cells.
(From Huvos, A. G.: Primary malignant fibrous histiocytoma of bone. Clinicopathologic study of 18
patients. N. Y. State J. Med., 76:552–559, 1976.)

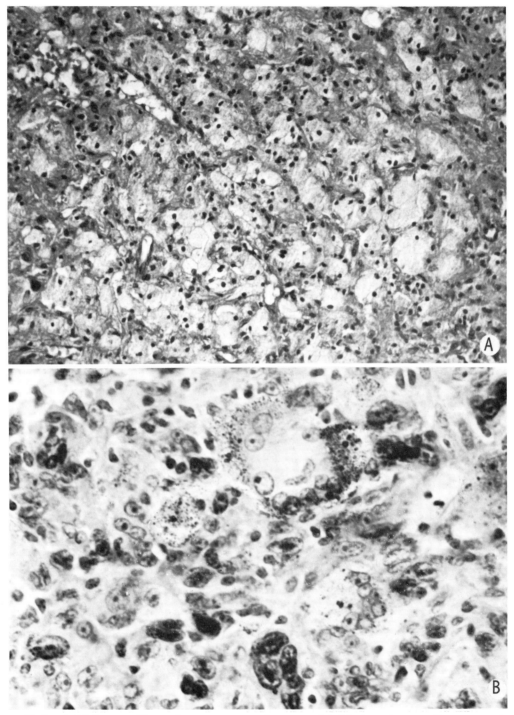

Figure 20-9. A, Malignant fibrous histiocytoma with a typical field of xanthoma cells. B, Huge lipid-laden Touton-type giant cells. (Hematoxylin-eosin stain. Magnification ×200.) (From Huvos, A. G.: Primary malignant fibrous histiocytoma of bone. Clinicopathologic study of 18 patients. N. Y. State J. Med., 76:552–559, 1976.)

brous histiocytomas have a storiform, matted histologic appearance. Evidence of histiocytic function, manifested by hemosiderin ingestion, erythrophagocytosis, and lipid deposition are features of fibrous histiocytoma and are not seen in fibrosarcoma. An occasional high-grade anaplastic fibrosarcoma may show multinucleated tumor giant cells similar to histiocytic tumors, but in purely fibrous growths, they appear adjacent to remnants of fibroblastic spindle cells exhibiting herringbone pattern. The presence of tumor giant cells and the absence of a storiform pattern support a diagnosis of high-grade fibrosarcoma.

Metastatic carcinoma arising in the renal parenchyma may be confused with malignant fibrous histiocytoma of bone both histologically and clinically. Many of the patients with primary or secondary malignant fibrous histiocytomas are in the same age group affected by metastatic carcinoma, especially from the lung and often presenting with pathologic fractures. The actual radiographic features of metastatic carcinoma and fibrous histiocytoma are identical, and, to add to the uncertainty, many of the metastatic renal carcinomas appear in the proximal humerus, which is also a favored primary site for malignant fibrous histiocytoma. The histologic distinction between malignant fibrous histiocytoma and markedly spindly metastases from a primary renal cell carcinoma is quite difficult, since an intense, occasionally whorled, spindle cell reaction may be seen around the granular or clear cells of a renal cell carcinoma. In such instances, there is a superficial resemblance to xanthomatous cells seen in malignant fibrous histiocytoma. Laboratory studies, including intravenous pyelogram or selective angiography or arteriography of the kidney, usually help to rule out a primary renal lesion.

The separation of primary malignant giant cell tumor and fibrous histiocytoma is difficult, since these lesions may share overlapping microscopic characteristics. The character of the giant cells may make differential diagnosis between malignant fibrous histiocytoma and primary malignant giant cell tumor practical. In giant cell tumors, the giant cells are of the osteoclastic multinucleated variety, so-called epulis type, and the nuclei appear to be benign. In malignant fibrous histiocytomas, the giant cells show bizarre, pleomorphic nuclei, and they are occasionally multinucleated and surrounded by vacuolated, foamy cytoplasm. They are most often the Touton type. In the frankly malignant primary giant cell tumors of bone, also designated Grade III lesions, the stromal character is usually, but not exclusively, that of a definite spindle cell fibrosarcoma with a typical herringbone pattern and a few residual benign giant cells. The strict separation of malignant fibrous histiocytomas of bone from malignant giant cell tumors, or occasionally from anaplastic osteogenic sarcomas with a prominent giant cell component, on limited biopsy material may at times be difficult, artificial, and not feasible.

TREATMENT AND PROGNOSIS

The histologic examination of these tumors shows them to be malignant, and their aggressive nature is confirmed by their subsequent biologic behavior. Most of the tumors destroy bone, break through the cortex, and extend into surrounding soft tissues. Amputation, disarticulation, and hemipelvectomy are the preferred methods of treatment. Radiation may be employed and may occasionally effect a clinical cure, especially if the lesion is predominantly histiocytic with only a slight fibrous component. Rarely, preoperative multidrug multicycle aggressive chemotherapy has been administered with beneficial results. This preoperative aggressive chemotherapy regimen consists of high dose methotrexate with citrovorum factor rescue, doxorubicin hydrochloride (Adriamycin), and vincristine; this is the therapeutic management now employed at our institution for children and young adults with osteogenic sarcoma (See Chapter 5). Subsequent to this therapy, patients undergo an *en bloc* resection of the tumor with immediate prosthetic bone replacement.

The five year survival rate at Memorial Hospital was 67 per cent (Fig. 20–10). It is of note that within two years the survival rate decreases precipitously. There were two long-time survivors, 19 and 20 years old respectively, after treatment at Me-

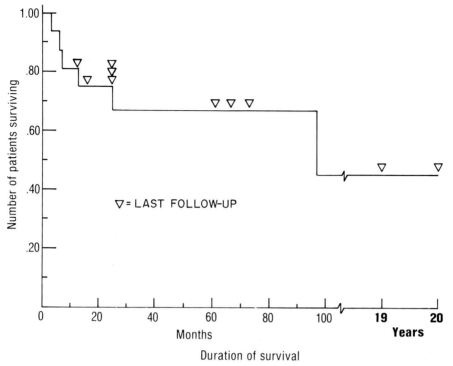

Figure 20–10. Survival after treatment of 16 patients at Memorial Hospital. (From Huvos, A. G.: Primary malignant fibrous histiocytoma of bone. Clinicopathologic study of 18 patients. N. Y. State J. Med., 76:552–559, 1976.)

morial Hospital.[14] In the series reported by Spanier, 11 of the 13 patients died of disease within four years. The average survival was 19 months and, therefore, these lesions are considered to be lethal at that medical center.[41] In contradistinction to these data, the Mayo Clinic reports 10 of their 19 patients surviving over five years, and four remained alive longer than 15 years. Three patients died six to seven years following definitive therapy.[5]

In none of the cases studied at Memorial Hospital and the Mayo Clinic did metastases to the regional nodes occur.[5, 14] In the series reported by Spanier, 3 of 11 patients who died of metastases, had their tumor spread to regional nodes.[41] Another case arising in the maxilla revealed cervical lymph node metastases.[38] The most common sites of blood-borne metastases were the lungs and other bones.

REFERENCES

1. Albright, J., Terry, B., Baker, R., et al.: Mandibular juvenile fibrous histiocytoma with ossification. A case report. J. Maxillofac. Surg., 4:120–123, 1976.
2. Blitzer, A., Lawson, W., and Biller, H. F.: Malignant fibrous histiocytoma of the head and neck. Laryngoscope, 87:1479–1499, 1977.
3. Cappa, A. P. J., and Veneroni, G.: Histocytic tumors of the soft tissues. Tumori, 55:9–25, 1969.
4. Cole, A. T., Straus, F. H., and Gill, W. B.: Malignant fibrous histiocytoma: an unusual inguinal tumor. J. Urol., 107:1005–1007, 1972.
5. Dahlin, D. C., Unni, K. K., and Matsuno, T.: Malignant (fibrous) histiocytoma of bone — fact or fancy? Cancer, 39:1508–1516, 1977.
6. Feldman, F., and Lattes, R.: Primary malignant fibrous histiocytoma (fibrous xanthoma) of bone. Skeletal Radiol., 1:145–160, 1977.
7. Feldman, F., and Norman, D.: Intra- and extraosseous malignant histiocytoma (malignant fibrous xanthoma). Radiology, 104:497–508, 1972.
8. Fisher, E. R., and Vuzevski, V. D.: Cytogenesis of schwannoma (neurilemoma), neurofibroma, dermatofibroma, and dermatofibrosarcoma as revealed by electron microscopy. Am. J. Clin. Pathol., 49:141–154, 1968.
9. Fretzin, D. F., and Helwig, E. B.: Atypical fibroxanthoma of the skin. A clinicopathologic study of 140 cases. Cancer, 31:1541–1552, 1973.
10. Fu, Y. S., Gabbiani, G., Kaye, G. I., et al.: Malignant soft tissue tumors of probable histiocytic origin (malignant fibrous histiocytomas): gener-

al considerations and electron microscopic and tissue culture studies. Cancer, 35:176–198, 1975.

11. Galli, S. J., Weintraub, H. P., and Proppe, K. H.: Malignant fibrous histiocytoma and pleomorphic sarcoma in association with medullary bone infarcts. Cancer, 41:607–619, 1978.

12. Guccion, J. G., and Enzinger, F. M.: Malignant giant cell tumor of soft parts. An analysis of 32 cases. Cancer, 29:1518–1529, 1972.

13. Hubbard, L. F., and Burton, R. I.: Malignant fibrous histiocytoma of the forearm: report of a case and review of the literature. J. Hand Surg., 2:292–296, 1977.

14. Huvos, A. G.: Primary malignant fibrous histiocytoma of bone. Clinicopathologic study of 18 patients. N. Y. State J. Med., 76:552–559, 1976.

15. Inada, O., Yumoto, T., Furuse, K., et al.: Ultrastructural features of malignant fibrous histiocytoma of bone. Acta Pathol. Jpn., 26:491–501, 1976.

16. Jee, A., Domboski, M., and Milobsky, S. A.: Malignant fibrohistiocytoma of the maxilla presenting with endodontically involved teeth. Oral Surg., 45:464–469, 1978.

17. Kahn, L. B.: Retroperitoneal xanthogranuloma and xanthosarcoma (malignant fibrous xanthoma). Cancer, 31:411–422, 1973.

18. Kauffman, S. L., and Stout, A. P.: Histiocytic tumors (fibrous xanthoma and histiocytoma) in children. Cancer, 14:469–482, 1961.

19. Kempson, R. L., and Kyriakos, M.: Fibroxanthosarcoma of the soft tissues. A type of malignant fibrous histiocytoma. Cancer, 29:961–976, 1972.

20. Kyriakos, M., and Kempson, R. L.: Inflammatory fibrous histiocytoma. An aggressive and lethal lesion. Cancer, 37:1584–1606, 1976.

21. Leite, C., Goodwin, J. W., Sinkovics, J. G., et al.: Chemotherapy of malignant fibrous histiocytoma. A Southwest Oncology Group report. Cancer, 40:2010–2014, 1977.

22. Lombardi, L., Pilotti, S., Carbone, A., et al.: The ultrastructure of malignant fibrous histiocytoma (case report). Tumori, 63:387–396, 1977.

23. Meares, E. M., Jr., and Kempson, R. L.: Fibrous histiocytoma of the scrotum in an infant. J. Urol., 110:130–132, 1973.

24. Merkow, L. P., Frich, J. C., Jr., Slifkin, M., et al.: Ultrastructure of a fibroxanthosarcoma (malignant fibroxanthoma). Cancer, 28:372–383, 1971.

25. Michael, R. H., and Dorfman, H. D.: Malignant fibrous histiocytoma associated with bone infarcts. Report of a case. Clin. Orthop., 118:180–183, 1976.

26. Mirra, J. M., Bullough, P. G., Marcove, R. C., et al.: Malignant fibrous histiocytoma and osteosarcoma in association with bone infarcts. Report of four cases, two in caisson workers. J. Bone Joint Surg. [Am.], 56:932–940, 1974.

27. Mirra, J. M., Gold, R. H., and Marafiote, R.: Malignant (fibrous) histiocytoma arising in association with a bone infarct in sickle-cell disease: coincidence or cause-and-effect? Cancer, 39:186–194, 1977.

28. Newland, R. C., Harrison, M. A., and Wright, R. G.: Fibroxanthosarcoma of bone. Pathology, 7:203–208, 1975.

29. O'Brien, J. E., and Stout, A. P.: Malignant fibrous xanthomas. Cancer, 17:1445–1455, 1964.

30. Ozzello, L., Stout, A. P., and Murray, M. R.: Cultural characteristics of malignant histiocytomas and fibrous xanthomas. Cancer, 16:331–344, 1963.

31. Palma, L. D., Gaeta, J. F., Kenny, G. M., et al.: Perirenal fibrous xanthoma: unusual retroperitoneal tumor. Diagnosis and treatment. J. Surg. Oncol., 2:45–53, 1970.

32. Pear, B. L.: The histiocyte in radiology. With case reports of retroperitoneal xanthogranuloma and malignant fibrous xanthoma. Am. J. Roentgenol. Radium Ther. Nucl. Med., 110:159–165, 1970.

32a. Perlmutter, S., McSweeney, J., Watson, R. C., et al.: Angiographic spectrum of malignant fibrous histiocytomas. (Unpublished data.)

33. Rice, D. H., Batsakis, J. G., Headington, J. T., et al.: Fibrous histiocytomas of the nose and paranasal sinuses. Arch. Otolaryngol., 100:398–401, 1974.

34. Riser, W. H., Brody, R. S., and Biery, D. N.: Bone infarctions associated with malignant bone tumors in dogs. J. Am. Vet. Med. Assoc., 160:411–421, 1972.

35. Rosas-Uribe, A., Ring, A. M., and Rappaport, H.: Metastasizing retroperitoneal fibroxanthoma (malignant fibroxanthoma). Cancer, 26:827–831, 1970.

36. Saito, R., and Caines, M. J.: Atypical fibrous histiocytoma of the humerus. A light and electron microscopic study. Am. J. Clin. Pathol., 68:409–415, 1977.

37. Shearer, W. T., Schreiner, R. L., Ward, S. P., et al.: Benign nasal tumor appearing as neonatal respiratory distress. First reported case of nasopharyngeal fibrous histiocytoma. Am. J. Dis. Child., 126:238–241, 1973.

38. Slootweg, P. J., and Müller, H.: Malignant fibrous histiocytoma of the maxilla. Report of a case. Oral Surg., 44:560–566, 1977.

39. Solomon, M. P., and Sutton, A. L.: Malignant fibrous histiocytoma of the soft tissues of the mandible. Oral Surg., 35:653–660, 1973.

40. Soule, E. H., and Enriquez, P.: Atypical fibrous histiocytoma, malignant fibrous histiocytoma, malignant histiocytoma, and epithelioid sarcoma. A comparative study of 65 tumors. Cancer, 30:128–143, 1972.

41. Spanier, S. S.: Malignant fibrous histiocytoma of bone. Orthop. Clin. North Am., 8:947–961, 1977.

42. Spanier, S. S., Enneking, W. F., and Enriquez, P.: Primary malignant fibrous histiocytoma of bone. Cancer, 36:2084–2098, 1975.

43. Spector, G. J., and Ogura, J. H.: Malignant fibrous histiocytoma of the maxilla. A report of an unusual lesion. Arch. Otolaryngol., 99:385–387, 1974.

44. Tamarit Montesinos, L. V., and Sánchez Cara, V.: Xantogranuloma oseo solitario malignizado. Informe de un caso con transformacion fibrosarcomatosa. Patologia, 6:123–130, 1973.

45. Taxy, J. B., and Battifora, H.: Malignant fibrous histiocytoma. An electron microscopic study. Cancer, 40:254–267, 1977.

46. Taylor, H. B., and Helwig, E. B.: Dermatofibrosarcoma protuberans. A study of 115 cases. Cancer, 15:717–725, 1962.
47. Townsend, G. L., Neel, H. B., Weiland, L. H., et al.: Fibrous histiocytoma of the paranasal sinuses. Report of a case. Arch. Otolaryngol., 98:51–52, 1973.
48. Webber, W. B., and Wienke, E. C.: Malignant fibrous histiocytoma of the mandible. Case report. Plast. Reconstr. Surg., 60:629–634, 1977.
49. Weiss, S. W., and Enzinger, F. M.: Myxoid variant of malignant fibrous histiocytoma. Cancer, 39:1672–1685, 1977.
50. Yumoto, T., Mori, Y., Inada, O., et al.: Malignant fibrous histiocytoma of bone. Acta Pathol. Jpn., 26:295–309, 1976.

21

EWING'S SARCOMA

DEFINITION

*Ewing's sarcoma is a primitive malig-
nant tumor of bone characterized by uniform, densely packed small cells with
round nuclei but without distinct cytoplasmic borders or prominent nucleoli.
The tumor cells may be derived from the
connective tissue framework of the bone
marrow.*

It is believed that Lücke, in 1866, was
the first to recognize this tumor.[92] Hildebrand, in 1890,[58] and Marckwald, in 1894
and 1895,[96] reported several well-
documented cases. In the United States in
1905, Howard and Crile mentioned 23 instances, four of which were studied by
them.[61] In 1916, Symmers and Vance, following Marckwald's suggestion concerning
histogenesis, emphasized the close resemblance of this bone tumor to multiple
myeloma.[152] In 1921, Ewing drew renewed
attention to this special form of primary
malignant bone tumor, which he popularized and designated "diffuse endothelioma" or "endothelial myeloma."[26, 35-37, 149]

Ewing's sarcoma of bone is by now
widely accepted as an independent entity,
a distinctive primary malignant tumor of
bone. Uncertainty still persists, however,
regarding its histogenesis and the cell of
origin. Controversy about the existence of
the disease as a true clinicopathologic entity distinct from metastatic neuroblastoma
or non-Hodgkin's lymphoma seems to
have been resolved; it is not just a syndrome complex, as was suggested by
Willis.[25, 67, 167] The question of metastatic
carcinoma is raised particularly with older
persons, and every effort should be made
to exclude the possibility of an occult or
clinically silent primary lesion else-
where.[59]

Distinctive histologic criteria are now
recognized, although the diagnosis of
some of the cases still causes some difficulty, even among experienced pathologists. In a recent British study of 40 cases
of "malignant round cell tumors of bone,"
five pathologists made a careful analysis of
these lesions. Cell outline, nuclear staining, nuclear pleomorphism, conspicuous
nucleoli, reticulin pattern, and intracellular glycogen were the histologic features
selected for this evaluation. They concluded that, based on these histologic features,
it is reasonable to distinguish between
Ewing's sarcoma and non-Hodgkin's lymphoma, although a considerable number of
tumors are not typical of either group.[6]

INCIDENCE

Ewing's sarcoma makes up approximately 10 per cent of the total number of pri-

mary malignant bone tumors occurring in Sweden, in contrast to the 14.2 per cent reported by the Netherlands Committee on Bone Tumours.[83] The mean annual incidence of Ewing's sarcoma per million population is 0.6 in England and 0.8 in Sweden.[83, 84, 124]

There is a significant difference in the racial incidence of this tumor. Blacks in both the United States and Africa are genetically resistant to Ewing's sarcoma and only rarely are they affected by it.[46, 54, 73, 89, 166] This is useful in the differential diagnosis and is an important etiologic consideration.

An interesting *familial aggregation* of Ewing's sarcoma has been described in two pairs of sisters.[63, 64, 68]

There are several case reports of Ewing's sarcoma occurring spontaneously in dogs[32, 136] and being experimentally induced with mesothorium in rabbits.[141]

SIGNS AND SYMPTOMS

Many of the patients with Ewing's sarcoma have slight to moderate fever, anemia, leukocytosis, and increased sedimentation rate on admission to hospital. These earliest symptoms of intermittent fever and leukocytosis have been noticed and commented on by many observers. Some even ascribe prognostic significance to these parameters by claiming that they are sinister portents.[88]

Pain and swelling are the most common symptoms. About two thirds of the patients complain of intermittent pain, its intensity varying from dull to severe, that usually becomes persistent at least one month prior to diagnosis. Visible or palpable tender swelling of rapidly increasing size is apparent in most patients. The size and consistency of the soft tissue swelling are quite variable. The larger the tumor, the softer and more fluctuant it becomes. A rapid growth rate from the onset, often followed by spontaneous improvement with quiescent periods lasting for a few weeks or many months, adds to the difficulty in diagnosing or even suspecting a tumor.[107] Local temperature elevation with dilated veins and associated tenderness accompany the lesion, thereby suggesting an inflammatory condition. Location in a rib is often associated with a pleural effusion. In mandibular lesions, paresthesia of lips and chin may be experienced.

Ewing's sarcoma arising in the innominate bone may demonstrate neurologic symptoms owing to involvement of the sacral plexus. Symptoms of neurogenic bladder caused by secondary invasion of Ewing's sarcoma originating in the sacrum or innominate bone may be noted.[131]

AGE AND SEX DISTRIBUTION

Ewing's sarcoma has a unique predilection for children and adolescents and is quite uncommon in people over the age of 30 years (Fig. 21–1). More than 80 per cent of the tumors occur in the first two decades of life. Those occurring in patients under the age of five years or over the age of 30 years should be accepted with reluctance. The youngest patient reported was five months old,[24] and the oldest was 83 years.[9] In younger children, metastatic neuroblastoma or, in older patients, non-Hodgkin's lymphoma or metastatic bronchial carcinoma should seriously be considered (Fig. 21–2). Glass and Fraumeni, analyzing 482 American children with Ewing's sarcoma, found the peak incidence in girls between 5 and 9 years of

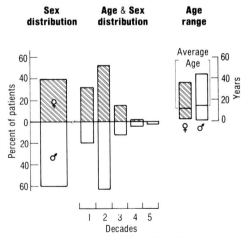

Ewing's Sarcoma   1949 - 1973
167 Pts.   (♂ = 101, ♀ = 66)

Figure 21–1. Age and sex distribution of 167 patients studied at Memorial Hospital from 1949 through 1973.

**Age Distribution of Patients
with Ewing's Sarcoma and
Non-Hodgkin's Lymphoma of Bone**

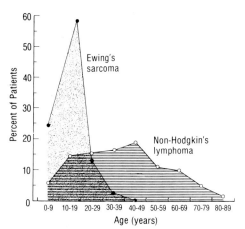

Figure 21-2. Age distribution of patients with Ewing's sarcoma and non-Hodgkin's lymphoma of bone studied at Memorial Hospital.

EWING'S SARCOMA
1949 - 1973

Skeletal Distribution of 167 Cases

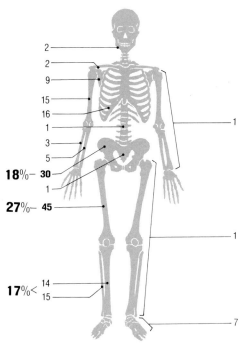

Figure 21-3. Skeletal distribution of 167 cases studied at Memorial Hospital from 1949 through 1973.

age and in boys from 10 to 14 years.[54] This dimorphism somewhat resembles the sex incidence of osteogenic sarcoma patients. Of the 167 patients with Ewing's sarcoma studied at Memorial Hospital from 1949 through 1973, males outnumbered females slightly (Fig. 21-1).

LOCATION

Skeletal distribution of 167 cases studied at Memorial Hospital showed that the long tubular bones were the most often affected. Among these osseous sites, the femur was involved in 27 per cent of the cases. The second most common regions among the long bones were the tibia and fibula (17 per cent together) and the humerus (9 per cent). Accordingly, the lower extremities are most frequently involved with Ewing's sarcoma. Among the flat bones, the pelvis was involved in 18 per cent of the cases (Fig. 21-3). In a report from Tata Memorial Hospital in Bombay, a predominance of primary involvement in the flat bones was noted.[9, 162] In contrast to the classic teaching and general belief that Ewing's sarcoma is predominantly located in the midshaft, the majority of the cases at Memorial Hospital were situated at or near the end of the long bones (diameta-

physis). Less often, the ribs (10 per cent),[13] vertebrae,[34] feet,[11, 33] and craniofacial bones are affected. This tumor occurs more frequently in the mandible (horizontal ramus preferred) than in the maxilla.[10, 15, 16, 20, 27, 62, 111, 119, 130]

RADIOGRAPHIC FEATURES

The characteristic presentation of a Ewing's sarcoma involving a long bone includes symmetrical, fusiform outline; soft tissue extension of tumor; mottled, moth-eaten-appearing internal pattern of bone destruction; poorly defined margins; and parallel, onionskin, periosteal reaction (Fig. 21-4). The appearance of the patchy, mottled, medullary bone destruction is sometimes likened to "cracked ice" (Fig. 21-5).

In the past, the radiographic image was considered to be pathognomonic of Ewing's sarcoma when, in a patient in the

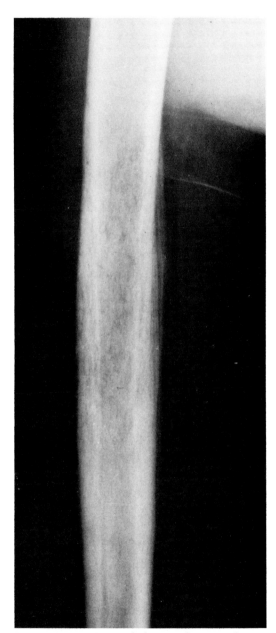

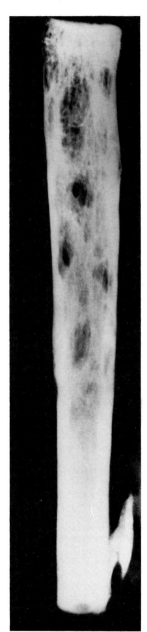

Figure 21–4. Typical humeral Ewing's sarcoma with moth-eaten-appearing medullary bone destruction and periosteal lamellation in a 25-year-old woman.

Figure 21–5. Specimen radiograph of a resected Ewing's sarcoma of the radius in a 16-year-old girl, showing patchy geographic-type bone destruction imitating angiosarcoma of bone.

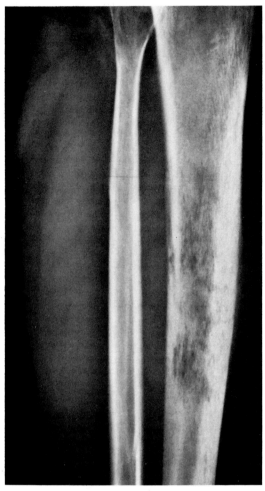

Figure 21–6. Typical diaphyseal Ewing's sarcoma of the right tibia in a 16-year-old boy, with mottled medullary bone involvement and cortical spread.

first two decades of life, the diaphysis of a long tubular bone, especially in the lower limb, showed destructive changes with a typical periosteal reaction in the form of multiple vertical layers, the so-called "onion-peel" reaction (Fig. 21–6). Many subsequent studies have demonstrated that neither the distribution of lesions nor their radiographic appearance is absolutely diagnostic for Ewing's sarcoma, and at best, only a presumptive diagnosis can be made, with histologic confirmation required in all cases.[40] Pathologic fracture is noted in approximately 5 per cent of the cases.[2]

Figure 21–7 describes and compares sequentially the radiographic *progression of disease* in both non-Hodgkin's lymphoma and Ewing's sarcoma of bone. In Ewing's sarcoma, an "onion-peel" periosteal lamellation is initially present in a diaphyseal location. Subsequently, a moth-eaten-appearing cortical destruction develops, with tumor extension in the spongiosa. Spontaneous fracture may result, in addition to bulky soft tissue involvement. In non-Hodgkin's lymphomas, the original "onion-peel" periosteal lamellation is followed by coarsely nodular cortical and some medullary bone destruction with a moth-eaten radiologic appearance. With further progression of the disease, spotty sclerosis and extensive medullary bone destruction may be noted with enhanced periosteal bone and spicule formation. The advancing disease manifests with marked cortical and medullary bone destruction characterized radiographically by a coarse stranded appearance. Very infrequently, bulky soft tissue involvement by tumor may be noted.

The scapula is a relatively uncommon site for Ewing's sarcoma (5 per cent).[147] In the nine cases studied radiographically at Memorial Hospital, there was a permeative or geographic type of bone destruction with a soft tissue mass (Fig. 21–8). Periosteal reaction was rare, and osteoblastic changes were quite infrequent but could be dramatic in a rare case.

Predominantly sclerotic lesions are extremely rare in central diaphyseal locations but may be seen occasionally with those located in the metaphysis. The central diaphyseal location, which is generally considered to be the classic presentation, constituted only about half the tumors in the long bones studied at Memorial Hospital.[144] Both centrally placed and eccentrically situated metaphyseal tumors have been encountered. In most of these cases the epiphysis is still open, as noted by Sherman and Soong,[144] providing some barrier to tumor permeation, but several instances of epiphyseal extension have been demonstrated. Metaphyseal lesions, as already noted, reveal an increased tendency for sclerotic intralesional changes and for brisk periosteal reactions of both lamellated and perpendicular type. Occasionally, the tempo of tumor growth is rapidly progressive and no appreciable reactive bone deposition within the lesion is noted. Such tumors are completely radio-

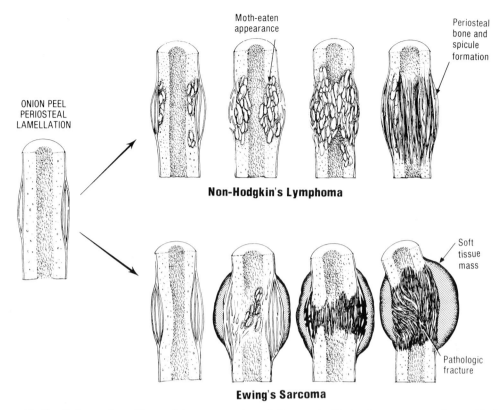

ONION PEEL PERIOSTEAL LAMELLATION

Moth-eaten appearance

Periosteal bone and spicule formation

Non-Hodgkin's Lymphoma

Soft tissue mass

Pathologic fracture

Ewing's Sarcoma

Figure 21–7. Schematic radiographic progression of disease in Ewing's sarcoma and non-Hodgkin's lymphoma of bone. (Modified from Uehlinger, E., Botsztejn, Ch., and Schinz, H. R.: Ewingsarkom und Knochenretikulosarkom. Klinik, Diagnose und Differentialdiagnose. Oncologia, *1*:193–245, 1948.)

lucent. The peculiarity of Ewing's sarcoma arising in a rib seems to be a prominent asymmetric intrathoracic soft tissue extension with a relatively slight extrathoracic soft tissue involvement. A huge intrathoracic aneurysmal bone cyst that destroys a rib and is associated with a pleural effusion in a child or adolescent may mimic a Ewing's sarcoma.[65]

Ewing's sarcoma arising in flat bones does not provide sufficiently diagnostic radiographic features to permit positive identification, since the lesions may be predominantly lytic, sclerotic, or mixed.

Periosteal Bone Formation

The parallel, laminated, onionskin radiographic presentation, usually several layers thick, is caused by the splitting and thickening of the cortex by the tumor cells. This pattern, although quite striking in Ewing's sarcoma, is not specific for this disease. The layering is usually continuous with reactive ossification in the form of Codman's triangles. Osteomyelitis, osteogenic sarcoma, or malignant lymphoma involving bones may show such an appearance.

The sunray pattern of periosteal bone formation in Ewing's sarcoma has been variously characterized as "radiating spicules of bone," "perpendicular new bone formation," "transverse striae," "radial spiculation of the cortex," and "groomed whiskers effect."[50] Some believe that these "trimmed whiskers" are thinner and more hairlike than those seen in osteogenic sarcoma.[52] It should be emphasized that these perpendicular trabeculae are not pathognomonic for Ewing's sarcoma, since they have been recorded in metastatic neuroblastoma, renal carcinoma, and even more frequently in osteogenic sarcoma.

The soft tissue mass adjacent to the intraosseous portion of the tumor is almost

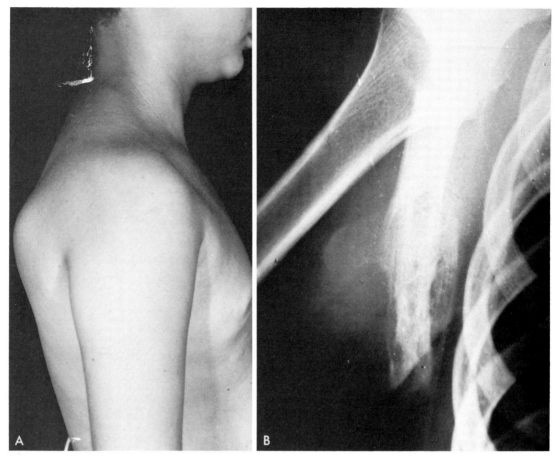

Figure 21–8.   *A,* Scapular Ewing's sarcoma with bulky soft tissue mass. *B,* Characteristic moth-eaten-appearing osseous destruction and periosteal onion-peel reaction in a young boy.

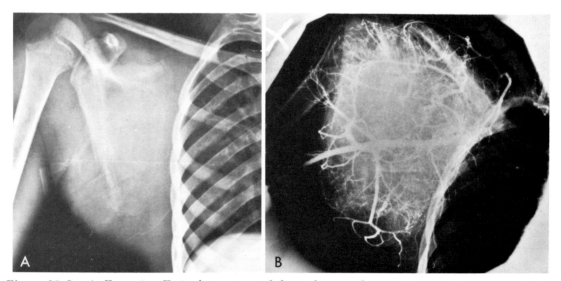

Figure 21–9.   *A,* Extensive Ewing's sarcoma of the right scapula in a 20-year-old woman with *B*: marked vascular markings. (Courtesy of Dr. J. Smith.)

always present, showing a poorly delineated mass without any significant degree of calcific deposits except for tiny occasional flecks in close proximity to the area of periosteal reaction (Fig. 21–8B).[144]

In some of the midshaft lesions, irregular saucerized cortical defect was noted with the central area of depression directed outward with occasional peripheral scalloping.

Angiography is useful in the diagnosis of Ewing's sarcoma. In about 90 per cent of the cases, hypervascularization is noted, with pathologic tortuous arteries present in approximately half of the cases examined.[159] The extensive vascular tumor staining diffusely involves the entire lesional tissue (Fig. 21–9). Arteriography is especially valuable in defining the extent of the soft tissue involvement.[79]

The clinical picture as well as the radiographic presentation of a Ewing's sarcoma may mimic osteomyelitis.[106] Constant, rather severe, pain, local tenderness, and swelling with concurrent fever and leukocytosis may be present in both. Both conditions may involve the metaphysis, although Ewing's sarcoma is somewhat more frequent in the midshaft. The motheaten pattern of bone destruction and reactive ossification are equally frequent in both diseases, making definite roentgen separation highly illusory.

PATHOLOGIC FEATURES

In very early stages, while the tumor is still intraosseous, the consistency of the tissue is firm. When cortical breakthrough is present, the lesional tissue, especially the extraosseous component, is soft, friable, and markedly hemorrhagic with areas of spongy and small cystic degeneration (Fig. 21–10). In later stages, involvement of soft parts is invariably present to some degree, showing an ill-defined mass encircling or enveloping the involved portion of the bone (Fig. 21–11). The overlying skin may be ulcerated.

Metastatic spread of Ewing's sarcoma to the lungs is one of the most frequently encountered types of secondary involvement. The metastatic deposits are multiple, subpleural, and intrapulmonary and

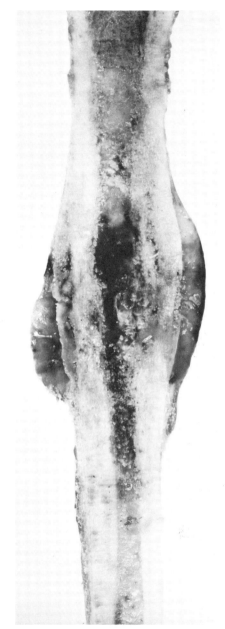

Figure 21–10. Ewing's sarcoma of midfemur in a 21-year-old woman, with soft spongy tumor showing intramedullary and soft tissue components.

may be readily separated from the surrounding pulmonary parenchyma. In addition to the lungs and pleura, the skeleton and the lymph nodes are sites of involvement by metastatic Ewing's sarcoma.[88, 98, 156]

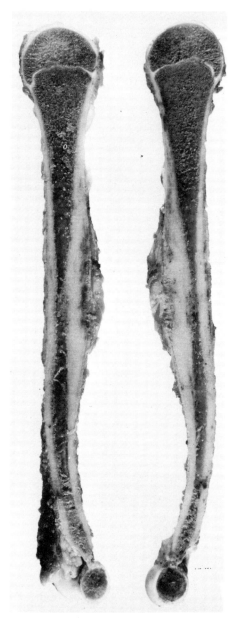

Figure 21-11. Amputation specimen of a Ewing's sarcoma of the midhumerus in an 11-year-old girl with eccentric soft tissue involvement.

HISTOLOGIC FEATURES

The histologic criteria for diagnosis have undergone some changes since Ewing's original description of the cell type as a small polygonal cell with pale cytoplasm, a small hyperchromatic nucleus, and an ill-defined cellular border (Figs. 21–12, 21–13, and 21–14).[35-37] He also recognized

that the cells tended to be arranged in compact broad sheets; at least in some foci, they are arranged around larger vascular spaces, giving the tumor a "perithelial" arrangement. Occasionally, a rosette or pseudorosette formation is noted (Fig. 21–15).[44] Experience has shown that the diagnosis of Ewing's sarcoma should not be made on histologic sections alone unless special stains are available and radiographs, as well as clinical history, are provided.

Cytologic examination shows at least two cell populations with transitional cellular forms.[137] Some of the cells have a larger, lightly stained, finely granular nucleus with a pale, ill-defined cytoplasm. Other cells show small, darker staining, but finely dispersed, nuclear chromatin feltwork with a rim of moderately well-delineated cytoplasm. In an occasional case, spindly cellular forms may be encountered intermixed with typical tumor cells.

In the histologic sections studied, the silver reticulin fibers are confined to the vascular septa with no penetration of cell groups or individual cells (Figs. 21–16 and 21–17). This presentation differs from non-Hodgkin's lymphoma of bone. Detailed studies by Salzer-Kuntschik, of the Vienna Bone Tumor Registry, revealed that retrospective cytologic and cytochemical examinations of round cell sarcomas of bone do not yield uniform results, although these tumors can be separated into several cytologic groups. The studies also revealed that glycogen demonstration by periodic acid–Schiff (PAS) and diastase reactions and the presence of peroxidase reaction are not uniform throughout the lesional tissue. The various types of esterases with and without sodium fluoride or acid and alkaline phosphatase reactions did not yield similar cytochemical behavior among the 18 cases examined. Significantly, her findings showed that a positive glycogen reaction after diastase digestion is not a foolproof criterion for the classification of "round cell sarcomas" of bone.[137-139]

In 1959, Schajowicz pointed out the presence of glycogen in the cytoplasm of Ewing's sarcoma cells.[140] The glycogen content of so-called endotheliomas was already known when Driessen, in 1893, described a glycogen-rich endothelioma.[31]

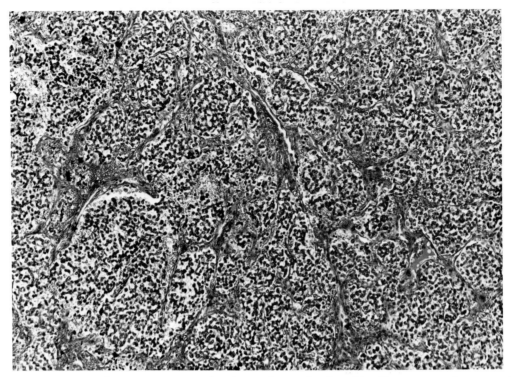

Figure 21–12. Ewing's sarcoma arranged in large clusters bordered by fibrous septa. (Hematoxylin-eosin stain. Magnification ×80.)

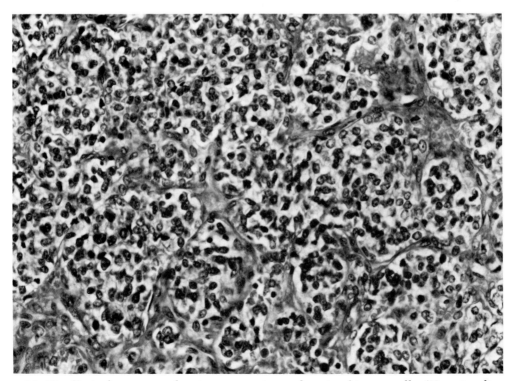

Figure 21–13. Ewing's sarcoma showing compact round nests of tumor cells. (Hematoxylin-eosin stain. Magnification ×125.)

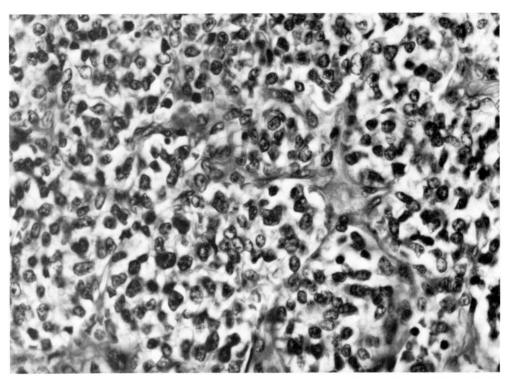

Figure 21–14. Ewing's sarcoma growing randomly. The tumor cells overlap and have ill-defined cellular borders but well-delineated nuclear outlines. (Hematoxylin-eosin stain. Magnification ×500.)

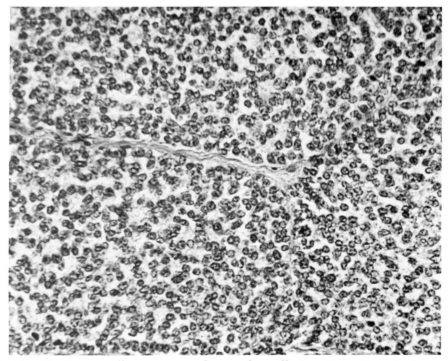

Figure 21–15. The tumor cells are arranged around capillaries. Note attempt at pseudorosette formation imitating neuroblastoma. (Hematoxylin-eosin stain. Magnification ×125.)

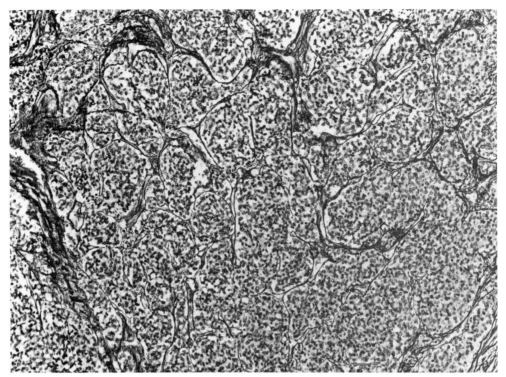

Figure 21–16. Silver impregnation technique delineates reticulin fibers that outline fibrous septa but are completely lacking around single tumor cells. (Wilder's stain. Magnification × 80.)

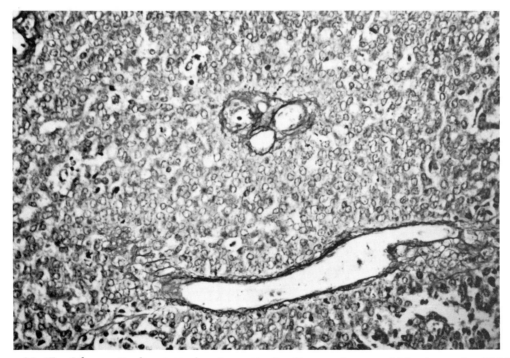

Figure 21–17. Silver reticulin stain showing reticulin fibers only around blood vessels. (Wilder's stain. Magnification × 250.)

The periodic acid–Schiff's stain shows, both on formalin-fixed tissue specimens and on air-dried touch preparation taken from the tumor, PAS-positive glycogen granules in the cytoplasm, which is sensitive to diastase digestion.[140] In an occasional case, false positive glycogen reaction may be noted when macrophages associated with tumor cells show PAS-positive diastase-resistant material. A positive glycogen stain helps to support this diagnosis, although a negative reaction does not rule out a Ewing's sarcoma. In approximately 5 to 10 per cent of the cases, no glycogen may be demonstrable on repeated histochemical examination. It should also be noted that monocytic and myelocytic leukemias secondarily involving the bone marrow may give a false positive, coarsely granular, glycogen reaction.[85, 86] Recent data from the Bristol Bone Tumour Registry, in addition to a solitary case report, described glycogen deposition in histologically proved neuroblastoma cells.[123, 158] Price demonstrated five glycogen-positive neuroblastomas out of 27 examined. Four of these cases were proved by autopsy examination.[123] As early as 1939, veritable soft tissue tumors with the light-microscopic and ultramicroscopic characteristics of Ewing's sarcoma of bone were described.[121] Larger series and individual case reports with ultrastructural analysis have confirmed that extraskeletal and osseous lesions are identical.[1, 153, 165]

The histologic interpretation of the biopsy material in Ewing's sarcoma may be greatly hampered and obscured by the generally poor quality of the tumor tissue, especially if there is widespread necrosis or poor preservation of the tumor cells, imitating necrotic leukocytes. Secondary acute or chronic inflammatory cell infiltrate with areas of tumor necrosis may obscure the true nature of the lesion. It is absolutely essential that an exact histologic diagnosis is established, for there are several other pathologic conditions that have been misdiagnosed as Ewing's sarcoma, including non-Hodgkin's lymphoma, embryonal rhabdomyosarcoma, poorly differentiated osteogenic sarcoma, and eosinophilic granuloma. To compound the diagnostic difficulties, both embryonal rhabdomyosarcoma and osteogenic sarcoma cells can show large amounts of glycogen. In fact, Ewing's sarcoma is a frequently imitated tumor, mimicked by benign and malignant conditions.

Embryonal rhabdomyosarcoma may involve the bone by direct extension, but if one evaluates the exact location of the tumor, the radiographic pattern of destruction, and the variability of the tumor cells, this error will be made only rarely. Rare osteogenic sarcomas, especially in young children, are quite often highly undifferentiated and may have the radiographic appearance identical to that of Ewing's sarcoma. In these undifferentiated or poorly differentiated osteogenic sarcomas, the osteoid production is quite inconspicuous, and many histologic sections must be examined before positive identification of tumor osteoid can be made. In these instances, the individual tumor cells may show great variation in size and shape. Some of the cases of poorly differentiated osteogenic sarcoma, the so-called small cell type, were originally diagnosed as Ewing's sarcoma with reactive bone formation.[50] In general, patients with Ewing's sarcoma and those with non-Hodgkin's lymphoma primarily involving a single bone have a different age distribution. In an occasional case, however, primary lymphomas in children may arise in a single bone. In such an unusual case, glycogen stains may be of help, since they are consistently negative; also, the tumor shows marked variation in its cellular makeup.

Once neuroblastoma is suspected, the diagnosis can usually be confirmed by biochemical analysis of catecholamines and their metabolites, which are secreted by these tumors. The specificity of the tests for the urinary excretion of HMPG (3-methoxy 4-hydroxyphenylethylene glycol), VMA (vanillylmandelic acid), HVA (homovanillic acid), and the metanephrines is over 90 per cent, thereby permitting a near fail-safe diagnosis.

The histologic diagnosis, as discussed above, may be quite difficult if one is to consider only examining limited tissue samples. It is also important to study the clinical presentation, the radiographic appearance of the tumor, and so on before arriving at the final, definitive diagnosis. The more important differential diagnostic features of small cell sarcomas in children are listed in Table 21–1.

TABLE 21–1.   Differential Diagnosis of Small Cell Sarcoma of Bone in Children

Ewing's Sarcoma	Non-Hodgkin's Lymphoma
Most common in second decade (but frequently occurs below 10 years of age)	No age or race predilection in children
Rare in Negroes	Long bones most common (femur and tibia)
Pain is most common presenting symptom	Diffuse metaphyseal lesion, usually mixed osteolytic and osteosclerotic areas
Flat bones (ribs, scapula, pelvis) are common sites	Lymphadenopathy and splenomegaly may be present
Femur is most common site	Early diffuse bone marrow involvement in children
Diaphyseal lesion in long bones	Reticulum fibers demonstrable with special stain
Diffuse osteolytic lesion of entire shaft	Cell nuclei somewhat larger and rounder than in Ewing's sarcoma
Large soft tissue mass (originating in bone)	Cytoplasmic border more distinct than in Ewing's sarcoma
May give positive stain for glycogen granules (PAS)	

Metastatic Neuroblastoma	Embryonal Rhabdomyosarcoma
Usually in children less than 5 years of age	Lesions of the trunk and extremity can frequently involve bone
Long bones are frequently symmetrically involved	Usually presents with soft tissue swelling rather than pain as the predominant symptom
Lytic lesions can be very extensive with a paucity of soft tissue mass	The soft tissue mass usually invades bone secondarily
Bone marrow aspiration can show clumps of extrinsic cells ("rosettes")	Systemic symptoms are rare
Presence of primary tumor; abnormal intravenous pyelogram or paraspinal mass	Lesions in the head and neck area are usually primary, not metastatic
Urine may be positive for vanillylmandelic acid and/or catecholamines	Cells have a predominance of pink cytoplasm occasionally exhibiting striations on higher magnification (rhabdomyoblast)

(From Rosen, G.: Management of malignant bone tumors in children and adolescents. Pediatr. Clin. North Am., 23:183–213, 1976.)

ULTRAMICROSCOPIC FEATURES AND HISTOGENESIS

Electromicroscopic examination reveals uniform, rather polygonal, small tumor cells with varying amounts of particulate glycogen in the cytoplasm and occasional typical or atypical desmosomal junctional complexes.[49, 60, 78, 90, 91, 105, 122, 127] Filamentous intracytoplasmic structures, but no viral particles, are present.[60, 154]

The exact histogenesis of Ewing's sarcoma remains uncertain even after numerous cytochemical and ultrastructural studies. Some ultrastructural interpretation, such as the work of Friedman and Gold, suggests that this tumor is a neoplasm of immature reticulum cells, i.e., of reticuloendothelial origin.[48] Others have raised the possibility that Ewing's sarcoma is derived from primitive and uncommitted mesenchymal supporting cells of bone marrow.[90, 91] Ultrastructural and tissue culture studies by Kadin and Bensch suggest the neoplastic cells to be of myelogenic derivation.[78] More recent data point to a transitional cell resembling both pericytes and vascular smooth muscle cells of the bone marrow[154] or of blood vessel origin.[122]

TREATMENT

The results of treatment, until very recently, have been uniformly poor, mainly because of the high frequency of diffuse osseous involvement, early metastases, and soft tissue extension by tumor. It is estimated that up to one third of the patients with Ewing's sarcoma have asymptomatic, and often clinically undetectable, microscopic metastases at the time of original diagnosis.[107] The great value of radioisotopic scanning is in the detection of small, otherwise unappreciated, bony, or, although less likely, pulmonary metastases. Total body scanning with minified images using ^{99m}Tc polyphosphate, ^{18}F, ^{87m}Sr, ^{75}Se methionine, or ^{67}Ga is most commonly employed (Fig. 21–18). They give proper resolution, reduced scanning time with short half-life, and low radiation dosage.

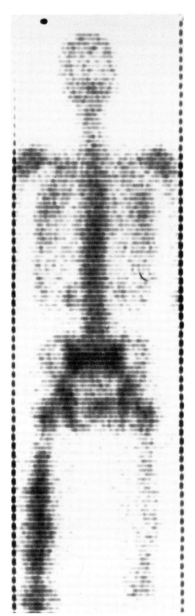

Figure 21–18. [18]F minified bone scan demonstrating a histologically proved Ewing's sarcoma diffusely involving the right lower extremity. (Courtesy of Dr. S. D. J. Yeh.)

In a comprehensive analysis of 435 cases, Bethge computed an average of 8.5 per cent five year survival rate, with a range from 4.8 per cent to 12.6 per cent. This study included pre-1938 data also.[8] Falk and Alpert calculated five year survival figures of 7.9 per cent on the basis of 944 cases collected from the literature.[39] The comparison of survival data from larger series of Ewing's sarcoma is greatly hampered by the fact that many studies lack strict histologic criteria by which the various authors chose their cases. Since most of the patients were to die of disseminated Ewing's sarcoma, Boyer and associates proposed local control of the primary lesion solely by irradiation to spare the trauma of ablative surgery.[12] The results from a single comprehensive cancer center are somewhat better. In 1967, Phillips and Higinbotham reported a 25 per cent five year survival rate of patients with Ewing's sarcoma at Memorial Hospital with the use of megavoltage radiation therapy to the entire involved bone.[115] It is of interest to note that many of these patients received adjuvant therapy with nitrogen mustard, dactinomycin, or Coley's toxin in combination with nitrogen mustard. All of these treatment regimens have incorporated some form of adjuvant chemotherapy in order to eradicate the microscopic foci of Ewing's sarcoma presumed to be present at the time of initial diagnosis. The Mayo Clinic achieved a five year survival rate of 16 per cent among 234 patients treated between the years 1912 and 1968.[125] Most of the survival data are based on the use of radiation therapy as the primary method of treatment, since the reported results seemed to be as good as, or even somewhat better than, those obtained by surgery alone. Radiation therapy, in addition, spared the patients amputation if they were to die from metastatic disease relatively soon. One of the main drawbacks of radiation therapy seemed to be that at least one third of the patients eventually exhibited local recurrence.[22, 41, 80, 94] The comprehensive retrospective analysis of cases treated at the Mayo Clinic presented further strong evidence in favor of primary surgical management of Ewing's sarcoma.[125] Among the patients with primary extremity lesions, 44.7 per cent of those treated by surgical means survived five years, in contrast to a 13.1 per cent five year survival rate after nonsurgical management. In this retrospective and nonrandomized study, no obvious preselection for favorable clinicopathologic characteristics could be identified, but still no definite and firm conclusions could be made. The controversy and the ongoing debate concerning primary surgery in preference to radiation therapy has been greatly complicated, but probably effectively eliminated, by the introduction of modern adjuvant chemotherapy as an additional routine therapeutic modality in the treatment of Ewing's sarcoma.[22, 66, 69, 72, 74, 94, 116, 135] The prognosis for patients with Ewing's sarcoma has now become considerably better. Multidrug multicycle aggressive chemotherapy combined with irradiation provides a two year survival rate in the 60 per cent range and an estimated five year survival rate of approximately 50 per cent.[116, 117] There is no question that, in many cases, this aggressive chemotherapy regimen does prevent microscopic occult metastases from becoming clinically manifest, and the patients under close observation show that true cures, not just temporary ones, may be achieved (Fig. 21–19).

The proclivity for local recurrence in Ewing's sarcoma may be somewhat reduced by increasing the radiation dose over 5000 rads in 25 fractions over a five week period.[22] Naturally, with these higher radiotherapeutic doses, the morbidity is also considerably enhanced. Analysis of this by Tefft and associates showed severe acute and late effects on the normal tissues if a combination of chemotherapy and radiation therapy for Ewing's sarcoma was given.[155] Unexpectedly serious and severe reaction to this combined treatment modality has been experienced, necessitating many interruptions for the patients so treated. The subsequently experienced late reactions also appeared to be more severe and protracted. This study demonstrated that the current radiation and chemotherapeutic regimens should be more defined, insuring that large volumes of normal tissue do not receive in excess of 5000 rads, and only a very small volume of tissue is exposed to more than this dose of radiation.

In a retrospective study, Lewis and his colleagues analyzed the long-term morbidity in 55 patients at Memorial Hospital with Ewing's sarcoma who survived two years or longer.[87] The lesions were located

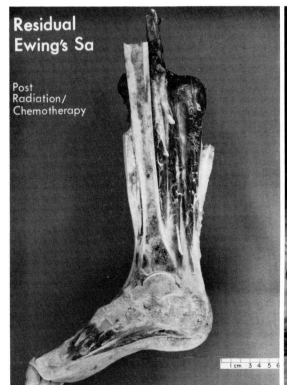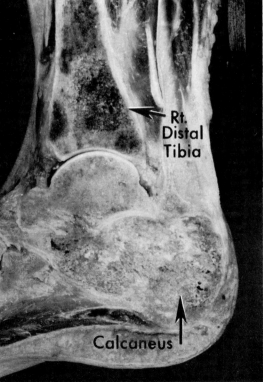

Figure 21–19.   Residual microscopic foci of Ewing's sarcoma found on serial sectioning after irradiation and chemotherapy (below knee amputation).

in the upper and lower extremities, the shoulder girdle, and the pelvis. This group of patients was treated either with surgery or radiation therapy combined with additional aggressive chemotherapy. Morbidity due to radiation therapy was graded as minimal, moderate, or severe as evidenced by the degree of shortening, deformity, and fibrosis or fracture of the involved bone. Disability of the patient was evaluated in view of whether a primary major amputation should have been the preferred choice of treatment. The complications associated with radiation therapy for lesions occurring in the pelvis included severe hemorrhagic cystitis and proctitis. In two of the patients treated with radiation therapy, a second osteogenic sarcoma appeared seven and nine years later respectively, probably related to the irradiation previously given at the site.

The delayed effects of radiation therapy, especially radiation-induced bone sarcoma, may be prevented by a more judicious use of radiation to spare normal soft tissues of the affected extremity. There is a recent trend toward a more liberal use of surgical excision of the primary tumor in patients with Ewing's sarcoma, especially in young children with lesions in the lower limb or in those with very bulky primary tumors. The surgical excision is not necessarily an amputation but may be limb-preserving with an *en bloc* resection of the tumor-bearing portion of the bone.

In the evaluation by Lewis and associates of these patients treated by irradiation, they also noted that the age of the patient and the site of the tumor definitely influenced both acute and late morbidity associated with radiation.[87] Severe growth impairment due to irradiation of the epiphyseal area is the most profound effect in children under the age of 12 years. In adults and in older children who have a mature skeleton, the site of the Ewing's sarcoma is very important. According to this study, radiation therapy may be employed for all tumors located in the upper extremity in patients of all ages. For tumors located in the lower extremity, both in adults and in older children, radiation therapy may be the treatment of choice. Ablative surgery is recommended for those children with limb lesions who are still growing and for all those patients whose tumors arose in the foot or in the distal end of the fibula. If pathologic frac-

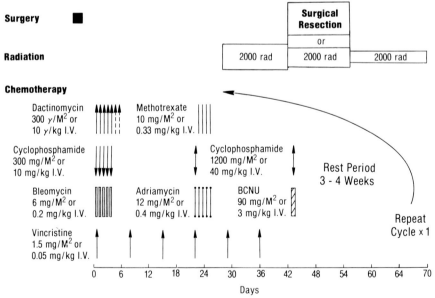

Figure 21–20. T-6 induction chemotherapy for Ewing's sarcoma as devised by Dr. G. Rosen. (From Rosen, G., Caparros, B., Mosende, C., et al.: Curability of Ewing's sarcoma and considerations for future therapeutic trials. Cancer, *41*:888–889, 1978.)

ture of a weight-bearing bone occurs, this also provides a definite indication for major surgery.

In 1978, a study from the Memorial Sloan-Kettering Cancer Center analyzed 20 previously untreated children with Ewing's sarcoma who were treated with surgery or radiation therapy (6000–7000 rads) for the primary tumor, in addition to a T-2 adjuvant chemotherapy protocol.[134, 135] Of these 20 children, 15 had no evidence of recurrent disease from 31 to 82 months, with a median of 46 months, from the start of treatment. The actuarial five year disease-free survival rate for this group of patients was 75 per cent. Evaluation of those who relapsed following adjuvant chemotherapy revealed that all recurrences occurred at the end of the second year or after T-2 chemotherapy ceased. Among the 23 patients who received so-called "curative" radiation therapy to their primary tumor, five (22 per cent) experienced local recurrence and six (26 per cent) had severe functional disability secondary to the combined radiation and the T-2 chemotherapy. Analysis of this experience culminated in the devising of a

more aggressive initial or "induction" chemotherapy (T-6) with a subsequent "maintenance" chemotherapy protocol (T-2) to effectively eradicate metastatic subclinical microfoci of Ewing's sarcoma, which are presumed to be present in most patients at the time of initial diagnosis (Figs. 21–20 and 21–21). This new aggressive approach advocates surgery alone or combined with moderate doses of radiation therapy, since experience has shown a predictably high risk of local recurrence in those with pelvic lesions and a high probability of functional debility in young children whose lesions arose in weight-bearing bones. Preliminary results, as reported by Rosen and associates, seem to be encouraging, with 11 of the 13 patients free of disease from 12 to 26 months.[134] In such lesions, the local recurrence rate is otherwise quite high.

THERAPEUTIC RECOMMENDATIONS[134]

1. A moderate dose of radiation therapy coupled with surgery is recommended for a primary Ewing's sarcoma occurring in

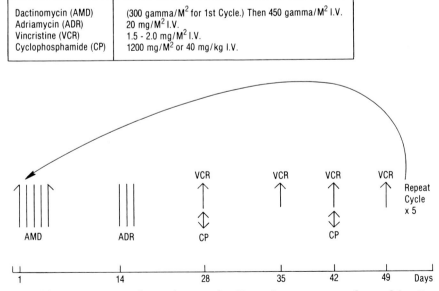

MAINTENANCE CHEMOTHERAPY FOR SOLID TUMORS (T - 2)

Dactinomycin (AMD)	(300 gamma/M^2 for 1st Cycle.) Then 450 gamma/M^2 I.V.
Adriamycin (ADR)	20 mg/M^2 I.V.
Vincristine (VCR)	1.5 - 2.0 mg/M^2 I.V.
Cyclophosphamide (CP)	1200 mg/M^2 or 40 mg/kg I.V.

Figure 21–21. T-2 maintenance chemotherapy for Ewing's sarcoma as devised by Dr. G. Rosen. (From Rosen, G., Caparros, B., Mosende, C., et al.: Curability of Ewing's sarcoma and considerations for future therapeutic trials. Cancer, *41*:888–889, 1978.)

the pelvis, where excessive irradiation would result in increased morbidity as far as bowel and bladder functions are concerned.

2. In young children whose lesions appear in the proximal femur, high-dose curative radiation therapy may result in increased morbidity manifested by flexion contractures. In such instances, moderate-dose radiation therapy to the involved bone, followed by resection of the tumor-bearing proximal femur, is recommended. Preoperative chemotherapy to reduce or eliminate soft tissue involvement by Ewing's sarcoma is indicated. The use of an artificial endoprosthesis for the replacement of the *en bloc* resected portion of the bone may be of use.

3. Children whose lesions involve the proximal tibia or distal femur, owing to the projected excessive discrepancy in leg length after irradiation and chemotherapy, should be treated with immediate amputation, rather than the combined therapeutic approach, for the control of the primary lesion and to secure proper ambulation.

4. In those patients whose lesions involve bones of the foot, effective radiation therapy is expected to result in extremely poor function with a pained gait; therefore, primary surgical treatment would be of benefit.

5. Lesions occurring in the rib, the fourth most common site of skeletal involvement, should be treated by preoperative chemotherapy, wide local surgical excision, and postoperative radiation therapy employing electron beam to avoid unnecessary irradiation of the underlying pulmonary tissues and heart.

6. Radiation therapy with a dose of 6000 to 7000 rads is recommended as the single mode of therapy directed to the entire tumor-bearing bone, employing shrinking fields to avoid irradiation of uninvolved normal soft tissues, for patients who have had their lesions in the long bones of the upper extremity. Similar treatment is advised for those lesions appearing in the lower extremities, where the projected shortening of the involved bone is not anticipated as being overly disabling.

7. The central nervous system is very rarely involved by Ewing's sarcoma as a clinically latent meningeal disease in spite of some reports to the contrary.[97, 100] Therefore, prophylactic irradiation to the skull, combined with intrathecal methotrexate, is contraindicated for asymptomatic patients.[132]

REFERENCES

1. Angervall, L., and Enzinger, F. M.: Extraskeletal neoplasm resembling Ewing's sarcoma. Cancer, 36:240–251, 1975.
2. Aufranc, O. E., Jones, W. N., and Turner, R. H.: Pathologic fracture of the proximal femur. J.A.M.A., 199:107–111, 1967.
3. Bacci, G., Figus, E., Cagnano, R., et al.: Association of local radiation therapy and systematic chemotherapy in the treatment of clinically localized Ewing's sarcoma. Minerva Med., 66:1263–1273, 1975.
4. Bacci, G., and Pagani, P. A.: Adjuvant chemotherapy in the treatment of Ewing tumor and osteosarcoma. Chir. Organi Mov., 62:491–506, 1975.
5. Baird, R. J., and Krause, V. W.: Ewing's tumour: A review of 33 cases. Can. J. Surg., 6:136–140, 1963.
6. Ball, J., Freedman, L., and Sissons, H. A.: Malignant round-cell tumours of bone: an analytical histological study from the Cancer Research Campaign's Bone Tumour Panel. Br. J. Cancer, 36:254–268, 1977.
7. Barden, R. P.: The similarity of clinical and roentgen findings in children with Ewing's sarcoma (endothelial myeloma) and sympathetic neuroblastoma. Am. J. Roentgenol. Radium Ther. Nucl. Med., 50:575–581, 1943.
8. Bethge, J. F. J.: Die Ewingtumoren oder Omoblastome des Knochens. Ergeb. Chir. Orthop., 39:327–425, 1955.
9. Bhansali, S. K., and Desai, P. B.: Ewing's sarcoma. Observations on 107 cases. J. Bone Joint Surg. [Am.], 45:541–553, 1963.
10. Blakemore, J. R., and Stein, M.: Primary Ewing's sarcoma of the mandible: report of a case. J. Oral Surg., 33:376–379, 1975.
11. Bonanone, V., and Cardani, R.: An unusual case of Ewing's tumour on the foot. Minerva Ortop., 24:441–447, 1973.
12. Boyer, C. W., Jr., Brickner, T. J., Jr., and Perry, R. H.: Ewing's sarcoma. Case against surgery. Cancer, 20:1602–1606, 1967.
13. Branson, J.: Ewing's tumour of rib. Australas. Radiol., 20:341–345, 1976.
14. Brereton, H. D., Simon, R., and Pomeroy, T. C.: Pretreatment serum lactate dehydrogenase predicting metastatic spread in Ewing's sarcoma. Ann. Intern. Med., 83:352–354, 1975.
15. Brocheriou, C., Guilbert, F., Rouchon, C., et al.: Ewing's sarcoma localised to the mandible — two cases. Rev. Stomatol., 75:877–884, 1974.
16. Brownson, R. J., and Cook, R. P.: Ewing's sarcoma of the maxilla. Ann. Otol. Rhinol. Laryngol., 78:1299–1304, 1969.
17. Buraczewski, J.: Problems connected with primary radiosensitive small-cell malignant tumors of bone. Nowotwory, Supplement:7–11, 1976.
18. Buraczewski, J., Borejko, M., Guzecki, A., et al.: Radiological symptomatology of primary malignant round cell radiosensitive bone tumors. Nowotwory, Supplement:47–61, 1976.

19. Bursell, S., and Gellerstedt, N.: Zur Kenntnis der primären, bösartigen Skelettgeschwülste von epitheliomorphem Typus. Zugleich einiges zur Endotheliomfrage. Upsala Läk. Fören., 43:91–100, 1937.

20. Carl, W., Schaaf, N. G., Gaeta, J., et al.: Ewing's sarcoma. Oral Surg., 31:472–478, 1971.

21. Červeňanský, J., and Kossey, P.: Round-cell bone sarcoma. Bratisl. Lek. Listy, 67:459–468, 1977.

22. Chabora, B. M., Rosen, G., Cham, W., et al.: Radiotherapy of Ewing's sarcoma. Local control with and without intensive chemotherapy. Radiology, 120:667–671, 1976.

23. Chan, P. Y. M., Gilbert, H. A., Stein, J. J., et al.: The role of early diagnosis and radiation therapy in the management of Ewing's sarcoma. Front. Rad. Ther. Onc., 10:141–151, 1975.

24. Coley, B. L., Higinbotham, N. L., and Bowden, L.: Endothelioma of bone (Ewing's sarcoma). Ann. Surg., 128:533–560, 1948.

25. Colville, H. C., and Willis, R. A.: Neuroblastoma metastases in bones, with a criticism of Ewing's endothelioma. Am. J. Pathol., 9:421–430, 1933.

26. Connor, C. L.: Endothelial myeloma, Ewing. Report of fifty-four cases. Arch. Surg., 12:789–829, 1926.

27. Crowe, W. W., and Harper, J. C.: Ewing's sarcoma with primary lesion in mandible: report of case. J. Oral Surg., 23:156–161, 1971.

28. Dabska, M.: Malignant round cell tumours of bone in the material of the Department of Pathology — Institute of Oncology in Warsaw. Nowotwory, Supplement:73–85, 1976.

29. Dahlin, D. C.: Is it worthwhile to differentiate Ewing's sarcoma and primary lymphoma of bone? In: Proceedings. National Cancer Conference, Seventh. Philadelphia, J. B. Lippincott Co., 1973, pp. 941–945.

30. Dahlin, D. C., Coventry, M. B., and Scanlon, P. W.: Ewing's sarcoma. A critical analysis of 165 cases. J. Bone Joint Surg. [Am.], 43:185–192, 1961.

31. Driessen, L. F.: Untersuchungen über glykogenreiche Endotheliome. Beitr. Pathol. Anat., 12:65–114, 1893.

32. Drieux, H., and Veretennikoff, S.: Diagnostic radiologique différentiel du sarcome d'Ewing et du sarcome de Parker-Jackson des os longs. Rec. Med. Vet., 142:37–45, 1966.

33. Dunn, E. J., Yuska, K. H., Judge, D. M., et al.: Ewing's sarcoma of the great toe. A case report. Clin. Orthop., 116:203–208, 1976.

34. Evans, J. E.: Ewing's tumour: uncommon presentation of an uncommon tumour. Med. J. Aust., 1:590–591, 1977.

35. Ewing, J.: Diffuse endothelioma of bone. Proc. N.Y. Path. Soc., 21:17–24, 1921.

36. Ewing, J.: Further report on endothelial myeloma of bone. Proc. N.Y. Path. Soc., 24:93–100, 1924.

37. Ewing, J.: A review of the classification of bone tumors. Surg. Gynecol. Obstet., 68:971–976, 1939.

38. Falk, S., and Alpert, M.: The clinical and roentgen aspects of Ewing's sarcoma. Am. J. Med. Sci., 250:492–508, 1965.

39. Falk, S., and Alpert, M.: Five year survival of patients with Ewing's sarcoma. Surg. Gynecol. Obstet., 124:319–324, 1967.

40. Feldman, F.: Round cell lesions of bone. In Margulis, A. R., and Gooding, C. A. (eds.): Diagnostic Radiology 1977. St. Louis, C. V. Mosby Co., 1977, pp. 437–454.

41. Fernandez, C. H., Lindberg, R. D., Sutow, W. W., et al.: Localized Ewing's sarcoma — treatment and results. Cancer, 34:143–148, 1974.

42. Fitzer, P. M., and Steffey, W. R.: Brain and bone scans in primary Ewing's sarcoma of the petrous bone. Case report. J. Neurosurg., 44:608–612, 1976.

43. Fleszarowa, I.: Radiological differential diagnosis of Ewing's sarcoma. Nowotwory, Supplement:63–71, 1976.

44. Foote, F. W., Jr., and Anderson, H. R.: Histogenesis of Ewing's tumor. Am. J. Pathol., 17:497–501, 1941.

45. Fossati-Bellani, F., Barni, S., Gasparini, M., et al.: Adriamycin, cytoxan and vincristine in the adjuvant treatment of localized Ewing's sarcoma. In Salmon, S. E., and Jones, S. E. (eds.): Adjuvant Therapy of Cancer. Amsterdam, Elsevier, 1977, pp. 373–380.

46. Fraumeni, J. F., Jr., and Glass, A. G.: Rarity of Ewing's sarcoma among U.S. Negro children. Letter to the editor. Lancet, 1:366–367, 1970.

47. Freeman, A. I., Sachatello, C., Gaeta, J., et al.: An analysis of Ewing's tumor in children at Roswell Park Memorial Institute. Cancer, 29:1563–1569, 1972.

48. Friedman, B., and Gold, H.: Ultrastructure of Ewing's sarcoma of bone. Cancer, 22:307–322, 1968.

49. Friedman, B., and Hanaoka, H.: Round-cell sarcomas of bone. A light and electron microscopy study. J. Bone Joint Surg. [Am.], 53:1118–1136, 1971.

50. Garber, C. Z.: Reactive bone formation in Ewing's sarcoma. Cancer, 4:839–845, 1951.

51. Gasparini, M., Barni, S., Lattuada, A., et al.: Ten years experience with Ewing's sarcoma. Tumori, 63:77–90, 1977.

52. Geschickter, C. F., and Maseritz, I. H.: Ewing's sarcoma. J. Bone Joint Surg., 21:26–39, 1939.

53. Gharpure, V. V.: Endothelial myeloma (Ewing's tumor of bone). Am. J. Pathol., 17:503–509, 1941.

54. Glass, A. G., and Fraumeni, J. F., Jr.: Epidemiology of bone cancer in children. J. Natl. Cancer Inst., 44:187–199, 1970.

55. Gouin, J. L.: Endothélioréticulosarcomes d'Ewing et réticulosarcomes. Rev. Prat., 19:2431–2439, 1969.

56. Haass, F., Jungblut, R., and Heinzler, F.: Die Strahlenbehandlung des Ewing-Sarkoms. Strahlentherapie, 140:133–142, 1970.

57. Heald, J. H., Soto-Hall, R., and Hill, H. A.: Ewing's sarcoma. Am. J. Roentgenol. Radium Ther. Nucl. Med., 91:1167–1171, 1964.

58. Hildebrand, Z. C.: Ueber das tubuläre Angiosarkom oder Endotheliom des Knochens. Dtsch. Z. Chir., 31:262–281, 1890–1891.

59. Hirsch, E. F., and Ryerson, E. W.: Metastases of the bone in primary carcinoma of the lung. A review of so-called endotheliomas of the bones. Arch. Surg., 16:1–30, 1928.

60. Hou-Jensen, K., Priori, E., and Dmochowski, L.: Studies on ultrastructure of Ewing's sarcoma of bone. Cancer, 29:280–286, 1972.

61. Howard, W. T., Jr., and Crile, G. W.: A contribution to the knowledge of endothelioma and

perithelioma of bone. Ann. Surg., *42*:358–393, 1905.

62. Hunsuck, E. E.: Ewing's sarcoma of the maxilla. Report of a case. Oral Surg., 25:923–928, 1968.

63. Huntington, R. W., Jr., Henkelmann, C. R., and Franklin, R.: Atypical Ewing tumor in the sister of a patient with Ewing's tumor. Clinical and autopsy findings. J. Bone Joint Surg. [Am.], *43*:572–574, 1961.

64. Huntington, R. W., Jr., Sheffel, D. J., Iger, M., et al.: Malignant bone tumors in siblings. Ewing's tumor and an unusual tumor, perhaps a variant of Ewing's tumor. A case report. J. Bone Joint Surg. [Am.], *42*:1065–1075, 1960.

65. Hurvitz, J. S., Harrison, M. R., and Weitzman, J. J.: Aneurysmal bone cyst mimicking Ewing's sarcoma of the rib. J. Pediatr. Surg., *12*:1067–1069, 1977.

66. Hustu, H. O., Holton, C., James, D., Jr., et al.: Treatment of Ewing's sarcoma with concurrent radiotherapy and chemotherapy. J. Pediatr., 73:249–251, 1968.

67. Hutchison, R.: On suprarenal sarcoma in children with metastases in the skull. Q. J. Med., *1*:33–41, 1907–1908.

68. Hutter, R. V. P., Francis, K. C., and Foote, F. W., Jr.: Ewing's sarcoma in siblings. Report of the second known occurrence. Am. J. Surg., *107*:598–603, 1964.

69. Jaffe, N., Traggis, D., Salian, S., et al.: Improved outlook for Ewing's sarcoma with combination chemotherapy (vincristine, actinomycin D and cyclophosphamide) and radiation therapy. Cancer, 38:1925–1930, 1976.

70. Jenkin, R. D. T.: Radiation treatment of Ewing's sarcoma and osteogenic sarcoma. Can. J. Surg., 20:530–536, 1977.

71. Jenkin, R. D. T., Rider, W. D., and Sonley, M. J.: Ewing's sarcoma: A retrospective analysis of treatment results at the Princess Margaret Hospital, Toronto, 1960–73, with particular reference to total body radiation. *In* Sinks, L. F., and Godden, J. O. (eds.): Conflicts in Childhood Cancer. An Evaluation of Current Management. New York, Alan R. Liss, Inc., 1975, pp. 265–277.

72 Jenkin, R. D., Rider, W. D., and Sonley, M. J.: Ewing's sarcoma. Adjuvant total body irradiation, cyclophosphamide and vincristine. Int. J. Radiat. Oncot. Biol. Phys., *1*:407–413, 1976.

73. Jensen, R. D., and Drake, R. M.: Rarity of Ewing's tumour in Negroes. Letter to the editor. Lancet, *1*:777, 1970.

74. Johnson, R., and Humphreys, S. R.: Past failures and future possibilities in Ewing's sarcoma. Experimental and preliminary clinical results. Cancer, 23:161–166, 1969.

75. Johnson, R. E., and Pomeroy, T. C.: Integrated therapy for Ewing's sarcoma. Am. J. Roentgenol. Radium Ther. Nucl. Med., *114*:532–535, 1972.

76. Johnson, R. E., and Pomeroy, T. C.: Evaluation of therapeutic results in Ewing's sarcoma. Am. J. Roentgenol. Radium Ther. Nucl. Med., *123*:583–587, 1975.

77. Johnson, R. E., Senyszyn, J. J., Rabson, A. S., et al.: Treatment of Ewing's sarcoma with local irradiation and systemic chemotherapy. A progress report. Radiology, 95:195–197, 1970.

78. Kadin, M. E., and Bensch, K. G.: On the origin of Ewing's tumor. Cancer, 27:257–273, 1971.

79. Kittredge, R. D.: Arteriography in Ewing's tumor. Radiology, 97:609–610, 1970.

80. Kotz, R., Kogelnik, H. D., Salzer-Kuntschik, M., et al.: Problems of local recurrence in patients with Ewing's sarcoma. Osterr. Z. Onkol., 4:7–12, 1977.

81. Kotz, R., Salzer, M., and Zwerina, H.: Evaluative analyses of the course the disease may take in tumor patients (with special reference to the Ewing-sarcoma). Osterr. Z. Onkol., 2:37–42, 1974.

82. Kotz, R., Salzer-Kuntschik, M., Zweymüller, K., et al.: Therapy and prognosis of the Ewing-Sarcoma. Osterr. Z. Onkol., *1*:15–22, 1974.

83. Larsson, S. E., Boquist, L., and Bergdahl, L.: Ewing's sarcoma. A consecutive series of 64 cases diagnosed in Sweden 1958–1967. Clin. Orthop., 95:263–272, 1973.

84. Larsson, S. E., and Lorentzon, R.: The geographic variation of the incidence of malignant primary bone tumors in Sweden. J. Bone Joint Surg. [Am.], 56:592–600, 1974.

85. Leder, L. D.: Cytochemical differentiation between normal and pathological mononuclear blood and bone marrow cells. Acta Histochem., 9 (Supplement):141–151, 1971.

86. Leinonen, E. A.: Cytochemical studies of acute leukemias. Acta Haematol., 43:219–227, 1970.

87. Lewis, R. J., Marcove, R. C., and Rosen, G.: Ewing's sarcoma: Functional effects of radiation therapy. J. Bone Joint Surg. [Am.], 59:325–331, 1977.

88. Lichtenstein, L., and Jaffe, H. L.: Ewing's sarcoma of bone. Am. J. Pathol., 23:43–77, 1947.

89. Linden, G., and Dunn, J. E.: Ewing's sarcoma in Negroes. Lancet, *1*:1171, 1970.

90. Llombart-Bosch, A., and Blache, R.: Studies on morphology and ultrastructure of Ewing's tumor of bone. Verh. Dtsch. Ges. Pathol., 58:459–466, 1974.

91. Llombart-Bosch, A., Blache, R., and Peydro-Olaya, A.: Ultrastructural study of 28 cases of Ewing's sarcoma: typical and atypical forms. Cancer, *41*:1362–1373, 1978.

92. Lücke, A.: Beiträge zur Geschwulstlehre. Virchows Arch. [Pathol. Anat.], 35:524–539, 1866.

93. Lumb, G., and Mackenzie, D. H.: Round-cell tumours of bone. Br. J. Surg., 43:380–389, 1956.

94. Macintosh, D. J., Price, C. H. G., and Jeffree, G. M.: Ewing's tumour. A study of behaviour and treatment in forty-seven cases. J. Bone Joint Surg. [Br.], 57:331–340, 1975.

95. Magnus, H. A., and Wood, H. L. C.: Primary reticulo-sarcoma of bone. J. Bone Joint Surg. [Br.], 38:258–278, 1956.

96. Marckwald, V. A.: Ein Fall von multiplem, intravasculärem Endotheliom in den gesammten Knochen des Skelets (Myelom, Angiosarcom). Virchows Arch. [Pathol. Anat.], *141*:128–152, 1895.

97. Marsa, G. W., and Johnson, R. E.: Altered pattern of metastasis following treatment of Ewing's sarcoma with radiotherapy and adjuvant chemotherapy. Cancer, 27:1051–1054, 1971.

98. Marsden, H. B., and Steward, J. K.: Ewing's tumours and neuroblastomas. J. Clin. Pathol., *17*:411–417, 1964.

99. McCormack, L. J., Orringer, H. B., and Phalen, G. S.: Primary "round cell" sarcomas of bone. Clin. Orthop., 7:47–56, 1956.

100. Mehta, Y., and Hendrickson, F. R.: CNS involvement in Ewing's sarcoma. Cancer, 33:859–862, 1974.

101. Millburn, L. F., O'Grady, L., and Hendrickson, F. R.: Radical radiation therapy and total body irradiation in the treatment of Ewing's sarcoma. Cancer, 22:919–925, 1968.

102. Mitra, S. R., and Banerjee, P.: Ewing's sarcoma. J. Indian Med. Assoc., 66:182–184, 1976.

103. Morgan, S. K., and Thurman, W. G.: Ewing's sarcoma in children. Lessons from 4 cases. Clin. Pediatr., 9:37–41, 1970.

104. Morton, J. J.: The treatment of Ewing's sarcoma of bone. In Pack, G. T., and Livingston, E. M. (eds.): Treatment of Cancer and Allied Diseases. Vol. III. New York, Paul B. Hoeber, Inc., 1940, pp. 2422–2436.

105. Nakayama, I., Tsuda, N., Muta, H., et al.: Fine structural comparison of Ewing's sarcoma with neuroblastoma. Acta Pathol. Jpn., 25:251–268, 1975.

106. Nance, C. L., Jr., Roberts, W. M., and Miller, G. R.: Ewing's sarcoma mimicking osteomyelitis. South. Med. J., 60:1044–1050, 1967.

107. Nesbit, M. E.: Ewing's sarcoma. CA, 26:174–180, 1976.

108. Nouri, M. M., and Hashemian, H.: Ewing's tumor. Review of 73 cases. Int. Surg., 60:478–481, 1975.

109. Oberling, Ch.: Les réticulosarcomes et les réticuloendothéliosarcomes de la moelle osseuse (sarcomes d'Ewing). Bull. Assoc. Fr. Cancer, 17:259–296, 1928.

110. Oberling, Ch., and Raileanu, C.: Nouvelles recherches sur les réticulosarcomes de la moelle osseuse (sarcomes d'Ewing). Bull. Assoc. Fr. Cancer, 21:333–347, 1932.

111. Oehlers, F. A. C.: A case of Ewing's tumor with primary lesion in the mandible. Br. Dent. J., 88:146–150, 1950.

112. Pearlman, A. W.: Growth rate investigation and tumor lethal dose in Ewing's sarcoma. Acta Radiol. [Ther.] (Stockh.), 12:57–70, 1973.

113. Perez, C. A., Razek, A., Tefft, M., et al.: Analysis of local tumor control in Ewing's sarcoma. Preliminary results of a cooperative intergroup study. Cancer, 40:2864–2873, 1977.

114. Phelan, J. T., and Cabrera, A.: Ewing's sarcoma. Surg. Gynecol. Obstet., 118:795–800, 1964.

115. Phillips, R. F., and Higinbotham, N. L.: Curability of Ewing's endothelioma of bone in children. J. Pediatr., 70:391–397, 1967.

116. Pomeroy, T. C., and Johnson, R. E.: Combined modality therapy of Ewing's sarcoma. Cancer, 35:36–47, 1975.

117. Pomeroy, T. C., and Johnson, R. E.: Integrated therapy of Ewing's sarcoma. Front. Rad. Ther. Onc., 10:152–166, 1975.

118. Pomeroy T. C., and Johnson, R. E.: Prognostic factors for survival in Ewing's sarcoma. Am. J. Roentgenol. Radium Ther. Nucl. Med., 123:598–606, 1975.

119. Potdar, G. G.: Ewing's tumor of the jaws. Oral Surg., 29:505–512, 1970.

120. Potdar, G. G.: Ewing's tumour. Clin. Radiol., 22:528–533, 1971.

121. Potozky, H., and Freid, J. R.: Ewing's tumor simulating sarcoma of soft-tissue origin. A clinical, pathological and radiotherapeutic study of 4 cases. Am. J. Cancer, 36:1–11, 1939.

122. Povysil, C., and Matejovsky, Z.: Ultrastructure of Ewing's tumour. Virchows Arch. [Pathol. Anat.], 374:303–316, 1977.

123. Price, C. H. G.: Discussion. In Price, C. H. G., and Ross, F. G. M. (eds.): Bone — Certain Aspects of Neoplasia. Philadelphia, F. A. Davis Co. (Butterworth), 1973, p. 204.

124. Price, C. H. G., and Jeffree, G. M.: Incidence of bone sarcoma in SW England, 1946–74, in relation to age, sex, tumour site and histology. Br. J. Cancer, 36:511–522, 1977.

125. Pritchard, D. J., Dahlin, D. C., Dauphine, R. T., et al.: Ewing's sarcoma. A clinicopathological and statistical analysis of patients surviving five years or longer. J. Bone Joint Surg. [Am.], 57:10–16, 1975.

126. Rapoport, A., Andrade Sobrinho, J., Carvalho, M. B., et al.: Ewing's sarcoma of the mandible. Oral Surg., 44:89–94, 1977.

127. Rice, R. W., Cabot, A., and Johnston, A. D.: The application of electron microscopy to the diagnostic differentiation of Ewing's sarcoma and reticulum cell sarcoma of bone. Clin. Orthop., 91:174–185, 1973.

128. Ridings, G. R.: Ewing's tumor. Radiol. Clin. North Am., 2:315–325, 1964.

129. Rivard, C. H., Duhaime, M., and Marton, D.: Sarcome d'Ewing. Union Med. Can., 105:874–877, 1976.

130. Roca, A. N., Smith, J. L., MacComb, W. S., et al.: Ewing's sarcoma of the maxilla and mandible. Study of 6 cases. Oral Surg., 25:194–203, 1968.

131. Rosen, G.: Management of malignant bone tumors in children and adolescents. Pediatr. Clin. North Am., 23:183–213, 1976.

132. Rosen, G.: Multidisciplinary management of Ewing's sarcoma. In Donaldson, M., and Seydel, H. G. (eds.): Trends in Childhood Cancer. New York, John Wiley & Sons, 1976, pp. 89–106.

133. Rosen, G.: Past experiences and future considerations with T-2 chemotherapy in the treatment of Ewing's sarcoma. In Management of Primary Bone and Soft Tissue Tumors. M. D. Anderson Hospital. Chicago, Year Book Medical Publishers, 1977, pp. 187–203.

134. Rosen, G., Caparros, B., Mosende, C., et al.: Curability of Ewing's sarcoma and considerations for future therapeutic trials. Cancer, 41:888–899, 1978.

135. Rosen, G., Wollner, N., Tan, C., et al.: Disease-free survival in children with Ewing's sarcoma treated with radiation therapy and adjuvant four-drug sequential chemotherapy. Cancer, 33:384–393, 1974.

136. Rudolph, R., Weiss, E., and Biel, M.: Multiple Ewing sarcoma in a dog. Zentralbl. Veterinaermed. [A], 16:426–437, 1969.

137. Salzer-Kuntschik, M.: Zum Problem der histologischen Diagnose "Ewing-Sarkom". Verh. Dtsch. Ges. Pathol., 56:629, 1972.

138. Salzer-Kuntschik, M.: Cytologic and cytochemical behavior of primary malignant bone tumors. In Grundmann, E. (ed.): Malignant Bone Tumors. New York, Springer-Verlag, 1976, pp. 145–156.

139. Salzer-Kuntschik, M., and Wunderlich, M.: Das

Ewing-Sarkom in der Literatur: Kritische Studien zur histomorphologischen Definition und zur Prognose. Arch. Orthop. Unfallchir., 71:297–306, 1971.

140. Schajowicz, F.: Ewing's sarcoma and reticulum-cell sarcoma of bone. With special reference to the histochemical demonstration of glycogen as an aid to differential diagnosis. J. Bone Joint Surg. [Am.], 41:349–356, 362, 1959.

141. Schürch, O., and Uehlinger, E.: Experimentelles Ewing-Sarkom nach Mesothoriumbestrahlung beim Kaninchen. Z. Krebsforsch, 45:240–251, 1937.

142. Schwenk, H. U., Hanssler, L., and Pesch, H. J.: On the individualized, combined therapy of Ewing's sarcoma. Med. Klin., 70:2069–2074, 1975.

143. Seeber, S., Gallmeier, W. M., Bruntsch, U., et al.: Recent advances in the treatment of Ewing's sarcoma. Dtsch. Med. Wochenschr., 99:883–887, 1974.

144. Sherman, R. S., and Soong, K. Y.: Ewing's sarcoma: its roentgen classification and diagnosis. Radiology, 66:529–539, 1956.

145. Sinkovics, J. G., Thota, H., Romero, J. J., et al.: Bone sarcomas: etiology and immunology. Can. J. Surg., 20:494–503, 1977.

146. Sinks, L. F., and Shah, N. K.: Adjunctive chemotherapy in Ewing's tumor: are controlled studies still essential? In Sinks, L. F., and Godden, J. O. (eds.): Conflicts in Childhood Cancer. An Evaluation of Current Management. New York, Alan R. Liss, Inc., 1975, pp. 279–282.

147. Smith, J., McLachlan, D. L., Huvos, A. G., et al.: Primary tumors of the clavicle and scapula. Am. J. Roentgenol. Radium Ther. Nucl. Med., 124:113–123, 1975.

148. Solarino, G., and Santacroce, G. C.: Ewing tumor: report on 20 cases. Chir. Organi Mov., 62:591–603, 1975.

149. Stout, A. P.: A discussion of the pathology and histogenesis of Ewing's tumor of bone marrow. Am. J. Roentgenol. Radium Ther. Nucl. Med., 50:334–342, 1943.

150. Swenson, P. C.: The roentgenologic aspects of Ewing's tumor of bone marrow. Am. J. Roentgenol. Radium Ther. Nucl. Med., 50:343–353, 1943.

151. Swierczewska-Strójwas, A., and Gajl, D.: Role of radiotherapy in the management of primary, radiosensitive bone tumors diagnosed as so-called Ewing's sarcoma. Nowotwory, Supplement:103–107, 1976.

152. Symmers, D., and Vance, M.: Multiple primary intravascular hemangio-endotheliomata of the osseous system associated with the symptoms of multiple myelomata, a lesion hitherto undescribed. Am. J. Med. Sci., 152:28–31, 1916.

153. Szakacs, J. E., Carta, M., and Szakacs, M. R.: Ewing's sarcoma, extraskeletal and of bone. Case report with ultrastructural analysis. Ann. Clin. Lab. Sci., 4:306–322, 1974.

154. Takahashi, K., Sato, T., and Kojima, M.: Cytological characterization and histogenesis of Ewing's sarcoma. Acta Pathol. Jpn., 26:167–190, 1976.

155. Tefft, M., Lattin, P. B., Jereb, B., et al.: Treatment of rhabdomyosarcoma and Ewing's sarcoma of childhood: Acute and late effects on normal tis-

sue following combination therapy with emphasis on the role of irradiation combined with chemotherapy. Cancer, 37:1201–1213, 1976.

156. Telles, N. C., Rabson, A. S., and Pomeroy, T. C.: Ewing's sarcoma: an autopsy study. Cancer, 41:2321–2329, 1978.

157. Treatment of Ewing's sarcoma. Editorial. Lancet, 2:391–392, 1977.

158. Triche, T. J., and Ross, W. E.: Glycogen-containing neuroblastoma with clinical and histopathologic features of Ewing's sarcoma. Cancer, 41:1425–1432, 1978.

159. Tzib, A. F., Bizer, V. A., and Mannanov, I. S.: Angio-lymphography in the diagnosis of Ewing's sarcoma and reticulosarcoma of the bone. Ortop. Travmatol. Protez., 12:43–48, 1977.

160. Uehlinger, E., Botsztejn, Ch., and Schinz, H. R.: Ewingsarkom und Knochenretikulosarkom. Klinik, Diagnose und Differentialdiagnose. Oncologia, 1:193–245, 1948.

161. Unander-Scharin, L.: On the tendency of Ewing's sarcoma to heal spontaneously, and on the alterations due to irradiation. Acta Orthop. Scand., 18:436–476, 1949.

162. Vohra, V. G.: Roentgen manifestations in Ewing's sarcoma. A study of 156 cases. Cancer, 20:727–733, 1967.

163. Voûte, P. A., van Dobbenburgh, O. A., and Burgers, J. M. V.: Ewing's sarcoma in children: results of the treatment in 11 children. Ned. Tijdschr. Geneeskd., 121:171–174, 1977.

164. Whitehouse, G. H., and Griffiths, G. J.: Roentgenologic aspects of spinal involvement by primary and metastatic Ewing's tumor. J. Can. Assoc. Radiol., 27:290–297, 1976.

165. Wigger, H. J., Salazar, G. H., and Blanc, W. A.: Extraskeletal Ewing sarcoma. An ultrastructural study. Arch. Pathol. Lab. Med., 101:446–449, 1977.

166. Williams, A. O.: Tumors of childhood in Ibadan, Nigeria. Cancer, 36:370–378, 1975.

167. Willis, R. A.: Metastatic neuroblastoma in bone presenting the Ewing Syndrome, with a discussion of Ewing's sarcoma. Am. J. Pathol., 16:317–333, 1940.

168. Winkler, K., and Landbeck, G.: Chemotherapy of Ewing's sarcoma and osteogenic sarcoma. Z. Kinderchir., 21:1–19, 1977.

169. Wroblowa, M., and Zomer-Drozda, J.: Clinical characteristic of cases of Ewing's sarcoma according to case records of patients examined in the Out-Patient Department of the Institute of Oncology in Warsaw in the years 1947–1973. Nowotwory, Supplement:37–46, 1976.

170. Wronkowski, Z.: Epidemiology of bone tumors including Ewing's sarcoma. Nowotwory, Supplement:13–19, 1976.

171. Zimbler, H., Robertson, G. L., Bartter, F. C., et al.: Ewing's sarcoma as a cause of the syndrome of inappropriate secretion of antidiuretic hormone. J. Clin. Endocrinol. Metab., 41:390–391, 1975.

172. Zucker, J. M., and Henry-Amar, M.: Therapeutic controlled trial in Ewing's sarcoma. Report on the results of a trial by the Clinical Cooperative Group on Radio- and Chemotherapy of E.O.R.T.C. Eur. J. Cancer, 13:1010–1023, 1977.

Tumors and Tumor-Like Lesions of Blood Vessels Arising in the Skeletal System
Chapters 22 and 23

22

HEMANGIOMA OF BONE (LYMPHANGIOMA. GLOMUS TUMOR. "DISAPPEARING BONE DISEASE.")

DEFINITION

Hemangioma is a benign lesion of bone composed of newly formed capillary, cavernous, or venous blood vessels. Some of these lesions are tumor-like malformations, hamartomas; others may be regarded as true neoplasms.

INCIDENCE

The first publication in the English literature mentioning cranial hemangioma goes back to the mid-19th century, when Toynbee reported a single case involving the parietal bone.[146, 147] In 1867, Virchow referred to Ammon's case of a one-month-old infant with a pulsating hemangioma of the sternum.[150]

In a painstaking examination of a large number of autopsies, an 11 per cent incidence of totally asymptomatic vertebral hemangiomas was noted.[70, 71, 125, 126, 145] There is, however, a wide disparity between this anatomic incidence and those hemangiomas that manifest clinical symptoms.

SIGNS AND SYMPTOMS

The vast majority of hemangiomas at any osseous site are asymptomatic.

The rare clinical complaint of hemangioma of long bones is characterized by vague, insidious pain that attracts initial attention. This pain gradually becomes constant and throbbing, without any alleviation or cessation, even temporarily. Localized swelling is rarely encountered and is only present in cases in which the lesion extends into surrounding soft tissues.

The initial complaints of patients with symptomatic vertebral hemangiomas are localized pain and muscle spasm. Neurologic complications may dominate the clinical picture with compression of the nerve roots, the spinal cord, or the cauda equina.[10, 64, 96, 98, 107] This may be the direct result of an involved, and therefore enlarged, deformed vertebra encroaching upon the spinal cord. Symptomatic hemangiomas of the vertebral bodies associated with neurologic manifestations are usually located in the mid-thoracic region, where the diameter of the spinal canal is small.[123] Hemangioma, with or without secondary hematoma, may also extend into extradural space, thereby giving symptoms of cord compression.[84] Rarely, compression fracture and collapse of the affected vertebra may be experienced.[13, 15, 53, 64] This may result in kyphosis or scoliosis.[46] These structural deformities, however, may result simply because of the presence of hemangiomatous involvement of a single vertebral body at the apex of the spinal curve.[20, 40, 46] The neurologic manifestations are characterized by hyperesthesia, hypesthesia, radiculitis, and even a transverse myelitis.

Hemangiomas of the jaws may present with gingival bleeding from the neck of teeth in the involved area, loose teeth, and localized anesthesia of the skin or oral mucosa innervated by the corresponding mental or infraorbital nerve branches.

Post-traumatic mandibular fractures may cause arteriovenous shunts.[65]

CLINICAL IMPORTANCE

The clinical significance of hemangiomas occurring in the maxilla and mandible is their intimate proximity to the teeth, which may render tooth extraction, even of loose ones, a dangerous procedure, resulting in a profuse and exsanguinating fatal hemorrhage.[20, 91, 136]

Symptomatic vertebral hemangiomas may masquerade as "disk problems," and laminectomy may be hazardous because unanticipated hemorrhage from the affected bone may be profuse and hard to control. The bleeding may originate from the intraosseous portion of large dilated hemangiomatous vessels, from the soft tissue component, or from an anomalous large vessel draining or feeding the lesion.

Various types of hemangiomas of bones may be seen in the manifold angiomatous syndromes ("systematized hemangiomatosis") in which not only the skeletal system but also many other sites and organs may be involved (Fig. 22–1).[4, 17, 18, 22, 31, 33, 38, 48, 57, 66, 67, 73, 79, 83, 87, 101, 103, 113, 122, 128, 135, 138, 154]

A case of consumptive coagulopathy characterized by hypofibrinogenemia and thrombocytopenia has been described as being associated with multiple cavernous hemangiomas of the vertebral bodies in a 13-year-old boy with scoliosis.[89] A rare example of a patient with Klippel-Trenaunay-Weber syndrome presenting with paraplegia due to compression by thoracic vertebral and epidural cavernous hemangiomas has been noted.[51]

LOCATION

The most common site for hemangioma of the skeleton is in the spine, especially in the thoracic region.[72, 107, 114] Extraspinal location is relatively rare, with the craniofacial bones, the humerus, and the bones of the feet and hands being affected (in descending order of frequency). The rela-

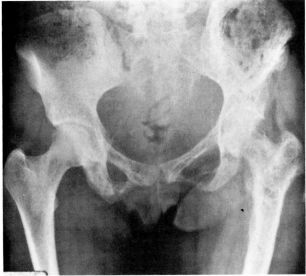

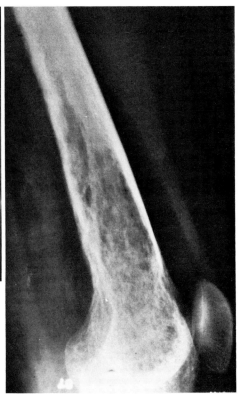

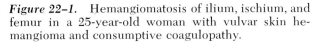

Figure 22–1. Hemangiomatosis of ilium, ischium, and femur in a 25-year-old woman with vulvar skin hemangioma and consumptive coagulopathy.

tive number of cases involving different osseous sites varies with the orientation and the referral pattern of the medical center and the main interest of the investigator. For instance, Töpfer described 41 cases, 29 of which occurred in the skull.[145]

Among the craniofacial bones, the skull, the mandible, and the maxilla are involved (in descending order of frequency). Gamez-Araujo and associates estimated the number of mandibular hemangiomas reported to be approximately 50, with considerably fewer maxillary lesions.[11, 44] In a series of 25 cases of lesions located in the skull, frontal localization was more frequent, in contrast to other studies in which the parietal region predominated.[3, 77, 145]

The rarity of hemangiomas arising in extracranial or extraspinal osseous sites is underscored by the fact that only 15 such cases were found before 1930.[24]

AGE AND SEX DISTRIBUTION

The incidence of hemangiomas seems to increase with age,[125, 126] and their occur-

rence after middle age is more frequent. Clinically, however, the symptomatic cases seem to attract attention in younger adults. Occasionally, children may also be affected. These essentially vague guidelines apply to both vertebral and calvarial hemangiomas.

Hemangiomas at all skeletal sites appear to be slightly more common in women. In a study of 25 cases involving the skull, however, a male to female ratio of 2:1 was found.[3, 77]

RADIOGRAPHIC FEATURES

Radiographic examination of vertebral lesions reveals axial sclerotic strands caused by vertical linear reactive ossification arranged around areas of rarefied hemangiomatous lesional tissue. The tumor usually involves primarily the vertebral body, with secondary extension into the laminae, pedicles, and transverse or spinous processes. Direct involvement into disk spaces or even into adjacent ribs may be present. The affected pedicles become poorly defined, thereby mimicking de-

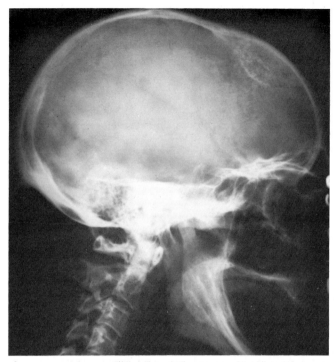

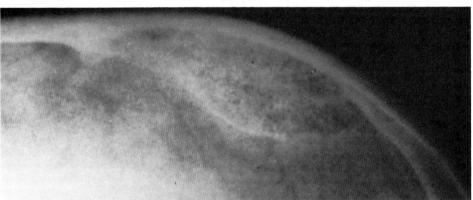

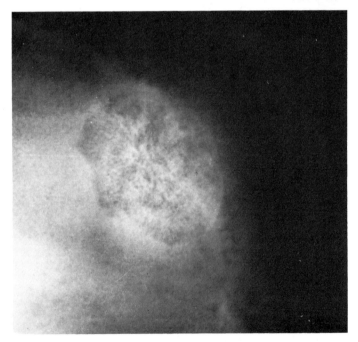

Figure 22–2. Cavernous hemangioma of skull showing slight convexity of the outer table. Radiographs reveal finely mottled osteoporosis resembling foam rubber with spicules of bone radiating from the surface producing a striated "sunburst" appearance.

struction by metastatic tumor. In occasional cases, expansion or even actual enlargement of the vertebrae, particularly the neural arches, may be observed.[96] There, widening of the pedicles and thickening of the laminae are the features.

In most cases, the plain radiographs are quite characteristic and the diagnosis is never in doubt. The ill-defined involvement of the pedicles may imitate destruction by metastatic cancer. Less characteristic bone involvement with a paravertebral soft tissue mass may suggest spinal tuberculosis. Routine radiographic examination may fail to reveal the presence of a vertebral hemangioma, and tomography is necessary to demonstrate intact cortices or actual bony expansion. Once vertebral collapse supervenes, the radiographic findings are not diagnostic. It should be kept in mind that disintegration of a vertebra is a rare and late complication of a hemangioma but is relatively common in metastatic cancer. The coarse trabeculation is more pronounced at the periphery, accompanied by vertebral expansion and, in rare cases, may mimic monostotic Paget's disease. Polyostotic involvement and high serum alkaline phosphatase values rule out hemangioma.

Direct injection of contrast medium into the calvarial hemangiomas is the best method to adequately visualize the lesion.[3] The radiographic presentation of calvarial hemangiomas is characterized by spicules of bone radiating from the center of the lesion toward the periphery, the so-called "sunburst" pattern. On lateral views, a bulge is clearly shown, with numerous radiopaque spicules projecting at right angles toward the surface, the so-called "sunray" effect (Fig. 22–2).

The differential diagnosis of hemangiomas of the skull should include a rare example of sclerosing osteogenic sarcoma or, more infrequently, a meningioma eliciting secondary hyperostosis and spiculation. Insidious progression and a long clinical history mitigate heavily against a sarcoma.

Mandibular and maxillary lesions show an irregular osteolytic defect with a lobulated, multicystic appearance. Fine vertical striations or trabeculations within this cystic area produce a "soap bubble" type of presentation.

Arteriovenous aneurysmal shunts in the jaws display a small radiolucent area that, if located adjacent to the root of a tooth, results in the preoperative clinical impression of a cyst.[29, 32, 59]

Hemangiomas of long bones are usually located toward the end of the diaphysis. The cortical contours of the affected area are characteristically bulging but are not eroded. A loculated, cystic appearance with delicate trabeculations that may appear as a honeycomb is often seen (Fig. 22–1). Rarely, a coarsening of these osseous trabeculae may be featured, situated at direct angles to the cortex ("sunburst" appearance). In the flat bones, these heavy trabecular markings may characterize the radiographic presentation from the very onset.

PATHOLOGIC FEATURES

On *gross examination*, a brownish-red, well-delineated lesion, approximately 1 cm in diameter, is seen in the vertebral body, either originating in the marrow spaces or arising in the periosteum with secondary resorption of the underlying bone. The center of the lesion is less rich in osseous trabeculae than the normal bone. According to Makrycostas, asymptomatic spinal hemangiomas are more likely to be multiple than solitary.[94] The body of the vertebra is the preferential location of primary involvement with secondary extension into the arch or the transverse process. Large hemangiomas of the vertebrae are rare, usually symptomatic, and produce marked bulging of the cortical contours. Hemangiomas involving the skull arise in the diploë, with subsequent progressive extension and erosion of the inner and outer tables. Bulging of the tables due to an enlarging hemangioma is usually more marked toward the outer surface. The sizes of the calvarial lesions range from 1.5 to 7 cm in greatest diameter. Hemangiomas of long bones reveal bulging contours, with the cortex largely or totally intact (Fig. 22–3). The lesions there are loculated with delicate partitions.

In vertebral hemangiomas, *microscopically*, the lesional tissue is characterized by a sparsely cellular osseous trabecular tissue with the individual bony trabeculae

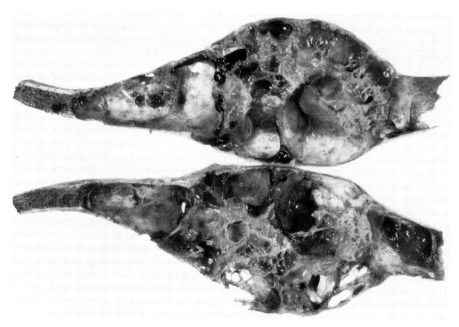

Figure 22-3. Cross section of a typical cavernous hemangioma of rib with expanded contours and loculated inner structure separated by delicate septa.

being relatively thick (Fig. 22–4). This thickening probably compensates for the corresponding scarcity of the resorbed trabeculae of bone in the lesional tissue (Fig. 22–5). The vascular component may be of the capillary, the cavernous, or the venous type. Microscopically, the capillary hemangiomas are characterized by lobules of capillary channels with occasional larger feeding vessels. The lining endothelial cells are small, flat, uniform, and inconspicuous. Mitotic figures are easily encountered. The cavernous type of hemangiomas are composed of multiple, large, thin-walled, dilated, blood-filled vascular spaces lined by flattened endothelial cells. The venous type display small, thick-

walled, venous vessels intermixed with arterioles, capillaries, or large caliber feeding vessels uniformly lined by small, inconspicuous endothelial cells.

Arteriovenous shunts are postulated by some authors in occasional hemangiomas.[15, 99] In the rare instances in which clinically arteriovenous anastomoses are strongly suspected, microscopically, a vast array of arteries and veins with walls of varying thicknesses is usually demonstrated.[29, 32, 59, 65]

In calvarial hemangiomas, the intimate intermixture of hemangiomatous, congested, vascular spaces and the bony trabeculae is found. This osseous supporting network most probably represents secondary

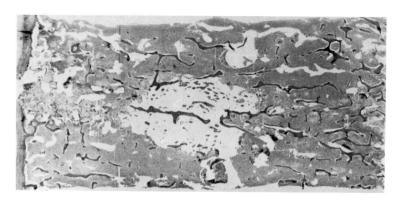

Figure 22-4. Hemangioma of vertebra incidentally discovered at autopsy. (Hematoxylin-eosin stain. Magnification ×10).

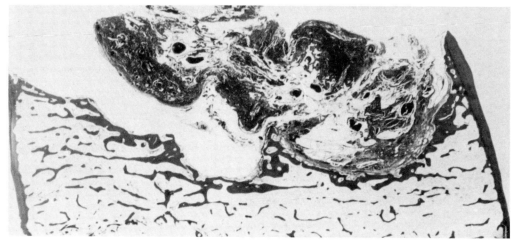

Figure 22–5. Hemangioma next to or in vertebral bone. Note pressure erosion of bony trabeculae.

reactive ossification elicited by the hemangioma. In many microscopic fields, the proliferating vascular channels lie directly next to these osseous trabeculae, but less frequently, they may be separated by a band of fibrous connective tissue.

TREATMENT

Primary surgical intervention in the form of laminectomy followed by irradiation is advocated by some and may yield good results.[8, 15, 24] An excessive morbidity and mortality as high as 25 per cent has been reported to follow laminectomy and is due to profuse hemorrhage.[95] Clinical workup of these cases should include, in addition to routine radiographs, preoperative spinal angiography, which not only establishes or confirms the diagnosis but also outlines the vascular channels contributing to or draining the lesion.[96] The extraosseous extent of the tumor may also be established.[55, 96] Because of the hazards of excessive hemorrhage, laminectomy should be used only for decompression of the cord.[89] Hemangiomas seem to be radiosensitive, and a dose of 3000 to 4000 rads is recommended.[42, 43, 52, 106] It should be remembered that, although irradiation effectively relieves the symptoms, the radiographic appearance of the lesion remains essentially unchanged.[95] Transthoracic ligation of the segmental arteries followed by irradiation and spinal fusion were successfully employed for a case of vertebral hemangioma associated with scoliosis.[23]

An exclusively surgical approach is advocated for calvarial hemangiomas, with total *en bloc* excision of the lesion surrounded by uninvolved bony tissue.[77]

LYMPHANGIOMA

Lymphangioma is an extremely rare benign lesion of bone composed of newly formed lymph vessels, usually in the form of dilated cystic spaces. The lesions may be progressive and multifocal.

It is known, at least since 1911, that lymphangiomas can arise in the skeletal system.[157] These extremely rare lesions may be solitary or multifocal, and they may be restricted to bones or to an association with other nonosseous sites, such as spleen or liver that can form a disseminated disease complex.[6, 16, 25, 31, 41, 57, 58, 80, 110, 132, 157] This condition is usually discovered during childhood or infancy. Single or multiple cystic defects are seen in the bones involved. Histologically, the neoplastic quality of the lymphangiectatic vessels remains in doubt, but a progressive bone destruction resulting in skeletal deformities, pressure erosion of the bone, or extension into other vital structures characterizes the clinical course of this poorly understood disease. The presence of lymphoid tissue in the vascular channels, clear fluid in the lesions at operation, and total absence of blood point to this condition as being a lymphangioma rather than a hemangioma.

GLOMUS TUMOR

Glomus tumor (glomangioma or angioglomoid tumor) is a benign lesion of bone composed of rounded uniform cells intimately associated with vascular structures and derived from the neuromyoarterial glomus.

The occurrence of glomus tumors primarily arising in the osseous system and not secondarily eroding bone originating in the adjacent soft tissues is extremely rare.

Most of the authentic cases have been noted to arise within the terminal phalanx.[27, 37, 85, 133, 141] In a case studied by the author, however, the tumor occurred in the midshaft of the femur of a 70-year-old retired physician with hypophosphatemia and normal serum calcium value. One case occurred in the pubic bone in a 9-year-old girl.[142] This tumor invaded and destroyed bone and adjacent soft tissues. Local surgical excision and irradiation yielded a six year recurrence-free cure.

REFERENCES

1. Abbott, W. D.: Angioma of the skull. Ann. Surg., 106:1100–1105, 1937.
2. Abbott, W. D.: Angioma of the skull. Ann. Surg., 113:306–311, 1941.
3. Agnoli, A. L., Kirchhoff, D., and Eggert, H.: Roentgenographic findings in hemangioma of the skull. Radiologe, 18:37–41, 1978.
4. André, J. M., Picard, L., and Kissel, P.: Systematised angiodysplasias. Classification, nosology. J. Neuroradiol., 1:3–45, 1974.
5. Anspach, W. E.: Sunray hemangioma of bone: with special reference to roentgen signs. J.A.M.A., 108:617–620, 1937.
6. Asch, M. J., Cohen, A. H., and Moore, T. C.: Hepatic and splenic lymphangiomatosis with skeletal involvement: Report of a case and review of the literature. Surgery, 76:334–339, 1974.
7. Askenasy, H., and Behmoaram, A.: Neurological manifestations in haemangioma of the vertebrae. J. Neurol. Neurosurg. Psychiatry, 20:276–284, 1957.
8. Bailey, P., and Bucy, P. C.: Cavernous hemangioma of the vertebrae. J.A.M.A., 92:1748–1751, 1929.
9. Bansal, V. P., Singh, R., Grewal, D. S., et al.: Haemangioma of the patella. A report of two cases. J. Bone Joint Surg. [Br.], 56:139–141, 1974.
10. Barnard, L., and Van Nuys, R. G.: Primary haemangioma of the spine. Ann. Surg., 97:19–25, 1933.
11. Baum, S. M., Pochaczevsky, R., Sussman, R., et al.: Central hemangioma of the maxilla. J. Oral Surg., 30:885–892, 1972.
12. Bell, K. A., and Simon, B. K.: Chylothorax and lymphangiomas of bone: unusual manifestations of lymphatic disease. South. Med. J., 71:459–460, 1978.
13. Bell, R. L.: Hemangioma of a dorsal vertebra with collapse and compression myelopathy. J. Neurosurg., 12:570–576, 1955.
14. Ben-Menachem, Y., and Epstein, M. J.: Posttraumatic capillary hemangioma of the hand. A case report. J. Bone Joint Surg. [Am.], 56:1741–1743, 1974.
15. Bergstrand, A., Hook, O., and Lidvall, H.: Vertebral haemangiomas compressing the spinal cord. Acta Neurol. Scand., 39:59–66, 1963.
16. Bickel, W. H., and Broders, A. C.: Primary lymphangioma of the ilium. Report of a case. J. Bone Joint Surg., 29:517–522, 1947.
17. Blanco Tuñon, J., and Perez Gonzalez, F.: Angiomatosis of the metacarpal skeleton. Hand, 9:88–91, 1977.
18. Bower, L. E., Ditkowsky, S. P., Klien, B. A., et al.: Arteriovenous angioma of mandible and retina with pronounced hematemesis and epistaxis. Am. J. Dis. Child., 64:1023–1029, 1942.
19. Bridger, M. W. M.: Haemangioma of the nasal bones. J. Laryngol. Otol., 90:191–200, 1976.
20. Broderick, R. A., and Round, H.: Cavernous angioma of the maxilla. Fatal haemorrhage after teeth extraction. Lancet, 2:13–15, 1933.
21. Brodsky, R. H.: Cavernous haemangioma of the right side of the mandible. Dent. Cosmos., 73:1076–1081, 1931.
22. Brower, A. C., Culver, J. E., Jr., and Keats, T. E.: Diffuse cystic angiomatosis of bone. Report of 2 cases. Am. J. Roentgenol. Radium Ther. Nucl. Med., 118:456–463, 1973.

23. Bucknill, T., Jackson, J. W., Kemp, H. B. S., et al.: Haemangioma of a vertebral body treated by ligation of the segmental arteries. Report of a case. J. Bone Joint Surg. [Br.], 55:534–539, 1973.

24. Bucy, P. C., and Capp, C. C.: Primary hemangioma of bone. With special reference to roentgenologic diagnosis. Am. J. Roentgenol. Radium Ther. Nucl. Med., 23:1–33, 1930.

25. Bullough, P. G., and Goodfellow, J. W.: Solitary lymphangioma of bone. A case report. J. Bone Joint Surg. [Am.], 58:418–419, 1976.

26. Campanacci, M., Cenni, F., and Giunti, A.: Angectasie, amartomi, e neoplasmi vascolari dello scheletro. ("Angiomi," emangioendotelioma, emangiosarcoma.) Chir. Organi Mov., 58:472–498, 1970.

27. Carroll, R. E., and Berman, A. T.: Glomus tumors of the hand. Review of the literature and report of twenty-eight cases. J. Bone Joint Surg. [Am.], 54:691–703, 1972.

28. Catalano, D.: Treatment of vertebral angiomas. G. Ital. Chir., 11:1037–1048, 1955.

29. Clay, R. C., and Blalock, A.: Congenital arteriovenous fistulas in the mandible. Surg. Gynecol. Obstet., 90:543–546, 1950.

30. Cohen, J., and Cashman, W. F.: Hemihypertrophy of lower extremity associated with multifocal intraosseous hemangioma. Clin. Orthop., 109:155–165, 1975.

31. Cohen, J., and Craig, J. M.: Multiple lymphangiectases of bone. J. Bone Joint Surg. [Am.], 37:585–596, 1955.

32. Cook, T. J., and Zbar, M. J.: Arteriovenous aneurysm of the mandible. Oral Surg., 15:442–445, 1962.

33. Dadash-Zadeh, M., Czapek, E. E., and Schwartz, A. D.: Skeletal and splenic hemangiomatosis with consumption coagulopathy; response to splenectomy. Pediatrics, 57:803–807, 1976.

34. Davies, D.: Cavernous hemangioma of the mandible. Plast. Reconstr. Surg., 33:457–461, 1964.

35. Davis, E., and Morgan, L. R.: Hemangioma of bone. Arch. Otolaryngol., 99:443–445, 1974.

36. Dorfman, H. D., Steiner, G. C., and Jaffe, H. L.: Vascular tumors of bone. Hum. Pathol., 2:349–376, 1971.

37. Dumont, J.: Glomus tumour of the fingers. Can. J. Surg., 18:542–544, 1975.

38. Eie, N.: Multiple primary haemangiomata in the bones of the extremities. Acta Orthop. Scand., 18:219–226, 1948–1949.

39. Erös, G.: Multiples Hämangiom der Schädelknochen. Zentralbl. Allg. Pathol., 43:532–538, 1928.

40. Fairbank, T.: Haemangioma of bone. Practitioner, 177:707–711, 1956.

41. Falkmer, S., and Tilling, G.: Primary lymphangioma of bone. Acta Orthop. Scand., 26:99–110, 1956.

42. Ferber, L., and Lampe, I.: Hemangioma of vertebra associated with compression of the cord. Response to radiation therapy. Arch. Neurol., 47:19–29, 1942.

43. Fuchs, G.: Zur Röntgentherapie des Wirbelangioms. Arch. Geschwulstforsch., 9:1–6, 1955.

44. Gamez-Araujo, J. J., Toth, B. B., and Luna, M. A.: Central hemangioma of the mandible and maxilla: Review of a vascular lesion. Oral Surg., 37:230–238, 1974.

45. Geschickter, C. F., and Maseritz, I. H.: Primary hemangioma involving bones of the extremities. J. Bone Joint Surg., 20:888–900, 1938.

46. Ghormley, R. K., and Adson, A. W.: Hemangioma of vertebrae. J. Bone Joint Surg., 23:887–895, 1941.

47. Glanzmann, Ch., Rush, M., and Horst, W.: Irradiation of vertebral angiomas: results in 62 patients during the years 1939 to 1975. Strahlentherapie, 153:552–525, 1977.

48. Glassy, F. J.: Visceral and bony hamartomatous angiomatosis with fibrinolysis. Wis. Med. J., 59:263–269, 1960.

49. Goidanich, I. F., and Campanacci, M.: Vascular hamartomata and infantile angioectatic osteohyperplasia of the extremities. A study of 94 cases. J. Bone Joint Surg. [Am.], 44:815–842, 1962.

50. Goldstein, M. R., Benchimol, A., Cornell, W., et al.: Chylopericardium with multiple lymphangioma of bone. N. Engl. J. Med., 280:1034–1037, 1969.

51. Gourie-Devi, M., and Prakash, B.: Vertebral and epidural hemangioma with paraplegia in Klippel-Trenaunay-Weber syndrome. Case report. J. Neurosurg., 48:814–817, 1978.

52. Gramiak, R., Ruiz, G., and Campeti, F. L.: Cystic angiomatosis of bone. Radiology, 69:347–353, 1957.

53. Griep, K.: Wirbelangiom und Unfall. Roentgenpraxis, 14:26–28, 1942.

54. Gutierrez, R. M., and Spjut, H. J.: Skeletal angiomatosis: report of three cases and review of the literature. Clin. Orthop., 85:82–97, 1972.

55. Hacker, H., and Alonso, A.: Die angiographische Darstellunge eines Wirbelkörperhämangioms. Fortschr. Geb. Roentgenstr. Nuklearmed., 111:581–583, 1969.

56. Hadders, H. N., and Rinsma, S. G.: Capillary haemangioma of the fibula giving rise to severe clinical manifestations. Arch. Chir. Neerl., 7:257–264, 1955.

57. Harris, R., and Prandoni, A. G.: Generalized primary lymphangiomas of bone: report of case associated with congenital lymphedema of forearm. Ann. Intern. Med., 33:1302–1313, 1950.

58. Hayes, J. T., and Brody, G. L.: Cystic lymphangiectasis of bone: a case report. J. Bone Joint Surg. [Am.], 43:107–117, 1961.

59. Hayton-Williams, D. S.: Arteriovenous aneurysm simulating a mandibular cyst. Oral Surg., 8:21–26, 1955.

60. Hekster, R. E. M., Luyendijk, W., and Tan, T. I.: Spinal-cord compression caused by vertebral haemangioma relieved by percutaneous catheter embolisation. Neuroradiology, 3:160–164, 1972.

61. Higinbotham, N. L., and Coley, B. L.: Vascular tumors of bone. Am. Acad. Orthop. Surg., 5:34–46, 1948.

62. Hitzrot, J. M.: Haemangioma cavernosum of bone. Ann. Surg., 65:476–482, 1917.

63. Holmes, E. M., Sweet, W. H., and Kelemen, G.:

Hemangiomas of the frontal bone. Report of 3 cases. Ann. Otol. Rhinol. Laryngol., 61:45–61, 1952.

64. Holta, O.: Hemangioma of the cervical vertebra with fracture and compression myelomalacia. Acta Radiol., 23:423–430, 1942.

65. Howe, G. L., and Wilson, J. S. P.: Traumatic arterio-venous aneurysm occurring as a complication of a mandibular fracture: case report. Br. J. Oral Surg., 2:54–58, 1964.

66. Hoyt, W. F., and Cameron, R. B.: Racemose angioma of the mandible, face, retina and brain: report of case. J. Oral Surg., 26:596–601, 1968.

67. Jacobs, J. E., and Kimmelstiel, P.: Cystic angiomatosis of the skeletal system. J. Bone Joint Surg. [Am.], 35:409–420, 1953.

68. James, J. N.: Cavernous haemangioma of the mandible. Proc. R. Soc. Med., 57:797–799, 1964.

69. Johnson, E. W., Jr., Ghormley, R. K., and Dockerty, M. B.: Hemangiomas of the extremities. Surg. Gynecol. Obstet., 102:531–538, 1956.

70. Junghanns, H.: Über die Häufigkeit gutartiger Geschwülste in den Wirbelkörpern (Angiome, Lipome, Osteome). Arch. Klin. Chir., 169:204–212, 1932.

71. Junghanns, H.: Hämangiom des 3. Brustwirbelkörpers mit Rückenmarkkompression. Laminektomie. Heilung. Arch. Klin. Chir., 169:321–330, 1932.

72. Kagan, E. M.: On the problem of haemangiomas of the bone skeleton. Vestn. Roentgenol. Radiol., 3:17–24, 1960.

73. Karlin, C. A., and Brower, A. C.: Multiple primary hemangiomas of bone. Am. J. Roentgenol. Radium Ther. Nucl. Med., 129:162–164, 1977.

74. Karshner, R. G., Rand, C. W., and Reeves, D. L.: Epidural hemangioma associated with hemangioma of the vertebrae: report of a case. Arch. Surg., 39:942–951, 1939.

75. Kats, V. A., Yagubov, A. S., and Lavnikova, G. A.: Light and electron microscopy in determination of histogenesis of vascular tumours. Arkh. Patol., 39:34–40, 1977.

76. Kelemen, G., and Holmes, E. M.: Cavernous haemangioma of the frontal bone. J. Laryngol. Otol., 72:557–563, 1948.

77. Kirchhoff, D., Eggert, H. R., and Agnoli, A L.: Cavernous angiomas of the skull. Neurochirurgia, 21:53–62, 1978.

78. Kleinsasser, O., and Albrecht, H.: Die Hämangiome und Osteohämangiome der Schädelknochen. Langenbecks Arch. Chir., 285:115–133, 1957.

79. Koblenzer, P. J., and Bukowski, M. J.: Angiomatosis (hamartomatous hem-lymphangiomatosis). Report of a case with diffuse involvement. Pediatrics, 28:65–76, 1961.

80. Kopperman, M., and Antoine, J. E.: Primary lymphangioma of the calvarium. Am. J. Roentgenol. Radium Ther. Nucl. Med., 121:118–120, 1974.

81. Krepp, S.: Über ein Knochenhämangio-Lipom. Zentralbl. Chir., 90:1674–1677, 1965.

82. Krueger, E. G., Sobel, G. L., and Weinstein, C.: Vertebral hemangioma with compression of spinal cord. J. Neurosurg., 18:331–338, 1961.

83. LaDow, C. S., Henefer, E. P., and McFall, T. A.: Central hemangioma of the maxilla, with von Hippel's disease: report of case. J. Oral Surg., 22:252–259, 1964.

84. Lang, E. F., and Peserico, I. L.: Neurologic and surgical aspects of vertebral hemangiomas. Surg. Clin. North Am., 40:817–823, 1960.

85. Lattes, R., and Bull, D. C.: A case of glomus tumor with primary involvement of bone. Ann. Surg., 127:187–191, 1948.

86. Laws, I. M.: Pulsating hemangiomata of the jaws. Br. J. Oral Surg., 5:222–229, 1967–1968.

87. Lidholm, S. O., Lindbom, Å., and Spjut, H. J.: Multiple capillary hemangiomas of the bones of the foot. Acta Pathol. Microbiol. Scand., 51:9–16, 1961.

88. Loxley, S. S., Thiemeyer, J. S., Jr., and Ellsasser, J. C.: Periosteal hemangioma. A report of two cases. Clin. Orthop., 85:151–154, 1972.

89. Lozman, J., and Holmblad, J.: Cavernous hemangiomas associated with scoliosis and a localized consumptive coagulopathy. A case report. J. Bone Joint Surg. [Am.], 58:1021–1024, 1976.

90. Lund, B. A., and Dahlin, D. C.: Hemangiomas of the mandible and maxilla. J. Oral Surg., 22:234–242, 1964.

91. Macansh, J. D., and Owen, M. D.: Central cavernous hemangioma of the mandible: report of cases. J. Oral Surg., 30:293–296, 1972.

92. Mackenzie, D. H.: Intraosseous glomus tumors: Report of two cases. J. Bone Joint Surg., [Br.], 44:648–651, 1962.

93. Mahnke, P. F.: Klassification, Histogenese und pathologische Anatomie der Hämangiome und Lymphangiome. Z. Aerztl. Fortbild. (Jena), 63:474–478, 1969.

94. Makrycostas, K.: Über das Wirbelangiom, -lipom und -osteom. Virchows Arch. [Pathol. Anat.], 265:259–303, 1927.

95. Manning, H. J.: Symptomatic hemangioma of the spine. Radiology, 56:58–65, 1951.

96. McAllister, V. L., Kendall, B. E., and Bull, J. W. D.: Symptomatic vertebral haemangiomas. Brain, 98:71–80, 1975.

97. McIntyre, N. G., Brebner, D. M., and Gluckman, J.: Primary cavernous haemangioma of the frontal bone. A case report. S. Afr. Med. J., 52:537–538, 1977.

98. Melot, C. J., Brihaye, J., Jeanmart, L., et al.: Les hemangiomes du rachis cervical. Acta Radiol. [Diagn.] (Stockh.), 5:1067–1078, 1966.

99. Moe, P. J.: Haemangioma columnae, mediastini and dorsi. Nord. Med., 64:1224–1227, 1960.

100. Moore, J. A., and Pearce, J. M.: Hemangioma of the nasal bone. Report of a case. Ann. Otol. Rhinol. Laryngol., 65:1012–1019, 1956.

101. Moseley, J. E., and Starobin, S. G.: Cystic angiomatosis of bone: manifestation of a hamartomatous disease entity. Am. J. Roentgenol. Radium Ther. Nucl. Med., 91:1114–1120, 1964.

102. Najman, E., Fabecic-Sabadi, V., and Temmer, B.: Lymphangioma in the inguinal region with cystic lymphangiomatosis of bone. J. Pediatr., 71:561–566, 1967.

103. Nehrkorn, O., and Wolfert, E.: Generalisierte Knochenhämangiomatose mit Lungenbeteili-

gung. Fortschr. Geb. Roentgenstr. Nuk-learmed., *104*:107–112, 1966.

104. Nelson, D. A.: Spinal cord compression due to vertebral angiomas during pregnancy. Arch. Neurol., *11*:408–413, 1964.

105. Nixon, G. W.: Lymphangiomatosis of bone demonstrated by lymphangiography. Am. J. Roentgenol. Radium Ther. Nucl. Med., *110*:582–586, 1970.

106. Otero Luna, J., and Aragon de la Cruz, G.: Radiotherapy of osseous angiomas. Critical study on its indication. Rev. Clin. Esp., *144*:367–373, 1977.

107. Perman, E.: On haemangiomata in the spinal column. Acta Chir. Scand., *61*:91–105, 1927.

108. Pusey, R. F.: Mandibular central haemangioma. Br. J. Oral Surg., 5:25–32, 1967.

109. Reeves, D. L.: Vertebral hemangioma with compression of the spinal cord. J. Neurosurg., *21*:710–712, 1964.

110. Reilly, B. J., Davidson, J. W., and Bain, H.: Lymphangiectasis of the skeleton. A case report. Radiology, *103*:385–386, 1972.

111. Resnick, D., and Oliphant, M.: Hemophilia-like arthropathy of the knee associated with cutaneous and synovial hemangiomas. Report of 3 cases and review of the literature. Radiology, *114*:323–326, 1975.

112. Rimondini, P., and Ferri, G. R.: Hemangiomas of the nasal bone. Otorinolaringol. Ital., 37:210–225, 1969.

113. Ritchie, G., and Zeier, F. G.: Hemangiomatosis of the skeleton and the spleen. J. Bone Joint Surg. [Am.], 38:115–122, 1956.

114. Robbins, L. R., and Fountain, E. N.: Hemangioma of cervical vertebras with spinal-cord compression. N. Engl. J. Med., 258:685–687, 1958.

115. Rolain, G., Olive, D., Marchal, C., et al.: Étude radiologique d'angiomes multiples hépatiques et osseux chez un nourrison. J. Radiol. Electrol. Med. Nucl., 59:109–111, 1978.

116. Rondier, J., Cayla, J., Chevrot, A., et al.: Les angiomatoses osseuses diffuses. Rev. Rhum. Mal. Osteoartic., 44:347–353, 1977.

117. Rosenquist, C. J., and Wolfe, D. C.: Lymphangioma of bone. J. Bone Joint Surg. [Am.], 50:158–162, 1968.

118. Sargent, E. N., Reilly, E. B., and Posnikoff, J.: Primary hemangioma of the skull. Case report of an unusual tumor. Am. J. Roentgenol., 95:874–879, 1965.

119. Sauvegrain, J., Parsa, G., Aicardi, J., et al.: Intraosseous lymphangiectasia and congenital lymphedema. Ann. Radiol., 16:1–10, 1973.

120. Schajowicz, F., Aiello, C. L., Francone, M. V., et al.: Cystic angiomatosis (hamartous haemolymphangiomatosis) of bone. A clinicopathological study of three cases. J. Bone Joint Surg. [Br.], 60:100–106, 1978.

121. Schettler, D., Bock, W. J., and Fiebach, B. J.O.: Methode der artefiziellen Embolisierung und Blockresektion bei ausgedehntem, ossarem Angiom des Oberkiefers. Fortschr. Kiefer, Gesichtschir., 22:189–191, 1977.

122. Schmmel, D. H., Moss, A. A., and Korobkin, M.: Use of abdominal arteriography in assessing diffuse skeletal haemangiomatosis. Br. J. Radiol., 47:142–144, 1974.

123. Schlezinger, N. S., and Ungar, H.: Hemangioma of the vertebra with compression myelopathy. Am. J. Roentgenol. Radium Ther. Nucl. Med., 42:192–216, 1939.

124. Schmidt, M. B.: Allgemeine Pathologie und pathologische Anatomie der Knochen. Fibrome, Myxome, Angiome. Ergeb. Pathol., 7:158–161, 1902.

125. Schmorl, G.: Die pathologische Anatomie der Wirbelsäule. Verh. Dtsch. Orthop. Ges., 21:3–41, 1927.

126. Schmorl, G., and Junghanns, H.: The Human Spine in Health and Disease. 2nd ed. New York, Grune & Stratton, 1971, p. 325.

127. Scott, P. W. B., Silvers, D. N., and Helwig, E. B.: Proliferating angioendotheliomatosis. Arch. Pathol., 99:323–326, 1975.

128. Seckler, S. G., Rubin, H., and Rabinowitz, J. G.: Systemic cystic angiomatosis. Am. J. Med., 37:976–986, 1964.

129. Sherman, M. S.: Capillary hemangioma of bone. Arch. Pathol., 38: 158–161, 1944.

130. Sherman, R. S., and Wilner, D.: The roentgen diagnosis of hemangioma of bone. Am. J. Roentgenol. Radium Ther. Nucl. Med., 86:1146–1159, 1961.

131. Shklar, G., and Meyer, I.: Vascular tumors of the mouth and jaws. Oral Surg., 19:335–358, 1965.

132. Shopfner, C. E., and Allen, R. P.: Lymphangioma of bone. Radiology, 76:449–453, 1961.

133. Siegel, M. W.: Intraosseous glomus tumor. A case report. Am. J. Orthop., 9:68–69, 1967.

134. Siegelman, S. S., Frankel, T. N., and Lewin, M. L.: Hemangioma of the nasal bone: Report of a case. Arch. Otolaryngol., 88:269–272, 1968.

135. Singh, R., Grewal, D. S., Bannerjee, A. K., et al.: Haemangiomatosis of the skeleton. Report of a case. J. Bone Joint Surg. [Br.], 56:136–138, 1974.

136. Smith, H. W.: Hemangioma of the jaws. Review of literature and report of a case. Arch. Otolaryngol., 70:579–587, 1959.

137. Smith, R. A.: Central hemangioma of the maxilla. Aust. Dent. J., 17:117–119, 1972.

138. Spjut, H. J., and Lindbom, Å.: Skeletal angiomatosis. Report of two cases. Acta Pathol. Microbiol. Scand., 55:49–58, 1962.

139. Steiner, G. M., Farman, J., and Lawson, J. P.: Lymphangiomatosis of bone. Radiology, 93:1093–1098, 1969.

140. Sugiura, I.: Tibial periosteal hemangioma. Clin. Orthop., 106:242–244, 1975.

141. Sugiura, I.: Intra-osseous glomus tumour. A case report. J. Bone Joint Surg. [Br.], 58:245–247, 1976.

142. Tang, T. T., Zuege, R. C., Babbitt, D. P., et al.: Angioglomoid tumor of bone. J. Bone Joint Surg. [Am.], 58:873–876, 1976.

143. Thomas, A.: Vascular tumors of bone. A pathological and clinical study of twenty-seven cases. Surg. Gynecol. Obstet., 74:777–795, 1942.

144. Topazian, R. G.: Central hemangioma of the mandible: Report of a case. Oral Surg., 18:1–6, 1964.

145. Töpfer, D.: I. Über ein infiltrierend wachsendes Hämangiom der Haut und multiple Kapil-

larektasien der Haut und inneren Organe. II. Zur Kenntnis der Wirbelangiome. Frankf. Z. Pathol., 36:337–345, 1928.

146. Toynbee, J.: An account of two vascular tumours developed in the substance of bone. Lancet, 2:676, 1845.

147. Toynbee, J.: Aneurism by anastomosis, in the substance of the parietal bones. Lancet, 1:230, 1847.

148. Trommer, B.: Zur Lehre der Hämangiome der Wirbelsäule. Frankf. Z. Pathol., 22:313–316, 1919–1920.

149. van den Bosch, J., van Damme, B., Baert, A., et al.: Diffuse skeletal haemangiomatosis with visceral haemangiomas. Ned. Tijdschr. Geneeskd., 119:1669–1674, 1975.

150. Virchow, R.: Die Krankhaften Geschwülste. Vol. 3. Berlin, Hirschwald, 1867, pp. 306–496.

151. Waldron, R. L., II, and Zeller, J. A.: Diffuse skeletal hemangiomatosis with visceral involvement. J. Can. Assoc. Radiol., 20:119–123, 1969.

152. Walker, E. A., Jr., and McHenry, L. C.: Primary hemangioma of the zygoma. Arch. Otolaryngol., 81:199–203, 1965.

153. Wallace, S.: Dynamics of normal and abnormal lymphatic systems as studied with contrast media. Cancer Chemother. Rep., 52:31–58, 1968.

154. Wallis, L. A., Asch, T., and Maisel, B. W.: Diffuse skeletal hemangiomatosis. Report of 2 cases and review of literature. Am. J. Med., 37:545–563, 1964.

155. Weinstein, I., Yamanaka, H., and Fuchihata, H.: Resection and reconstruction of the mandible for removal of a central hemangioma. Oral Surg., 16:2–13, 1963.

156. Winterberger, A. R.: Radiographic diagnosis of lymphangiomatosis of bone. Radiology, 102:321–324, 1972.

157. Wrede, L.: Ueber Lymphangiome im Knochen. Beitr. Klin. Chir., 73:213–225, 1911.

158. Wyke, B. D.: Primary hemangioma of the skull. A rare cranial tumor. Am. J. Roentgenol. Radium Ther. Nucl. Med., 61:302–316, 1946.

159. Zsebök, Z.: Klavikulahemangiom. Fortschr. Geb. Roentgenstr. Nuklearmed., 87:131–132, 1957.

"DISAPPEARING BONE DISEASE"

Massive osteolysis is a rare disease of unknown etiology that is characterized by the usually spontaneous and progressive destruction and disappearance of one or more bones. Synonyms abound: massive osteolysis, essential osteolysis, vanishing bone disease, disappearing bone disease, phantom bone disease, Gorham's disease, Jackson-Gorham's disease, spontaneous absorption of bone, and progressive atrophy of bone. This disorder was described in 1838 and in 1872 when a "a boneless arm," i.e., absorption of the humerus following fracture, was noted.[3, 7] Our basic understanding of this condition has advanced very little, although by now about 100 cases involving almost every bone or combination of bones have been reported. Some, but definitely not all, cases reveal multiple hemangiomas confined either to a single bone or to a number of contiguous bones without any skip areas of osseous involvement.[33] The soft tissue involvement is restricted to regions directly adjacent to the bone lesions.

No sexual predilection is discernible, but most of the cases occur in children or in adults under the age of 40 years. Frequently, a history of recent trauma can be elicited. In Kümmell's disease, a wedging collapse of a vertebral body (vertebra plana) due to a linear fracture, which is often not demonstrable in roentgenographs taken immediately after the initial trauma, is seen. After a second, often minor, traumatic incident, the vertebral body disintegrates. One wonders whether this disease is, in fact, related to the idiopathic massive osteolysis as described above.

There have been unsuccessful attempts at filling the dilated vascular channels by angiographic means.[37, 42] Other physicians however, have succeeded by injecting contrast medium directly into the lesion.[29, 33]

REFERENCES

1. Abel, M. S., and Smith, G. R.: The case of the disappearing pelvis. Radiology, 111:105–106, 1974.

2. Abell, J. M., Jr., and Badgley, C. E.: Disappearing bone disease. J.A.M.A., 177:771–773, 1961.

3. Absorption of the humerus after fracture. Boston Med. Surg. J. N.S., 10:245–247, 1872.

4. Aston, J. N.: A case of massive osteolysis of the femur. J. Bone Joint Surg. [Br.], 40:514–518, 1958.

5. Aulich, A., Schindler, E., and Kretzschmar, K.: Zur röntgenologischen Differentialdiagnose von Osteolysen der Schädelbasis. Radiologe, 18:62–68, 1978.

6. Beals, R. K., and Bird, C. B.: Carpal and tarsal

osteolysis. A case report and review of the literature. J. Bone Joint Surg. [Am.], 57:681–686, 1975.

7. A boneless arm. Boston Med. Surg. J., 18:368–369, 1838.

8. Branch, H. E.: Acute spontaneous absorption of bone. Report of a case involving a clavicle and a scapula. J. Bone Joint Surg., 27:706–710, 1945.

9. Branco, F., and da Silva Horta, J.: Notes on a rare case of essential osteolysis. J. Bone Joint Surg. [Br.], 40:519–527, 1958.

10. Bullough, P. G.: Massive osteolysis. N.Y. State J. Med., 71:2267–2278, 1971.

11. Butler, R. W., McCance, R. A., and Barrett, A. M.: Unexplained destruction of the shaft of the femur in a child. J. Bone Joint Surg. [Br.], 40:487–493, 1958.

12. Campbell, J., Almond, H. G. A., and Johnson, R.: Massive osteolysis of the humerus with spontaneous recovery. Report of a case. J. Bone Joint Surg. [Br.], 57:238–240, 1975.

13. Case records of the Massachusetts General Hospital. Case 16-1964. N. Engl. J. Med., 270:731–736, 1964.

14. Caulet, T., Fandre, M., Adnet, J. J., et al.: Ostéolyse massive scapulo-cléido-costale. Ann. Anat. Pathol., 13:177–199, 1968.

15. D'Amico, J. A., Hoffman, G. C., and Dyment, P. G.: Klippel-Trénaunay syndrome associated with chronic disseminated intravascular coagulation and massive osteolysis. Cleve. Clin. Q., 44:181–188, 1977.

16. De Sèze, S., and Hubault, A.: Ostéolyse essentielle scapulo-thoraco-brachiale. Rev. Rhum. Mal. Osteoartic., 23:517–523, 1956.

17. Donaldson, J. R., and Marshall, C. E.: Massive osteolysis. Indian J. Surg., 24:136–140, 1962.

18. El-Mofty, S.: Atrophy of the mandible (massive osteolysis). Oral Surg., 31:690–700, 1971.

19. Ellis, D. J., and Adams, T. O.: Massive osteolysis: report of case. J. Oral Surg., 29:659–663, 1971.

20. Fine, R. D., and Gonski, A.: Angiomatous osteolysis of the skull vault. Med. J. Aust., 2:867–869, 1977.

21. Fornasier, V. L.: Haemangiomatosis with massive osteolysis. J. Bone Joint Surg. [Br.], 52:444–451, 1970.

22. Frame, B., Herrera, L. F., Mitchell, D. C., et al.: Massive osteolysis and tumoral calcinosis. Am. J. Med., 50:408–412, 1971.

23. Gorham, L. W.: Circulatory changes associated with osteolytic and osteoblastic reactions in bone. The possible mechanism involved in massive osteolysis: An experimental study. Arch. Intern. Med., 105:199–216, 1960.

24. Gorham, L. W., and Stout, A. P.: Massive osteolysis (acute spontaneous absorption of bone, phantom bone, disappearing bone). Its relation to hemangiomatosis. J. Bone Joint Surg. [Am.], 37:985–1004, 1955.

25. Gorham, L. W., Wright, A. W., Schultz, H. H., et al.: Disappearing bones: A rare form of massive osteolysis. Report of two cases, one with autopsy findings. Am. J. Med., 17:674–682, 1954.

26. Grepl, J., and Kudrmann, J.: Osteolýza kosti nártu, metartzů a článků prstů při hemangioendoteliomu. Periferní forma procesu blízká Gorhamovu-Stoutovu syndromu. Cesk. Radiol., 30:118–124, 1976.

27. Halaby, F. A., and Di Salvo, E. I.: Osteolysis: A complication of trauma. Report of 2 cases. Am. J. Roentgenol. Radium Ther. Nucl. Med., 94:591–594, 1965.

28. Halliday, D. R., Dahlin, D. C., Pugh, D. G., et al.: Massive osteolysis and angiomatosis. Radiology, 82:637–644, 1964.

29. Hambach, R., Pujman, J., and Malý, V.: Massive osteolysis due to hemangiomatosis. Report of a case of Gorham's disease with autopsy. Radiology, 71:43–47, 1958.

30. Hampton, J., and Arthur, J. F.: Massive osteolysis affecting the mandible. Br. Dent. J., 120:538–541, 1966.

31. Imbert, J. C., and Picault, C.: Ostéolyse massive idiopathic ou maladie de Jackson-Gorham. A propos d'une nouvelle observation (Mémoire). Rev. Chir. Orthop., 60:73–80, 1974.

32. Iyer, G. V., and Nayar, A.: Massive osteolysis of the skull. Case report. J. Neurosurg., 43:92–94, 1975.

33. Johnson, P. M., and McClure, J. G.: Observations on massive osteolysis. A review of the literature and report of a case. Radiology, 71:28–42, 1958.

34. Jones, G. B., Midgley, R. L., and Smith, G. S.: Massive osteolysis — disappearing bones. J. Bone Joint Surg. [Br.], 40:494–501, 1958.

35. Kery, L., and Wouters, H. W.: Massive osteolysis. Report of two cases. J. Bone Joint Surg. [Br.], 52:452–459, 1970.

36. Leriche, R.: A propos des ostéolyses d'origine indéterminée. Mem. Acad. Chir., 63:418–421, 1937.

37. Milner, S. M., and Baker, S. L.: Disappearing bones. J. Bone Joint Surg. [Br.], 40:502–513, 1958.

38. Phillips, R. M., Bush, O. B., Jr., and Hall, H. D.: Massive osteolysis (phantom bone, disappearing bone). Report of a case with mandibular involvement. Oral Surg., 34:886–896, 1972.

39. Sage, M. R., and Allen, P. W.: Massive osteolysis. Report of a case. J. Bone Joint Surg. [Br.], 56:130–135, 1974.

40. Steenhuis, D. G., and Nauta, J. H.: Osteolyse der ganzen Mandibula durch chronische Entzündung. Roentgenpraxis, 8:607–609, 1936.

41. Thoma, K. H.: A case of progressive atrophy of the facial bones with complete atrophy of the mandible. J. Bone Joint Surg., 15:494–501, 1933.

42. Thompson, J. S., and Schurman, D. J.: Massive osteolysis. Case report and review of literature. Clin. Orthop., 103:206–211, 1974.

43. Tilling, G.: The vascular anatomy of long bones. A radiological and histological study. Acta Radiol., 160:(Supplement) 1–107, 1958.

44. Torg, J. S., and Steel, H. H.: Sequential roentgenographic changes occurring in massive osteolysis. J. Bone Joint Surg. [Am.], 51:1649–1655, 1969.

45. Touraine, R, Bernard, J. P., Troullier, J. P., et al.: Chylothorax et maladie de Gorham. J. Fr. Med. Chir. Thorac., 25:315–326, 1971.

46. Tyler, T., and Rosenbaum, H. D.: Idiopathic multicentric osteolysis. Am. J. Roentgenol. Radium Ther. Nucl. Med., 126:23–31, 1976.

23

ANGIOSARCOMA OF BONE

DEFINITION

Malignant hemangioendothelioma of bone is a neoplasm characterized by the formation of irregular anastomosing vascular channels lined by one or several layers of atypical endothelial cells having an anaplastic, immature appearance. The tumors may be solitary (unifocal) or multicentric (multifocal) (Fig. 23–1).

SYNONYMS

There is considerable confusion in the literature about the great variety of names given to this tumor. This lesion has also been referred to as angiosarcoma, angioendothelioma, malignant angioma, angiofibrosarcoma, hemangiosarcoma, hemangioblastoma, angioblastic sarcoma, hemangioendothelioblastoma, malignant angioblastoma, hemangioendotheliosarcoma, intravascular endothelioma, and multiple endothelioma.

HISTORICAL ASPECTS

The concept of a primary malignant tumor of bone predominantly composed of neoplastic blood vessels is not new, but the detailed histologic criteria for the diagnosis remained poorly established in spite of several attempts by late 19th and 20th century authors. The appearance of erythrocytes in groups of tumor acini was sufficient for a diagnosis of endothelioma, and numerous reports are not acceptable by today's standards. Some of the reported cases turned out to be metastatic carcinomas of renal origin[49] or were poorly differentiated sarcomas of prominent vascularity; others would now be diagnosed as Ewing's sarcoma.[22, 41] The eight examples reported by Bucy and Capp appear to be no more than hemangiomas of bone.[6] There are several well-documented case reports accompanied by a review of the pertinent world literature, but it is very difficult to establish the exact number of bona fide cases, since many have less than adequate documentation.[7, 27, 32, 37, 43, 44, 56, 57]

In 1908, Mallory was the first to use the term hemangioendothelioma.[50] It was Kolodny, in 1926, who studied the cases of the Registry of Bone Sarcoma and identified the two original instances of hemangioendothelioma of bone.[46] The classic study by Thomas in 1942 laid the modern foundation for our knowledge of vascular tumors of bone.[77] He not only outlined the benign tumors but also studied the malignant tumors of vascular origin. He pro-

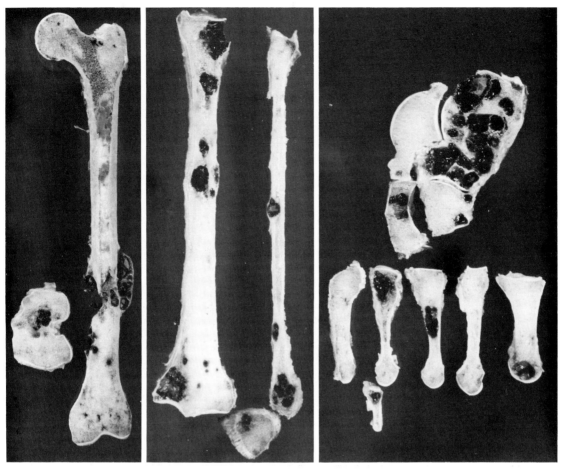

Figure 23–1. Multifocal hemangioendothelioma in a 45-year-old man, extensively involving bones of the right lower extremity and extending into soft tissues adjacent to mid-femur. Popliteal lymph nodes showed metastases. Hemipelvectomy provided the patient with a 7 year cure.

posed the division of malignant vascular tumors into angioendotheliomas, in which the endothelial cell is the proliferating neoplastic unit, and malignant angioma, in which the blood vessel is involved in the vasoformative neoplastic properties of the lesion. In 1943, Stout refined our understanding of both benign and malignant hemangioendotheliomas and defined the latter as a tumor of blood vessels characterized by atypical endothelial cell proliferation with vasoformative properties associated with the delicate reticulin fiber network and an exaggerated tendency for interanastomosing vascular lumen formation.

Particular confusion has arisen from the use of the term angiosarcoma to describe a malignant lesion of vascular origin. Correctly employed, it is a generic term for malignant vascular tumors, which include hemangioendotheliomas as well as hemangiopericytomas. When analyzing the published literature on hemangioendotheliomas of bone, one is immediately struck by the fact that, in the absence of adequate photomicrographs or radiographs, the inclusion or exclusion of certain cases was quite arbitrary.[43, 44] Also, the experience of the investigator reporting a case may be quite limited with these rare tumors of bone.

INCIDENCE

Malignant hemangioendothelioma of bone is a rare tumor. A 1965 review of the literature yielded only 34 cases.[7] The tally of acceptably well-documented hemangioendotheliomas yields 90 to 100 cases, with the unifocal examples outnumbering the multifocal presentation by a ratio of 2:1. These tumors represent less than 1 per cent of primary malignant bone tumors reported by the Netherlands Committee on Bone Tumours and 0.5 per cent of those registered at the Mayo Clinic.[16, 58] The Swedish Cancer Registry estimated the incidence to be 0.86 per cent, with annual occurrence for the population of Sweden calculated at approximately one case per 14,000,000 people.[47]

Hemangioendotheliomas have been induced in animals under experimental conditions by strontium-90, thorium-228, and, rarely, plutonium-239.[1, 2, 4] (See Chapter 9 for details.) Hemangioendothelioma involving the tibia and the soft tissues of the leg has been reported in an 84-year-old man, developing 30 years after metallic fixation for a nonhealing fracture.[19] Angiosarcoma may develop in chronic osteomyelitis.[59]

SIGNS AND SYMPTOMS

The tumors usually produce dull local pain and tenderness with some swelling. Vertebral presentation is accompanied by nerve root pain. The duration of symptoms is quite variable and ranges from a few weeks to many years, with an average of five months.[60] Soft tissue mass or pathologic fracture are rarely encountered as presenting signs. A unique case involving the iliac bone presenting with pulsations and a bruit has been noted.[34] On rare occasions, a primary skeletal presentation may ultimately prove to be a metastasis from a yet hidden hepatic angiosarcoma.[15]

LOCATION

As already noted, hemangioendotheliomas may present with multifocal osseous involvement or may affect a single bone as a solitary lesion (Figs. 23–2 and 23–3). Multifocal lesions may be monostotic or polyostotic and almost exclusively involve a single limb or cluster in one anatomic region (Figs. 23–1 and 23–2). For the 39 solitary lesions studied at Memorial Hos-

Hemangioendothelioma of Bone

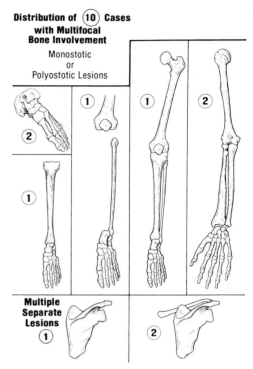

Distribution of ⑩ Cases with Multifocal Bone Involvement

Monostotic or Polyostotic Lesions

Multiple Separate Lesions

Figure 23–2. Skeletal distribution of 10 hemangioendotheliomas with multifocal bone involvement, studied at Memorial Hospital. The tally includes both monostotic and polyostotic lesions. All lesions are on the right side.

pital, the tibia, the humerus, the pelvic bones, and the femur were the most common bones involved (Fig. 23–3). The multifocal osseous involvement in 10 cases is depicted in Figure 23–2. It is of some interest to note that most multifocal lesions were on the right side.

AGE AND SEX DISTRIBUTION

Hemangioendothelioma of bone can occur at any age. It has been recorded in children and in mature adults, with the age ranging from 10 to 75 years in patients at Memorial Hospital.[24] The average age was 43 years among women and 32 years among men. Patients affected by multifocal disease are, on the average, 10 years younger than those with unifocal lesions. Multifocal disease is much more frequent among males, in contrast to solitary bone involvement, for which the sex incidence is equal.

HEMANGIOENDOTHELIOMA OF BONE
Distribution of 39 Cases with
Solitary Bone Involvement
(single lesions)

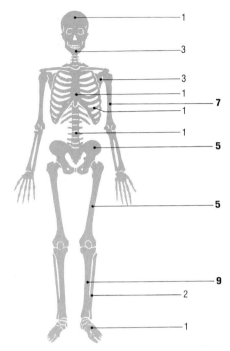

Figure 23–3. Skeletal distribution of 39 hemangioendotheliomas with solitary (unifocal) bone involvement, treated or seen in consultation at Memorial Hospital.

RADIOGRAPHIC FEATURES

The lesions may appear in the long or short tubular bones or involve the flat bones and tend to be in metaphyseal locations (Fig. 23–4). Only rarely are diaphyseal locations noted (Fig. 23–5).[42] These tumors are purely osteolytic with expansile contours and minimal periosteal reaction (Fig. 23–6). The overlying cortex is partially or totally eroded, with an occasional zone of sclerosis surrounding the tumor. The borders vary from well-demarcated and even to irregular and indistinct. Radiologic features of intralesional new bone formation have been described in a case arising in the mandible.[68] The radiographic appearance of solitary hemangioendotheliomas of bone is completely nonspecific and definite identification seems unlikely. Solitary plasmacytoma, medullary fibrosarcoma, or an osteolytic metastasis from an unknown primary tumor are commonly considered.

In multifocal presentation with small "punched out" areas, the diagnostic accuracy is quite considerable. The lesions here are clustered in a single limb or in a single anatomic region (Figs. 23–1 and 23–4). In general, they are small, measuring 1 to 2 cm in diameter, and appear to be well-circumscribed. Occasionally, they may be considerably larger, showing well-defined septum formation imitating a metastatic lesion from a primary renal cancer.

Angiography

Angiographic studies clearly outline the extent of most lesions, although in some only ill-defined areas of increased tumor staining may be noted. In general, the distally located lesions exhibit more bone destruction and have an abnormal vascular pattern.[70] However, the proximally located hemangioendotheliomas, both multifocal and solitary, reveal only slight vascular abnormalities with minimal tumor staining, which goes hand in hand with relatively minor osseous destruction. Most of the lesions are diffusely vascular, but there is no evidence of arteriovenous shunting, although prominent large sinusoidal filling may be seen. The arteriographic examination clearly outlined extension of the tumor into the surrounding soft tissues. In the differential diagnosis of highly vascular lesions of bone, the arteriographic appearance of metastatic renal or thyroid carcinoma or the solitary form of plasma cell myeloma may show similar vascular tumor staining characteristics.

PATHOLOGIC FEATURES

On *gross examination*, the lesions are soft, fleshy, and highly vascular and have an appearance of an organizing blood clot or sponge rubber (Fig. 23–7). The tumor nodules are of varying size but appear to be well-delineated and occasionally raised and are located in the cortex or the medulla. Periosteal or adjacent soft tissue extension may be noted.[10]

Microscopically, a varied spectrum of appearances is noted, but the vast majority of the tumors display characteristic features. In the smallest lesions, a pronounced proliferation of capillaries domi-

Text continued on page 367

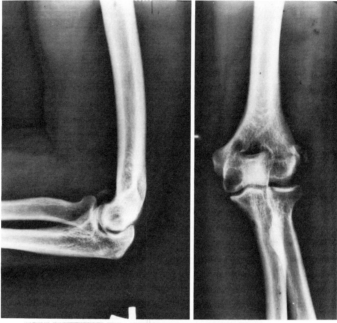

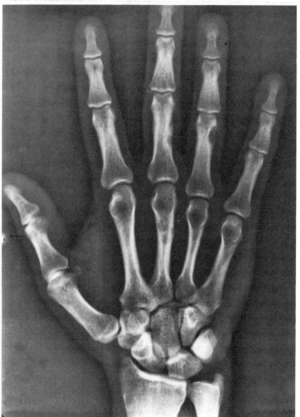

Figure 23–4. Multifocal hemangioendothelioma involving bones of the hand and arm in a 26-year-old man. Note lytic "punched out" lesions.

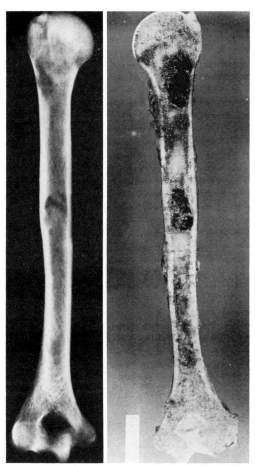

Figure 23–5. Multifocal hemangioendothelioma showing two separate lesions (upper and midshaft) of the right humerus in a 36-year-old man. Two curettages followed by forequarter amputation resulted in the patient being disease-free for over three years.

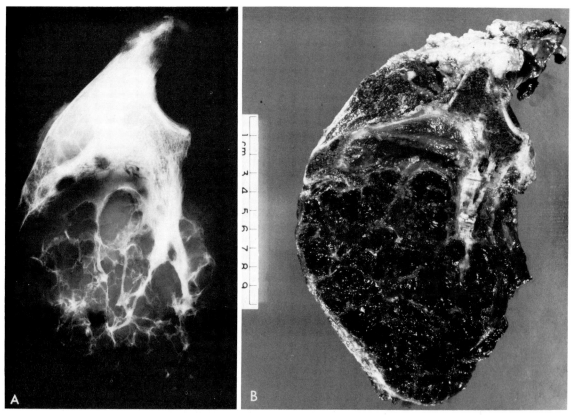

Figure 23-6. A, Specimen radiograph of the scapula showing extensive, lytic honeycombed destruction by hemangioendothelioma in a 32-year-old man. (From Smith, J., McLachlan, D. L., Huvos, A. G., et al.: Primary tumors of the clavicle and scapula. Am. J. Roentgenol. Radium Ther. Nucl. Med., *124*:113–123, 1975.) *B*, The hemorrhagic soft tumor destroys bone and extends into adjacent soft tissues. (Courtesy of Dr. R. C. Marcove.)

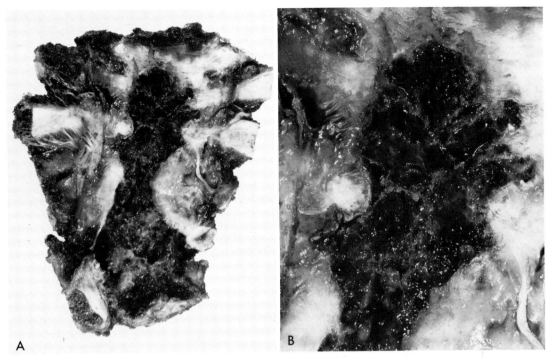

Figure 23–7. Hemangioendothelioma of sternum in a 29-year-old male. The markedly hemorrhagic soft tumor involves the entire sternum and extends microscopically into one rib. Total sternectomy and partial resection of the left clavicle for discontinuous tumor involvement yielded long-term cure.

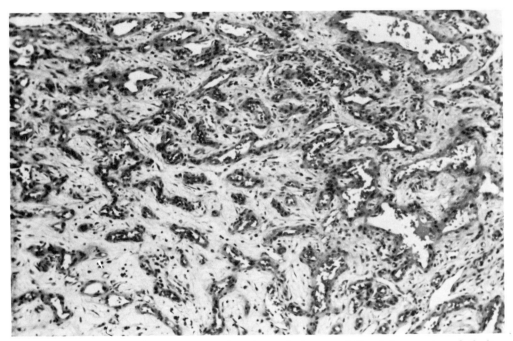

Figure 23–8. Diffusely proliferating vascular channels in a multifocal hemangioendothelioma of bone. Note deceptively benign features. (Hematoxylin-eosin stain. Magnification × 50.)

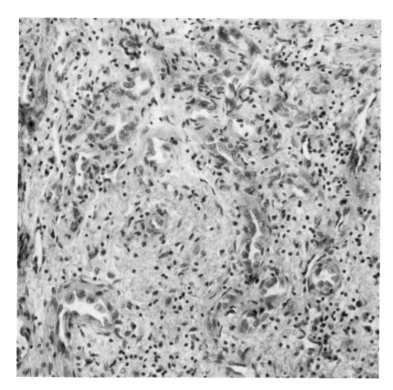

Figure 23–9. Marked vascular proliferation with prominent and quite atypical lining cells in a multifocal hemangioendothelioma of bone. Note the slight sprinkling of eosinophils in the background. (Hematoxylin-eosin stain. Magnification × 80.)

nates the picture (Fig. 23–8). The cells of the endothelial lining are plump, pleomorphic, and hyperchromatic, but their neoplastic quality remains in doubt. The surrounding stroma is infiltrated by identical tumor cells, however. As the lesions enlarge, the peripheral areas continue to show the inconspicuous but freely anastomosing vascular proliferation while the center of the tumor becomes clearly sarcomatous. The interanastomosing vascular channels are lined by markedly pleomorphic endothelial cells with hyperchromatic nuclei and prominent nucleoli (Fig. 23–9). The cytoplasm is always abundant and has an acidophilic staining reaction and occasional granularity due to the deposited hemosiderin granules. A striking resemblance to hepatocytes is suggested. Mitotic activity appears to be moderate. The loose stroma regularly exhibits cells similar to those lining the vascular channels. These findings are especially evident in large destructive lesions. In some of the cases, a definite intravascular papillary proliferation composed of endothelial cells lining connective tissue projections is noted.

The clinically *unifocal* lesions reveal marked anaplasia of both the lining and stromal endothelial cells with atypical mitoses pointing to a diagnosis of a high-grade sarcoma (Fig. 23–10). These cases may require multiple histologic sections and special staining methods, notably silver reticulin preparations, to discover the hidden vasoformative properties within the anaplastic tumors. In *multifocal* osseous involvement, the lesions are composed of a multitude of vascular spaces lined by increased numbers of uniform large endothelial cells with pink cytoplasm, and evenly dispersed nuclear chromatin pattern. Similar tumor cells are seen infiltrating the loose stroma. Cellular pleomorphism and anaplasia are rare exceptions in multifocal osseous lesions but are the rule in unifocal presentation. A conspicuous reactive cellular infiltration by eosinophils may be seen intermingled with the tumor cells (Fig. 23–9). A recent study of large numbers of hemangioendotheliomas of bone, both unifocal and multifocal, revealed that, in general, solitary clinical presentation goes hand in hand with high-grade sarcomatous histologic features and that multifocal lesions are microscopically less malignant, i.e., better differentiated. The ultrastructural features of a heman-

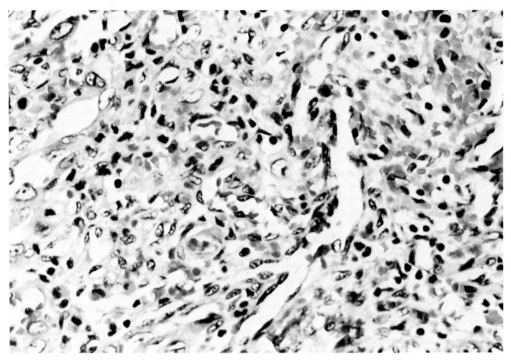

Figure 23–10. The neoplastic vascular spaces are lined by markedly atypical cells similar to those infiltrating the surrounding stroma in a unifocal hemangioendothelioma of bone. (Hematoxylin-eosin stain. Magnification × 200.)

gioendothelioma of bone have been reported.[71]

The *histologic differential diagnosis*, especially on initial examination of biopsy material, most often includes the diagnosis of aneurysmal bone cyst. On closer scrutiny, it becomes apparent that in aneurysmal bone cyst none of the neoplastic cells appear in the stroma between the proliferating vascular channels. In hemangioendotheliomas of bone, one does not find the metaplastic bone formation that is so characteristic of aneurysmal bone cysts. A study of hemangioendotheliomas of bone at the Mayo Clinic also revealed that aneurysmal bone cysts tend to involve adjacent soft tissues as a vascular proliferation, as does a pseudosarcomatous fasciitis, in contradistinction to malignant vascular tumors that invade in solid masses.[79] Telangiectatic osteogenic sarcoma may also be considered, but the presence of osteoid directly produced by the sarcoma cells clearly rules out a high-grade hemangioendothelioma.[23] In occasional cases, a superficial resemblance to metastatic renal carcinoma or round cell liposarcoma may be seen. It is good to remember that any highly vascular forms of carcinoma showing sinusoidal blood spaces are difficult to distinguish from a hemangioendothelioma.

TREATMENT

Major amputation or total resection remains the cornerstone of the treatment of malignant hemangioendotheliomas of bone, whether the lesion is multifocal or solitary. *En bloc* resection of the involved bone with endoprosthetic replacement is a treatment of great promise.[21] For tumors located in the vertebral body or the skull, radiation therapy is the preferred method of treatment, with long-term cures reported in individual cases.[30, 33, 56, 57, 62] In sternal lesions, if the entire bone is involved, total resection of the sternum is often necessary. Ox fascia and Marlex mesh are preferred for reconstruction of the bony defect (Fig. 23–7).[52, 64]

PROGNOSIS

Based on histologic appearance, Dorfman and associates have attempted to subdivide malignant vascular tumors of bone into two groups in order to predict prognosis.[18] These authors have described the well-differentiated tumors as hemangioendotheliomas, in contradistinction to the poorly differentiated variants described as angiosarcomas. The clinical data provided is too scanty, however, and the exact histologic criteria used to establish this subdivision do not permit testing of the prognostic validity. Another attempt at predicting prognosis has been made at the Mayo Clinic.[79] In this study, malignant vascular tumors of bone have been grouped into increasing histologic grades of malignancy, which appears to influence the outcome of the disease. In several clinicopathologic studies at Memorial Hospital, there has been a distinct difference in the clinical behavior of those tumors that were multifocal and those that were solitary.[24, 36, 60] Patients with a single hemangioendothelioma of bone had a much worse prognosis, with only 18 per cent surviving five years and 35 per cent succumbing to their disease within one year.[24] Those patients who had multifocal lesions fared much better. Eight of 10 patients survived five years, and only one patient died of disease in two years.

HEMANGIOPERICYTOMA OF BONE

Hemangiopericytoma is a malignant tumor characterized by the proliferation of rather uniform, round, oval, or spindle-shaped pericytic cells arranged around irregular vascular spaces lined by a single layer of endothelial cells. Increased numbers of mitoses are noted.

The occurrence of hemangiopericytoma

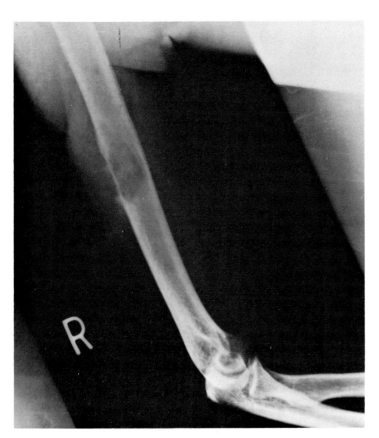

Figure 23–11. Hemangiopericytoma of mid-diaphyseal portion of humerus in a 39-year-old man showing a well-demarcated lytic defect.

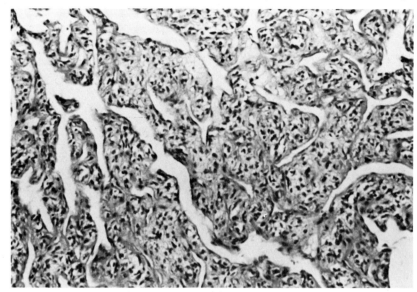

Figure 23–12. Hemangiopericytoma with a classic pattern demonstrating irregular vascular channels surrounded by round to spindly pericytic cells. (Hematoxylin-eosin stain. Magnification × 50.)

originating in bone is very infrequent.[13, 20, 24, 25, 31, 48, 51, 60, 67, 79] Six patients with histologically proved lesions were studied at Memorial Hospital.[24] Their ages ranged from 15 to 48 years and the sexes were equally represented. Pain was the most common presenting complaint, its duration ranging from a few weeks to over a year. The femur and the humerus were affected in two cases each; the scapula and the pelvis were involved in single examples. In two instances, soft tissue exten-

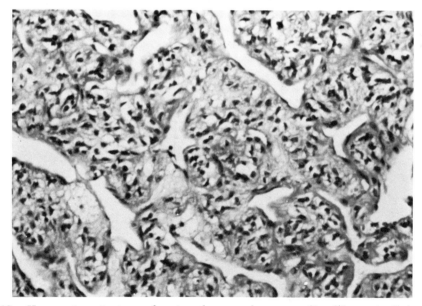

Figure 23–13. Hemangiopericytoma showing the vascular spaces lined by a single layer of inconspicuous endothelial cells and stromal pericytic cells of variable shapes and sizes. (Hematoxylin-eosin stain. Magnification × 80.)

sion by tumor was noted, and in one, pathologic fracture of the humerus complicated the clinical course.

Radiographic examination reveals a destructive lesion with cortical erosion and reactive ossification. The contours of the involved portion of bone may be expanded (Fig. 23–11).

Histologically, the lesions were characterized by proliferating vasoformative channels lined by a single layer of attenuated endothelial cells and spindly, round, or oval cells, the so-called pericytes of Zimmermann (Figs. 23–12 and 23–13). These cells have ample eosinophilic cytoplasm and vary only insignificantly in size or shape in low-grade malignant lesions. In high-grade malignant variants, the pericytic tumor cells show marked variation in size and shape and loose cellular cohesion and reveal multiple mitotic figures.

Before accepting the diagnosis of prima-ry hemangiopericytoma of bone, it behooves one to remember that some carcinomas sometimes exhibit a peritheliomatous growth pattern and occasionally reveal a loose reticulin feltwork cloaking clusters of neoplastic epithelial cells.

Treatment modalities at Memorial Hospital included preoperative radiation therapy coupled with major surgical excision or amputation and chemotherapy. Three patients died of widely disseminated hemangiopericytoma, and one was alive with clinically apparent disease six years after radiation therapy and vaccine treatment. One patient is alive without evidence of disease 15 years after radiation therapy and subtotal scapulectomy and nine years after excision of solitary pulmonary metastasis. One patient with a mid-humeral lesion recently underwent excision with fibula graft followed by chemotherapy (Fig. 23–11).

KAPOSI'S SARCOMA OF BONE

Osseous involvement in disseminated Kaposi's sarcoma and secondary invasion of bone by a soft tissue lesion are well-recognized complications in this disease.[17, 35, 55, 61, 76] The bones most commonly involved, usually by asymmetrically distributed lesions, are the fibula, tibia, radius, and ulna.[61] The characteristic radiographic changes include areas of rarefaction progressing to "rubbed out" loss of bony trabeculation, central medullary cyst formation, and cortical destruction.[17, 55, 61]

REFERENCES

1. Ash, P., and Loutit, J. F.: The ultrastructure of skeletal haemangiosarcomas induced in mice by strontium-90. J. Pathol., *122*:209–218, 1977.
2. Benjamin, S. A., Hahn, F. F., Chiffelle, T. L., et al.: Occurrence of hemangiosarcomas in beagles with internally deposited radionuclides. Cancer Res., *35*:1745–1755, 1975.
3. Berger, A.: Hemangiosarcoma of mandible (metastatic?). Ann. Dent., *1*:15–20, 1942.
4. Boone, C. W.: Malignant hemangioendotheliomas produced by subcutaneous inoculation of Balb/3T3 cells attached to glass beads. Science, *188*:68–70, 1975.
5. Brindley, G. V., Jr.: Primary malignant tumors of the chest wall (excluding primary cutaneous neoplasms). Ann. Surg., *153*:684–696, 1961.
6. Bucy, P. C., and Capp, C. S.: Primary hemangioma of bone. With special reference to roentgenologic diagnosis. Am. J. Roentgenol. Radium Ther. Nucl. Med., *23*:1–33, 1930.
7. Bundens, W. D., Jr., and Brighton, C. T.: Malignant hemangioendothelioma of bone. Report of two cases and review of the literature. J. Bone Joint Surg. [Am.], *47*:762–772, 1965.
8. Campanacci, M., Cenni, F., and Giunti, A.: Angectasie, amartomi, e neoplasmi vascolari dello scheletro. ("Angiomi," emangioendotelioma, emangiosarcoma.) Chir. Organi Mov., *58*:472–498, 1970.
9. Carter, J. H., Dickerson, R. and Needy, C.: Angiosarcoma of bone: A review of the literature and presentation of a case. Ann. Surg., *144*:107–117, 1956.
10. Case records of the Massachusetts General Hospital. Case 43521. N. Engl. J. Med., *257*:1283–1287, 1957.
11. Case records of the Massachusetts General Hospital. Case 46092. N. Engl. J. Med., *262*:467–473, 1960.
12. Cayla, J., Roger, M., Rondier, J., et al.: Les hémangioendothéliomes malins osseux. Rev. Rhum. Mal. Osteoartic., *44*:354–358, 1977
13. Cenni, F.: Manifestazioni scheletriche in un caso di "sarcoma idiopatico" di Kaposi. Chir. Organi Mov., *55*:3–14, 1966.

14. Chow, R. W., Wilson, C. B., and Olsen, E. R.: Angiosarcoma of the skull. Report of a case and review of the literature. Cancer, 25:902–906, 1970.

15. Couderc, P., Panh, M. H., Pasquier, B., et al.: Angiosarcome osseux révélateur d'une tumeur hépatique chez un travailleur exposé au chlorure de vinyle. Sem. Hop. Paris, 52:31–32, 1976.

16. Dahlin, D. C.: Bone Tumors. 2nd ed. Springfield, Illinois, Charles C Thomas, 1967, pp. 100–109.

17. Davies, A. G. M.: Bone changes in Kaposi's sarcoma: An analysis of 15 cases occurring in Bantu Africans. J. Fac. Radiol., 8:32–40, 1956.

18. Dorfman, H. D., Steiner, G. C., and Jaffe, H. L.: Vascular tumors of bone. Hum. Pathol., 2:349–376, 1971.

19. Dube, V. E., and Fisher, D. E.: Hemangioendothelioma of the leg following fixation of the tibia. Cancer, 30:1260–1266, 1972.

20. Dunlop, J.: Primary haemangiopericytoma of bone. Report of two cases. J. Bone Joint Surg. [Br.], 55:854–857, 1973.

21. Dunlop, J.: Malignant hemangioendothelioma of bone. Case report of en bloc resection and prosthetic hip replacement. J. Bone Joint Surg. [Am.], 59:832–834, 1977.

22. Ewing, J.: Review and classification of bone sarcomas. Arch. Surg., 4:485–533, 1922.

23. Farr, G. H., Huvos, A. G., Marcove, R. C., et al.: Telangiectatic osteogenic sarcoma: a review of twenty-eight cases. Cancer, 34:1150–1158, 1974.

24. Farr, G. H., Huvos, A. G., Smith, J., et al.: Angiosarcoma of bone. (In preparation.)

25. Fathie, K.: Hemangiopericytoma of the thoracic spine: Case report. J. Neurosurg., 32:371–374, 1970.

26. Feigl, W., Denk, H., Davidovits, A., et al.: Blood group isoantigens in human benign and malignant vascular tumors. Virchows Arch. [Pathol. Anat.], 370:323–332, 1976.

27. Fienberg, R., and Baehr, F. H.: Hemangioendothelioma of tibia with metastasis to the popliteal artery. Arch. Pathol., 31:811–818, 1941.

28. Freilich, E. B., and Coe, G. C.: Angiosarcoma. Case report and review of the literature. Am. J. Cancer, 26:269–275, 1936.

29. Gandhi, R. K., Kinare, S. G., Parulkar, G. B., et al.: Hemangiosarcoma (malignant hemangioendothelioma) of the mandible in a child. Oral Surg., 22:359–362, 1966.

30. Garcia-Moral, C. A.: Malignant hemangioendothelioma of bone. Review of world literature and report of two cases. Clin. Orthop., 82:70–79, 1972.

31. Gerner, R. E., Moore, G. E., and Pickren, J. W.: Hemangiopericytoma. Ann. Surg., 179:128–132, 1974.

32. Geschickter, C. F., and Maseritz, I. H.: Primary hemangioma involving bones of the extremities. J. Bone Joint Surg., 20:888–900, 1938.

33. Glenn, J. N., Reckling, F. W., and Mantz, F. A.: Malignant hemangioendothelioma in a lumbar vertebra. A rare tumor in an unusual location. J. Bone Joint Surg. [Am.], 56:1279–1282, 1974.

34. Gordon-Taylor, G., and Wiles, P.: Pulsating angio-endothelioma of the innominate bone treated by hindquarter amputation. J. Bone Joint Surg. [Br.], 31:410–413, 1949.

35. Gorham, L. W.: Kaposi's sarcoma involving bone, with particular attention to angiomatous components of the tumor in relation to osteolysis. Arch. Pathol., 76:456–463, 1963.

36. Hartmann, W. H., and Stewart, F. W.: Hemangioendothelioma of bone. Unusual tumor characterized by indolent course. Cancer, 15:846–854, 1962.

37. Hauser, H.: Angiosarcoma of bone. Am. J. Roentgenol. Radium Ther. Nucl. Med., 42:656–662, 1939.

38. Hauser, E. D. W., and Constant, G. A.: Skeletal hemangioendothelioma. A case report. J. Bone Joint Surg. [Am.], 30:517–521, 1948.

39. Henny, F. A.: Angiosarcoma of maxilla in a 3 month old infant: report of a case. J. Oral Surg., 7:250–252, 1949.

40. Higinbotham, N. L., and Coley, B. L.: Vascular tumors of bone. Am. Acad. Orthop. Surg., 5:34–46, 1948.

41. Howard, W. T., and Crile, G. W.: A contribution to the knowledge of endothelioma and perithelioma of bone. Ann. Surg., 42:358–393, 1905.

42. Kaczurba, M.: Radiological pattern of primary malignant bone neoplasms of vascular origin. Pol. Przegl. Radiol., 41:111–117, 1977.

43. Khanna, S. D., Pandove, S. P., and Chander, J.: Haemangioendothelioma — a histologic study of 30 cases. Ind. J. Cancer, 8:269–277, 1971.

44. Khanna, S. D., and Saigal, R. K.: Malignant haemangioendothelioma of bone. (Clinical-pathological report of 15 cases and review of literature.) Indian J. Surg., 36:144–146, 1974.

45. Kinkade, J. M.: Angiosarcoma of the petrous portion of the temporal bone. Ann. Otol. Rhinol. Laryngol., 57:235–240, 1948.

46. Kolodny, A.: Angio-endothelioma of bone. Arch. Surg., 12:854–866, 1926.

47. Larsson, S. E., Lorentzon, R., and Boquist, L.: Malignant hemangioendothelioma of bone. J. Bone Joint Surg. [Am.], 57:84–89, 1975.

48. Legré, G., Payan, H., and Aubert, M.: Osseous hemangiopericytoma. Rev. Chir. Orthop., 52:551–559, 1966.

49. Lutz, J. F., and Pusch, L. C.: Angio-endothelioma of bone. J.A.M.A., 113:1009–1012, 1939.

50. Mallory, F. B.: The results of the application of special histological methods to the study of tumors. J. Exp. Med., 10:575–593, 1908.

51. Marcial-Rojas, R. A.: Primary hemangiopericytoma of bone. Review of the literature and report of the first case with metastases. Cancer, 13:308–311, 1960.

52. Martini, N., Huvos, A. G., Smith, J., et al.: Primary malignant tumors of the sternum. Surg. Gynecol. Obstet., 138:391–395, 1974.

53. McGee, A. R., Penny, S. F., and Chetwynd, J. B.: Hemangioendotheliosarcoma of bone. J. Can. Assoc. Radiol., 5:13–16, 1954.

54. Milgram, J. W., and Riley, L. H., Jr.: Hemangioendothelioma of the proximal part of the humerus. A case report. J. Bone Joint Surg. [Am.], 54:1543–1547, 1972.

55. Morgan, C. L., and Gehweiler, J. A.: Kaposi's sarcoma in bone: a case report with unusual radiographic findings and an abnormal radioisotope scan. Rev. Interam. Radiol., 1:37–41, 1976.

56. Morgenstern, P., Olivetti, R. G., and Westing, S. W.: Five year cure in a case of malignant hemangioendothelioma of bone treated with

roentgen rays. Am. J. Roentgenol. Radium Ther. Nucl. Med., 83:1083–1086, 1960.

57. Morgenstern, P., and Westing, S. W.: Malignant hemangioendothelioma of bone. Fourteen-year follow-up in a case treated with radiation alone. Cancer, 23:221–224, 1969.

58. Netherlands Committee on Bone Tumours: Radiological Atlas of Bone Tumours. Vol. 1. Baltimore, Williams & Wilkins, 1966, pp. 191–193.

59. Olmi, R., and Rubbini, L.: Hemangiosarcoma developed in a chronic osteomyelitis of the tibia. Chir. Organi Mov., 61:765–768, 1975.

60. Otis, J., Hutter, R. V. P., Foote, F. W., Jr., et al.: Hemangioendothelioma of bone. Surg. Gynecol. Obstet., 127:295–305, 1968.

61. Palmer, P. E. S.: The radiological changes of Kaposi's sarcoma. In Ackerman, L. V., and Murray, J. F. (eds.): Symposium on Kaposi's Sarcoma. Basel, S. Karger, 1963.

62. Pearlman, A. W.: Hemangioendothelial sarcoma of bone: the role of irradiation and tumor growth studies. Bull. Hosp. Joint Dis., 33:135–149, 1972.

63. Pindborg, J. J., and Philipsen, H. P.: Malignant angioblastoma of the bone. A case occurring in the mandible. Acta Pathol. Microbiol. Scand., 49:408–416, 1960.

64. Pollak, A.: Angiosarcoma of the sternum. Am. J. Surg., 77:522–527, 1949.

65. Pritchard, J. E.: A case of haemangioendothelioma of bones of the wrist. Can. Med. Assoc. J., 24:689–692, 1931.

66. Röhrl, W.: Angiosarkom des Knochens mit multiplen Metastasen. Roentgenpraxis, 13:389–391, 1941.

67. Sage, H. H., and Salman, I.: Malignant hemangiopericytoma in the area of a previous ameloblastoma of the mandible. Oral Surg., 26:275–283, 1968.

68. Singh, J., Sidhu, B. S., and Kanta, S.: Hemangioendothelioma of the mandible: report of case. J. Oral Surg., 35:673–674, 1977.

69. Smith, J., McLachlan, D. L., Huvos, A. G., et al.: Primary tumors of the clavicle and scapula. Am. J. Roentgenol. Radium Ther. Nucl. Med., 124:113–123, 1975.

70. Smith, J., Watson, R. C., Farr, G. H., et al.: Multicentric malignant hemangioendothelioma of bone — a radiological diagnosis. (Unpublished data.)

71. Steiner, G. C., and Dorfman, H. R.: Ultrastructure of hemangioendothelial sarcoma of bone. Cancer, 29:122–135, 1972.

72. Stjernvall, L.: Vertebral angiosarcoma: A case report. Acta Orthop. Scand., 41:165–168, 1970.

73. Stone, R. S.: Angiosarcoma and myeloma; 2 unusual cases. Am. J. Roentgenol. Radium Ther. Nucl. Med., 22:153–155, 1929.

74. Stout, A. P.: Hemangio-endothelioma: a tumor of blood vessels featuring vascular endothelial cells. Ann. Surg., 118:445–464, 1943.

75. Sweterlitsch, P. R., Torg, J. S., and Watts, H.: Malignant hemangioendothelioma of the cervical spine: A case report. J. Bone Joint Surg. [Am.], 52:805–808, 1970.

76. Templeton, A. C.: Studies in Kaposi's sarcoma. Postmortem findings and disease patterns in women. Cancer, 30:854–867, 1972.

77. Thomas, A.: Vascular tumors of bone. A pathological and clinical study of twenty-seven cases. Surg. Gynecol. Obstet., 74:777–795, 1942.

78. Toto, P. D., and Lavieri, J.: Primary hemangiosarcoma of the jaw. Oral Surg., 12:1459–1463, 1959.

79. Unni, K. K., Ivins, J. C., Beabout, J. W., et al.: Hemangioma, hemangiopericytoma, and hemangioendothelioma (angiosarcoma) of bone. Cancer, 27:1403–1414, 1971.

80. Warner, W. P., and Singleton, A. C.: A case of angio-endothelioma of bone with haemothorax due to pleural metastases. Can. Med. Assoc. J., 29:610–612, 1933.

81. Wells, H. G.: The relation of multiple vascular tumors of bone to myeloma. Arch. Surg., 2:435–442, 1921.

24

CHORDOMA

DEFINITION

Chordoma is a malignant tumor arising from developmental remnants of the notochord in the axial skeleton and is characterized by a lobular arrangement of the lesional tissue with highly vacuolated, so-called physaliferous, cells and ample mucoid intercellular material.

HISTORICAL ASPECTS

In 1857, Virchow named the unique jelly-like excrescences at Blumenbach's clivus "ecchondrosis physalifora," believing them to be cartilaginous growths,[134] and in 1858, Müller was the first to postulate that they were persisting notochordal relics, naming them "ecchordosis physalifora."[97] Müller's thesis was not generally accepted until 1894, however, when Ribbert, basing his studies on the doctoral dissertation of H. Steiner, established their derivation beyond doubt and coined the term "chordoma."[112] Ribbert, and also Congdon 43 years later, produced similar lesions experimentally in rabbits by piercing the anterior intervertebral ligaments with a needle and allowing the escape of nucleus pulposus.[28, 113] The possibility that chordomas may be related to injury has since been suggested.[106] In 1926, Stewart

and Morin suggested that these benign heterotopic vestiges, which some incorrectly refer to as benign chordomas, give rise to the development of true neoplasms — chordomas.[128] These benign remnants and a vertebral chordoma have been found in the same patient.[18] Investigations by Horwitz in 1941, based on studies by others,[3, 72, 85, 87, 96,120] established that "chordoma arises from the aberrant chordal vestiges rather than from the chordal remnants within the nucleus pulposus of the intervertebral disk."[68] Yet it must be stated that truly neoplastic spheno-occipital chordomas may arise in such persisting notochordal residues.

DEVELOPMENTAL CONSIDERATIONS OF THE NOTOCHORD

During the earliest period of embryologic development, before the mesodermal somites appear (presomite embryo), the caudally moving Hensen's node (primitive knot) gives rise to cells that migrate forward between the ectoderm and endoderm to constitute the notochord. At this stage, cells develop from the sides of the primitive streak, as well as from Hensen's node, to form the paraxial mesoderm. Simultaneously, the notochordal cells are placed axially around a poorly fashioned canal that advances to penetrate the endoderm. This ill-formed tubular channel soon breaks down, and a rodlike notochord emerges that, after its separation from the endoderm, tends to lie between the ectoderm and the endoderm.[65] This early intimate relationship between the three primary germ layers stimulated considerable discussion as to which blastodermic germ cell layer produced the notochord. Geschickter and Copeland, among others, maintained that the notochord is of endodermal derivation.[49] Lichtenstein and Robbins believed that both ectoderm and mesoderm contribute to the dual origin of the notochord, which, in turn, is reflected by the cellular features of chordoma.[83, 115] Whatever the case, the notochord represents a unique and specific tissue. It attains complete maturation in the 11 mm embryo, since the vertebrae reach their maximum number of 42 at this stage of development.[68] During the early phases of

cartilage and bone formation, which eventually establish the vertebral body, the notochord is enmeshed within its ossification center and undergoes gradual obliteration due to intravertebral tension. The disappearance of the notochord within the vertebral bodies becomes an established fact during the second month of embryonal life. The marked kinking and coiling of the notochord, on the other hand, accompanied by branching and budding, results in gradual displacement of notochordal tissue to the periphery of the sacrococcygeal portion of the spine.[68] These ectopic deposits of cells may survive and proliferate well into adult life. Microscopic foci of notochordal remnants have been found in the peripheral portions of the vertebral bodies in adults, and such tissue, both well preserved and degenerated, also remains in the sacrum and the coccyx[120] (Fig. 24–1). The central portion of the intervertebral disk, which contains notochor-

NOTOCHORDAL REMNANTS AND SUBSEQUENT CHORDOMA

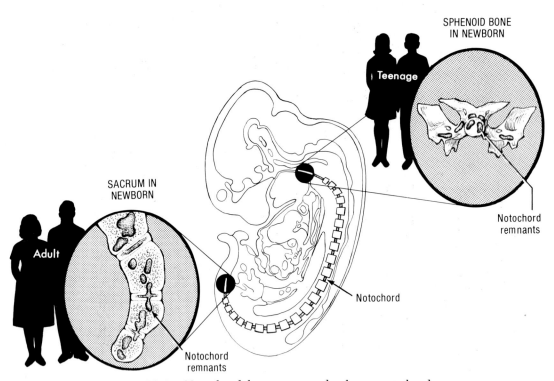

Figure 24–1.   Notochordal remnants and subsequent chordoma.

dal tissue in the form of nucleus pulposus, persists for an indefinite period of time.

During the sixth week of intrauterine life, the notochord substantially involutes at its cranial end and retracts from the infundibular process of the pituitary gland. During this regression, twists and curls with thickenings occur, resulting in clusters of notochordal vestiges frequently entangled in the vicinity of the spheno-occipital synchondrosis or in the basiocciput (Fig. 24–1). On rare occasions, the notochord may even progress in a ventral direction into the pharyngeal wall, where this peculiar interaction between pharyngeal epithelium and notochord stimulates cellular proliferation.[72]

INCIDENCE

Chordomas are relatively infrequent tumors; approximately 1000 cases have been reported, with an estimated overall incidence of 1 per cent of all malignant bone tumors. Some specialized major medical referral centers report an unusually high incidence of 4 per cent. Compilation of reported cases of cranial chordomas up to the year 1970 yields 234 examples.[82] From 1949 through 1973, 89 patients with histologically verified chordomas were seen at Memorial Hospital.

SIGNS AND SYMPTOMS

The signs and symptoms vary with the location and extent of the tumor. Sacrococcygeal presentation is associated with pain in the lower back or localized to the sacrum or coccyx that is present for over a year preceding the diagnosis. The quality of pain is not characteristic and is variously described as dull, sharp, constant, and intermittent. As pointed out by Sundaresan and associates, the pain is so uncharacteristic and insidious that it is often ignored by both patient and physician, thereby causing considerable delay (more than a year) in diagnosis.[129] Scores of patients are initially treated for degenerative disk problems, coccydynia, or hemorrhoids for a considerable length of time, and even removal of a suspected pilonidal cyst may be planned before the true nature of the lesion is discovered. Delay in diagnosis results when patients with lumbar (L_{1-2}) lesions experience pain in the hip, knee, groin, or sacroiliac region. Intra-abdominal presentation obscures the origin of the tumor, and only after an unnecessary exploratory laparotomy is its origin in the spine realized. Paraparesis of the patient may lead to a prompt identification of a thoracic chordoma. Spasticity may occur with cervical and thoracic lesions, while involvement of the cauda equina results in flaccidity. The history of previous trauma to the lower back, sufficiently severe to require medical attention, is provided by up to 50 per cent of all patients (15 per cent at Memorial Hospital) with sacrococcygeal chordomas.[82] Almost all of these patients (95 per cent) are male. On occasion, stress urinary and fecal incontinence, or constipation, may be the first symptom. Sometimes, slowly increasing pelvic and low back pain, accompanied by dyspareunia, results in the patient's referral to a gynecologist.[36] Rectal dysfunction was noted as an initial symptom in 42 per cent of the patients.[129]

Headache, sometimes present for years, is the first and by far the single most frequent symptom of *cranial chordomas* and is present in over 80 per cent of the cases. The pain, the quality of which is perceived as dull and constant by the patient, is usually generalized but may be experienced in the posterior skull or the neck. Signs of chiasmal compression are quite frequent and may be characterized by endocrine disturbances (amenorrhea or impotence, polydipsia, cachexia, weight gain, decrease in libido, and diabetes insipidus) or by intermittent multiple cranial neuropathies of insidious and gradually progressive character. These cranial nerve signs are often unilateral (more often on the left side) or asymmetrically bilateral; symmetrical bilateral nerve palsies are unusual.[52, 82, 118]

Chordomas presenting in the *nasopharynx* manifest with symptoms of mechanical obstruction or nasal stuffiness and purulent or bloody nasal discharge before neurologic manifestations become obvious. A palpable or visible nasopharyngeal mass is frequently noted.

LOCATION

Chordomas arise anywhere in the vertebral column, from the region of the spheno-occipital synchondrosis to the tip of the coccyx.

Among the 89 patients with chordomas studied at Memorial Hospital from 1949 through 1973, 66 cases (74 per cent) were located in the sacrococcygeal region, 15 (17 per cent) involved the vertebral column at a higher level, and 8 (9 per cent) were situated in the spheno-occipital area (Fig. 24–2). The number of cases actually treated at this institution naturally is smaller.[66, 129]

Analysis of the cases reported in the literature reveals that approximately 50 per cent arise in the sacrum, 35 per cent in the clivus, and 15 per cent in the true vertebrae.[35, 39, 43, 87, 136–138] Chordomas in the paranasal sinuses and nasal cavities or involving the nasopharynx are extremely rare, and only a few cases have been reported.[1, 9, 12, 102, 114, 144]

AGE AND SEX DISTRIBUTION

The ages of the 89 patients studied at Memorial Hospital ranged from 2.5 to 74 years, with the fifth to seventh decades of life predominating (Fig. 24–3). Patients with spheno-occipital chordomas were younger, with a predominance in the second to fifth decades of life, in contradistinction to those with sacrococcygeal lesions (Fig. 24–1). The mean age of patients with sacrococcygeal tumors was 56 years; those with chordomas originating in other vertebral locations had a mean age of 47 years.[129] The average age of female patients was about six years younger than that of male patients.[133]

In general, there is a slight increase in the male to female ratio in the reported series for all sites. Among the cases collected from the literature, no clear predominance of either sex could be discerned among patients with cranial chordomas.[82]

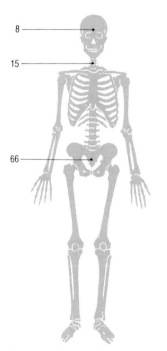

CHORDOMA
1949 - 1973
Skeletal Distribution of 89 Cases

Figure 24–2. Skeletal distribution of 89 chordomas studied, but not necessarily treated, at Memorial Hospital from 1949 through 1973.

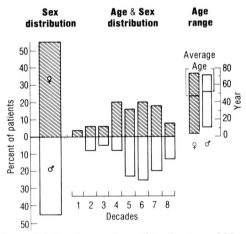

Chordoma · 1949 - 1973
89 Pts. (♂ = 40, ♀ = 49)

Figure 24–3. Age and sex distribution of 89 patients studied at Memorial Hospital from 1949 through 1973. This number includes those seen only in consultation.

ASSOCIATED DISEASES

The association of a clival chordoma with a spongioblastoma[27] and a meningioma of the falx[109] has been noted. Willis mentions the occurrence of a coccygeal chordoma with skeletal osteochondromatosis.[140] The simultaneous appearance of chordomas in twins (classified as autosomal recessive phenotypes) has also been noted.[42] An instance of a familial nasopharyngeal chordoma in successive generations of direct lineage has been confirmed.[78] The occurrence of a spinal (D_3) meningioma and a parasellar chordoma,[38] in addition to a case of nasopharyngeal chordoma and an intracranial aneurysm,[12] has been reported.

RADIOGRAPHIC FEATURES

Radiographic examination is the single most important diagnostic procedure in both cranial and spinal chordomas. The most significant roentgenologic feature of vertebral lesions studied at Memorial Hospital was the asymmetric destruction of a single vertebra with an adjacent soft tissue mass. In other studies, and also in some cases at Memorial Hospital, multiple adjoining vertebral destructions were a more consistent finding (Fig. 24–4).[70, 107, 133] The initial lytic vertebral destruction sparing the intervertebral disk spaces ultimately reveals secondary osteosclerotic changes predominantly at the periphery of the lesion. There has been controversy generated by several studies over whether these sclerotic changes are indeed present and are, in fact, diagnostic of vertebral chordomas.[107, 109, 122, 133, 143] The question of disk space involvement also remains a matter of opinion. Although some radiologists clearly state that vertebral disks are not involved on radiographic examination,[2, 74, 122] others demonstrate unmistakable narrowing of the disk spaces and irregularity of the opposing vertebral end plates in the majority of the patients.[107] In sacral chordomas, massive destruction of several segments is seen, with a soft tissue mass placed anterior to the sacrum (Fig. 24–5).

Myelographic evaluation on a routine basis in both vertebral and sacral lesions will reveal intraspinal epidural extension of the tumor mass even in the absence of neurologic symptoms. Paravertebral soft tissue involvement may be adequately demonstrated by intravenous pyelography, ultrasound, arteriography, venography, or CT scanning.[129] These studies usually reveal the main tumor bulk to be present anterior to the vertebral bodies. Foci of calcification within the soft tissue mass may be seen and are probably due to extensive tumor necrosis.

In many intracranial chordomas, destruction of the dorsum and the floor of the sella, the posterior clinoid processes, the clivus, the apices of both the petrous bone and the sphenoid is present. Progression of the tumor results in a usually purely osteolytic destruction of the base of the skull in the midline with poorly defined eroded edges without reactive ossification.[84] If the lesion extends into the nasopharynx, a contrasting shadow between tumor and air can be seen.[133] Intralesional calcifications may be noted and do not rule out a diagnosis of chordoma.

Carotid and vertebral angiograms have been found to be useful to outline the displacement of the internal carotid artery in the petrosal and cavernous sinus segments and to determine the intracranial extent of tumor in relation to the internal carotid and basilar arterial systems.

PATHOLOGIC FEATURES

Grossly, chordomas are well-demarcated, lobulated, partially translucent lesions varying in size, usually from about 2 to 15 cm in diameter (Fig. 24–6). Often, a fibrous cleavage plane, a pseudocapsule, surrounds the lesion, providing an explanation for less than adequate primary surgical removal. This apparent encapsulation is usually evident only in the soft tissues and is completely lacking in the region of the bone extension by tumor, where the osseous destruction and infiltration are poorly defined. Intact but elevated periosteum covers sacral lesions. Intracranial chordomas are considerably better delineated than those arising in the sacrococcygeal region. The surface varies from clearly rough to smooth. The consistency is also variable from soft, jelly-like, and gelatinous to hard and cartilage-like. Cra-

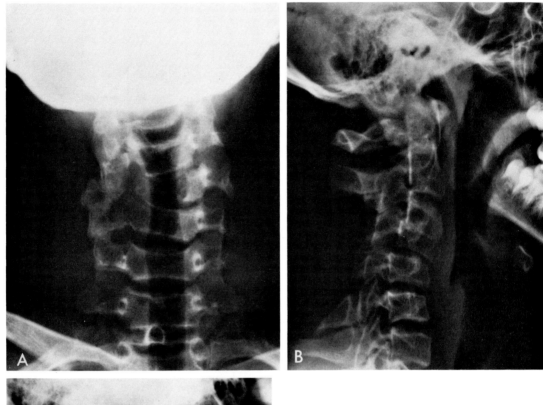

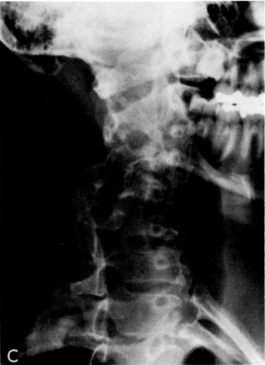

Figure 24-4. Cervical chordoma in a 14-year-old boy with increasing difficulty of neck motion and pain of one year duration. Radiation therapy with shielding of the spinal cord resulted in a disease-free period of 5½ years. *A* and *B*, Following C_4–C_6 laminectomy. *C*, 32 months after radiation therapy. (Courtesy of Drs. G. J. D'Angio and B. Hilaris.)

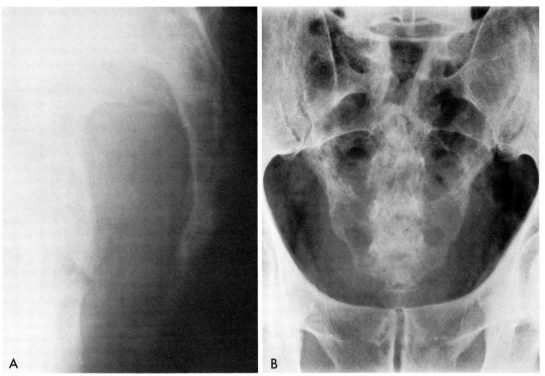

Figure 24–5. Chordoma of sacrum with lateral (*A*) and anteroposterior (*B*) radiographs showing a smoothly irregular destruction of the sacrum and large continuous soft tissue mass.

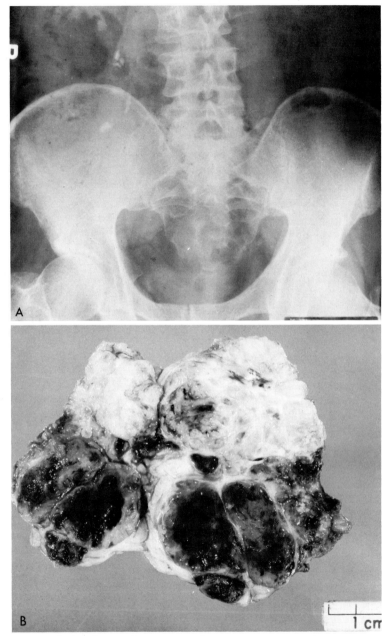

Figure 24-6. *A*, Typical chordoma of sacrum with massive osseous destruction. *B*, The resected specimen reveals a lobulated tumor with solid, gray-white, and distinct hemorrhagic areas.

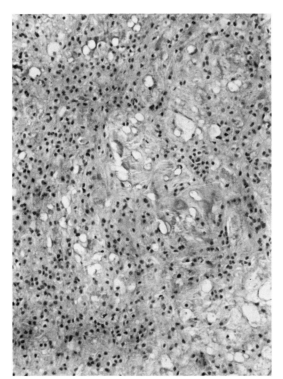

Figure 24-7. Diffuse sheetlike arrangement of chordoma cells. No lobular architecture is discernible. (Hematoxylin-eosin stain. Magnification ×50.)

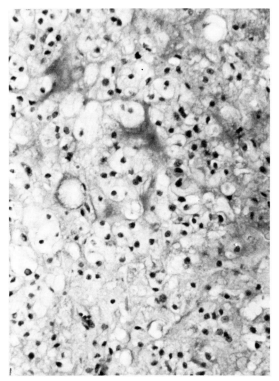

Figure 24-8. Chordoma cells with variation in size and marked cytoplasmic vacuolization. (Hematoxylin-eosin stain. Magnification ×80.)

nial chordomas are primarily situated extradurally, but by destroying the basal dura they secondarily lie intradurally.

An overall uniformity of *microscopic composition* prevails in most tumors, although considerable variability in architecture or cytologic details may be encountered in an occasional case (Figs. 24–7, 24–8, and 24–9). Microscopically, the lesions are characterized by a distinctly lobular framework formed by solid structures of physaliferous (derived from the Greek word meaning bubble or drop) frothy cells with ample vacuolated cytoplasm and the more common "signet ring" type of cells in which the nucleus is displaced to one side by one or two vacuoles (Figs. 24–10, 24–11, and 24–12). A densely thick layer of fibrous trabecular investment may be seen that is focally incomplete and is often infiltrated by tumor cells. The fibrous septa carry the vascular channels, for the central areas of the tumor lobules seem to be avascular. An occasional feature of these fibrous divisions is a dense infiltration of lymphocytes.[63] This incomplete encapsula-

tion and the microscopic involvement by strands and columns of chordoma cells at some distance from the main tumor mass may at least partially explain the high local recurrence rate or, more properly put, the high persistence rate of this neoplasm. The mucinous character is quite obvious and represents the most characteristic diagnostic feature. The intracytoplasmic mucus droplets vary greatly in size, and a positive-staining reaction for both glycogen and mucin may be demonstrated. The smaller, better preserved tumor nodules exhibit oval or polygonal cells in close proximity to each other, showing a striking resemblance to adenocarcinoma cells with mucin production. The larger tumor lobules show ample extracellular stromal mucin production with only a few tumor cells scattered about, especially in the peripheral areas. A marked variation in nuclear size and chromatin is featured with binucleate forms and multinucleated tumor giant cells. Mitotic figures are rarely discerned. Cellular anaplasia and increasing mitotic rate do

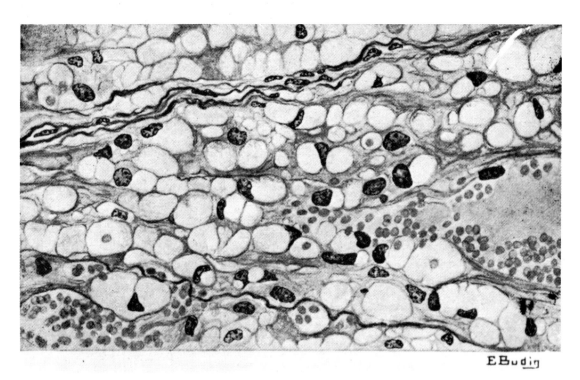

Figure 24–9.   Chordoma of coccyx showing vacuolated signet ring type of tumor cells. Note the delicate stroma and the hemorrhages. (Masson's trichrome preparation.) (Original drawing from Piraud, G.: La Notochorde; Embryologie Générale et Expérimentale, Vestiges et Tumeurs. Paris, Lefrançois, 1933.)

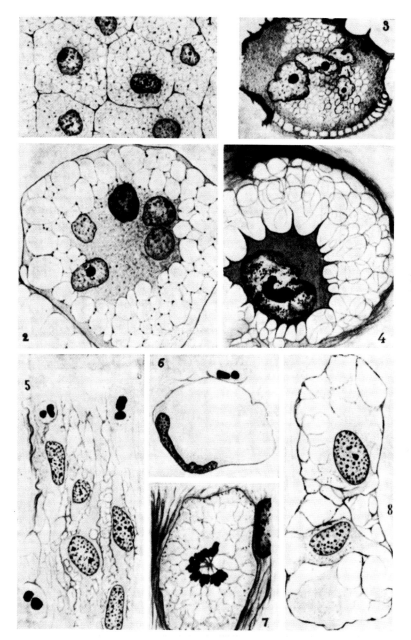

Figure 24–10. An imposing array of various chordoma cells with manifold structural patterns of vacuolization. (From Piraud, G.: La Notochorde; Embryologie Générale et Expérimentale, Vestiges et Tumeurs. Paris, Lefrançois, 1933.)

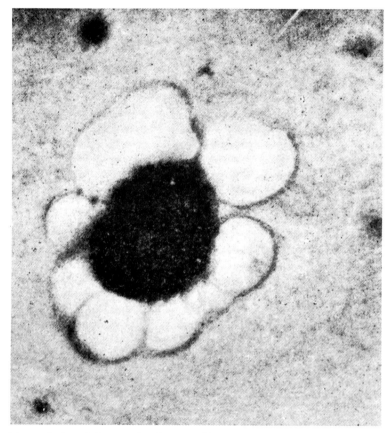

Figure 24–11. Typical physaliferous chordoma cell presenting as a stylized flower. (From Piraud, G.: La Notochorde; Embryologie Générale et Expérimentale, Vestiges et Tumeurs. Paris, Lefrançois, 1933.)

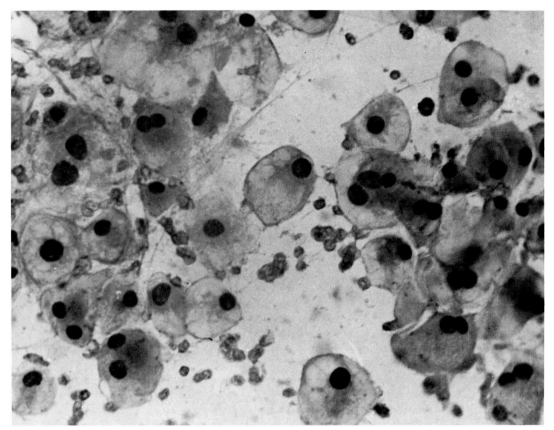

Figure 24-12. Air-dried hematoxylin and eosin stained aspiration smear of a chordoma showing clusters of large mononuclear cells with sharply defined cell borders and cytoplasmic vacuoles. (Magnification × 450.)

not seem to presage a more virulently progressive biologic behavior. The tumor's infiltrating capacity is well-documented by the frequent finding of clusters or columns of chordoma cells invading between the muscle bundles and along nerve trunks.

Clinically recurrent lesions, or those that were treated by irradiation, may show a prominent component of a spindle cell sarcoma, thereby obscuring the true morphologic identity of the tumor.[63, 79, 80]

In the differential diagnosis, benign mixed tumors of salivary glands (pleomorphic adenoma) or heavily mucin-producing signet ring adenocarcinomas of the rectosigmoid colon may occasionally be considered. The key to the correct diagnosis is in the examination of several histologic sections, in addition to the careful evaluation of the clinical details.

In 1968, Falconer and associates advanced the idea that chordomas arising at the basicranium may possess cartilaginous features.[38] They felt that both of these tumors, i.e., chondromas and chordomas, may originate from remnants of the notochord at the skull base and may, occasionally, be mistaken for one another. Based on a study of six cases, Zöch denied the existence of hybrid chordomas with a cartilaginoid component, since he maintained the origin of chondromas at the base of the skull to be from chondrocranial cartilage and not from notochordal residues.[147] The occurrence of "chondroid chordomas" was subsequently confirmed by others.[64, 114] In these tumors, in addition to typical areas of chordoma, an abundant cartilaginous component may be present. Merging microscopic fields are seen, varying from scattered foci of benign hyaline cartilage to fields of typical chondrosarcoma. In an occasional case, the diagnostic decision as to whether the case at hand is a chordoma or a chondrosarcoma may be quite difficult and arbitrary. The explanation of this phenomenon may be related to the fact that during intrauterine development, notochordal foci have been found in the occipital area of the chondrocranium of the pig embryo.[124] The tendency for both intracellular and extracellular mucin production and the usual lack of calcification in chordomas help to distinguish them from cartilaginous tumors. According to Crawford,[31] chondromas show a positive staining reaction with phosphotungstic acid hematoxylin (PTAH) and are readily impregnated by silver reticulin. These histochemical reactions leave chordomas largely unaffected. These special stains were not found to be useful in other studies.[9, 114]

In 1948, F.W. Stewart described a curious soft tissue tumor as "chordoid tumor," and in 1951, Laskowski named a similar tumor "parachordoma."[34] The lesions histologically resemble chordomas but tend to arise adjacent to tendons and synovia or next to osseous structures. Their exact histogenesis is still a matter of controversy.

The thought-provoking embryologic considerations and the much discussed histogenesis of chordomas have stimulated numerous excellent *electron microscopic studies.*[16, 21, 37, 46, 47, 50, 67a, 75, 79, 98, 101, 105, 125, 131, 132, 145] These have emphasized the ultrastructural similarities of the tumor cells to those of the primitive notochord and also have underlined the belief that chordomas are derived from one distinct cell type. Various stages of cellular differentiation and activity from the small nonvacuolated stellate cells to the large vacuolated physaliferous variety can be discerned. By using the electron microscope, it becomes evident that the intracellular vacuoles demonstrated by light microscopy to be so characteristic of this tumor are, in fact, extracellular spaces enclosed by cytoplasmic processes.[47] The intracytoplasmic vacuolization seems to be derived from rough endoplasmic reticulum,[46, 50] from smooth endoplasmic reticulum,[98, 125] or, according to Erlandson and associates, from both.[37] Electron microscopic studies also reveal the cytoplasmic vacuoles of chordoma cells to be identical with the extracellular material, suggesting the means by which the particular synthetic and secretory functions are conducted.[16, 50, 105, 125] Horten and Montague underlined the not unexpectedly similar ultrastructural features shared by the developing notochord, the ecchordosis, and the chordoma cells.[67a] Ecchordosis physaliphora exhibits features of an actively proliferating tumor, namely extensive Golgi apparatus, large numbers of mitochondria, and endoplasmic reticulum.[67a]

TREATMENT

The treatment of chordomas varies according to their location. Vertebral lesions are infrequently amenable to complete removal and, by necessity, are treated by decompression laminectomy, with excision of the major bulk of the tumor involving bone, soft tissues, and extradural space. This limited surgical excision is routinely accompanied by postoperative radiation therapy to attempt to allay the almost certain local recurrence. Sacrococcygeal tumors are best treated by major surgical excision if the second sacral segment is uninvolved.[35] This is often followed by irradiation. Localio and associates advocate an abdominosacral resection for sacrococcygeal tumors.[86]

Simply stated, the problem is that patients with small, surgically completely resectable lesions are quite rare and that the majority will present with bulky tumors of unresectable dimensions. A heroic surgical intervention, hemicorporectomy, has been recommended for those chordomas situated below the second lumbar segment when the tumor is not resectable by any other means.[91, 94] Although some physicians may find this superradical approach surgically expedient, many patients may consider it emotionally unacceptable and, perhaps, unjustified. Patients deemed to be essentially inoperable should undergo radical radiation therapy once the histologic diagnosis is established.

The treatment of intracranial chordomas, all in all, is quite discouraging, since the operative mortality is substantial and the total removal of the lesion is rarely attainable. This relegates the treatment to being essentially palliative. Microsurgical techniques may improve this bleak assessment.

The evaluation of the beneficial effects of radiotherapy is hampered by the great variation in the techniques employed in the past.[27, 38, 57, 66, 74, 96, 103, 104, 109, 141, 143] The guidelines for radiation therapy depend on the aim of the treatment, i.e., whether it is given as a primary radical curative measure or is for palliation only. Doses of 6000 to 7000 rads delivered in six to 10 weeks are recommended for radical treatment, and 4000 to 5000 rads in four to six weeks is used for palliative purposes. Recurrent chordomas may also be treated by irradiation (Fig. 24–4), but the dose will be dependent on whether previous radiation was already given, the dose factors, and the state of the surrounding normal tissues. More modern and improved methods of irradiation, such as the wedge-filter techniques to adapt the beam, and rotation therapy employing gravity-oriented blocks to spare such vital organs as the spinal cord or to protect normal surrounding tissues (the Proimos device) have been proposed and hold great hope to control this disease.[76]

The stereotactic implantation of radioactive seeds, such as yttrium-90 and radiogold, has been tried in order to control intracranial chordomas, but the results are tentative and more experience is needed before this method of treatment can be fairly evaluated.[82, 148]

Chemotherapy employing single or a combination of agents is employed to treat recurrent or disseminated disease but seems to provide poor results.[43, 74] Radioactive sulfur-35 therapy has been attempted but yielded only questionable benefits.[92]

PROGNOSIS

Although the majority of chordomas are slow-growing, progressively enlarging tumors with a propensity for local recurrence, at least 5 per cent and as many as 43 per cent will eventually metastasize.[23, 35, 39, 44, 66, 87, 135] These usually blood-borne metastases most commonly will involve the lungs, liver, bone, lymph nodes, and regional soft tissues.[23] In the series of 54 patients studied by Sundaresan, 11 of 18 vertebral chordomas and 10 of 36 sacral tumors manifested metastases

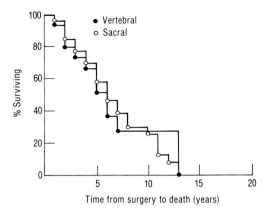

Figure 24–13. Survival rates of 54 patients with chordomas at Memorial Hospital. Eighteen vertebral and 36 sacrococcygeal tumors. (From Sundaresan, N., Galicich, J. H., Chu, F. C. H., et al.: Spinal chordomas: a clinical review. J. Neurosurg.) (in press)

uniformly throughout the course of disease.[129] The discovery of metastases spanned from 1 to 10 years after initial diagnosis. Prolonged survival, even in the face of widespread metastases, is not unprecedented.

The results of treatment were analyzed in 54 patients with spinal chordomas studied at Memorial Hospital.[129] The likelihood of survival for patients with sacrococcygeal and vertebral lesions is demonstrated in Figure 24–13. The median survival for both groups of patients was approximately six years. Five year survival rates were 66 per cent for those with sacrococcygeal tumors and 50 per cent for those with vertebral presentation (Fig. 24–13). The ten year survival rate for patients with sacral chordomas was 40 per cent. The risk of dying from disease remains constant throughout the follow-up period.

The prognosis seems to be independent of the age or sex of the patient. It is important to point out that only 4 of the original 54 patients treated at Memorial Hospital were entirely disease-free for five or more years, and 2 of these patients eventually succumbed to their disease after 17 and 20 years respectively.[129] The effect of the various treatment modalities, and their influence on survival, is compared in Figure 24–14. It is shown that those patients who received surgical excision coupled with radiation therapy and those who were treated solely with a radical surgical approach have fared equally.

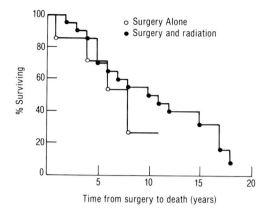

Figure 24-14. The effect of various treatment modalities on the survival of patients with chordomas at Memorial Hospital. (From Sundaresan, N., Galicich, J. H., Chu, F. C. H., et al.: Spinal chordomas: A clinical review. J. Neurosurg.) (in press)

The study of chordomas at the skull base by Heffelfinger and colleagues suggests a marked difference in survival between patients with typical chordomas and those with "chondroid chordomas."[64] The average survival time for 19 patients with "chondroid chordomas" was 15.8 years, as compared to 4.1 years for those 36 patients who had typical chordomas, despite similar treatment regimens.

Careful analysis of survival data, both from Memorial Hospital and from many other medical centers, confirms the impression that chordoma is a capricious and inscrutable tumor. A wide spectrum of behavior is exhibited, from insidious and indolent growth to rapidly progressive and virulent disease with massive recurrence and widespread dissemination.

REFERENCES

1. Adams, W. S.: A case of chordoma of the right frontal sinus. J. Laryngol. Otol., 62:93–95, 1948.
2. Adson, A. W., Kernohan, J. W., and Woltman, A. W.: Cranial and cervical chordomas. A clinical and histologic study. Arch. Neurol. Psychiatr., 33:247–261, 1935.
3. Alézais, H., and Peyron, A.: Sur l'histogenese et l'origine des chordomes. C. R. Acad. Sci. (Paris), 174:419–421, 1922.
4. Anderson, W. B., and Meyers, H. I.: Multicentric chordoma. Report of a case. Cancer, 21:126–128, 1968.
5. Ariel, I. M., and Verdu, C.: Chordoma: an analysis of 20 cases treated over a 20 year span. J. Surg. Oncol., 7:27–44, 1975.
6. Bach, S. T.: Cervical chordoma. Report of a case and a brief review of the literature. Acta Otolaryngol., 69:450–456, 1970.
7. Baker, H. W., and Coley, B. L.: Chordoma of lumbar vertebra. J. Bone Joint Surg. [Am.], 35:403–408, 1953.
8. Bassi, P., Sanna, G., and Bassi, L.: Radioterapia del cordoma del clivo. Radiobiol. Radioter. Fis. Med., 25:223–239, 1970.
9. Batsakis, J. G., and Kittleson, A. C.: Chordomas. Otorhinolaryngologic presentation and diagnosis. Arch. Otolaryngol., 78:168–175, 1963.
10. Beaugié, J. M., Mann, C. V., and Butler, E. C. B.: Sacrococcygeal chordoma. Br. J. Surg., 56:586–588, 1969.
11. Becker, L. E., Yates, A. J., Hoffman, H. J., et al.: Intracranial chordoma in infancy. Case report. J. Neurosurg., 42:349–352, 1975.
12. Berdal, P., and Myhre, E.: Cranial chordomas involving the paranasal sinuses. J. Laryngol. Otol., 78:906–919, 1964.
13. Birrell, J. H. W.: Chordomata. A review of nineteen cases of chordomata including five vertebral cases. Aust. N. Z. J. Surg., 22:258–267, 1953.
14. Botticelli, A., Ravetto, C., Pozzi, F., et al.: Sul cordoma sacro-coccigeo. Aspetti istomorfologici e istochimici. Arch. De Vecchi Anat. Patol., 53:577–596, 1968.
15. Burghele, T., Vlad, C., and Ioachim, H.: Le chordome sacrococcygien. J. Chir., 75:241–247, 1958.
16. Cancilla, P., Morecki, R., and Hurwitt, E. S.: Fine structure of a recurrent chordoma. Arch. Neurol., 11:289–295, 1964.
17. Capelli, A., Jasonni, V., and Pizzoferrato, A.: Profilo morfologico ed istochimico dei cordomi. Arch. Ital. Anat. Ist. Patol., 42:46–92, 1968.
18. Cappell, D. F.: Chordoma of the vertebral column with three new cases. J. Pathol. Bacteriol., 31:797–814, 1928.
19. Castellano, G. C., and Johnston, H. W.: Intrathoracic chordoma presenting as a posterior mediastinal tumor. South. Med. J., 68:109–112, 1975.
20. Cermak, I.: Clinical course of an intracranial chordoma. Wien. Z. Nev. Grenzg., 9:320–329, 1954.
21. Cesarini, J. P., and Bonneau, H.: A propos de l'étude ultrastructurale d'un chordome sacré. Arch. Anat. Pathol., 19:95–102, 1971.
22. Chalmers, J., and Coulson, W. F.: A metastasising chordoma. J. Bone Joint Surg. [Br.], 42:556–559, 1960.
23. Chalmers, J., and Heard, B. E.: A metastasising chordoma: a further note. J. Bone Joint Surg. [Br.], 54:526–529, 1972.
24. Chebysheva, A. Z., and Kiselev, A. V.: Morphological diagnosis of chordomas in children. Arkh. Patol., 38(7):69–71, 1976.
25. Clay, A., Dupont, A., and Gosselin, B.: Observation anatomoclinique d'un chordome lombaire avec métastases viscérales multiples. Arch. Anat. Pathol., 17:111–114, 1969.
26. Coley, G. M., Otis, R. D., and Clark, W. E., II: Multiple primary tumors including bilateral breast cancers in a man with Klinefelter's syndrome. Cancer, 27:1476–1481, 1971.

27. Congdon, C. C.: Benign and malignant chordomas. A clinicoanatomical study of twenty-two cases. Am. J. Pathol., 28:793–821, 1952.

28. Congdon, C. C.: Proliferative lesions resembling chordoma following puncture of nucleus pulposus in rabbits. J. Natl. Cancer Inst., 12:893–907, 1952.

29. Conley, J. J., and Clairmont, A. A.: Some aspects of cervical chordoma. Trans. Am. Acad. Ophthalmol. Otolaryngol., 84:145–147, 1977.

30. Corradini, E.: Morfologia del cordoma, con particolare riferimento alla citochimica. Arch. De Vecchi Anat. Patol., 33:471–489, 1960.

31. Crawford, T.: The staining reactions of chordoma. J. Clin. Pathol., 11:110–113. 1958.

32. Crikelair, G. F., and McDonald, J. J.: Nasopharyngeal chordoma. Plast. Reconstr. Surg., 16:138–144, 1955.

33. Crowe, G. G., and Muldoon, P. B. Ll.: Thoracic chordoma. Thorax, 6:403–407, 1951.

34. Dabska, M.: Parachordoma. A new clinicopathologic entity. Cancer, 40:1586–1592, 1977.

35. Dahlin, D. C., and MacCarty, C. S.: Chordoma. A study of fifty-nine cases. Cancer, 5:1170–1178, 1952.

36. Drukker, B. H., Lee, C. Y., and Kim, T. W.: Sacral chordoma. A rare cause of chronic pelvic and low-back pain. Obstet. Gynecol., 49:(Supplement):64s–66s, 1977.

37. Erlandson, R. A., Tandler, B., Lieberman, P. H., et al.: Ultrastructure of human chordoma. Cancer Res., 28:2115–2125, 1968.

38. Falconer, M. A., Bailey, I. C., and Duchen, L. W.: Surgical treatment of chordoma and chondroma of the skull base. J. Neurosurg., 29:261–275, 1968.

39. Faust, D. B., Gilmore, H. R., Jr., and Mudgett, C. S.: Chordomata: a review of the literature with report of a sacrococcygeal case. Ann. Intern. Med., 21:678–698, 1944.

40. Firooznia, H., Pinto, R. S., Lin, J. P., et al.: Chordoma: radiologic evaluation of 20 cases. Am. J. Roentgenol. Radium Ther. Nucl. Med., 127:797–805, 1976.

41. Fletcher, E. M., Woltman, H. W., and Adson, A. W.: Sacrococcygeal chordomas. A clinical and pathologic study. Arch. Neurol. Psychiatr., 33:283–299, 1935.

42. Foote, R. F., Ablin, G., and Hall, W.: Chordoma in siblings. Calif. Med., 88:383–386, 1958.

43. Forti, E., and Venturini, G.: Contributo alla conoscenza delle neoplasie notocordali. Riv. Anat. Patol. Oncol., 17:317–396, 1960.

44. Fox, J. E., Batsakis, J. G., and Owano, L. R.: Unusual manifestations of chordoma. A report of two cases. J. Bone Joint Surg. [Am.], 50:1618–1628, 1968.

45. Freier, D. T., Stanley, J. C., and Thompson, N. W.: Retrorectal tumors in adults. Surg. Gynecol. Obstet., 132:681–686, 1971.

46. Friedmann, I., Harrison, D. F. N., and Bird, E. S.: The fine structure of chordoma with particular reference to the physaliphorous cell. J. Clin. Pathol., 15:116–125, 1962.

47. Fu, Y. S., Pritchett, P. S., and Young, H. F.: Tissue culture study of a sacrococcygeal chordoma with further ultrastructural study. Acta Neuropathol., 32:225–233, 1975.

48. Gentil, F., and Coley, B. L.: Sacrococcygeal chordoma. Ann. Surg., 127:432–455, 1948.

49. Geschickter, C. F., and Copeland, M. M.: Tumors of Bone. 3rd ed. Philadelphia, J. B. Lippincott Co., 1949, p. 651.

50. Gessaga, E. C., Mair, W. G. P., and Grant, D. N.: Ultrastructure of a sacrococcygeal chordoma. Acta Neuropathol., 25:27–35, 1973.

51. Giambelli, E., Felici, A., Allegri, C., et al.: Two cases of chordoma of the sacrum. Minerva Chir., 32:1133–1140, 1977.

52. Givner, I.: Ophthalmologic features of intracranial chordoma and allied tumors of the clivus. Arch. Ophthalmol., 33:397–403, 1945.

53. Glotzer, S., and Stapen, M. H.: Chordoma of the sacrum. N. Y. State J. Med., 56:1656–1658, 1956.

54. Goidanich, I. F., and Battaglia, L.: Cordoma. (Considerazioni su cinque casi a localizzazione vertebrale e sacrococcigea). Chir. Organi Mov., 42:323–364, 1955.

55. Graf, L.: Sacrococcygeal chordoma with metastases. Arch. Pathol., 37:136–139, 1944.

56. Gray, S. W., Singhabhandu, B., Smith, R. A., et al.: Sacrococcygeal chordoma: Report of a case and review of the literature. Surgery, 78:573–582, 1975.

57. Greenwald, C. M., Meaney, T. F., and Hughes, C. R.: Chordoma — uncommon destructive lesion of cerebrospinal axis. J.A.M.A., 163:1240–1244, 1957.

58. Gregorius, F. K., and Batzdorf, U.: Removal of thoracic chordoma by staged laminectomy and thoracotomy: a case report. Am. Surg., 43:631–634, 1977.

59. Güthert, H.: Über Chordome der Wirbelsäule. Z. Krebsforsch., 48:557–577, 1939.

60. Guthkelch, A. N., and Williams, R. G.: Anterior approach to recurrent chordomas of the clivus. Technical note. J. Neurosurg., 36:670–672, 1972.

61. Hagenlocher, H. U., and Ciba, K.: Radiological aspects of cervical chordomas. Fortschr. Geb. Roentgenstr. Nuklearmed., 125:228–232, 1976.

62. Hale, J. E.: Sacrococcygeal chordoma. Proc. R. Soc. Med., 70:276–278, 1977.

63. Harvey, W. F., and Dawson, E. K.: Chordoma. Edinburgh Med. J., 48:713–730, 1941.

64. Heffelfinger, M. J., Dahlin, D. C., MacCarty, C. S., et al.: Chordomas and cartilaginous tumors at the skull base. Cancer, 32:410–420, 1973.

65. Heuser, C. H.: A presomite embryo with a definite chorda canal. Contrib. Embryol. (Carnegie Inst.), 23:251–267, 1932.

66. Higinbotham, N. L., Phillips, R. F., Farr, H. W., et al.: Chordoma. Thirty-five-year study at Memorial Hospital. Cancer, 20:1841–1850, 1967.

67. Holtzer, H.: An experimental analysis of the development of the spinal column. Part II. The dispensability of the notochord. J. Exp. Zool., 121:573–591, 1952.

67a. Horten, B. C., and Montague, S. R.: Human ecchordosis physaliphora and chick embryonic notochord. A comparative electron microscopic study. Virchows Arch. [Pathol. Anat.], 371:295–303, 1976.

68. Horwitz, T.: Chordal ectopia and its possible re-

lationship to chordoma. Arch. Pathol., *31*:354–362, 1941.

69. Horwitz, T.: The Human Notochord. A Study of its Development and Regression, Variations and Pathologic Derivative, Chordoma. Indianapolis, Limited Private Printing, 1977.

70. Hsieh, C. K., and Hsieh, H. H.: Roentgenologic study of sacrococcygeal chordoma. Radiology, 27:101–108, 1936.

71. Hübener, K. H., and Klott, K. J.: Chordoma lumbalis. Fortschr. Geb. Roentgenstr. Nuklearmed., *128*:373–374, 1978.

72. Huber, G. C.: On the relation of the chorda dorsalis to the anlage of the pharyngeal bursa or median pharyngeal recess. Anat. Rec., 6:373–404, 1912.

73. Iurato, S., and Leonardelli, G. B.: Il profilo istomorfologico e istochimico del cordoma rinofaringeo. Tumori, *42*:559–575, 1956.

74. Kamrin, R. P., Potanos, J. N., and Pool, J. L.: An evaluation of the diagnosis and treatment of chordoma. J. Neurol. Neurosurg. Psychiatry, *24*:157–165, 1964.

75. Kay, S., and Schatzki, P. F.: Ultrastructural observations of a chordoma arising in the clivus. Hum. Pathol., 3:403–413, 1972.

76. Kelley, C. D., Reid, A., Simpson, L. D., et al.: The Proimos device: a gravity oriented blocking system for use in external radiation therapy. Clin. Bull., 6:107–113, 1976.

77. Kendall, B. E., and Lee, B. C. P.: Cranial chordomas. Br. J. Radiol., *50*:687–698, 1977.

78. Kerr, W. A., Allen, K. L., Haynes, D. R., et al.: Familial nasopharyngeal chordoma. Letter to the editor. S. Afr. Med. J., *49*:1584, 1975.

79. Kishikawa, H., and Tanaka, K.: Chordoma — report of an autopsy case with fibrosarcoma. Acta Pathol. Jpn., *24*:299–308, 1974.

80. Knechtges, T. C.: Sacrococcygeal chordoma with sarcomatous features (spindle cell metaplasia). Am. J. Clin. Pathol., *53*:612–616, 1970.

81. Knysh, I. T.: Chordomas of sacrol-coccygeal vertebrae. Khirurgiia (Mosk.), *51*:79–83, 1975.

82. Krayenbühl, H., and Yaşargil, M. G.: Cranial chordomas. Prog. Neurol. Surg., 6:380–434, 1975.

83. Lichtenstein, L.: Bone Tumors. 4th ed. St. Louis, C. V. Mosby Co., 1972, p. 336.

84. Lim, G. H. K.: Clivus chordoma with unusual bone sclerosis and brainstem invasion. A case report with review of the radiology of cranial chordomas. Australas. Radiol., *19*:242–250, 1975.

85. Linck and Warstat: Zur Kenntniss der malignen Chordome in der Sacro-Coccygealregion, zugleich ein Beitrag zur Frage der Genese und Lokalisation maligner Chordome überhaupt. Beitr. Klin. Chir., *127*:612–626, 1922.

86. Localio, S. A., Francis, K. C., and Rossano, P. G.: Abdominosacral resection of sacrococcygeal chordoma. Ann. Surg., *166*:394–402, 1967.

87. Mabrey, R. E.: Chordoma: a study of 150 cases. Am. J. Cancer, *25*:501–516, 1935.

88. MacCarty, C. S., Dahlin, D. C., and Heffelfinger, M. J.: Chordomas of the neural axis. *In*: Vinken, P. J., and Bruyn, G. W. (eds.): Handbook of Clinical Neurology. Vol. 19. Tumours of the Spine and Spinal Cord, Part I. New York, American Elsevier, 1975, pp. 287–292.

89. MacCarty, C. S., Waugh, J. M., Coventry, M. B., et al.: Sacrococcygeal chordomas. Surg. Gynecol. Obstet., *113*:551–554, 1961.

90. MacCarty, C. S., Waugh, J. M., Mayo, C. W., et al.: The surgical treatment of presacral tumors: a combined problem. Mayo Clin. Proc., *27*:73–84, 1952.

91. Maroske, D., and Hupe, K.: Sacrococcygeal chordoma. Radical operation, a problem. Chirurg., *48*:118–122, 1977.

92. Mayer, K., Pentlow, K. S., Marcove, R. C., et al.: Sulfur-35 therapy of chondrosarcoma and chordoma. *In* R. P. Spencer (ed): Therapy in Nuclear Medicine. New York, Grune & Stratton, 1978, pp. 185–192.

93. Meaney, T. F., Greenwald, C. M., and Phalen, G. S.: Chordoma. Clin. Orthop., 7:103–112, 1956.

94. Miller, T. R., Mackenzie, A. R., Randall, H. T., et al.: Hemicorporectomy. Surgery, *59*:988–993, 1966.

95. Montella, L., and Molino, D.: Contribution to study of sacrococcigeal chordoma. Rass. Int. Clin. Ter., *53*:238–247, 1973.

96. Montgomery, A. H., and Wolman, I. J.: Sacrococcygeal chordomas in children. Am. J. Dis. Child., *46*:1263–1281, 1933.

97. Müller, H.: Über das Vorkommen von Resten der Chorda dorsalis bei Menschen nach der Geburt und über ihr Verhältniss zu den Gallertgeschwülsten am Clivus. Z. Rationelle Med., 2:202–229, 1858.

98. Murad, T. M., and Murthy, M. S. N.: Ultrastructure of a chordoma. Cancer, *25*:1204–1215, 1970.

99. Paavolainen, P., and Teppo, L.: Chordoma in Finland. Acta Orthop. Scand., *47*:46–51, 1976.

100. Papadimitriou, K., Nakopoulou, L., Billalis, D., et al.: A chordoma of sacrococcygeal region as a cause of nephrotic syndrome. Zentralbl. Allg. Pathol., *120*:500–504, 1976.

101. Pardo Mindan, F. J., Canadell, J. M., Herranz, P., et al.: Sarcoma cordoide de fémur. Estudio a microscopio óptico y electrónico de un caso. Rev. Med. Univ. Navarra, *19*:133–141, 1975.

102. Pastore, P. N., Sahyoun, P. F., and Mandeville, F. B.: Chordoma of the maxillary antrum and nares. Report of a case clinically resembling Hodgkin's disease first diagnosed by biopsy of a cervical node. Arch Otolaryngol., *50*:647–658, 1949.

103. Pearlman, A. W., and Friedman, M.: Radical radiation therapy of chordoma. Am. J. Roentgenol. Radium Ther. Nucl. Med., *108*:333–341, 1970.

104. Pearlman, A. W., Singh, R. K., Hoppenstein, R., et al.: Chordoma: combined therapy with radiation and surgery: case report and new operative approach. Bull. Hosp. Joint Dis., *33*:47–57, 1972.

105. Pena, C. E., Horvat, B. L., and Fisher, E. R.: The ultrastructure of chordoma. Am. J. Clin. Pathol., *53*:544–551, 1970.

106. Peyron, A., and Mellissinos, J.: Chordome, tumeur traumatique. Ann. Med. Légale, *15*:478–488, 1935.

107. Pinto, R. S., Lin, J. P., Firooznia, H., et al.: The osseous and angiographic manifestations of vertebral chordoma. Neuroradiology, 9:231–241, 1975.

108. Piraud, G.: La Notochorde; Embryologie Générale et Expérimentale, Vestiges et Tumeurs. Paris, Lefrançois, 1933.

109. Poppen, J. L., and King, A. B.: Chordoma: experience with thirteen cases. J. Neurosurg., 9:139–163, 1952.

110. Prignitz, R., and Tauber, R.: The sacrococcygeal chordoma in the infancy. Strahlentherapie, 149:368–374, 1975.

111. Rasmussen, T. B., Kernohan, J. W., and Adson, A. W.: Pathologic classification, with surgical consideration, of intraspinal tumors. Ann. Surg., 111:513–530, 1940.

112. Ribbert, H.: Ueber die Ecchondrosis physalifora sphenooccipitalis. Zentralbl. Allg. Pathol., 5:457–461, 1894.

113. Ribbert, H.: Ueber die experimentelle Erzeugung einer Ecchondrosis physalifora. Verh. Dtsch. Kongr. Inn. Med., 13:455–464, 1895.

114. Richter, H. J., Batsakis, J. G., and Boles, R.: Chordomas: Nasopharyngeal presentation and atypical long survival. Ann. Otol. Rhinol. Laryngol., 84:327–332, 1975.

115. Robbins, S. L.: Lumbar vertebral chordoma. Arch. Pathol., 40:128–132, 1945.

116. Rosenqvist, H., and Saltzman, G. F.: Sacrococcygeal and vertebral chordomas and their treatment. Acta Radiol., 52:177–193, 1959.

117. Saegesser, F., Zoupanos, G., and Gloor, E.: Chordomes. Helv. Chir. Acta., 40:107–128, 1973.

118. Sassin, J. F.: Intracranial chordoma. In Vinken, P. J., and Bruyn, G. W. (eds.): Handbook of Clinical Neurology. Vol. 18. Tumours of the Brain and Skull, Part III. New York, American Elsevier, 1975, pp. 151–164.

119. Schechter, M. M., Liebeskind, A. L., and Azar-Kia, B.: Intracranial chordomas. Neuroradiology, 8:67–82, 1974.

120. Schwabe, R.: Untersuchungen über die Rückbildung der Bandscheiben im menschlichen Kreuzbein. Virchows Arch. [Pathol. Anat.], 287:651–713, 1933.

121. Seaton, R. W., and Weaver, E. N.: The chordoma. Va. Med. Mon., 89:34–38, 1962.

122. Sennett, E. J.: Chordoma: its roentgen diagnostic aspects and its response to roentgen therapy. Am. J. Roentgenol. Radium Ther. Nucl. Med., 69:613–622, 1953.

123. Shaw, J. F., Hamilton, T., and Thompson, D.: Chordoma presenting as a scrotal swelling. J. R. Coll. Surg. Edinb., 23:100–103, 1978.

124. Slípka, J.: Relationship of the notochord to development of the skull basis. Folia Morphol. (Praha), 22:244–246, 1974.

125. Spjut, H. J., and Luse, S. A.: Chordoma: an electron microscopic study. Cancer, 17:643–656, 1964.

126. Steckler, R. M., and Martin, R. G.: Sacrococcygeal chordoma. Am. Surg., 40:579–581, 1974.

127. Stewart, M. J.: Malignant sacrococcygeal chordoma. J. Pathol. Bacteriol., 25:40–62, 1922.

128. Stewart, M. J., and Morin, J. E.: Chordoma: a review, with report of a new sacrococcygeal case. J. Pathol. Bacteriol., 29:41–60, 1926.

129. Sundaresan, N., Galicich, J. H., Chu, F. C. H., et al.: Spinal chordomas: a clinical review. J. Neurosurg. (In press.)

130. Tewfik, H. H., McGinnis, W. L., Nordstrom, D. G., et al.: Chordoma. Evaluation of clinical behavior and treatment modalities. Int. J. Radiat. Oncol. Biol. Phys., 2:959–962, 1977.

131. Thiery, J. P., Mazabraud, A., Mignot, J., et al.: Electron microscopic study of a sacral chordoma. Characterization of various evolutive stages of the tumoral cells. Ann. Anat. Pathol., 22:193–204, 1977.

132. Tripier, M. F., Hassoun, J., and Toga, M.: Étude ultrastructurale d'un chordome. J. Neurol. Sci., 25:361–370, 1975.

133. Utne, J. R., and Pugh, D. G.: The roentgenologic aspects of chordoma. Am. J. Roentgenol. Radium Ther. Nucl. Med., 74:593–608, 1955.

134. Virchow, R. L. K.: Untersuchungen über die Entwickelung des Schädelgrundes im gesunden und krankhaften Zustande und über den Einfluss derselben auf Schädelform, Gesichtsbildung und Gehirnbau. Berlin, G. Reimer, 1857, p. 128.

135. Wang, C. C., and James, A. E., Jr.: Chordoma: Brief review of the literature and report of a case with widespread metastases. Cancer, 22:162–167, 1968.

136. Wellinger, Cl.: Rachidial chordoma — I. Review of the literature since 1960. Rev. Rhum. Mal. Osteoartic., 42:109–116, 1975.

137. Wellinger, Cl.: Rachidial chordoma — II. Review of the literature since 1960. Rev. Rhum. Mal. Osteoartic., 42:195–204, 1975.

138. Wellinger, Cl.: Rachidial chordoma — III. Review of the literature since 1960. Rev. Rhum. Mal. Osteoartic., 42:287–295, 1975.

139. Willis, R. A.: Sacral chordoma with widespread metastases. J. Pathol. Bacteriol., 33:1035–1043, 1930.

140. Willis, R. A.: Pathology of Tumours. 4th ed. Philadelphia, F. A. Davis Co. (Butterworths), 1967.

141. Windeyer, B. W.: Chordoma. Proc. R. Soc. Med., 52:1088–1100, 1959.

142. Windle-Taylor, P. C.: Cervical chordoma: report of a case and the technique of transoral removal. Br. J. Surg., 64:438–441, 1977.

143. Wood, E. H., Jr., and Himadi, G. M.: Chordomas: A roentgenologic study of sixteen cases previously unreported. Radiology, 54:706–716, 1950.

144. Wright, D.: Nasopharyngeal and cervical chordoma — some aspects of their development and treatment. J. Laryngol. Otol., 81:1337–1355, 1967.

145. Wyatt, R. B., Schochet, S. S., Jr., and McCormick, W. F.: Ecchordosis physaliphora. An electron microscopic study. J. Neurosurg., 34:672–677, 1971.

146. Yarom, R., and Horn, Y.: Sacrococcygeal chordoma with unusual metastases. Cancer, 25:659–662, 1970.

147. Zöch, K.: Chordome der Schädelbasis. Eine klinisch-morphologische Studie über sechs Fälle. Schweiz. Arch. Neurol. Neurochir. Psychiatr., 105.293–321, 1969.

148. Zoltán, L., and Fényes, I.: Stereotactic diagnosis and radioactive treatment in a case of sphenooccipital chordoma. J. Neurosurg., 17:888–900, 1960.

25

SKELETAL MANIFESTATIONS OF MALIGNANT LYMPHOMAS AND LEUKEMIAS

PRIMARY NON-HODGKIN'S LYMPHOMA OF BONE

DEFINITION

Primary non-Hodgkin's lymphoma of bone is a rare extranodal lymphoma histologically identical with others arising in lymphoid or soft tissues but presenting initially as a localized solitary bone lesion.

The classification of neoplastic diseases of the hematopoietic and lymphoid tissues is in a state of flux.[47] It is not feasible at present, therefore, to propose a uniformly accurate, scientific, and clinically tested classification or nomenclature for non-Hodgkin's lymphomas that is acceptable to all, or even to a majority. Since only a few studies employing modern staging techniques and histologic studies dealing with lymphomas presenting in bone are available, in order to avert controversy, this author will not subclassify or subdivide these lesions into various histologic or cy-

tologic types here. Some of the tumors have been referred to in the past as "lymphosarcoma," "reticulum cell sarcoma," or "reticulosarcoma." It may be assumed that non-Hodgkin's lymphoma is arising from bone if "thorough" workup of the patient does not reveal any other evidence of disease. Coley and associates laid down the rather arbitrary rule that there should be a minimal interval of six months between the onset of symptoms related to the primary disease and the development of eventual regional or distant spread of lymphoma.[14, 30, 78]

Over the years, the strict criteria for exclusion or inclusion of a case and the thoroughness of the clinical and laboratory workup required underwent remarkable changes. The minimal requirement seems to be a radiographic skeletal survey and palpation of regional or distant lymph nodes. Some of the investigators, however, disregard regional lymph node involvement and include these cases in their study of primary lymphomas of bone.[30, 70]

HISTORICAL ASPECTS

That malignant lymphomas arise primarily in bones has been known since at least 1901.[95] The reliable and consistent separation of reticulum cell sarcoma of bone from Ewing's sarcoma was largely accomplished by Oberling in 1928[59] and by Oberling and Raileanu in 1932.[60] The attempts at segregation of these two entities remained less than completely successful, for, in 1972, they seemed to require renewed clarification and prompted the question, Is it worthwhile to differentiate Ewing's sarcoma and primary lymphoma of bone?[19] Some questioned the feasibility of separating this tumor from Ewing's sarcoma, however.[49] Parker and Jackson, in 1939, studied 17 cases of primary reticulum cell sarcoma of bone and established it as a distinct clinicopathologic presentation separate from the generalized form of this disease.[61] This study established that the lesions were predilecting long bones of the extremities, with a solitary bone being involved. Also, the patients were under the age of 40 years, and the disease appeared to run a more favorable course, showing a relatively good prognosis. These results contrasted sharply with those of Craver and Copeland, who, in 1934, studied 17 examples of disseminated reticulum cell sarcoma with osseous involvement.[18] The patients in this study were older and exhibited polyostotic involvement with a preference for the spine and pelvis, in addition to having a much poorer prognosis. The characteristic radiographic features of primary reticulum cell sarcoma of bone, based on a substantial number of well-documented cases, were first described by Sherman and Snyder in 1947.[76]

INCIDENCE

Some 5 to 25 per cent of non-Hodgkin's lymphomas arise in extranodal sites, one of the more frequent being the skeletal system.[13, 33, 82] Primary malignant lymphoma of bone constitutes about 5 per cent of all malignant bone tumors[14] and 2.5 per cent of all bone tumors.[41, 42] The osseous system is secondarily involved in about 30 per cent of malignant lymphomas.[13]

The development of modern, more accurate staging procedures, such as lymphangiogram, bone marrow and percutaneous liver biopsies, bone scanning, and total body scanning, has reduced the number of examples fit for the category of primary osseous lymphoma. Nevertheless, the fact remains that a rare and distinct group of primary lymphomas of bone that appears to have a good overall prognosis exists.

Retrospective appraisal of previously reported series of cases is made difficult by the inclusion of patients with Hodgkin's disease[5, 79] or by the exclusion of those who developed evidence of dissemination within six months of the initial diagnosis.[5, 14, 30, 43, 78]

SIGNS AND SYMPTOMS

Localized pain is the most consistent initial complaint and is present in almost all patients. The pain is experienced as dull, aching, intermittent, and quite nonspecific and is often unresponsive to conservative supportive measures.[92] Palpable mass or soft tissue swelling is demonstrable in many. The history of trauma is obtained from many patients and probably serves to call attention to the lesion. The apparent general good health of the patient is vividly contrasted with the frequently extensive bone destruction.[30, 61] Tenderness, local heat, and elevated temperature are infrequent findings. In lesions presenting in the jaws, hard swelling associated with pain and symptoms of nerve involvement are noted. Loosening of the teeth is a common finding. Approximately 50 per cent of the patients report symptoms related to the lesion for longer than a year, and about 10 per cent have these complaints for more than three years. In spite of a predominantly lytic type of osseous destruction, pathologic fracture is not a common finding. In about 20 per cent of cases, however, it may complicate the disease. Joint pain with effusion may also be a presenting symptom.[35, 78, 79]

LOCATION

Practically all bones may give rise to non-Hodgkin's lymphoma. The femur (25 per cent) and the pelvic bones (19 per cent) are the most common sites of involvement (Fig. 25–1). The bones of the lower extremity are affected in over 30 per cent of the cases, and the humerus accounts for 9 per cent of the lesions. This tumor infrequently arises in the most peripheral portions of the upper extremity distal to the elbow but is more common in bones below the knee. The incidence of lymphoma in the appendicular as compared to the axial skeleton is greatly increased to a ratio of 2:1 or even 3:1. This is remarkable since, in 1934, Craver and Copeland remarked on the presence of a reverse relationship in the bone involvement of generalized lymphoma.[18] The skeletal distribution of cases in Figure 25–1 reveals several examples of multifocal osseous involvement in the absence of lymph node disease.

Lymphomas presenting in the maxillary antrum, the fifth most common location of extranodal head and neck lymphomas, may, in fact, have arisen in the bone rather than from the lining of the antrum,[8, 12, 22, 32] but this is hard to prove. The mandible may be the site of a primary lymphoma.[2, 4, 10, 21, 27, 36, 54, 63, 80]

AGE AND SEX DISTRIBUTION

Primary non-Hodgkin's lymphoma can occur at any age, but it is more frequent after the second decade of life and is extremely rare in young children, thus the age distribution differs significantly from Ewing's sarcoma (see Fig. 21–2). The mean age of the 116 patients studied at Memorial Hospital was 38 years (35 years for men and 46 years for women), the range being from 1 to 81 years (Fig. 25–2). The one-year-old infant had a diffuse, poorly differentiated, lymphocytic type of lymphoma with a leukemic "conversion." The peak incidence in this study was in the fifth decade of life, with a plateau-like age distribution over several decades of

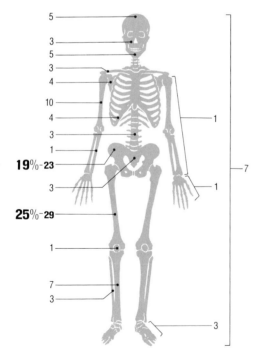

NON-HODGKIN'S LYMPHOMA OF BONE
1949 - 1973
Skeletal Distribution of 116 Cases

Figure 25–1. Skeletal distribution of 116 cases of non-Hodgkin's lymphoma of bone studied at Memorial Hospital from 1949 through 1973.

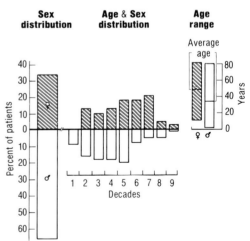

Non-Hodgkin's Lymphoma of Bone
1949 - 1973
116 Pts. (♂ = 77, ♀ = 39)

Figure 25–2. Age and sex distribution of 116 patients with non-Hodgkin's lymphoma of bone studied at Memorial Hospital from 1949 through 1973.

adulthood (Fig. 25–2). There were 77 male patients and 39 female patients, a ratio of almost 2:1 (Fig. 25–2). Among 35 cases reported from Western India, this tumor occurred five times more frequently in males than in females.[66]

RADIOGRAPHIC FEATURES

The radiographic appearance is quite variable and, except for its malignant features, is often not sufficiently characteristic to permit a definite diagnosis. The typical, but often partially altered, radiographic progression of osseous involvement is depicted in Figure 21–7 and is compared with that of Ewing's sarcoma. In non-Hodgkin's lymphoma, the earliest radiographic features show destruction of the medullary portion of the bone in the dia-

physis, with the initially small areas of cancellous bone erosion progressively coalescing into larger fields of involvement (Fig. 25–3). The incipient, slight onionskin type of periosteal lamellation gradually progresses and goes hand in hand with a coarsely nodular cortical bone destruction.

When the intramedullary portion of the lesion erodes or penetrates the adjacent cortex, the periosteum is stimulated to lay down new bone in an effort to strengthen the weakened cortex. Periosteal reactive bone formation and spiculation may be prominent features (Fig. 25–4). Coarse stranded cortical and medullary bone erosion characterizes advanced disease. Foci of intralesional sclerosis may be present. The progression of cortical destruction initially reveals a permeative appearance that later advances to larger areas of permeative-type involvement or to a moth-

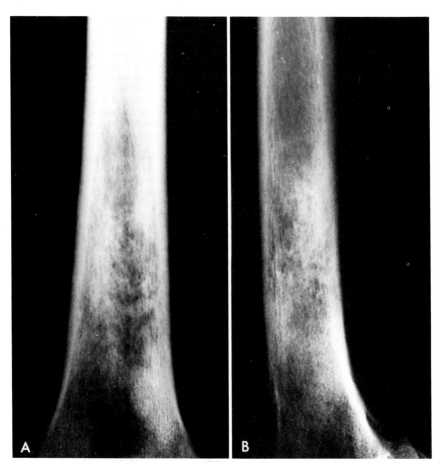

Figure 25–3. Non-Hodgkin's lymphoma involving mid-femur in a 49-year-old woman. The roentgenographs show a lytic, mottled permeative type of destruction in the shaft.

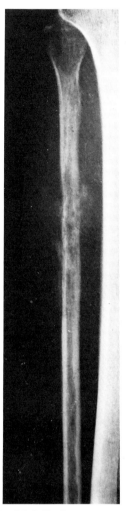

Figure 25-4. Mid-fibular non-Hodgkin's lymphoma in a 55-year-old woman revealing a mixed lytic and sclerotic destructive lesion with periosteal and soft tissue extension. The differential diagnosis here includes metastatic carcinoma and osteogenic sarcoma.

eaten-appearing pattern (Fig. 25–5).[78] In later stages, the frankly destructive disease produces a complete disruption of the cortical outline. Usually, at this stage, a soft tissue mass can be demonstrated, representing direct extension of tumor through cortex and periosteum (Fig. 25–6).[96] In acute and subacute osteomyelitis, the cortex of the affected long tubular bone may be thickened, and the medullary cavity is similarly the site of reparative new bone formation. This radiographic appearance may pose diagnostic problems, and one

may misread the picture as indicating the presence of a tumor, particularly a malignant lymphoma or an osteogenic sarcoma. Marked reactive intralesional sclerosis may be seen, on occasion, and is frequently misinterpreted as consistent with metastatic carcinoma.

All together, many of the radiographic features of non-Hodgkin's lymphoma arising in bones are not sufficiently distinctive to permit the recognition of the individual lesion with ease and absolute certainty. In cases in which the lymphoma involves a single bone, especially a long tubular bone, the area of osseous destruction in the radiograph may strongly suggest an eosinophilic granuloma. This diagnostic quandary is magnified in cases in which several bones are involved, since the radiographs may reveal identical appearances in lymphomas, multifocal eosinophilic granulomas, and metastatic tumors to the skeleton.

PATHOLOGIC FEATURES

Histologically, the tumor cells in the so-called reticulum cell sarcoma variant are large, often produce argyrophilic fibrils, and may exhibit phagocytosis. A conspicuous variation in cellular and nuclear shapes is noted. The cellular borders are well-demarcated, with the cytoplasm pale and abundant. The intercellular reticulin fibers, when present, completely envelop the individual cells. Nuclear outlines are ovoid or often indented. Lysozyme production and fluoride-inhibited nonspecific esterase activity point, in some of the tumors, to histiocytic derivation. Other tumors reveal a diffuse, poorly differentiated, lymphocytic; a mixed lymphocytic-histiocytic; or a diffuse, undifferentiated, pleomorphic, lymphomatous neoplastic cell proliferation.[67] Whatever the cytologic subclassification of these lymphomas, the tumor cells always grow in a diffuse manner. In none of the cases studied at Memorial Hospital could a nodular pattern of growth be identified. In one example reported, a nodular lymphoma appeared to arise in the mandible.[54] So far, no modern studies exist employing immunologic techniques such as cell surface markers to

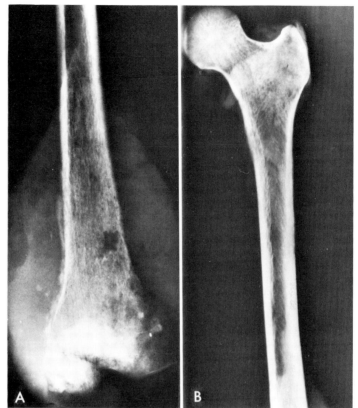

Figure 25–5. Specimen radiographs reveal (*A*) a focally sclerotic ill-defined radiolucent non-Hodgkin's lymphoma of the distal femur with a moth-eaten-appearing pattern in a 25-year-old woman. *B*, Multiple patchy medullary areas of bone destruction present in the upper portion of the femur.

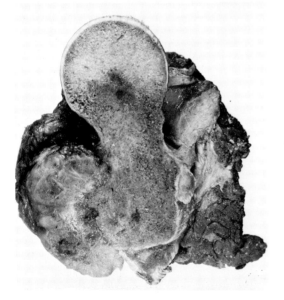

Figure 25–6. Non-Hodgkin's lymphoma arising in the left femoral neck of a 38-year-old man. The hemorrhagic soft medullary tumor extends through the cortex into adjacent soft tissue.

identify special groups with similar clinical features among the lymphomas presenting in bone.[17, 55, 98]

In the histologic differential diagnosis, especially in children, Ewing's sarcoma is always a strong consideration (see Fig. 21–1). In general, the nuclei of the tumor cells in lymphomas appear to be somewhat larger and rounder and the cytoplasmic borders more distinct than in Ewing's sarcoma; there is also marked variation in the cellular makeup in many of the malignant lymphomas.

Silver impregnation techniques exaggerate the reticulin fibers surrounding individual cells or penetrating small groups of cells, a characteristic finding emphasized by many investigators.[5, 19, 20, 72] We met with mixed success using this method since, in some of the poorly differentiated small cell lesions, where one needs most help, the cells lacked these fibers entirely.

Transitional forms, gradations between an undifferentiated lymphoma and Ewing's sarcoma as discussed by Dahlin,[20] were not recognized in the cases studied at Memorial Hospital. The distinction between these two entities, especially relying on necrotic, poorly preserved, histologic material, may cause formidable difficulties. It is helpful to remember that glycogen is present in the cytoplasm of Ewing's sarcoma cells and that reticulin fibers are at least focally absent from many undifferentiated lymphomas and from Ewing's sarcoma. The demonstration of glycogen in the tumor cells, even in small specimens obtained by aspiration biopsy and smears, is the single most useful parameter in the exclusion of a malignant lymphoma.[72]

The histologic separation of chronic osteomyelitis from a non-Hodgkin's lymphoma of bone may be greatly impeded or concealed by the poor preservation of the tissue, especially if there is extensive necrosis and the tumor cells mimic necrotic leukocytes. Secondary acute or chronic inflammatory cell infiltration with foci of tumor necrosis may obscure the true identity of the lesion.

The pathologist is sometimes confronted with a rare eosinophilic granuloma in which the vast majority of the cells are histiocytes and only a few eosinophils are present, so that confusion with a histiocytic type of lymphoma is a real possibility.[45]

Another pitfall is presented by the difficult histologic distinction between chronic osteomyelitis and a mixed histiocytic-lymphocytic lymphoma in a small biopsy specimen, especially when lymphocytes are plentiful.[80]

In rare cases of chronic myeloid leukemia involving osseous sites as well as lymph nodes, the clinical manifestations and light microscopic features may mimic malignant lymphomas. These cases are frequently misinterpreted as showing a histiocytic type of lymphoma, so-called "reticulum cell sarcoma." In order to avoid this diagnostic pitfall, the microscopist should try to identify eosinophilic myelocytes and employ the naphthol-AS-D chloracetate-esterase reaction in tissue section, findings present only in a leukemic involvement.

TREATMENT AND PROGNOSIS

In general, a tumor dose of 4500 to 5000 rads of megavoltage radiation delivered in four to five weeks, employing shrinking fields to avoid irradiation of uninvolved normal soft tissues, is recommended.[11, 43, 92] It should be remembered that the entire bone, including articular surfaces and adjacent soft tissues, must be included in the field of irradiation since, based on roentgenograms of this disease, one habitually underestimates the extent of osseous involvement. Local tumor recurrence was observed in 43 per cent of 46 patients reported by Shoji and Miller, who claimed that whole bone irradiation produced better control than using restricted fields.[78]

A moderate-dose radiation therapy followed by surgery and adjuvant chemotherapy should be considered for primary non-Hodgkin's lymphoma arising in the pelvic girdle, where excessive irradiation would cause increased morbidity as far as intestinal and bladder functions are concerned.[69]

Major amputation as the primary approach to treatment is not recommended and is usually reserved for those extensive lesions that fail to respond to proper radiation therapy. A combination of radiotherapy and adjuvant chemotherapy is advisable, even in those instances when no regional or distant spread of disease is evident.[97]

Even under the influence of aggressive

systemic multidrug multicycle chemotherapy, the patient may rapidly develop meningeal involvement by non-Hodgkin's lymphoma similar to that seen in acute lymphoblastic leukemia.[69] Prior to the use of central nervous system prophylactic treatment, six out of eight patients developed meningeal lymphomatous disease.[97] These results have prompted the revision of the treatment protocol of non-Hodgkin's lymphoma, which now incorporates prophylactic intrathecal chemotherapy.[97]

The effectiveness of treating apparently localized disease with surgery, irradiation, or a combination of both appears to be significantly dependent on the actual extent of involvement. Shoji and Miller proposed to correlate prognosis with the radiographic features of the affected bone.[78] The analysis of survival following radiation therapy for primary osseous lymphoma with regional lymph node involvement yielded only one of four survivors for five years.[92] In the same series of 16 patients receiving radiation therapy as the primary method of treatment, with or without amputation, 10 survived five or more years without disease.[92]

Soft tissue extension of the primarily intraosseous lymphoma seems to impart a worse prognosis if it appears in patients with long tubular bone involvement but appears not to affect the clinical outcome of disease when it involves flat bones.[78] Others found the local response to treatment to be more related to tumor bulk than to its osseous site.[48]

It is generally agreed by most investigators that lymphoma arising in bone has an apparently better prognosis than disseminated disease involving bone.[5, 14, 19, 20, 61, 78] The five and 10 year end results without evidence of disease are approximately 48 per cent and 33 per cent respectively.[30] In contrast to this relatively favorable prognosis, Dolan, based on a study of eight patients, reported early dissemination of disease resulting in the deaths of seven treated by radiation therapy.[25] The explanation of this perplexing inconsistency may lie in the lack of thorough staging procedures in several studies or simply in a sampling bias owing to relatively few cases. For instance, careful staging of 14 patients with clinically primary lymphomas of bone, who were studied at the National Cancer Institute, showed extensive stage IV disease in 12 of these patients.[67]

Miller and Nicholson reviewed the end results of malignant lymphoma of bone treated by bacterial toxins (Coley's toxin) singly or in association with surgery or radiotherapy or a combination of the two.[53] The results of their careful analysis of the many factors that may affect prognosis suggest that the toxin-treated patients enjoyed a consistently and significantly better five year survival rate (64 per cent) than those who received only surgery, radiotherapy, or both.

The spread of disease favors other bones, regional and distant lymph nodes, and the liver, spleen, and kidneys, in order of descending frequency.[48] The incidence of pulmonary involvement varies greatly. The Bristol Bone Tumour Registry in England reports none, while others find it to be present in about 20 per cent of cases.[48, 53, 57] The relative rarity of lung involvement in disseminated lymphoma contrasts vividly with its high incidence in more than half the patients with Ewing's sarcoma.

SO-CALLED "BURKITT'S TUMOR" IN THE JAWS

A peculiar B-cell type of lymphoma, often referred to as Burkitt's tumor, is found most often in the jaws of African children and has attracted considerable interest. It was originally described clinically in 1901 and in 1904 by Albert Cook at the Church Missionary Society's Hospital at Mengo, Uganda, and, in 1958, was better defined as a clinical syndrome by Dennis Burkitt, a British surgeon working at the Mulago Hospital in Kampala, Uganda.[1, 7] As originally described, the tumor affects mainly children, the median age being seven years, but the ages can range from three to 60 years. In Africa, the chief presenting symptoms refer to the mandible and maxilla in about 60 per cent of the cases, with abdominal masses caused by ovarian, mesenteric, or retroperitoneal involvement in approximately 30 per cent of the patients. Peripheral lymph nodes, the spleen, and the liver are rarely involved with the presenting features. In Africa, a unique geographical distribution related to temperature and rainfall but independent of racial or tribal background was noted. Serologic and virologic studies have pointed to the Epstein-

Barr virus (EBV) genome as being associated with many, but not all, African cases, perhaps as a passenger virus.[39]

Among American patients, the abdominal masses are predominantly featured (75 per cent), and the facial manifestations are quite rare. Maxillary presentation is twice as common as lesions in the mandible are.[1] Both the buccal and palatal surfaces of the alveolar bone are involved at the same time, with secondary invasion of the antrum and the orbit. Mandibular lesions more often present on the buccal aspect and are followed by a lingual extension.[99]

Radiographically, the earliest changes include the loss of continuity of the lamina dura around the roots of teeth, usually in the molar region. Osteolytic medullary bone destruction is noted and characterized by complete loss or marked distortion of the normal cancellous bony pattern.[94] The advanced lesion may appear as a multifocal medullary bone expansion and destruction, with cortical erosion and extension into adjacent soft tissues. In later stages, large multilocular destructions may be seen. In the differential diagnosis, osteomyelitis is the most important consideration, often giving rise to misinterpretation. Osteomyelitis of the jaw treated by antibiotics is particularly difficult, well nigh impossible, to distinguish from an incipient lymphomatous involvement.[94]

Histologically, the lesion is considered to be a B-cell type of diffusely growing, poorly differentiated lymphocytic lymphoma. The cytoplasms of the tumor cells are intensely basophilic (pyroninophilic) and may contain lipid droplets (sudanophilia). Histiocytes containing cell debris are often mixed in with the tumor cells, giving the appearance of the so-called "starry sky." Whether these histologic features are indeed specific or pathognomonic is far from certain.

REFERENCES

1. Adatia, A. K.: Burkitt's tumour in the jaws. Br. Dent. J., 120:315–326, 1966.
2. Appel, P. W.: Reticulum-cell sarcoma in the jaws. Report of two cases. Oral Surg., 26:92–95, 1968.
3. Banerjee, P., Mookerjee, C. L., Mitra, S. R., et al.: Primary malignant lymphoma of bones. J. Indian Med. Assoc., 66:12–14, 1976.
4. Blum, T., Kaletsky, T., and Gettinger, R.: Agranulocytosis and lymphosarcoma with lesions in the mandibular third molar region. Arch. Clin. Oral Pathol., 4:378–383, 1940.
5. Boston, H. C., Jr., Dahlin, D. C., Ivins, J. C., et al.: Malignant lymphoma (so-called reticulum cell sarcoma) of bone. Cancer, 34:1131–1137, 1974.
6. Boyes, J. G., Jr.: Primary reticulum cell sarcoma of the femur: 12-year follow-up after radiation therapy and pathologic fracture. South. Med. J., 67:335–339, 1974.
7. Burkitt, D.: A sarcoma involving the jaws in African children. Br. J. Surg., 46:218–223, 1958.
8. Calman, H. I.: Lymphosarcoma of the maxilla. Oral Surg., 6:232–236, 1953.
9. Campbell, J. B., Reeder, M. M., and Sewell, J.: Lymphoma cutis with osseous involvement. Radiology, 103:99–100, 1972.
10. Campbell, R. L., Kelly, D. E., and Burkes, E. J., Jr.: Primary reticulum-cell sarcoma of the mandible. Review of the literature and report of a case. Oral Surg., 39:918–928, 1975.
11. Case records of the Massachusetts General Hospital. Case 28-1971. N. Engl. J. Med., 285:166–173,1971.
12. Catlin, D.: Surgery for head and neck lymphomas. Surgery, 60:1160–1166, 1966.
13. Coles, W. C., and Schulz, M. D.: Bone involvement in malignant lymphoma. Radiology, 50:458–462, 1948.
14. Coley, B. L., Higinbotham, N. L., and Groesbeck, H. P.: Primary reticulum-cell sarcoma of bone. Summary of 37 cases. Radiology, 55:641–658, 1950.
15. Cook, H. P.: Oral lymphomas. Oral Surg., 14:690–704, 1961.
16. Correlation Conferences in Radiology and Pathology. Rosen, R. A., and Kadish, A. (eds.): Holes in the head. N.Y. State J. Med., 75:584–586, 1975.
17. Cossman, J., Schnitzer, B., and Deegan, M. J.: Immunologic surface markers in non-Hodgkin's lymphomas. Am. J. Pathol.,87:19–32, 1977.
18. Craver, L. F., and Copeland, M. M.: Lymphosarcoma in bone. Arch. Surg., 28:809–824, 1934.
19. Dahlin, D. C.: Is it worthwhile to differentiate Ewing's sarcoma and primary lymphoma of bone? In Proceedings Seventh National Cancer Conference. Philadelphia, J. B. Lippincott Co., 1973, pp. 941–945.
20. Dahlin, D. C.: Primary malignant lymphoma (reticulum cell sarcoma) of bone. In Price, C. H. G., and Ross, F. G. M. (eds.): Bone — Certain Aspects of Neoplasia. Philadelphia, F. A. Davis Co. (Butterworths), 1973, pp. 207–215.
21. Darlington, C. G., and Lefkowitz, L. I.: A pathological study of "so called" dental tumors. Am. J. Clin. Pathol., 6:330–348, 1936.
22. Dechaume, M., Grellet, M., Payen, J., et al.: Tumeurs réticulaires malignes à localisation unique monomaxillaire. Rev. Stomatol., 58:587–594, 1957.
23. Denaut, M., Parmentier, R., Yernault, J. C., et al.: Primary reticulum cell sarcoma of a rib. Report of 2 cases. Acta Tuberc. Pneumol. Belg., 66:390–400, 1975.
24. Dietz, R.: Unusual localization of a reticulum cell sarcoma in the area of the clavicular epiphysis. Strahlentherapie, 151:222–227, 1976.

25. Dolan, P. A.: Reticulum cell sarcoma of bone. Am. J. Roentgenol. Radium Ther. Nucl. Med., 87:121–127, 1962.

26. Edwards, J. E.: Primary reticulum cell sarcoma of the spine. Report of a case with autopsy. Am. J. Pathol., 16:835–844, 1940.

27. Ellis, D. J., and Winslow, J. R.: Reticulum-cell sarcoma of the mandible. Report of a case. Oral Surg., 42:570–577, 1976.

28. Fanale, S. J., and McCauley, H. B.: Lymphosarcoma of dental interest: Report of a case. J. Oral Surg., 3:186–193, 1945.

29. Fayemi, A. O., Gerber, M. A., Cohen, I., et al.: Myeloid sarcoma. Review of the literature and report of a case. Cancer, 32:253–258, 1973.

30. Francis, K. C., Higinbotham, N. L., and Coley, B. L.: Primary reticulum cell sarcoma of bone. Report of 44 cases. Surg. Gynecol. Obstet., 99:142–146, 1954.

31. Frank, V. H., and Pratt, C. I., Jr.: A lymphosarcoma with metastasis. J. Oral Surg., 9:19–24, 1951.

32. Freedman, L. J.: Primary lymphosarcoma of the hard palate. Am. J. Roentgenol. Radium Ther. Nucl. Med., 43:702–705, 1940.

33. Freeman, C., Berg, J. W., and Cutler, S. J.: Occurrence and prognosis of extranodal lymphomas. Cancer, 29:252–260, 1972.

34. Friedman, B., and Hanaoka, H.: Round-cell sarcomas of bone. A light and electron microscopic study. J. Bone Joint Surg. [Am.], 53:1118–1136, 1971.

35. Fripp, A. T., and Sissons, H. A.: A case of reticulosarcoma (reticulum-cell sarcoma) of bone. Br. J. Surg., 42:103–107, 1954.

36. Gerry, R. G., and Williams, S. F.: Primary reticulum-cell sarcoma of the mandible. Oral Surg., 8:568–581, 1955.

37. Hande, K. R., Reimer, R. R., and Fisher, R. T.: Comparison of nodal primary versus extranodal primary histiocytic lymphoma. Cancer Treat. Rep., 61:999–1000, 1977.

38. Harrigan, W. F., Butler, F. S., and Schaffer, A. B.: Reticulum cell sarcoma of chin. J. Oral Surg., 12:210–214, 1954.

39. zur Hausen, H.: Oncogenic herpes viruses. Biochem. Biophys. Acta, 417:25–53, 1975.

40. Hustu, H. O., and Pinkel, D.: Lymphosarcoma, Hodgkin's disease and leukemia in bone. Clin. Orthop., 52:83–93, 1967.

41. Ivins, J. C., and Dahlin, D. C.: Reticulum-cell sarcoma of bone. J. Bone Joint Surg. [Am.], 35:835–842, 1953.

42. Ivins, J. C., and Dahlin, D. C.: Malignant lymphoma (reticulum cell sarcoma) of bone. Proc. Mayo Clin., 38:375–385, 1963.

43. Jack, G. A.: Radiotherapy of reticulum cell sarcoma of bone. Radiol. Clin. Biol., 40:230–242, 1971.

44. Khanolkar, V. R.: Reticulum-cell sarcoma of bone. Arch. Pathol., 46:467–476, 1948.

45. Kotner, L. M.: Episodic pain in the thigh. J.A.M.A., 218:1820–1821, 1971.

46. Lambert, A., and Stout, A. P.: Reticulum-cell sarcoma of a rib. Report of a case with an 18-year symptom-free survival. Arch. Surg., 81:107–111, 1960.

47. Lukes, R. J., and Collins, R. D.: A functional approach to the classification of malignant lym-phoma. Recent Results Cancer Res., 46:18–30, 1974.

48. Macintosh, D. J., Price, C. H. G., and Jeffree, G. M.: Malignant lymphoma (reticulosarcoma) in bone. Clin. Oncol., 3:287–300, 1977.

49. Magnus, H. A., and Wood, H. L. C.: Primary reticulo-sarcoma of bone. J. Bone Joint Surg. [Br.], 38:258–278, 1956.

50. McCormack, L. J., Ivins, J. C., Dahlin, D. C., et al.: Primary reticulum-cell sarcoma of bone. Cancer, 5:1182–1192, 1952.

51. McDonald, C. R., and Paine, C. J.: Extranodal lymphoma with an unusual constellation of features. South. Med. J., 68:1177–1179, 1975.

52. Medill, E. V.: Primary reticulum-cell sarcoma of bone. J. Fac. Radiol., 8:102–117, 1956.

53. Miller, T. R., and Nicholson, J. T.: End results in reticulum cell sarcoma of bone treated by bacterial toxin therapy alone or combined with surgery and/or radiotherapy (47 cases) or with concurrent infection (5 cases). Cancer, 27:524–547, 1971.

54. Mincey, D. L., and Warnock, M. L.: Primary malignant lymphoma of mandible: report of a case. J. Oral Surg., 32:221–224, 1974.

55. Morris, M. W., and Davey, F. R.: Immunologic and cytochemical properties of histiocytic and mixed histiocytic-lymphocytic lymphomas. Am. J. Clin. Pathol., 63:403–414, 1975.

56. Mukadum, F. K., and Pinto, J. M.: Radiology in primary reticulum cell sarcoma of bone (a review of 53 cases). Indian J. Cancer, 12:170–178, 1975.

57. Newall, J., and Friedman, M.: Reticulum-cell sarcoma. Radiology, 97:99–102, 1970.

58. Ngan, H., and Preston, B. J.: Non-Hodgkin's lymphoma presenting with osseous lesions. Clin. Radiol., 26:351–356, 1975.

59. Oberling, Ch.: Les réticulosarcomes et les réticuloendothéliosarcomes de la moelle osseuse (sarcomes d'Ewing). Bull. Assoc. Fr. Cancer, 17:259–296, 1928.

60. Oberling, Ch., and Raileanu, C.: Nouvelles recherches sur les réticulosarcomes de la moelle osseuse (Sarcomes d'Ewing). Bull. Assoc. Fr. Cancer, 21:333–347, 1932.

61. Parker, F., Jr., and Jackson, H., Jr.: Primary reticulum cell sarcoma of bone. Surg. Gynecol. Obstet., 68:45–53, 1939.

62. Pear, B. L.: Skeletal manifestations of the lymphomas and leukemias. Semin. Roentgenol., 9:229–240, 1974.

63. Penhale, K. W.: Primary lymphosarcoma of the mandible. J. Oral Surg., 1:84–88, 1943.

64. Piltz, J., and Pietkiewicz, D.: Reticulosarcoma of bone with metastases to the genital tract. Ginekol. Pol., 45:475–479, 1974.

65. Pinck, R. L., Levitt, L. M., Pichel, R., et al.: Primary reticulum cell sarcoma of the femur. Am. J. Surg., 100:753–756, 1960.

66. Potdar, G. G.: Primary reticulum-cell sarcoma of bone in Western India. Br. J. Cancer, 24:48–55, 1970.

67. Reimer, R. R., Chabner, B. A., Young, R. C., et al.: Lymphoma presenting in bone. Results of histopathology, staging, and therapy. Ann. Intern. Med., 87:50–55, 1977.

68. Rice, R. W., Cabot, A., and Johnston, A. D.: The application of electron microscopy to the diag-

nostic differentiation of Ewing's sarcoma and reticulum cell sarcoma of bone. Clin. Orthop., *91*:174–185, 1973.

69. Rosen, G.: Management of malignant bone tumors in children and adolescents. Pediatr. Clin. North Am., 23:183–213, 1976.

70. Rubin, S. A., and Himmelfarb, E.: Malignant lymphoproliferative disorder with unusual osseous abnormalities. A case report. J. Can. Assoc. Radiol., 25:251—253, 1974.

71. Sarrazin, D., Schweisguth, O., and Hourtella, F. G.: Radiotherapy of reticulum cell sarcoma of bone; technique and result. Ann. Roentgenol., *10*:401–418, 1967.

72. Schajowicz, F.: Ewing's sarcoma and reticulum-cell sarcoma of bone: with special reference to the histochemical demonstration of glycogen as an aid to differential diagnosis. J. Bone Joint Surg. [Am.], *41*:349–356, 1959.

73. Schick, A., and Ladd, A. T.: Lymphosarcoma showing unusual bone manifestations. Am. J. Roentgenol. Radium Ther. Nucl. Med., 79:638–642, 1958.

74. von Schowingen, R. S.: Primary reticulum cell sarcoma of bone. Am. J. Surg., 97:41–49, 1957.

75. Seldin, H. M., Seldin, S. D., and Rakower, W.: Oral lymphosarcoma. J. Oral Surg., *12*:3–15, 1954.

76. Sherman, R. S., and Snyder, R. E.: The roentgen appearance of primary reticulum cell sarcoma of bone. Am. J. Roentgenol. Radium Ther. Nucl. Med., 58:291–306, 1947.

77. Sherman, R. S., and Wolfson, S. L.: Roentgen diagnosis of lymphosarcoma and reticulum cell sarcoma in infancy and childhood. Am. J. Roentgenol. Radium Ther. Nucl. Med., 86:693–701, 1961.

78. Shoji, H., and Miller, T. R.: Primary reticulum cell sarcoma of bone. Significance of clinical features upon the prognosis. Cancer, 28:1234–1244, 1971.

79. Short, J. H.: Malignant lymphoma (reticulum cell sarcoma) of bone. Radiography, *43*:139–143, 1977.

80. Steg, R. F., Dahlin, D. C., and Gores, R. J.: Malignant lymphoma of the mandible and maxillary region. Oral Surg., *12*:128–141, 1959.

81. Strange, V. M., and de Lorimier, A. A.: Reticulum-cell sarcoma primary in the skull. A report of three cases. Am. J. Roentgenol. Radium Ther. Nucl. Med., 71:40–50, 1954.

82. Sugarbaker, E. D., and Craver, L. F.: Lymphosarcoma. A study of 196 cases with biopsy. J.A.M.A., *115*:17–23, 1940.

83. Szutu, C., and Hsieh, C. K.: Primary reticulum

cell sarcoma of bone: Report of two cases with bone regeneration following reontgenotherapy. Ann. Surg., *115*:280–291, 1942.

84. Tillman, H. H.: Malignant lymphomas involving the oral cavity and surrounding structures. Report of twelve cases. Oral Surg., *19*:60–72, 1965.

85. Tomich, C. E., and Shafer, W. G.: Lymphoproliferative disease of the hard palate: A clinicopathologic entity. A study of twenty-one cases. Oral Surg., 39:754–768, 1975.

86. Topolnicki, W., and White, R. J.: Primary reticulum cell sarcoma of the skull. Response to irradiation. Cancer, 24:569–573, 1969.

87. Uehlinger, E., Botsztejn, C., and Schinz, H. R.: Ewingsarkom und Knochenretikulosarkom. Klinik, Diagnose und Differentialdiagnose. Oncologia, *1*:193–245, 1948.

88. Ullrich, D. P., and Bucy, P. C.: Primary reticulum cell sarcoma of the skull. Am. J. Roentgenol. Radium Ther. Nucl. Med., 79:653–657, 1958.

89. Valls, J., Muscolo, D., and Schajowicz, F.: Reticulum-cell sarcoma of bone. J. Bone Joint Surg. [Br.], *34*:588–598, 1952.

90. Van Slyck, E. J.: The bony changes in malignant hematologic disease. Orthop. Clin. North Am., 3:733–744, 1972.

91. Wang, C. C.: Treatment of primary reticulum-cell sarcoma of bone by radiation. N. Engl. J. Med., 278:1331–1332, 1968.

92. Wang, C. C., and Fleischli, D. J.: Primary reticulum cell sarcoma of bone: with emphasis on radiation therapy. Cancer, 22:994–998, 1968.

93. Watanabe, T.: Bone lesions of malignant lymphoma. Nippon Acta Radiol., 35:111–118, 1975.

94. Whittaker, L. R.: The radiological appearance of Burkitt's tumour involving bone. Aust. Radiol., *13*:307–310, 1969.

95. Wieland, E.: Studien über das primär multipel auftretende Lymphosarcom der Knochen. Virchows Arch. [Pathol. Anat.], *166*:103–157, 1901.

96. Wilson, T. W., and Pugh, D. G.: Primary reticulum cell sarcoma of bone, with emphasis on roentgen aspects. Radiology, 65:343–351, 1955.

97. Wollner, N., Burchenal, J. H., Lieberman, P. H., et al.: Non-Hodgkin's lymphoma in children. Med. Pediatr. Oncol., *1*:235–263, 1975.

98. Yam, L. T., Tavassoli, M., and Jacobs, P.: Differential characterization of the "reticulum cell" in lymphoreticular neoplasms. Am. J. Clin. Pathol., *64*:171–179, 1975.

99. Ziegler, J. L., Wright, D. H., and Kyalwazi, S. K.: Differential diagnosis of Burkitt's lymphoma of the face and jaws. Cancer, 27:503–514, 1971.

SKELETAL CHANGES OF ACUTE AND CHRONIC LEUKEMIAS IN CHILDREN AND ADULTS

The initial complaints of pain and tenderness in a child with a still undiscovered acute leukemia may refer to the various long bones and joints.[9, 10, 12, 20, 23, 25, 26, 32, 33, 34, 39, 41, 42] Familiarity with the radiographic changes in bones in this condition should facilitate arriving promptly at a proper diagnosis, even if only approximately 50 per cent of the patients with leukemia will show any osseous abnormalities. The earliest radiographic alterations are characterized by slender transverse radiolucent zones in the epiphyseal-diaphyseal areas of long tubular bones (Fig. 25–7). These areas are the most active sites of endochondral skeletal maturation. The alterations preferentially involve the knee region but may extend later into other long bones as well.[3, 4, 31, 34] According to Erb[13] and Follis and Park,[14] the reasons for these radiolucent juxtaepiphyseal zones may lie

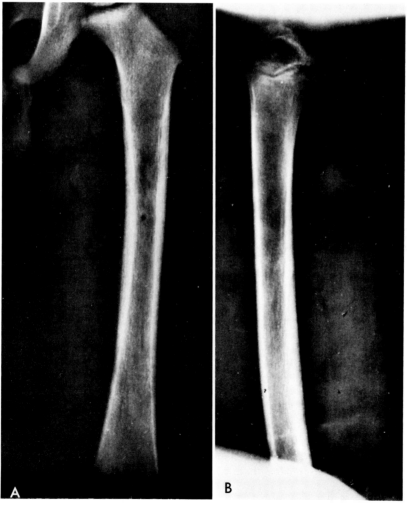

Figure 25–7.   Scattered spotty radiolucent and radiopaque bone destruction with lamellar periosteal reaction and cortical thickening in a 3½-year-old boy with acute lymphoid leukemia. The differential diagnosis here includes Ewing's sarcoma. (Courtesy of Dr. E. L. Coffey, Jr.)

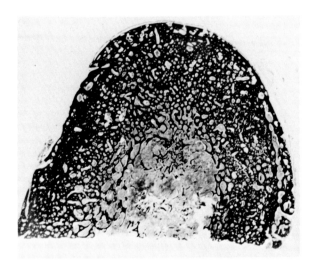

Figure 25–8. Marked leukemic osteosclerosis with the haversian system distended by tumor cells. Subperiosteal bone deposition is noted. (Cross-section, Hematoxylin-eosin stain. Magnification × 10.)

in the presence of a dense leukemic cellular infiltrate compressing and thwarting the singularly unstable osseous trabecular tissue in this region, or perhaps the poor general condition of the patients suppresses endochondral bone activity. During remission, these changes may regress.[11] Jaffe has pointed out that the transverse radiolucent zones are not only seen in leukemic children but also may be encountered in scurvy and after severe nonleukemic illnesses.[18]

As the leukemic process fulminates, the metaphyseal regions show increasing fields of rarefaction with focal cortical erosion manifested by several round or oval "punched out" radiolucent areas. In this stage of lytic destruction, serious consideration should be given to metastases from a neuroblastoma. Periosteal new bone formation may also be a prominent feature. This is produced by invasion and elevation of the periosteum, the leukemic infiltrate reaching the periosteum via the broadened and penetrated haversian system (Fig. 25–8).[29] In occasional cases, the paradoxical reaction of osteosclerosis may occur, manifested by increased radiopacity lacking any signs of periosteal new bone formation or rarefied radiolucent osseous changes (Fig. 25–9).[2, 15, 16, 18, 24, 28, 37, 38, 43]

Acute leukemia in adults often lacks osseous manifestations and is rarely the source of clinicopathologic concern. During the course of dissemination, a malignant lymphoma may show a leukemic marrow conversion, thereby also manifesting some skeletal abnormalities.[17] On the other hand, similar osseous changes of mild generalized osteoporosis may be seen in chronic lymphoid or myeloid leukemia.[6, 8] The porotic alterations go hand in hand with distinct or confluent areas of radiolucencies and small intermittent zones of radiopacity.[22, 35] Periosteal new bone formation is only rarely seen. According to Apitz, the focal leukemic marrow necrosis seen on light microscopic examination not only is accompanied by necrotic bony trabeculae in the spongiosa but

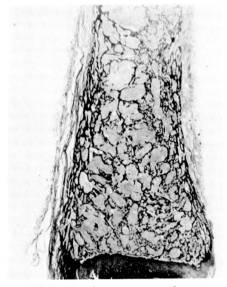

Figure 25–9. Leukemic osteosclerosis in an adult with a closely meshed thickened spongy trabecular pattern seen in a longitudinal full-bone section. (Hematoxylin-eosin stain. Magnification × 6.)

also may extend into the adjacent cortex.[1] Similar to those seen in children, the radiographic osseous changes in adults may reveal diffuse osteosclerosis involving several bones.[7, 19, 27, 28, 36-38, 43, 44]

REFERENCES

1. Apitz, K.: Über Knochenveränderungen bei Leukämie. Virchows. Arch. [Pathol. Anat.], 302:301–322, 1938.
2. Assmann, H.: Beiträge zur osteosklerotischen Anämie. Beitr. Pathol. Anat. Allg. Pathol., 41:565–595, 1907.
3. Baty, J. M., and Vogt, E. C.: Bone changes of leukemia in children. Am. J. Roentgenol. Radium Ther. Nucl. Med., 34:310–314, 1935.
4. Bender, I. B.: Bone changes in leucemia. Am. J. Orthod., 30:556–563, 1944.
5. Brünner, J. M., Gudbjerg, G. E., and Iversen, T.: Skeletal lesions in leukaemia in children. Acta Radiol., 49:419–424, 1958.
6. Campbell, E., Jr., Maldonado, W., and Suhrland, G.: Painful lytic bone lesion in an adult with chronic myelogenous leukemia. Cancer, 35:1354–1356, 1975.
7. Carpenter, G., and Flory, C. M.: Chronic nonleukemic myelosis: report of a case with megakaryocytic myeloid splenomegaly, leukoerythroblastic anemia, generalized osteosclerosis and myelofibrosis. Arch. Intern. Med., 67:489–508, 1941.
8. Chabner, B. A., Haskell, C. M., and Canellos, G. P.: Destructive bone lesions in chronic granulocytic leukemia. Medicine, 48:401–410, 1969.
9. Craver, L. F., and Copeland, M. M.: Changes of the bones in the leukemias. Arch. Surg., 30:639–646, 1935.
10. Curtis, A. B.: Childhood leukemias: osseous changes in jaws on panoramic dental radiographs. J. Am. Dent. Assoc., 83:844–847, 1971.
11. deCastro, L. A., Kuhn, J. P., Freeman, A. I., et al.: Complete remodeling of the vertebrae in a child successfully treated for acute lymphocytic leukemia (ALL). Cancer, 40:398–401, 1977.
12. Dresner, E.: The bone and joint lesions in acute leukaemia and their response to folic acid antagonists. Q. J. Med., 19:339–352, 1950.
13. Erb, I. H.: Bone changes in leukaemia. Part II. Pathology. Arch. Dis. Child., 9:319–326, 1934.
14. Follis, R. H., Jr., and Park, E. A.: Some observations on the morphologic basis for the roentgenographic changes in childhood leukemia. Bull. Hosp. Joint Dis., 12:67–73, 1951.
15. Fresen, O.: On osteomyelosclerosis. Acta Pathol. Jpn., 11:87–108, 1961.
16. Goldberg, A., and Seaton, D. A.: The diagnosis and management of myelofibrosis, myelosclerosis and chronic myeloid leukaemia. Clin. Radiol, 11:266–270, 1960.
17. Hustu, H. O., and Pinkel, D.: Lymphosarcoma, Hodgkin's disease and leukemia in bone. Clin. Orthop. 52:83–93, 1967.
18. Jaffe, H. L.: Skeletal manifestations of leukemia and malignant lymphoma. Bull. Hosp. Joint Dis., 13:217–238, 1952.
19. Jordan, H. E., and Scott, J. K.: A case of osteosclerosis with extensive extramedullary hemopoiesis and a leukemic blood reaction. Arch. Pathol., 32:895–909, 1941.
20. Kalayjian, B. S., Herbut, P. A., and Erf, L. A.: The bone changes of leukemia in children. Radiology, 47:223–233, 1946.
21. Massimo, L., Comelli, A., and Astaldi, A., Jr.: A study of the incidence of malformations and of familial neoplastic diathesis in children with leukemia and other malignancies. Gaslini, 6:74–77, 1974.
22. Nesbitt, J., and Roth, R. E.: Solitary lytic bone lesions in an adult with chronic myelogenous leukemia. Radiology, 64:724–726, 1955.
23. Nixon, G. W., and Gwinn, J. L.: The roentgen manifestations of leukemia in infancy. Radiology, 107:603–609, 1973.
24. Oechslin, R. J.: Osteomyelosklerose und Skelett. Acta Haematol. (Basel), 16:214–234, 1956.
25. O'Hara, A. E.: Roentgenographic osseous manifestations of the anemias and the leukemias. Clin. Orthop., 52:63–82, 1967.
26. Patrassi, G.: Zerstörungsvorgänge am Skelett im Verlauf leukämischer Erkrankungen. Beitr. Pathol. Anat. Allg. Pathol., 86:643–662, 1931.
27. Pettigrew, J. D., and Ward, H. P.: Correlation of radiologic, histologic, and clinical findings in agnogenic myeloid metaplasia. Radiology, 93:541–548, 1969.
28. Pitcock, J. A., Reinhard, E. H., Justus, B. W., et al.: A clinical and pathological study of seventy cases of myelofibrosis. Ann. Intern. Med., 57:73–84, 1962.
29. Poynton, F. J., and Lightwood, R.: Lymphatic leukaemia, with infiltration of periosteum simulating acute rheumatism. Lancet, 1:1192–1194, 1932.
30. von Rohr, K.: Myelofibrose und Osteomyelosklerose (Osteomyeloretikulose-Syndrom). Acta Haematol. (Basel), 15:209–234, 1956.
31. Silverman, F. N:The skeletal lesions in leukemia; clinical and roentgenographic observations in 103 infants and children with a review of the literature. Am. J. Roentgenol. Radium Ther. Nucl. Med., 59:819–844, 1948.
32. Silverstein, M. N., and Kelly, P. J.: Leukemia with osteoarticular symptoms and signs. Ann. Intern. Med., 59:637–645, 1963.
33. Simmons, C. R., Harle, T. S., and Singleton, E. B.: The osseous manifestations of leukemia in children. Radiol. Clin. North Am., 6:115–130, 1968.
34. Snelling, C. E., and Brown, A.: Bone changes in leukaemia. Part I. Clinical and roentgenological. Arch. Dis. Child., 9:315–318, 1934.
35. Spengler, D. M., Leiberg, O. U., and Bailey, R. W.: Rapid diaphyseal destruction. An unusual osseous manifestation of chronic granulocytic leukemia. Clin. Orthop., 115:231–235, 1976.
36. Stodtmeister, R., and Sandkühler, S.: Knochenmarkatrophie und Knochenmarkfibrose. Dtsch. Med. Wochenschr., 76:1431–1433, 1951.
37. Sussman, M. L.: Myelosclerosis with leukoerythroblastic anemia. Am. J. Roentgenol. Radium Ther. Nucl. Med., 57:313–320, 1947.
38. Sussman, M. L.: Skeletal changes associated with diseases of the blood. Bull. N.Y. Acad. Med., 26:763–778, 1950.
39. Thomas, L. B., Forkner, C. E., Jr., Frei, E., et al.:

Skeletal lesions of acute leukemia. Cancer, *14*:608–621, 1961.

40. Townsend, S. R.: A single myeloid bone tumour associated with a blood picture of chronic myelocytic leukaemia. Can. Med. Assoc. J., *40*:352–354, 1939.

41. Van Slyck, E. J.: The bony changes in malignant hematologic disease. Orthop. Clin. North Am., 3:733–744, 1972.

42. Willson, J. K. V.: The bone lesions of childhood

leukemia. A survey of 140 cases. Radiology, 72:672–681, 1959.

43. Wolf, C.: Über einen Fall von osteosklerotischer Pseudoleukämie. Beitrag zur Frage der Osteosklerosen. Beitr. Pathol. Anat. Allg. Pathol., 89:151–182, 1932.

44. Wyatt, J. P., and Sommers, S. C.: Chronic marrow failure, myelosclerosis and extramedullary hematopoiesis. Blood, 5:329–347, 1950.

OSSEOUS MANIFESTATIONS OF HODGKIN'S DISEASE. PRIMARY HODGKIN'S DISEASE OF BONE

INCIDENCE

The incidence of osseous involvement in Hodgkin's disease varies greatly, depending on whether the data reported are based on clinical material or supported by an autopsy.[20] The clinical incidence is described as being about 10 to 20 per cent.[31, 58, 66] Based on autopsy findings, the frequency of bone involvement is much higher and varies from 34 per cent[79] to 78 per cent.[73]

The osseous involvement may appear late in the course of the disease in some patients and quite early in others. The question as to whether Hodgkin's disease can, or does, arise primarily in bone is not an easy one to answer. Some refute such an occurrence by stating that bone involvement can only occur either by hematogenous dissemination (stage IV disease) or by direct extension of nodal or soft tissue lesions (so-called local extranodal spread).

Abdominal, bipedal lymphangiography and inferior venacavography only became uniformly available as reliable tools for clinical staging of Hodgkin's disease after 1960.[76] Surgical staging with exploratory laparotomy became popular somewhat later.[30] The absence of these studies, or the lack of radioisotopic workups like bone and liver or gallium scans, makes it difficult, if not impossible, to reliably gauge the extent of involvement and whether the disease is indeed arising in a single bone.[23] Osseous

involvement may be assessed by the use of radiography,[28, 31, 35] scintiscan,[84] or biopsy examination of the bone marrow.[20, 32, 67, 69,83] Clinically, in Hodgkin's disease, primary osseous presentation in the absence of peripheral lymphadenopathy or splenic enlargement is usually insufficient evidence, without the above-mentioned studies, to classify a bone lesion as unquestionably the site of origin. An arbitrary six month symptom-free period between the discovery of the bony tumor and the appearance of other sites of involvement may suffice for some but may be deemed less than compelling proof by many others. These and other reservations make the concept of primary Hodgkin's disease of bone hard to prove. Primary osseous Hodgkin's disease does occur but is very rare and difficult to verify.

Many published articles report reasonably well-documented cases of Hodgkin's disease with apparently primary bone lesions in the absence of nodal involvement.[2, 4, 6, 8, 22, 28, 29, 34, 38, 45, 46, 48, 49, 51, 52, 54, 63, 72, 73, 77, 78]

SIGNS AND SYMPTOMS

Pain is the most common presenting symptom, often directed toward the affected bone, but entirely asymptomatic lesions are not unusual. Often, the pain precedes the roentgenographically inapparent involvement by several months. In general, lytic lesions are more likely to be symptomatic than are sclerotic ones.[75] Sometimes, alcohol consumption precipitates bone pain.[3, 9, 11, 15, 42] Radiating pain is associated with sacroiliac disease; neurologic signs may accompany vertebral lesions with spinal cord compression. Pathologic fractures may be seen with weight-bearing bone tumors or those involving ribs. Painless bone lesions have been described.[66]

LOCATION

In clinically manifested skeletal involvement, Hodgkin's disease preferentially involves the vertebral column with the bodies being primarily altered. The vertebral processes, pedicles, laminae, or spine are involved less often. In particular, the lower thoracic and upper lumbar regions are affected. The innominate bone and its iliac portion, the sternum, the scapula, the ribs, and the femur are involved, in order of decreasing frequency. The mandible is rarely the site of involvement.[25, 28, 73, 74]

RADIOGRAPHIC FEATURES

The true incidence of radiographically demonstrable osseous involvement is not fully known. The rate of occurrence varies from a low of 8.3 per cent[73] to 9.6 per cent[31] to a high of 23 per cent.[40] Consider-

able bone marrow replacement may be present without corresponding cortical erosion. This paradoxical occurrence usually accompanies the lymphocyte-depleted form of the disease.[65, 67]

The bone destruction of Hodgkin's disease may be of the lytic, sclerotic, or mixed variety. According to the findings of Granger and Whitaker, 75 per cent of the lesions are lytic, 15 per cent sclerotic, and 5 per cent mixed and the remaining 5 per cent show only a periosteal reaction.[31] In two thirds of the patients, the lesions are multifocal, and their appearance may vary in the same patient.[65]

Radiographically, a predominantly osteolytic destructive process is usually seen that most frequently involves a vertebral body or several adjacent ones with resulting eventual collapse (Fig. 25–10). Involvement of the vertebral processes, pedicles, laminae, and spine is much less common. Scalloping of the anterior or lateral aspects of a vertebral body is a well-recognized but rare finding.[65] In rare instances, a pronounced sclerotic reaction, both patchy and diffuse, may be featured, culminating in the appearance of an "ivory" vertebra.[36] It has become increasingly clear that, especially in a child, the wedging collapse of a vertebral body, suggesting vertebra plana (also called Calvé's disease) most often results from an eo-

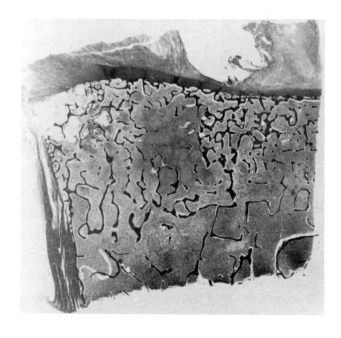

Figure 25–10. Patchy destruction of the third lumbar vertebra in a patient with Hodgkin's disease. The vertebral disk remains uninvolved. (Hematoxylin-eosin stain. Magnification ×5.)

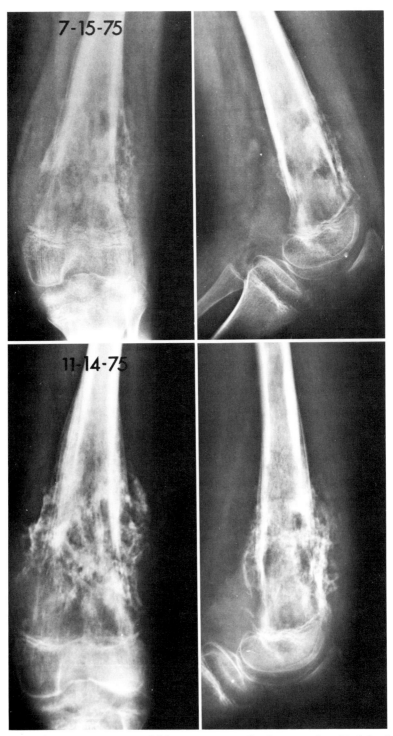

Figure 25–11. Rapidly progressing painful lesion eventually diagnosed as Hodgkin's disease in the distal femur of a 13-year-old boy. Marked periosteal reaction with mixed lytic and sclerotic bone destruction. (Courtesy of Drs. R. C. Marcove and G. Rosen.)

sinophilic granuloma and not from Hodgkin's disease.[14, 27, 41, 44, 60, 86] Naturally, this diagnosis becomes much more obvious if a paraspinal soft tissue mass is present. Hodgkin's disease tends to spare the vertebral discs.

Prominent calcification affecting the longitudinal spinal ligaments accompanied by abutting vertebral sclerosis may be seen even in the absence of treatment.[21] Osteosclerotic lesions changing into osteolytic destruction usually accompany progressive disease. Sclerosis may be an initial finding or may be the result of treatment, especially radiation.[65, 82]

The reason that the bone reacts with such peculiar osteosclerotic changes, which go hand in hand with the connective tissue replacement of the marrow spaces, is not entirely clear. This process is often referred to as osteomyelosclerosis. The pathogenesis of this occurrence is far from clear. It seems that the gradual replacement of the marrow spaces by neoplastic cells slowly incites a fibrous tissue proliferation that eventually results in the replacement of the myeloid elements. The bony trabeculae react to the progressive marrow involvement by increased bone production either by heightened osteoblastic activity or by conversion of the fibrous connective tissue first into primitive and then into mature calcified bone.[26, 61]

A radiolucent destruction characterizes the involvement of a flat bone, usually the pelvis. Sharply demarcated, "punched out" radiolucent lesions of varying sizes are evident. Intermittent areas of osteosclerosis are noted, especially parallel to the sacroiliac joints. Pear suggested that this finding may represent contiguous extension by overlying involved iliac lymph nodes.[65] Paget disease–like pelvic osseous changes, characterized by compact cortical broadening and a mixed type of destruction, may be seen.

In long tubular bones, the lytic destruction of the spongiosa extends into adjacent cortex and may incite a mild or occasionally luxuriant periosteal bone reaction (Fig. 25–11). This aspect of periosteal new bone formation was emphasized by Granger and Whitaker, who demonstrated it in one third of their cases.[31] Mixed osteolytic and osteoblastic lesions in the long bones may be featured prominently.

The costal and sternal involvement may be manifested by osseous expansion accompanied by a lamellated or spiculated periosteal reaction. Mandibular lesions present with well-delimited radiolucent areas related to the apices of teeth with loss of the lamina dura.[25]

HISTOLOGIC FEATURES

In Hodgkin's disease, typical Sternberg-Reed cells and mononuclear cells with similar nuclear characteristics form the neoplastic components.[53] These are intimately associated with a variety of inflammatory cells that may often form the major portion of the lesion. The classic picture of Hodgkin's disease, the mixed cellularity type (and this is the most common variant seen in those arising in bones), is characterized by Sternberg-Reed cells or mononuclear cells with corresponding nuclear features, in addition to many lymphocytes and histiocytes. The inflammatory and reactive components of the lesion are composed of eosinophilic and neutrophilic mature granulocytes, plasma cells, and lymphocytes. The eosinophilic component and the reactive histiocytes may be prominent features, which presents a problem when making a diagnostic distinction between eosinophilic granuloma and Hodgkin's disease. The time-honored adage should be kept in mind: If tissue examination of a bone lesion, particularly in a middle-aged or elderly patient but also occasionally in an adolescent, suggests that one might be dealing with an eosinophilic granuloma, there is still a good probability that the lesion is, in fact, Hodgkin's disease.[41]

Attempts at aspiration biopsy of the posterior iliac crest often yield no diagnostic material. Needle biopsy, however, is usually more rewarding and brings forth a definitive diagnosis.

TREATMENT

The treatment and prognosis of Hodgkin's disease is directly related to the stage of the disease. In the rare localized osseous presentation, in the absence of nodal or other organ involvement with a negative staging laparotomy, radiotherapy should be given. A total therapeutic dose of 4000 to 5000 rads in four to five weeks, directed to the entire involved bone, should be planned in order to permanently eradicate the disease. Irradiation of the involved lymph nodes in higher stage disease and intensive multiple drug therapy sequentially employing doxorubicin hydrochloride (Adriamycin) followed by prednisone, procarbazine hydrochloride, and vincristine sulfate, in addition to cyclophosphamide, is recommended by Tan and associates.[76]

REFERENCES

1. Abrams, H. S.: The osseous system in Hodgkin's disease. Ann. Surg., *108*:296–304, 1938.
2. Abreu, E. F.: Un caso de Hodgkin de punto de partida periostico. Cir. Ortop. Traumatol., 5:277–280, 1937.
3. Alexander, D. A.: Alcohol-induced pain in Hodgkin's disease. Br. Med. J., 2:1376, 1953.
4. Arnold, H. S., Meese, E. H., D'Amato, N. A., et al.: Localized Hodgkin's disease presenting as a sternal tumor and treated by total sternectomy. Ann. Thorac. Surg., 2:87–93, 1966.
5. Beachley, M. C., Lau, B. P., and King, E. R.: Bone involvement in Hodgkin's disease. Am. J. Roentgenol. Radium Ther. Nucl. Med., 114:559–563, 1972.
6. Blount, W. P.: Hodgkin's disease: an orthopaedic problem. J. Bone Joint Surg., 11:761–770, 1929.
7. Bournons, J., and Jeanmart, L.: Les infiltrations osseuses de nature Hodgkinienne. J. Belge Radiol., 56:407–413, 1973.
8. Bouvier, M., Lejeune, E., Deplante, J. P., et al.: Hodgkin's disease beginning with ostalgic manifestations. J. Med. Lyon, 55:643–657, 1974.
9. Braun, W. E., and Shnider, B. I.: Alcohol-induced pain in Hodgkin's disease. J.A.M.A., *168*:1882–1885, 1958.
10. Busy, J., Lotte, J., and Pallardy, G.: Etude radiologique des localisations osseuses de la maladie de Hodgkin. J. Radiol. Electrol. Med. Nucl., 39:239–247, 1958.
11. Case records of the Massachusetts General Hospital. Case 7–1975. N. Engl. J. Med., 292:357–363, 1975.
12. Case records of the Massachusetts General Hospital. Case 8–1978. N. Engl. J. Med., 298:501–505, 1978.
13. Charache, H.: Tumors in one of homologous twins. Hodgkin's disease with primary skeletal manifestations. Am. J. Roentgenol. Radium Ther. Nucl. Med., 54:179–181, 1945.
14. Compere, E. L., Johnson, W. E., and Coventry, M. B.: Vertebra plana (Calvé's disease) due to eosinophilic granuloma. J. Bone Joint Surg. [Am.], 36:969–980, 1954.
15. Conn, H. O.: Alcohol-induced pain as a manifestation of Hodgkin's disease. Arch. Intern. Med., *100*:241–247, 1957.
16. Craver, L. F., and Copeland, M. M.: Changes in bone in Hodgkin's granuloma. Arch. Surg., 28:1062–1086, 1934.
17. De Seze, S., Lequesne, M., and Moghtader, R.: Le pincement diseal juxta-néoplasique contemporain des affections malignes du corps vertébral. Rev. Rheum. Mal. Osteoartic., 35:225–230, 1968.
18. De Seze, S., and Ordonneau, P.: Localisations osseuses dans la maladie de Hodgkin. Rev. Rheum. Mal. Osteoartic., 11:4–7, 1944.
19. Desprez-Curely, J. P., and Picard, J. D.: Aspects radiologiques des localisations osseuses au cours de la maladie de Hodgkin. Sem. Hop. Paris, 33:1482–1489, 1957.
20. Duhamel, G., Najman, A., and André, R.: Les localisations à la moelle osseuse de la maladie de Hodgkin — leur place dans l'évolution de la maladie. Etude par biopsie médullaire de 100 observations. Nouv. Presse Méd., 79:2305–2308, 1971.
21. Duncan, A. W.: Calcification of the anterior longitudinal vertebral ligaments in Hodgkin's disease. Clin. Radiol., 24:394–395, 1973.
22. Dyttert, V.: Primary osseous lymphogranuloma. A contribution. Neoplasma, 13:105–111, 1966.
23. Ferrant, A., Rodhain, J., Michaux, J. L., et al.: Detection of skeletal involvement in Hodgkin's disease: a comparison of radiography, bone scanning, and bone marrow biopsy in 38 patients. Cancer, 35:1346–1353, 1975.
24. Fisher, A. M., Kendall, B., and Van Leuven, B. D.: Hodgkin's disease: a radiological survey. Clin. Radiol., 13:115–127, 1962.
25. Forman, G. H., and Wesson, C. M.: Hodgkin's disease of the mandible. Br. J. Oral Surg., 7:146–152, 1970.
26. Fresen, O.: On osteomyelosclerosis. Acta Pathol., Jpn., 11:87–108, 1961.
27. Fripp, A. T.: Vertebra plana, J. Bone Joint Surg., [Br.], 40:378–384, 1958.
28. Fucilla, I. S., and Hamann, A.: Hodgkin's disease in bone. Radiology, 77:53–60, 1961.
29. Giraud and Lacorre: Les localisations osseuses cliniquement primitives de la maladie de Hodgkin. J. Radiol. Electrol. Med. Nucl., 31:583–586, 1950.
30. Glatstein, E., Guernsey, J. M., Rosenberg, S. A., et al.: The value of laparotomy and splenectomy in the staging of Hodgkin's disease. Cancer, 24:709–718, 1969.
31. Granger, W., and Whitaker, R.: Hodgkin's disease in bone, with special reference to periosteal reaction. Br. J. Radiol., 40:939–948, 1967.
32. Han, T., Stutzman, L., and Roque, A. L.: Bone marrow biopsy in Hodgkin's disease and other neoplastic diseases. J.A.M.A., 217:1239–1241, 1971.
33. Harder, J.: Über Knochenlymphogranulomatose. Fortschr. Geb. Roentgenstr. Nuklearmed., 93: 445–455, 1960.
34. Herscher, H.: Hodgkin's disease of bone marrow and liver without apparent involvement of lymph nodes. Am. J. Roentgenol. Radium Ther. Nucl. Med., 35:73–77, 1936.
35. Horan, F. T.: Bone involvement in Hodgkin's disease. A survey of 201 cases. Br. J. Surg., 56:277–281, 1969.
36. Hultén, O.: Ein Fall von "Elfenbeinwirbel" bei

Lymphogranulomatose. Acta Radiol., 8:245–251, 1927.

37. Hustu, H. O., and Pinkel, D.: Lymphosarcoma, Hodgkin's disease and leukemia in bone. Clin. Orthop., 52:83–93, 1967.

38. Inglesakis, J. A., Abbes, M., and Martin, E.: Maladie de Hodgkin a debut vertebral. Soc. Chir. Marseille, 15:77–84, 1963.

39. Jackson, H., and Parker, F., Jr.: Hodgkin's disease. II. Pathology. N. Engl. J. Med., 231:35–44, 1944.

40. Jackson, H., Jr., and Parker, F., Jr.: Hodgkin's disease. IV. Involvement of certain organs. N. Engl. J. Med., 232:547–559, 1945.

41. Jaffe, H. L.: Metabolic, Degenerative, and Inflammatory Diseases of Bones and Joints. Philadelphia, Lea & Febiger, 1972, p. 877.

42. James, A. H.: Hodgkin's disease with and without alcohol-induced pain. A clinical and histological comparison. Q. J. Med., 29:47–66, 1960.

43. Kaplan, H. S.: Contiguity and progression in Hodgkin's disease. Cancer Res., 31:1811–1813, 1971.

44. Kieffer, S. A., Nesbit, M. E., and D'Angio, G. J.: Vertebra plana due to histiocytosis X: serial studies. Acta Radiol. [Diagn.] (Stockh.), 8:241–250, 1969.

45. Kooreman, P. J., and Haex, A. J.: Hodgkin's disease of the skeleton. Acta Med. Scand., 115:177–196, 1943.

46. Krumbhaar, E. B.: Hodgkin's disease of bone marrow and spleen without apparent involvement of lymph nodes. Am. J. Med. Sci., 182:764–769, 1931.

47. Lamarque, P., Betoulieres, P., Pelissier, M., et al.: Au subjet des lésions osseuses de la maladie de Hodgkin. J. Radiol. Electrol. Med. Nucl., 34:695–699, 1953.

48. Lecanet, D., Bernageau, T., Basch, A., et al.: Les localisations osseuses de la maladie de Hodgkin. Ann. Radiol., 14:845–861, 1971.

49. LeDoux-Lebard, R., Marchand, J. H., and Lefebvre, J.: Localisation primitivement osseuse d'une lymphogranulomatose. Bull. Soc. Electr. Radiol. Med. France, 14:150–153, 1939.

50. Lefebre, R., and Laurain, J.: Maladie de Hodgkin à localisation osseuse primitive. Rev. Med. Nord-Est, 62:57–62, 1957.

51. Leger, L., Pineau, P., and Andrieux, J.: Localisations osseuses de la maladie de Hodgkin. Presse Méd., 60:1762–1766, 1952.

52. Livingston, S. K.: Hodgkin's disease of the skeleton without glandular involvement. A case report proved by autopsy. J. Bone Joint Surg., 17:189–194, 1935.

53. Lukes, R. J., and Butler, J. J.: The pathology and nomenclature of Hodgkin's disease. Cancer Res., 26:1063–1081, 1966.

54. Meher-Homji, D. R., DeSouza, L. J., Mohanty, B., et al.: Unusual sternal mass in Hodgkin's disease. J. Bone Joint Surg. [Am.], 54:402–404, 1972.

55. Moir, P. J., and Brockis, J. G.: Observations on bone lesions in Hodgkin's disease. Br. J. Surg., 36:414–417, 1949.

56. Montgomery, A. H.: Hodgkin's disease of bones. Ann. Surg., 87:755–766, 1928.

57. Moseley, J. E.: Patterns of bone change in the malignant lymphomas. J. Mt. Sinai Hosp., 29:463–503, 1962.

58. Musshoff, K.: Prognostic and therapeutic implications of staging in extranodal Hodgkin's disease. Cancer Res., 31:1814–1827, 1971.

59. Myers, C. E., Chabner, B. A., DeVita, V. T., et al.: Bone marrow involvement in Hodgkin's disease: pathology and response to MOPP chemotherapy. Blood, 44:197–204, 1974.

60. Nesbit, M. E., Kieffer, S., and D'Angio, G. J.: Reconstitution of vertebral height in histiocytosis X: A long-term follow up. J. Bone Joint Surg. [Am.], 51:1360–1368, 1969.

61. Oechslin, R. J.: Osteomyelosklerose und Skelett. Acta Haematol. (Basel), 16:214–234, 1956.

62. Olmer, J., Mongin, M., and Muratore, R.: Lésions osseuses au cours d'un paragranulome hodgkinien. Sang, 31:135–138, 1960.

63. Papillon, J., Croizat, P., Revol, L., et al.: Les localisations osseuses de la lymphogranulomatose maligne. J. Radiol. Electrol. Med. Nucl., 45:109–116, 1964.

64. Pavlovsky, A., Paterson Toledo, R., and Muscolo, D.: Linfogranulomatosis ósea: comentarios sobre 25 observaciones. Rev. Ortop. Traumatol., 3:136–157, 1944.

65. Pear, B. L.: Skeletal manifestations of the lymphomas and leukemias. Semin. Roentgenol., 9:229–240, 1974.

66. Perttala, Y., and Kijanen, I.: Roentgenologic bone lesions in lymphogranulomatosis maligna: analysis of 453 cases. Ann. Chir. Gynaecol. Fenn., 54:414–424, 1965.

67. Pris, J., Fabre, J., Corberand, J., et al.: Biopsies de moelle et maladie de Hodgkin. Nouv, Rev. Fr. Hematol., 13:410–415, 1973.

68. Properzi, E.: Manifestazioni scheletriche del linfogranuloma maligno. Radiol. Med. (Torino), 37:287–303, 1951.

69. Rosenberg, S. A.: Hodgkin's disease of the bone marrow. Cancer Res., 31:1733–1736, 1971.

70. Rosala, E., Schachter, A., and Georgesco, I.: Considérations radiologiques sur quelques localisations osseuses monovertébrales au cours de la lymphogranulomatose maligne. Presse Méd., 74:1051–1054, 1966.

71. Roussel, J., Schoumacher, P., Pernot, M., et al.: Considérations sur les localisations osseuses de la maladie de Hodgkin. J. Radiol. Electrol. Med. Nucl., 47:482–485, 1966.

72. Spencer, J., and Dresser, R.: Lymphoblastoma (Hodgkin's and sarcoma type) of bone. With a report of three cases simulating primary malignant tumor of bone. N. Engl. J. Med., 214:877–879, 1936.

73. Steiner, P. E.: Hodgkin's disease: incidence, distribution, nature and possible significance of lymphogranulomatous lesions in bone marrow; review with original data. Arch. Pathol., 36:627–637, 1943.

74. Stern, N. S., and Shensa, D. R.: Hodgkin's disease of the mandible: report of case. J. Oral Surg., 31:628–631, 1973.

75. Stuhlbarg, J., and Ellis, F. W.: Hodgkin's disease of bone. Favorable prognostic significance? Am. J. Roentgenol. Radium Ther. Nucl. Med., 93:568–572, 1965.

76. Tan, C., D'Angio, G. J., Exelby, P. R., et al.: The

changing management of childhood Hodgkin's disease. Cancer, 35:808–816, 1975.

77. Touzard, R. C.: A propos d'une localisation costale révélatrice d'une maladie de Hodgkin. J. Chir., 100:411–414, 1970.

78. Trompeter, J., and Rosen, G.: Primary Hodgkin's disease of bone in children and young adults. (In preparation.)

79. Uehlinger, E.: Über Knochen-Lymphogranulomatose. Virchows Arch. [Pathol. Anat.], 288:36–118, 1933.

80. Ultmann, J. E., Cunningham, J. K., and Gellhorn, A.: The clinical picture of Hodgkin's disease. Cancer Res., 26:1047–1060, 1966.

81. Van Slyck, E. J.: The bony changes in malignant hematologic disease. Orthop. Clin. North Am., 3:733–744, 1972.

82. Vieta, J. O., Friedell, H. L., and Craver, L. F.: A survey of Hodgkin's disease and lymphosarcoma in bone. Radiology, 39:1–15, 1942.

83. Webb, D. I., Ubogy, G., and Silver, R. T.: Importance of bone marrow biopsy in the clinical staging of Hodgkin's disease. Cancer, 26:313–317, 1970.

84. Weber, W. G., De Nardo, G. L., and Bergin, J. J.: Scintiscanning in malignant lymphomatous involvement of bone. Arch. Intern. Med., 121:433–437, 1968.

85. Wellens, P., and Jansen, W.: Considérations relatives aux lésions osseuses de la maladie de Hodgkin. J. Belge Radiol., 37:441–453, 1954.

86. Yabsley, R. H., and Harris, W. R.: Solitary eosinophilic granuloma of a vertebral body causing paraplegia. Report of a case. J. Bone Joint Surg. [Am.], 48:1570–1574, 1966.

26

MULTIPLE MYELOMA, INCLUDING SOLITARY OSSEOUS MYELOMA

DEFINITION

Multiple myeloma is a malignant tumor of plasma cells primarily characterized by widespread osteolytic bone destruction and often associated with refractory anemia, hypercalcemia, renal dysfunction, and decreased ability to resist infection. Amyloid deposition, derangement of coagulation, cryoglobulinemia, and elevated serum viscosity are less common features. "Myeloma" means marrow tumor.

HISTORICAL ASPECTS

Multiple myeloma has been recognized since the mid-19th century when, based on separate studies of the same patient, Dalrymple described the microscopic appearance of the bone lesions,[53] Bence Jones identified the protein excreted in the urine,[19] and Macintyre outlined the clinical findings.[150] In 1873, von Rustizky delineated in detail the clinicopathologic features of this disease.[259] Some refer to multiple myeloma as "Kahler's disease,"

after the late-19th century clinician from Prague whose seminal lectures were instrumental in the better understanding of the varied symptomatology of this condition.[112, 113]

INCIDENCE

Multiple myeloma is the most common neoplasm of bone in adults. It represents approximately half of all malignant bone tumors, and its incidence appears to be rising gradually. The National Cancer Survey in 1973 found an incidence of two to three myeloma cases per 100,000 people in the United States, which is about the same frequency as for Hodgkin's disease and chronic lymphoid leukemia. The Scandinavian countries also seem to have an increased rate of incidence, while this disease is quite rare in Japan. It is a matter of conjecture whether better diagnostic techniques or longer life expectancy have materially contributed to this apparently increased incidence or whether an absolute increase in myeloma cases has truly occurred. The rate of occurrence among

413

Jamaican blacks is augmented.[55, 255] This disease also affected prehistoric American Indians.[177]

In the United States, for both sexes, high rates of mortality due to multiple myeloma have been found to occur in Montana, the Dakotas, Minnesota, and Iowa.[161]

SIGNS AND SYMPTOMS

Pain is the cardinal initial symptom, suggesting neuralgia or arthritis, and is present in more than 75 per cent of the patients early in the course of the disease. The location of the pain varies widely, but it is usually felt in the pelvis, spine, and thoracic cage. Characteristically, this pain is mild and transient at first, seems unexplained, and is practically never associated with preceding injury. Pain is much more prevalent during the day, and the patients are more comfortable and usually without pain when in bed. Weight-bearing, exercise, and activity enhance the pain. Low back pain frequently conceals multiple myeloma, and the patients are often treated for herniated intervertebral disk problems, sciatica, or lumbago before the correct diagnosis is established. Soft tissue swelling is only present in about 10 per cent of the patients, and pathologic fractures are even less frequent as presenting symptoms but do occur later in approximately 20 per cent of the patients. Rarely, insignificant trauma may result in fractures, and spontaneous vertebral compression fractures are warning signs that should be heeded. Fractures often involve non-weight-bearing bones, especially the 5th to 12th ribs. Soft tissue involvement may be present to a considerable extent.[58] The delay between the earliest symptom and the diagnosis varies significantly and ranges from one month to three years, with an average of 13 months. In the more advanced stages of disease, there is excruciating pain due to multiple fractures, excessive weight loss, and anemia. The extensive involvement of the vertebrae and ribs or sternum may result in bizarre thoracic deformities, kyphoscoliosis, and shortening of stature by as much as five inches or more. With prompt diagnosis, more effective chemotherapy, and better overall management, these disfigurements have become less prevalent. An increased susceptibility to infection of all kinds complicates the clinical picture.[173] This may be related to a deficiency of both antibody production and activity, to the markedly decreased mobility of the patients, or even to the immunosuppressive, leukopenic effects of massive chemotherapy. Mandibular lesions may present with numbness of the lip or chin. Loosening of the teeth may be featured.

During the clinically asymptomatic or presymptomatic phase of myeloma, M-type serum and urine proteins may be detected with unexplained elevated erythrocyte sedimentation rate or persistent proteinuria.[192]

As a consequence of widespread bone destruction, the patients experience hypercalciuria, which, in the absence of adequate hydration, progresses into hypercalcemia and azotemia. Virtually all patients have normocytic and normochromic anemia during the course of the disease, more severely as the dissemination progresses. The anemia may also be macrocytic and is usually associated with a megaloblastic bone marrow. It is refractory to iron, B_{12}, folic acid, or liver administration. This is probably related to the marrow replacement by the tumor cells, increased destruction of erythrocytes, or other similar factors. Rouleaux formation by erythrocytes, as well as erythrocyte aggregation, also called "sludged blood," may be noted.[62] Elevated erythrocyte sedimentation rates and cryoglobulins are found in many patients with multiple myeloma. About 10 to 25 per cent of patients with classic multiple myeloma have generalized amyloidosis.[18] Hypercalcemia is common, and it may mimic hyperparathyroidism.[250]

Although the name "multiple myeloma" may imply that several autochthonous tumors have arisen either synchronously or metachronously in the bone marrow, in fact this disease process is the prime example of a clonal type of neoplasm that originated in cells in one solitary focus when the neoplastic transformation unfolded.[12, 41, 205] A considerable number of patients have definite serologic evidence of a monoclonal gamma spike before the onset of radiographically demonstrable bone destruction.[192] The striking resemblance of the M-type proteins during the preclinical and clinically apparent phases strongly indicates that this explanation is a correct one. An alternative reasonable consideration may invoke the presence of an initial autochthonous bone marrow or soft tissue myeloma clone subsequently metastasizing to other bones or nonosseous sites.

Occasionally, plasmacytomas arise in extraosseous sites, of which the upper respiratory tract is the most common. Some patients eventually show plasma cell lesions at other sites and may exhibit the clinical picture of a disseminated osseous multiple myeloma.[49, 58, 66, 269]

Patients who have had Gaucher's disease for a long time may develop polyclonal IgG elevations and myeloma.[202, 207] A number of patients with Paget's disease of bone have developed multiple myeloma.[26, 48, 76, 79, 85, 167, 208, 217, 226, 240, 241] Fanconi's syndrome in adults may be a manifestation of latent myeloma.[154]

A few reports on familial incidence have implicated some genetic factors in the pathogenesis of multiple myeloma.[153, 168, 188, 220, 267] Myeloma has also been noted in spouses.[128]

LOCATION

Any bone containing hematopoietic red marrow, and to a great extent yellow marrow as well, can harbor the nodules of multiple myeloma. The vertebral bodies, ribs, pelvic bones, and skull are the most frequently involved skeletal sites, but no bone is exempt from involvement. In many cases, it is difficult, well nigh impossible, to establish the initial site of skeletal involvement or to be certain whether the lesion actually began in bone or soft tissue.

Multiple myeloma involves the mandible and the maxilla in approximately 30 per cent of cases, but some investigators consider this estimate far too low.[38] Mandibular lesions are much more frequent than maxillary lesions. Any part of the mandible may be involved, but a slight preference for the molar and premolar areas, as well as the angle, is shown.[30, 34, 91, 141, 170, 242, 254, 266, 271,273] Multiple myeloma with small bone involvement is rare.[63, 246]

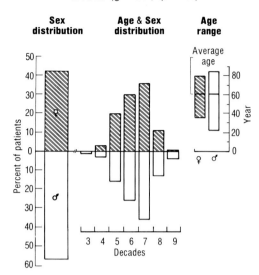

Figure 26–1. Age and sex distribution of 424 patients with plasma cell myeloma of bone seen at Memorial Hospital from 1949 through 1973.

AGE AND SEX DISTRIBUTION

Analysis of sex distribution for 424 patients studied at Memorial Hospital indicates a slightly increased male to female ratio, although there is a bias toward a higher incidence in females reported from Malmö, Sweden[260] (Fig. 26–1).

The onset of myeloma symptoms, in most cases, ranges from young adulthood to more advanced years. At Memorial Hospital, patients in their sixth and seventh decades of life were most frequently affected (Fig. 26–1). The average age of the patients, both male and female, was 60 years, with a range from early 20's to mid 80's. Women, as depicted in Figure 26–1, had a distinctly narrower age range. In the Swedish series, the peak incidence was from 70 to 80 years of age, and not one of the patients was under 40 years of age.[260] Only very few well-documented cases of myeloma have been described in patients under the age of 30 years.[44, 93, 243]

RADIOGRAPHIC FEATURES

Characteristically, myeloma presents with numerous predominantly osteolytic

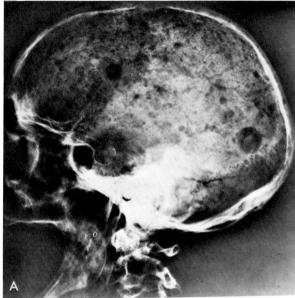

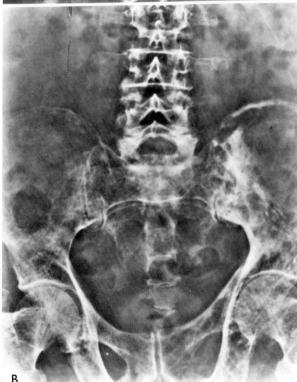

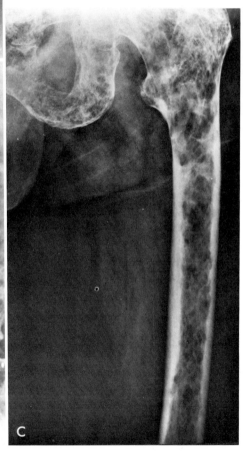

Figure 26–2. Multiple myeloma involving (A) the skull, (B) the pelvis, and (C) the left femur in a 74-year-old man. The typical osteolytic sharply defined round lesions are of variable size and become more confluent in the femur. Here, the endosteal surface of the cortex is eroded by tumor.

"punched out" areas of bone destruction with minimal or no periosteal reaction and slight thinning of the cortex (Fig. 26–2). These osteolytic lesions are frequently irregular and differ in size. Some sclerosis may be seen, usually at the periphery of the radiolucent lesions. In flat bones, the areas of bone destruction are frequently round or oval with no circumferential bone reaction. Myeloma involving the vertebral bodies presents with a structureless diffuse picture indistinguishable from osteoporosis of the spinal column. Exceptional cases of severe postmenopausal osteoporosis sometimes suggest diffuse myelomatosis involving the entire skeletal system. In long tubular bones, the lesions are circular or ovoid and may be quite extensive. Medullary bone destruction abuts the endosteal aspects of the cortex and imparts to it a wavy appearance (Fig. 26–3). Some of the intralesional areas of destruc-

tion have a fine meshwork-like structure. Especially in the mandible, myeloma may present as a slightly expansile, multilocular radiolucency simulating an ameloblastoma.[266] The cortex of the mandible is often perforated by the tumor. Calvarial lesions are typically radiolucent and sharply circumscribed but a rare "sunburst" type of presentation may also be seen.[195]

The "punched out" osteolytic bone lesions are the hallmark of multiple myeloma, the direct result of which is a state of severe negative calcium balance, which occasionally is reversible by corticosteroids. The exact mechanism by which the myeloma cells inflict this pronounced osteolytic damage is not known. Recent studies implicated an osteoclast-stimulating factor, a calcium-mobilizing polypeptide that may be responsible for activating the osteoclasts in the areas of bone resorption.[180] The serum alkaline

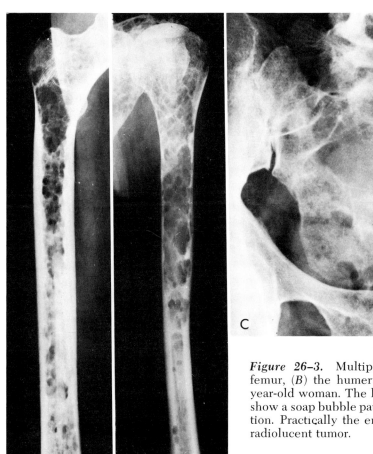

Figure 26–3. Multiple myeloma involving (A) the femur, (B) the humerus, and (C) the sacrum in a 49-year-old woman. The lesions in the long tubular bones show a soap bubble pattern of diffuse osteolytic destruction. Practically the entire sacrum is destroyed by the radiolucent tumor.

phosphatase of bone derivation remains generally normal throughout the entire course of the disease.

In most instances, osteolytic metastases from a carcinoma cannot be separated from the radiographic features of a multiple myeloma. Jacobson and colleagues have emphasized several features that help to alleviate this diagnostic dilemma.[107] The presence of a paraspinal soft tissue mass favors myeloma.[90] Osteoporosis associated with multiple myeloma is often more diffuse and pronounced than that seen in the relatively uninvolved osseous system in metastatic carcinoma. The lytic areas in the calvarium are more sharply delimited and more radiolucent in myeloma than in metastatic carcinoma. Early vertebral pedicle involvement characterizes metastatic carcinoma, although this is a late event in the course of multiple myeloma. This feature is referred to as the "vertebral pedicle sign."[107] An occasional case of skeletal echinococcosis may simulate multiple myeloma.

As already stressed, multiple myeloma presents almost exclusively with osteolytic lesions. There are occasional reports emphasizing bone sclerosis elicited by this disease, however.[29, 42, 59, 60, 94, 120, 162, 187, 222, 224] A definite association of progressive polyneuropathy and osteosclerotic myeloma was reported in a considerable number of patients.[69, 156] In 1970 and 1978, Waldenström outlined an atypical form of osteosclerotic myeloma associated with polyneuritis in younger patients.[261, 262] It is questionable whether the reported disease condition is truly a form of myeloma.

The sclerotic lesion of myeloma may be restricted to only one of the many otherwise typical osteolytic tumors, or, less often, it may represent a more generalized appearance of several regions of the osseous system. Typical "punched out" osteolytic lesions may change to osteosclerotic ones after systemic chemotherapy or in fields of irradiation. It should not be forgotten that osteoblastic metastases from an undetected primary lesion may mimic an osteosclerotic focus of myeloma. The widely disseminated form of osteosclerotic myeloma is not distinguishable from examples of myelofibrosis seen in polycythemia vera.

Kutcher and associates have stressed the value of angiography in calvarial myelomas.[122] Their review of the pertinent literature, in addition to the two cases they studied, revealed the lesions to be intensely vascular, although the tumor "blush" was less intense and of briefer duration than usually seen in meningiomas or metastases. In all cases, a prominent extracranial artery was present, directly supplying the lesion. Dural extension by tumor resulted in distorted and displaced intracranial blood vessels.

PATHOLOGIC FEATURES

On *gross examination* the appearance of the skeletal lesions reveals considerable variation. Most often, the marrow spaces are diffusely replaced by poorly defined, confluent, small tumor nodules of gelatinous consistency and dark red or brownish in color. These nodules usually reach the size of approximately 1 cm. Only in rare instances can one appreciate well-circumscribed tumor nodules in the marrow with interspersed uninvolved regions of spongiosa. As emphasized by Azar, the multiple "skipped" areas of discrete plasmacytic tumors seen on gross examination prove to be a continuous myelomatous infiltration of the bone marrow on close microscopic scrutiny.[12] In about 70 per cent of the cases, multiple myeloma reveals an extraosseous spread by the myeloma cells.[41]

The myeloma cells diffusely replace the marrow and destroy the bony trabeculae in addition to the cortex. An involved vertebral column is often rendered so pliable and soft that at autopsy it can be cut with ease and the vertebral bodies can be crushed without effort. This is the reason why the disease is also referred to as "mollities ossium."

Depending on the presence or absence of grossly recognizable extraskeletal tumors, multiple myeloma may be subdivided into three distinct stages: local intraosseous lesions, paraskeletal lesions with direct extension into adjacent soft tissues, and extraskeletal and presumably metastatic dissemination.[197] Pasmantier and Azar also found clear correlation between the gross stage of disease and the histologic grade of the myeloma cells. The better differentiated plasma cells appeared in the lower stages of disease and poorly differentiated tumor cell components appeared to be more prevalent in the most advanced stage of disease.[197] An exception to this simple and easily reproducible subdivision, however, is the occasional case with disseminated bone marrow involvement but relatively small intraosseous tumor. Other important prognostic factors seem to be the extent of myelomatous involvement of the entire skeleton as gauged by the skeletal survey, the levels of hemoglobin and serum calcium, and the abnormal protein levels in the serum as well as in the urine.[5, 56, 57]

MICROSCOPIC FEATURES

The lesions in multiple myeloma show a densely cellular tumor, the cells clustered in close aggregates, with the result that the cellular outlines are often not discernible (Fig. 26–4). The surrounding stroma is sparse and displays a delicate fibrous septa and reticulin meshwork dividing clusters

and sheets of tumor cells. Thin-walled blood vessels appear in the stroma with adjacent hemorrhages. The tumor cells closely mimic plasma cells and have a usually basophilic cytoplasm that acquires a distinctive rose-red color in methyl-green pyronine-stained preparations (Fig. 26–5). In some cases, the more immature plasmacytic cellular forms intermingle with other less differentiated plasmacytic reticulum cells (Figs. 26–6 and 26–7). By means of combined immunofluorescence techniques using fluorescein and rhodamine, a monoclonal immunoglobulin can be directly demonstrated in the myeloma cells.

Myeloma Cells and Their Function

The striking resemblance between myeloma cells and mature plasma cells was originally recognized by Wright at the turn of this century.[275] Subsequently, it became established that, although plasma cells and myeloma cells share some morphologic features, they are unlike in many important cytologic ways. Myeloma cells are

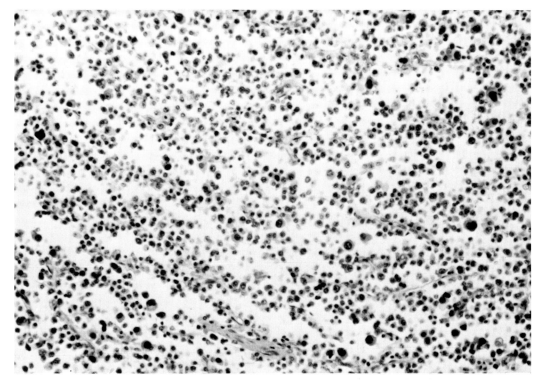

Figure 26–4. Loosely arranged diffuse sheet of myeloma cells. Note lack of vascularity and sparse stroma. (Hematoxylin-eosin stain. Magnification ×80.)

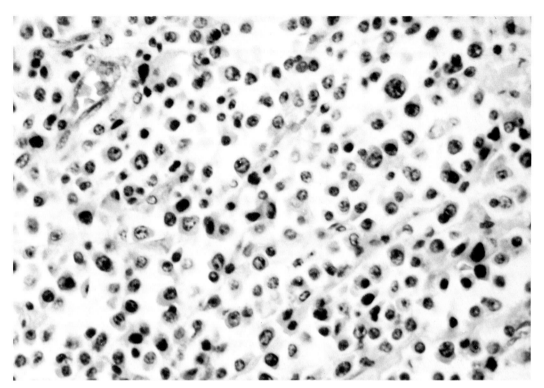

Figure 26–5. Myeloma cells with immature plasmacytic forms intermingling with more differentiated plasma cells (Hematoxylin-eosin stain. Magnification × 200.)

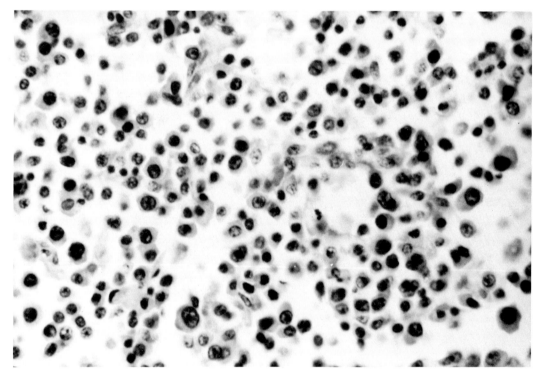

Figure 26–6. Clusters of typical myeloma cells intermixed with binucleate and giant tumor cells. (Hematoxylin-eosin stain. Magnification × 200.)

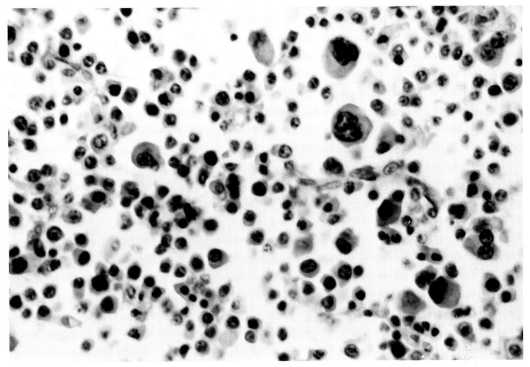

Figure 26–7. Bizarre tumor cell forms in a background of more characteristic myeloma cells. (Hematoxylin-eosin stain. Magnification × 600.)

generally larger than plasma cells and measure in excess of 20μ in widest diameter. The nuclear chromatin is more plentiful and widespread. The "cartwheel" or "spokewheel" nuclear appearance, also referred to as "Radkern," is absent, but prominent nucleoli or a solitary nucleolus frequently can be seen. The perinuclear halo, sometimes called the "Hof," representing the Golgi region is less conspicuous and often not discernible at all, especially on light microscopic examination. Intracellular, acidophilic, hyaline bodies, so-called Russell's bodies are rarely present. Pleomorphism and multinucleation are not necessarily diagnostic features of myeloma cells.

Myelomas may be classified into three histologic grades and accordingly may vary from the well-differentiated through the moderately differentiated to the poorly differentiated anaplastic variants. The well-differentiated myeloma cells are quite difficult to distinguish from normal or reactive plasma cells. The anaplastic myeloma cells, on the other hand, may mimic undifferentiated carcinomas, immunoblastic sarcomas, especially with B-type cell markers, and undifferentiated small cell sarcomas.

The plasma cells are primarily responsible for the production of immunoglobulins, the immunologically functioning proteins. Multiple plasma cell myeloma is most often accompanied by one of the five classes of serum proteins, IgG, IgA, IgM, IgD, and IgE, or light chain (Bence Jones) monoclonal immunoglobulin elaboration. A corresponding M-protein or polypeptide is demonstrable in the serum and urine by immunochemical techniques. In about half of the cases, IgG is elaborated, followed by IgA, Bence Jones light chain protein, and IgD.[58, 96, 98, 99, 196, 211] A solitary predominant protein is secreted and a narrow peak or spike is displayed on electrophoresis. In an occasional case of otherwise classic myeloma, no atypical immunoglobulin is demonstrated in the serum, but studies show these aberrant proteins to be present in the plasma cells without being relinquished into the circulation. In such instances, immunofluorescent demonstration of minute quantities of myeloma proteins may be feasible.[10] These rare cases are referred to as "nonsecretory" myeloma.[13, 81, 104, 231, 238]

In *plasma cell leukemia*, a diffuse infiltration of the bone marrow by plasma cells is present, accompanied by Bence Jones proteinuria and a monoclonal immunoglobulin secretion.[200, 211] The steady presence of increased numbers of plasma cells in the peripheral blood, the prompt appearance of bone marrow replacement similar to other types of acute leukemias, and the frequent generalized lymphadenopathy characterize this rare form of leukemia. These features and the absence of a distinct bone tumor separate plasma cell leukemia from multiple myeloma. Some of the patients with IgE myeloma, however, may show the pattern of plasma cell leukemia.

In multiple myeloma, in addition to there being circumscribed bone tumor formation, the proliferating plasma cells often diffusely infiltrate radiographically uninvolved bones, thereby making a diagnosis from a random bone marrow sample feasible. This condition is also referred to as "disseminated nonosteolytic myelomatosis."[12]

Examination of the bone marrow by aspiration or by biopsy is necessary for the diagnosis of myeloma. In most cases, sampling of the marrow from the iliac crest, sternum, or a vertebral body will demonstrate increased numbers of plasma cells, usually exceeding 5 to 10 per cent. When the relative proportion of the plasma cells reaches the 20 per cent level, especially when aggregates or sheets of plasma cells are noted, the diagnosis of myeloma is almost certain, particularly if the component cells are immature and have abnormal and often multinucleated forms.

It should be emphasized that multiple myeloma is a complex diagnosis that should not be entertained solely on general cytologic characteristics or the relative increase in the number of plasma cells. Clinical supporting data, radiographic examination, serum and urine electrophoresis, and immunoelectrophoresis are indivisible components of a fail-safe diagnosis.

Approximately 10 to 25 per cent of patients with classic multiple myeloma develop generalized *amyloidosis*.[18] These amyloid deposits predominantly occur in the cardiovascular system and the gastrointestinal tract, including the tongue, and less frequently, involve the kidneys, liver, spleen, and adrenal glands.[125] Traces of amyloid have been found in close relationship to myeloma cells, suggesting production of this substance by these cells.[117, 146, 227] Among 66 cases of multiple myeloma, Dahlin and Dockerty identified 14 instances in which amyloid could be demonstrated in the lesional tissue.[52] Amyloid tumors blended with immature plasma cells were described in the body of the sternum and ribs[61] as well as in the pelvis.[146] Macroglossia and carpal tunnel syndrome may be associated with amyloidosis.[2]

SOLITARY OSSEOUS MYELOMA

Solitary myeloma is a localized osseous tumor composed of a single focus of plasma cells.

This is an extremely rare occurrence, and only very few cases are acceptable.[14, 33, 74, 82, 140, 145, 164, 172, 182, 189, 198, 199, 251, 270, 276] The criteria for acceptance, as promulgated by Bichel and Kirketerp,[23] are

1. Histologic proof of the lesion
2. Complete skeletal survey ruling out the presence of other lesions
3. Negative marrow examination
4. Neither dysproteinemia nor Bence Jones proteinuria

The use of these criteria eliminates many of the purported cases, and, among the 27 examples reported up to 1938, only two fulfilled all requirements.[23] Others have restricted the acceptability of solitary myelomas to those cases that fail to show radiographic evidence of additional lesions for at least one year.[215, 268]

Considerable doubt remains as to whether the solitary form of myeloma truly exists. This diagnosis should be seriously entertained only with the full realization that the lesion may be a temporarily localized manifestation of an already disseminated, but not yet apparent, myeloma or that it may be the first appearance of an eventually generalizing process. The dissemination is quite unpredictable and may take a considerable length of time to materialize, but some remain localized nonetheless. Complete skeletal survey and immunologic and biochemical studies are necessary, both at the time of presentation and during the ensuing protracted follow-up period (lasting at least 10 years), to establish the true potential of a given lesion. Peripheral neuropathy does not necessarily rule out a solitary osseous myeloma.[82, 216, 229, 258]

Some believe that solitary plasmacytoma is a benign variant of myeloma or a plasmacytic pseudotumor, also referred to as a plasma cell granuloma.[1, 111, 158, 172] In questionable cases, the demonstration of monoclonal immunoglobulins in either the blood serum or the urine, or even better, in both, may clearly dramatize the true neoplastic nature of the lesion on hand, especially when the other clinicopathologic findings are not diagnostic.[105] It is of interest that in plasma cell granulomas, the plasma or preplasma cells are admixed with lymphocytes, leukocytes, macrophages, and fibroblasts, in addition to having a marked vascular proliferation.[157, 158] Quite frequently, there is an easily appreciable differentiation of the plasma cells in spite of their bi- or multinucleation. Russell's bodies are often seen in plasma cell granulomas, but their presence in myelomas is exceptional.

The solitary presentation is not only rare but also may be quite puzzling at times, since it may show a cystic trabeculated appearance not unlike a giant cell tumor.[74]

On the basis of 14 examples of well-documented solitary myelomas, Valderrama and Bullough emphasized the fact that even in the event of further dissemination the prognosis of these patients remains definitely better than that of those with initially multiple lesions.[257] The solitary tumors may spread by local extension through the cortex and periosteum into adjacent soft tissues. On histologic examination, the solitary lesion is inseparable from the multiple form, and, cytologically, the plasma cells reveal all stages of differentiation in both processes.

The most common sites of single bone involvement are the vertebral bodies, the bones of the pelvic and shoulder girdles, and, less frequently, the long tubular bones of the lower extremity.

These tumors should be treated by excision and irradiation. In some of the well-documented cases of solitary myeloma,

serum electrophoresis may reveal abnormal values, and M-type protein abnormalities are almost invariably present, but adequate surgical removal or radiation therapy results in the disappearance of these deranged protein tracings.[115, 132] The reappearance of abnormal electrophoretic values after therapy for solitary myeloma heralds the reactivation and progression of the quiescent disease process.[160]

TREATMENT AND PROGNOSIS

For many years a dire prognosis and pessimistic therapy characterized the treatment of multiple myeloma. In 1955, 52 per cent of the patients died within three months, and only three of 60 patients survived for two years.[36] From 1960 until recently, the average survival time of 17 months from clinical onset of disease was considered the yardstick for comparing subsequent studies using melphalan or sarcolysine as single drug agents.[25, 190, 203] In 1973, a series of 189 patients treated with a combination of melphalan and prednisone was reported by Costa and associates.[50] They achieved an average survival of 53 months in good-risk patients and 21 months in poor-risk ones.[50] This and other studies underscored the fact that although prednisone doubled the response rate, the median survival rate remained basically unaltered. Substituting cyclophosphamide for melphalan did not change the prognosis.[20, 165, 166] The triple alkylating agent regimen, including BCNU, cyclophosphamide, and melphalan with prednisone, even with additional azathioprine as a maintenance therapy, did not show any real advantage.[7]

Some of the improvements in survival were, to a large measure, due to better medical management and clarification of pathophysiologic mechanisms, since early deaths were often caused by overwhelming infections and renal failure.[62] A useful clinical staging system for myeloma was devised that facilitated dividing patients into distinctive prognostic groups.[56, 57] The separation proceeded according to the total tumor cell mass and the severity of the clinical signs or symptoms — the degree of anemia, the elevation of serum calcium, the extent of bone destruction, and the rate of paraprotein production. A newly developed, more sensitive radioimmunoassay for various myeloma genotypes (idiotypes) made the close follow-up of patients easily attainable.[67]

The first glimmer of a possible breakthrough in the treatment of myeloma was perceived by the Memorial Hospital myeloma team when they found that the triple alkylating agent and prednisone protocol could be improved by adding vincristine (M-2 protocol).[137] The updated follow-up results continue to register significantly improved survival times in patients treated with melphalan, prednisone, cyclophosphamide, vincristine, and BCNU (1,3-bis-(2-chloroethyl)-1-nitrosourea).[37] This five-drug regimen has achieved objective remissions for over 22 months in 40 of 46 previously untreated patients, most of whom had stage III severe multiple myeloma. The survival in this ongoing study has been markedly enhanced, even in those patients who did not respond to treatment with melphalan and prednisone. Improved survival results have also been achieved by the Southwest Oncology Group.[7] Treatment by irradiation as an adjuvant measure, coupled with immunotherapy, may be a reasonable addition in the foreseeable future. An unexpected spinoff is the fact that these studies resulted in the practical absence of leukemia accompanying multiple myeloma, which has been noted previously.[131, 142, 221, 228]

REFERENCES

1. Aherne, W. A.: The differentiation of myelomatosis from other causes of bone marrow plasmacytosis. J. Clin. Pathol., 11:326–329, 1958.
2. Akin, R. K., Barton, K., and Walters, P. J.: Amyloidosis, macroglossia, and carpal tunnel syndrome associated with myeloma. J. Oral Surg., 33:690–692, 1975.
3. Alexander, L. L., and Bennignhoff, D. L.: Familial multiple myeloma. J. Natl. Med. Assoc., 57:471–475, 1965.
4. Alexanian, R.: Plasma cell neoplasms. CA, 26:38–49, 1976.
5. Alexanian, R., Balcerzak, S., Bonnet, J. D., et al.: Prognostic factors in multiple myeloma. Cancer, 36:1192–1201, 1975.
6. Alexanian, R., Balcerzak, S., Gehan, E. A., et al.: Remission maintenance therapy for multiple myeloma. Arch. Intern. Med., 135:147–152, 1975.
7. Alexanian, R., Salmon, S., Bonnet, J., et al.: Com-

8. Ameis, A., Ko, H. S., and Pruzanski, W.: M components — a review of 1242 cases. Can. Med. Assoc. J., 114:889–895, 1976.
9. Anda, L.: Multiple myeloma. Acta Radiol., 33:515–528, 1950.
10. Arend, W. P., and Adamson, J. W.: Nonsecretory myeloma. Immunofluorescent demonstration of paraprotein within bone marrow plasma cells. Cancer, 33:721–728, 1974.
11. Azam, L., and Delamore, I. W.: Combination therapy for myelomatosis. Br. Med. J., 4:560–564, 1974.
12. Azar, H. A., and Potter, M. (eds.): Multiple Myeloma and Related Disorders. Vol. 1. New York, Harper & Row, 1973.
13. Azar, H. A., Zaino, E. C., Pham, T. C., et al.: "Non-secretory" plasma cell myeloma. Observations on 7 cases with electron microscopic studies. Am. J. Clin. Pathol., 58:618–629, 1972.
14. Baitz, T., and Kyle, R. A.: Solitary myeloma in chronic osteomyelitis. Report of case. Arch. Intern. Med., 113:872–876, 1964.
15. Barclay, W. R.: Multiple myeloma, melphalan, and neoplasia. J.A.M.A., 236:1612, 1976.
16. Batts, M., Jr.: Multiple myeloma. Review of forty cases. Arch. Surg., 39:807–823, 1939.
17. Bayrd, E. D.: The bone marrow on sternal aspiration in multiple myeloma. Blood, 3:987–1018, 1948.
18. Bayrd, E. D., and Bennett, W. A.: Amyloidosis complicating myeloma. Med. Clin. North Am., 34:1151–1164, 1950.
19. Bence Jones, H.: On a new substance occurring in the urine of a patient with mollities ossium. Philos. Trans. R. Soc. Lond. [Biol.], 1:55–62, 1848.
20. Bergsagel, D. E.: Plasma cell myeloma. Cancer, 30:1588–1594, 1972.
21. Bergsagel, D. E., and Pruzanski, W.: Treatment of plasma cell myeloma with cytotoxic agents. Arch. Intern. Med., 135:172–176, 1975.
22. Berman, H. H.: Waldenström's macroglobulinemia with lytic osseous lesions and plasma-cell morphology. Report of a case. Am. J. Clin. Pathol., 63:397–402, 1975.
23. Bichel, J., and Kirketerp, P.: Notes on myeloma. Acta Radiol., 19:487–503, 1938.
24. Björkholm, M., Holm, G., Mellstedt, H., et al.: Extensive nodular infiltration of extra-osseous tissues in human myelomatosis. A case report. Acta Med. Scand., 200:139–142, 1976.
25. Blokhin, N., Larionov, L., Perevodchikova, L., et al.: Clinical experiences with sarcolysin in neoplastic diseases. Ann. N.Y. Acad. Sci., 68:1128–1132, 1958.
26. Bouvenot, G., Paillas, J. E., and Carcassonne, Y.: Coexistence d'un myélome multiple et d'une maladie osseuse de Paget chez un même malade. Cah. Med., 15:273–278, 1974.
27. Brook, J., Prasad, R., Mathiala, R., et al.: Sequential therapy compared with combination therapy in multiple myeloma. Arch. Intern. Med., 135:163–171, 1975.
28. Bross, I. D. J., Viadana, E., and Pickren, J. W.:

The metastatic spread of myeloma and leukemias in men. Virchows Arch. [Pathol. Anat.], 365:91–101, 1975.

29. Brown, T. S., and Paterson, C. R.: Osteoclerosis in myeloma. J. Bone Joint Surg. [Br.], 55:621–623, 1973.

30. Bruce, K. W., and Royer, R. Q.: Multiple myeloma occurring in the jaws. A study of 17 cases. Oral Surg., 6:729–744, 1953.

31. Brunner, K. W.: Die Therapie des Plasmacytoms. Dtsch. Med. Wochenschr., 92:1505–1507, 1967.

32. Buonocore, E., Solomon, A., and Kerley, H. E.: Pseudomyeloma. Radiology, 95:41–46, 1970.

33. Calle, R., Graic, Y., Mazabraud, A., et al.: Plasmacytome osseux solitaire: à propos de quatre cas. Bull. Cancer, 59:395–404, 1972.

34. Calman, H. I.: Multiple myeloma. Report of a case first observed in the maxilla. Oral Surg., 5:1302–1311, 1952.

35. Canale, D. D., Jr., and Collins, R. D.: Use of bone marrow particle sections in the diagnosis of multiple myeloma. Am. J. Clin. Pathol., 61:382–392, 1974.

36. Carson, C. P., Ackerman, L. V., and Maltby, J. D.: Plasma cell myeloma. A clinical, pathologic and roentgenologic review of 90 cases. Am. J. Clin. Pathol., 25:849–888, 1955.

37. Case, D. C., Jr., Lee, B. J., III, and Clarkson, B. D.: Improved survival times in multiple myeloma treated with melphalan, prednisone, cyclophosphamide, vincristine and BCNU: M-2 protocol. Am. J. Med., 63:897–903, 1977.

38. Cataldo, E., and Meyer, I.: Solitary and multiple plasma-cell tumors of the jaws and oral cavity. Oral Surg., 22:628–639, 1966.

39. Chen, Y., Bhoopalam, N., Yakulis, V., et al.: Changes in lymphocyte surface immunoglobulins in myeloma and the effect of an RNA-containing plasma factor. Ann. Intern. Med., 83:625–631, 1975.

40. Christopherson, W. M., and Miller, A. J.: Re-evaluation of solitary plasma-cell myeloma of bone. Cancer, 3:240–252, 1950.

41. Churg, J., and Gordon, A. J.: Multiple myeloma. Lesions of the extra-osseous hematopoietic system. Am. J. Clin. Pathol., 20:934–945, 1950.

42. Clarisse, P. D. T., and Staple, T. W.: Diffuse bone sclerosis in multiple myeloma. Radiology, 99:327–328, 1971.

43. Cleary, B., Binder, R. A., Kales, A. N., et al.: Simultaneous presentation of acute myelomonocytic leukemia and multiple myeloma. Cancer, 41:1381–1386, 1978.

44. Clough, V., Delamore, I. W., and Whittaker, J. A.: Multiple myeloma in a young woman. Letter to the editor. Ann. Intern. Med., 86:117–118, 1977.

45. Coelho, I. M., Pereira, M. T., and Virella, G.: Analytical study of salivary immunoglobulins in multiple myeloma. Clin. Exp. Immunol., 17:417–426, 1974.

46. Cohen, D. M., Svien, H. J., and Dahlin, D. C.: Long-term survival of patients with myeloma of the vertebral column. J.A.M.A., 187:914–917, 1964.

47. Coley, W. B.: Multiple myeloma. Ann. Surg., 93:77–89, 1931.

48. Copelan, H. L.: Coexistence of multiple myeloma and Paget's disease of bone. Calif. Med., 101:118–120, 1964.

49. Correlation Conferences in Radiology and Pathology. Binet, E. F., and Markarian, B. (eds.): Left thigh mass. N.Y. State J. Med., 74:1798–1801, 1974.

50. Costa, G., Engle, R. L., Jr., Schilling, A., et al.: Melphalan and prednisone: an effective combination for the treatment of multiple myeloma. Am. J. Med., 54:589–599, 1973.

51. Craver, L. F., and Miller, D. G.: Multiple myeloma. CA, 16:142–155, 1966.

52. Dahlin, D. C., and Dockerty, M. B.: Amyloid and myeloma. Am. J. Pathol., 26:581–593, 1950.

53. Dalrymple, J.: On the microscopical character of mollities ossium. Dublin Q. J. Med. Sci., 2:85–95, 1846.

54. Davis, G. D., and Havens, F. Z.: Plasma cell myeloma of the mandible. Proc. Mayo Clin., 29:569–571, 1954.

55. Dörken, H., and Vollmer, I.: Die Epidemiologie des multiplen Myeloms-Untersuchung von 149 Fällen. Arch. Geschwulstforsch., 31:18–38, 1968.

56. Durie, B. G. M., and Salmon, S. E.: A clinical staging system for multiple myeloma. Correlation of measured myeloma cell mass with presenting clinical features, response to treatment, and survival. Cancer, 36:842–854, 1975.

57. Durie, B. G. M., and Salmon, S. E.: Evaluation and treatment of multiple myeloma and related disorders. Front. Rad. Ther. Onc., 10:170–177, 1975.

58. Edwards, G. A., and Zawadski, Z. A.: Extraosseous lesions in plasma cell myeloma. A report of six cases. Am. J. Med., 43:194–205, 1967.

59. Engels, E. P., Smith, R. C., and Krantz, S.: Bone sclerosis in multiple myeloma. Radiology, 75:242–247, 1960.

60. Evison, G., and Evans, K. T.: Bone sclerosis in multiple myeloma. Br. J. Radiol., 40:81–89, 1967.

61. Fadell, E. J., and Morris, H. C.: Amyloidoma presenting as a primary sternal tumor. Am. J. Surg., 108:75–79, 1964.

62. Farhangi, M., and Osserman, E. F.: The treatment of multiple myeloma. Semin. Hematol., 10:149–161, 1973.

63. Farman, J., and Degnan, T. J.: Multiple myeloma with small-bone involvement. N.Y. State J. Med., 76:990–992, 1976.

64. Feinleib, M., and MacMahon, B.: Duration of survival in multiple myeloma. J. Natl. Cancer Inst. 24:1259–1269, 1960.

65. Fishkin, B. G., and Spiegelberg, H. L.: Cervical lymph node metastasis as the first manifestation of localized extramedullary plasmacytoma. Cancer, 38:1641–1644, 1976.

66. Fruhling, L., and Chadli, A.: Le sarcome plasmocytaire extrasquelettique. Ann. Anat. Pathol., 8:317–376, 1963.

67. Gailani, S., Seon, B. K., Nussbaum, A., et al.: Radioimmunoassay for myeloma idiotype. J. Natl. Cancer Inst., 58.1553–1555, 1977.

68. Geschickter, C. F., and Copeland, M. M.: Multiple myeloma. Arch. Surg., 16:807–863, 1928.

69. Getaz, P., Handler, L., Jacobs, P., et al.: Osteosclerotic myeloma with peripheral neuropathy. S. Afr. Med. J., 48:1246–1250, 1974.

70. Ghadially, F. N., Lowes, N. R., and Mesfin, G. M.: Atypical glycogen deposits in a plasmacytoma: an ultrastructural study. J. Pathol., *122*:157–162, 1977.

71. Glenchur, H., Zinneman, H. H., and Hall, W. H.: A review of 51 cases of multiple myeloma. Emphasis on pneumonia and other infections as complications. Arch. Intern. Med., *103*:173–183, 1959.

72. Goldman, I. D., Gupta, V., White, J. C., et al.: Exchangeable intracellular methotrexate levels in the presence and absence of vincristine at extracellular drug concentrations relevant to those achieved in high-dose methotrexate-folinic acid "rescue" protocols. Cancer Res., *36*:276–279, 1976.

73. Gompels, B. M., Votaw, M. L., and Martel, W.: Correlation of radiological manifestations of multiple myeloma with immunoglobulin abnormalities and prognosis. Radiology, *104*:509–514, 1972.

74. Gootnick, L. T.: Solitary myeloma: review of sixty-one cases. Radiology, *45*:385–391, 1945.

75. Gordon, H., and Schneider, B.: Plasma-cell myeloma in child: report of case. Int. Clin., *4*:173–181, 1940.

76. Grader, J., and Moynihan, J. W.: Multiple myeloma and osteogenic sarcoma in a patient with Paget's disease. J.A.M.A., *176*:685–687, 1961.

77. Graham, R. C., Jr., and Bernier, G. M.: The bone marrow in multiple myeloma: correlation of plasma cell ultrastructure and clinical state. Medicine, *54*:225–243, 1975.

78. Griffiths, D. Ll.: Orthopaedic aspects of myelomatosis. J. Bone Joint Surg. [Br.], *48*:703–728, 1966.

79. Gross, R. J., and Yelin, G.: Multiple myeloma complicating Paget's disease. Am. J. Roentgenol. Radium Ther. Nucl. Med., *65*:585–589, 1951.

80. Grossman, R. E., and Hensley, G. T.: Bone lesion in primary amyloidosis. Am. J. Roentgenol. Radium Ther. Nucl. Med., *101*:872–875, 1967.

81. Guillan, R. A., Ranjini, R., Zelman, S., et al.: Multiple myeloma with hypogammaglobulinemia. Electron microscopic and chromosome studies. Cancer, *25*:1187–1192, 1970.

82. Gupta, S. P., and Prabhakar, B. R.: Peripheral neuropathy and solitary myeloma. Letter to the editor. Br. Med. J., *2*:1004, 1965.

83. Güthert, H., Wöckel, W., and Jänisch, W.: Zur Haufigkeit des Plasmazytoms und seiner Ausbreitung im Skelettsystem. Munch. Med. Wochenschr., *103*:1561–1564, 1961.

84. Halliday, D., Davey, F. R., Call, F., et al.: Identification of intracellular immunoglobulin in extramedullary myeloma. Arch. Pathol. Lab. Med., *101*:522–525, 1977.

85. Hanisch, C. M.: Paget's disease complicated by multiple myeloma. Bull. Hosp. Joint Dis., *11*:43–47, 1950.

86. Harding, W. G., II, and Kimball, T. S.: Solitary myeloma (plasmacytoma) of the femur: report of one case. Am. J. Cancer, *16*:1184–1192, 1932.

87. Haurani, F. I.: Effect of multiple myeloma and dysproteinemias on bone. Clin. Orthop., *52*:113–118, 1967.

88. Hayes, L. G., Plapp, F. V., Brewer, G. J., et al.: Electrophoresis of human multiple myeloma and Waldenström's macroglobulinemia sera in sodium dodecyl sulfate polyacrylamide gels. Clin. Chim. Acta, *66*:119–123, 1976.

89. Hayhoe, F. G. J., and Neuman, Z.: Cytology of myeloma cells. J. Clin. Pathol., *29*:916–922, 1976.

90. Heiser, S., and Schwartzman, J. J.: Variations in the roentgen appearance of the skeletal system in myeloma. Radiology, *58*:178–191, 1952.

91. Henderson, D., and Rowe, N. L.: Myelomatosis affecting the jaws. Br. J. Oral Surg., *6*:161–172, 1969.

92. Heremans, E. P., and Waldenström, J.: Cytology and electrophoretic pattern in myeloma. Acta Med. Scand., *170*:575–589, 1961.

93. Hewell, G. M., and Alexanian, R.: Multiple myeloma in young persons. Ann. Intern. Med., *84*:441–443, 1976.

94. Himmelfarb, E., Sebes, J., and Rabinowitz, J.: Unusual roentgenographic presentations of multiple myeloma. J. Bone Joint Surg. [Am.], *56*:1723–1728, 1974.

95. Hinds, E. C., Pleasants, J. E., and Bell, W. E.: Solitary plasma-cell myeloma of the mandible. Oral Surg., *9*:193–202, 1956.

96. Hobbs, J. R.: Paraproteins, benign or malignant? Br. Med. J., *3*:699–704, 1967.

97. Hobbs, J. R.: Immunocytoma o' mice an' men. Br. Med. J., *2*:67–72, 1971.

98. Hobbs, J. R., and Corbett, A. A.: Younger age of presentation and extra-osseous tumour in IgD myelomatosis. Br. Med. J., *1*:412–414, 1969.

99. Hobbs, J. R., Slot, G. M. J., Campbell, C. H., et al.: Six cases of gamma-D myelomatosis. Lancet, *2*:614–618, 1966.

100. Holt, J. M., and Robb-Smith, H. T.: Multiple myeloma: Development of plasma cell sarcoma during apparently successful chemotherapy. J. Clin. Pathol., *26*:649–659, 1973.

101. Hoogstraten, B., Costa, J., Cuttner, J., et al.: Intermittent melphalan therapy in multiple myeloma. J.A.M.A., *209*:251–253, 1969.

102. Huguley, C. M., Jr., Hammack, W. J., Chan, Y. K., et al.: Treatment of myeloma. Arch. Intern. Med., *135*:157–162, 1975.

103. Humphrey, R. L., Wright, J. R., Zachary, J. B., et al.: Renal transplantation in multiple myeloma. A case report. Ann. Intern. Med., *83*:651–653, 1975.

104. Hurez, D., Preud'Homme, J. L., and Seligmann, M.: Intracellular "monoclonal" immunoglobulin in nonsecretory human myeloma. J. Immunol., *101*:263–264, 1970.

105. Hyun, B. H., Kwa, D., Gabaldon, H., et al.: Reactive plasmacytic lesions of the bone marrow. Am. J. Clin. Pathol., *65*:921–928, 1976.

106. Jackson, H., Jr., Parker, F., Jr., and Bethea, J. M.: Studies of diseases of lymphoid and myeloid tissues. II. Plasmacytomata and their relation to multiple myelomata. Am. J. Med. Sci., *181*:169–180, 1931.

107. Jacobson, H. G., Poppel, M. H., Shapiro, J. H., et al.: The vertebral pedicle sign. A roentgen finding to differentiate metastatic carcinoma from multiple myeloma. Am. J. Roentgenol. Radium Ther. Nucl. Med., *80*:817–821, 1958.

108. Jacox, H. W., and Kahn, E. A.: Multiple myeloma with spinal cord involvement. Am. J. Roentgenol. Radium Ther. Nucl. Med., 30:201–205, 1933.

109. Jákó, J., Virágh, S., Boga, M., et al.: A case of IgD-lambda myeloma. Haematologia, 9:261–278, 1975.

110. Jancelewicz, Z., Takatsuki, K., Sugai, S., et al.: IgD multiple myeloma. Arch. Intern. Med., 135:87–93, 1975.

111. Johnson, L. C., and Meador, G. E.: The nature of benign "solitary myeloma" of bone. Bull. Hosp. Joint Dis., 12:298–313, 1951.

112. Kahler, O.: Zur Symptomatologie des multiplen Myeloms. Wien. Med. Presse, 30:209–213, 253–255, 1889.

113. Kahler, O.: Zur Symptomatologie des multiplen Myeloms. Beobachtung von Albumosurie. Prag. Med. Wochenschr., 14:4a, 5a, 1889.

114. Kalderon, A. E., Bogaars, H. A., Diamond, I., et al.: Ultrastructure of myeloma cells in a case with crystal-cryoglobulinemia. Cancer, 39:1475–1481, 1977.

115. Kaplan, G. A., and Bennett, J.: Solitary myeloma of the lumbar spine successfully treated with radiation. Report of a case. Radiology, 91:1017–1018, 1968.

116. Karle, H., Hansen, N. E., and Plesner, T.: Neutrophil defect in multiple myeloma. Scand. J. Haematol., 17:62–70, 1976.

117. Kavanaugh, J. H.: Multiple myeloma, amyloid arthropathy, and pathological fracture of the femur. A case report. J. Bone Joint Surg. [Am.], 60:135–137, 1978.

118. Kirsch, I. E.: Plasma-cell myeloma of bone, of over 12 years' duration. Med. Bull. Vet. Admin., 18:96–97, 1941.

119. Klein, H. O., and Lennartz, K. J.: Chemotherapy after synchronization of tumor cells. Semin. Hematol., 11:203–227, 1974.

120. Krainin, P., D'Angio, G. J., and Smelin, A.: Multiple myeloma with new bone formation. Arch. Intern. Med., 84:976–982, 1949.

121. Krajny, M., and Pruzanski, W.: Waldenström's macroglobulinemia: review of 45 cases. Can. Med. Assoc. J., 114:899–905, 1976.

122. Kutcher, R., Ghatak, N. R., and Leeds, N. E.: Plasmacytoma of the calvaria. Radiology, 113:111–115, 1974.

123. Kutushev, F. K.: Myelomatosis in girl 13 years old. Vestn. Khir., 74:75, 1954.

124. Kyle, R. A.: Multiple myeloma. Review of 869 cases. Mayo Clin. Proc., 50:29–40, 1975.

125. Kyle, R. A., and Bayrd, E. D.: "Primary" systemic amyloidosis and myeloma. Discussion of relationship and review of 81 cases. Arch. Intern. Med., 107:344–353, 1961.

126. Kyle, R. A., Bayrd, E. D., McKenzie, B. F., et al.: Diagnostic criteria for electrophoretic patterns of serum and urinary proteins in multiple myeloma. Study of one hundred and sixty-five multiple myeloma patients and of seventy-seven nonmyeloma patients with similar electrophoretic patterns. J.A.M.A., 174:245–251, 1960.

127. Kyle, R. A., and Elveback, L. R.: Management and prognosis of multiple myeloma. Mayo Clin. Proc., 51:751–760, 1976.

128. Kyle, R. A., Heath, C. W., Jr., and Carbone, P.: Multiple myeloma in spouses. Arch. Intern. Med., 127:944–946, 1971.

129. Kyle, R. A., Jowsey, J., Kelly, P. J., et al.: Multiple-myeloma bone disease. The comparative effect of sodium fluoride and calcium carbonate or placebo. N. Engl. J. Med., 293:1334–1338, 1975.

130. Kyle, R. A., Nobrega, F. T., and Kurland, L. T.: Multiple myeloma in Olmsted County, Minnesota, 1945–1964. Blood, 33:739–745, 1969.

131. Kyle, R. A., Pierre, R. V., and Bayrd, E. D.: Multiple myeloma and acute leukemia associated with alkylating agents. Arch. Intern. Med., 135:185–192, 1975.

132. Lane, S. L.: Plasmacytoma of the mandible. Oral Surg., 5:434–442, 1952.

133. Law, I. P., and Jones, C.: IgA myeloma and sternal fracture. Letter to the editor. J.A.M.A., 233:767–768, 1975.

134. Lawrence, J. H., and Wasserman, L. R.: Multiple myeloma: a study of 24 patients treated with radioactive isotopes (P^{32} and Sr^{89}). Ann. Intern. Med., 33:41–55, 1950.

135. Leb, L., Grimes, E. T., Balogh, K., et al.: Monoclonal macroglobulinemia with osteolytic lesions. Cancer, 39:227–231, 1977.

136. Lee, B. J., Pinsky, C. M., and Miller, D.: The management of plasma cell neoplasms. Med. Clin. North Am., 55:703–719, 1971.

137. Lee, B. J., Sahakian, G., Clarkson, B. D., et al.: Combination chemotherapy of multiple myeloma with Alkeran, Cytoxan, vincristine, prednisone, and BCNU. Cancer, 33:533–538, 1974.

138. Leoncini, D. L., and Korngold, L.: Multiple myeloma in 2 sisters. An immunochemical study. Cancer, 17:733–737, 1964.

139. Lergier, J. E., Jiménez, E., Maldonado, N., et al.: Normal pregnancy in multiple myeloma treated with cyclophosphamide. Cancer, 34:1018–1022, 1974.

140. Lewin, H., and Stein, J. M.: Solitary plasma cell myeloma with new bone formation. Am. J. Roentgenol. Radium Ther. Nucl. Med., 79:630–637, 1958.

141. Lewin, R. W., and Cataldo, E.: Multiple myeloma discovered from oral manifestations: report of case. J. Oral Surg., 25:68–72, 1967.

142. Lewis, E. B.: Leukemia, multiple myeloma, and aplastic anemia in American radiologists. Science, 142:1492–1494, 1963.

143. Lichtenstein, L., and Jaffe, H. L.: Multiple myeloma. A survey based on thirty-five cases, eighteen of which came to autopsy. Arch. Pathol., 44:207–246, 1947.

144. Lindström, F. D., Williams, R. C., Jr., and Brunning, R. D.: Thymoma associated with multiple myeloma. Arch. Intern. Med., 122:526–531, 1968.

145. Lipper, S., Kahn, L. B., and Hesselson, N.: Localised myeloma with osteogenesis and Russell body formation. S. Afr. Med. J., 49:2041–2045, 1975.

146. Lowell, D. M.: Amyloid-producing plasmacytoma of the pelvis. Case report and review of the literature. Arch. Surg., 94:899–903, 1967.

147. Lumb, G.: Solitary plasmocytoma of bone with renal changes. Br. J. Surg., 36:16–22, 1948.

148. Lumb, G.: The pathology of the myelomata (plasma cell tumours). Ann. R. Coll. Surg. Engl., 10:241–256, 1952.

149. Macdougall, L. G., Brown, J. A., Cohen, M. M., et al.: C-monosomy myeloproliferative syndrome: A case of 7-monosomy. J. Pediatr., 84:256–259, 1974.

150. Macintyre, W.: Case of mollities and fragilitas ossium accompanied with urine strongly charged with animal matter. Med. Chir. Soc. Trans., 33:211–232, 1850.

151. Maeda, K., Abesamis, C. M., Kuhn, L. M., et al.: Multiple myeloma in childhood. Report of a case with breast tumors as a presenting manifestation. Am. J. Clin. Pathol., 60:552–558, 1973.

152. Maldonado, J. E., Brown, A. L., Jr., Bayrd, E. D., et al.: Ultrastructure of the myeloma cell. Cancer, 19:1613–1627, 1966.

153. Maldonado, J. E., and Kyle, R. A.: Familial myeloma. Am. J. Med., 57:875–884, 1974.

154. Maldonado, J. E., Velosa, J. A., Kyle, R. A., et al.: Fanconi syndrome in adults. A manifestation of a latent form of myeloma. Am. J. Med., 58:354–364, 1975.

155. Mangalik, A., Lahiri Mazumdar, T. N., and Kasturi, J.: A case of solitary myeloma with a monoclonal spike in alpha-2 region responding to radiotherapy. J. Assoc. Physicians India, 24:865–868, 1976.

156. Mangalik, A., and Veliath, A. J.: Osteosclerotic myeloma and peripheral neuropathy. A case report. Cancer, 28:1040–1045, 1971.

157. Markel, S. F.: Plasma cell granuloma or myeloma. Letter to the editor. J.A.M.A., 220:278, 1972.

158. Markel, S. F., and Theros, E. G.: RPC of the month from the AFIP. Radiology, 95:679–686, 1970.

159. Martino, L. J., Yesger, V. L., and Taylor, J. J.: Growth of a plasma cell myeloma in lathyritic mice. Arch. Pathol., 99:536–539, 1975.

160. Maruyama, Y., and Thomson, J., Jr.: Radiotherapeutic response of plasma cell tumors associated with monoclonal gammopathy. Cancer, 26:110–113, 1970.

161. Mason, T. J., and McKay, F. W.: U.S. Cancer Mortality by County. Washington, D.C., DHEW Publication No. (NIH) 74–615, 1974.

162. Mathews, J. W., Jr., and Olivier, C. A.: Osteoblastic multiple myeloma. Case report. South. Med. J., 67:318, 360, 1974.

163. Mazzaferri, E. L., and Penn, G. M.: Kaposi's sarcoma associated with multiple myeloma. Report of a patient and review of the literature. Arch. Intern. Med., 122:521–525, 1968.

164. McLauchlan, J.: Solitary myeloma of the clavicle with long survival after total excision. Report of a case. J. Bone Joint Surg. [Br.], 55:357–358, 1973.

165. Medical Research Council's Working Party for Therapeutic Trials in Leukaemia: Myelomatosis: comparison of melphalan and cyclophosphamide therapy. Br. Med. J., 1:640–641, 1971.

166. Medical Research Council's Working Party for Therapeutic Trials in Leukaemia: Report on the first myelomatosis trial. Part I. Analysis of presenting features of prognostic importance. Br. J. Haematol., 24:123–139, 1973.

167. Mehbod, H., and Sweeney, W. M.: Multiple myeloma in Paget's disease. Letter to the editor. J.A.M.A., 177:531, 1961.

168. Meijers, K. A. E., de Leeuw, B., and Voormolen-Kálova, M.: The multiple occurrence of myeloma and asymptomatic paraproteinaemia within one family. Clin. Exp. Immunol., 12:185–193, 1972.

169. Mellstedt, H., Hammarström, S., and Holm, G.: Monoclonal lymphocyte population in human plasma cell myeloma. Clin. Exp. Immunol., 17:371–384, 1974.

170. Meloy, T. M., Jr., Gunter, J. H., and Sampson, D. A.: Mandibular lesion as first evidence of multiple myeloma. Am. J. Orthod., 31:685–689, 1945.

171. Meszaros, W. T.: The many facets of multiple myeloma. Semin. Roentgenol., 9:219–228, 1974.

172. Meyer, J. E., and Schulz, M. D.: "Solitary" myeloma of bone. A review of 12 cases. Cancer, 34:438–440, 1974.

173. Meyers, B. R., Hirschman, S. Z., and Azelrod, J. A.: Current patterns of infection in multiple myeloma. Am. J. Med., 52:87–92, 1972.

174. Mikulski, S. M.: Anion gap and myeloma. Letter to the editor. N. Engl. J. Med., 294:111–112, 1976.

175. Mill, W. B.: Radiation therapy in multiple myeloma. Radiology, 115:175–178, 1975.

176. Monta, L. E., and Ramanan, S. V.: Recurrent pulmonary embolism. A sign of multiple myeloma. J.A.M.A., 233:1192–1193, 1975.

177. Morse, D., Dailey, R. C., and Bunn, J.: Prehistoric multiple myeloma. Bull. N.Y. Acad. Med., 50:447–458, 1974.

178. Moseley, J. E.: Patterns of bone change in multiple myeloma. J. Mt. Sinai Hosp., 28:511–536, 1961.

179. Moss, R. L.: Multiple myeloma with maxillary myelomatous epulis and malignant pheochromocytoma. Report of a case. Oral Surg., 11:951–959, 1958.

180. Mundy, G. R., Raisz, L. G., Cooper, R. A., et al.: Evidence for the secretion of an osteoclast stimulating factor in myeloma. N. Engl. J. Med., 291:1041–1046, 1974.

181. Murray, T., Long, W., and Narins, R. G.: Multiple myeloma and the anion gap. N. Engl. J. Med., 292:574–575, 1975.

182. Naylor, A., and Chester-Williams, F. E.: Myelomata of bone. A review of 25 cases. Br. Med. J., 1:120–124, 1954.

183. Nelson, C. L., Jr., and Evarts, C. M.: Multiple myeloma with cord compression. Report of a case. J. Bone Joint Surg. [Am.], 50:305–310, 1968.

184. Nerenberg, S. T.: Gamma globulin studies of biopsy material and serum in solitary plasmacytoma of the spine. Cancer, 24:750–757, 1969.

185. Nilsson, K., Killander, D., Killander, J., et al.: Short-term tissue culture of two nonsecretory human myelomas. A morphological and functional study. Scand. J. Immunol., 5:819–828, 1976.

186. Norton, L., and Simon, R.: Tumor size, sensitivity to therapy, and design of treatment schedules. Cancer Treat. Rep., 61:1307–1317, 1977.

187. Odelberg-Johnson, O.: Osteosclerotic changes in myelomatosis; report of a case. Acta Radiol., 52:139–144, 1959.

188. Ogawa, M., Wurster, D. H., and McIntyre, O. R.: Multiple myeloma in one of a pair of monozygotic twins. Acta Haematol., 44:295–304, 1970.

189. Onofrio, B. M., and Svien, H. J.: Solitary and multiple vertebral myelomas. In Vinken, P. J., and Bruyn, G. W. (eds.): Handbook of Clinical Neurology. Vol. 20. Tumours of the Spine and Spinal Cord. Part II. New York, American Elsevier, 1976, pp. 9–18.

190. Osgood, E. E.: Survival time of patients with plasmacytic myeloma. Cancer Chemother. Rep., 9:1–10, 1960.

191. Osserman, E. F.: Multiple myeloma. Current clinical and chemical concepts. Am. J. Med., 23:283–309, 1957.

192. Osserman, E. F.: Natural history of multiple myeloma before radiological evidence of disease. Radiology, 71:157–174, 1958.

193. Osserman, E. F., and Takatsuki, K.: Plasma cell myeloma: Gamma globulin synthesis and structure. A review of biochemical and clinical data, with the description of a newly recognized and related syndrome, "H$^{\gamma-2}$-chain (Franklin's) disease." Medicine, 42:357–384, 1963.

194. Pankovich, A. M., and Griem, M. L.: Plasma-cell myeloma. A thirty-year follow-up. Radiology, 104:521–522, 1972.

195. Papavasiliou, C., Kalliterakis, E., Dodis, A., et al.: "Sonnenstrahlähnliche" Knochengeschwulst beim multiplen Myelom. Ther. Ggw., 111:252–258, 1972.

196. Paraskevas, F., Heremans, J., and Waldenström, J.: Cytology and electrophoretic pattern in $\gamma_{1A}(\beta_{2A})$ myeloma. Acta Med. Scand., 170:575–589, 1961.

197. Pasmantier, M. W., and Azar, H. A.: Extraskeletal spread in multiple plasma cell myeloma. A review of 57 autopsied cases. Cancer, 23:167–174, 1969.

198. Pasternack, J. G., and Waugh, R. L.: Solitary myeloma of bone. Ann. Surg., 110:427–436, 1939.

199. Paul, L. W., and Pohle, E. A.: Solitary myeloma of bone. Radiology, 35:651–667, 1940.

200. Pedraza, M. A.: Plasma-cell leukemia with unusual immunoglobulin abnormalities. Am. J. Clin. Pathol., 64:410–415, 1975.

201. Perry, M. C., and Kyle, R. A.: The clinical significance of Bence Jones proteinuria. Mayo Clin. Proc., 50:234–238, 1975.

202. Pinkhas, J., Djaldetti, M., and Yaron, M.: Coincidence of multiple myeloma with Gaucher's disease. Isr. J. Med. Sci., 1:537–540, 1965.

203. Pinsky, C. M., and Lee, B. J.: Melphalan in the treatment of multiple myeloma. Clin. Bull., 6:142–146, 1976.

204. Porter, R. R.: Structural studies of immunoglobulins. Science, 180:713–716, 1973.

205. Potter, M.: The developmental history of the neoplastic plasma cells in mice: A brief review of recent development. Semin. Hematol., 10:19–32, 1973.

206. Potter, M., and Boyce, C. R.: Induction of plasma-cell neoplasms in strain BALB/c mice with mineral oil and mineral oil adjuvants. Nature, 193:1086–1087, 1962.

207. Pratt, P. V., Estren, S., and Kochwa, S.: Immunoglobulin abnormalities in Gaucher's disease. Report of 16 cases. Blood, 31:633–640, 1968.

208. Price, C. H. G.: Myeloma occurring with Paget's disease of bone. Skeletal Radiol., 1:15–19, 1976.

209. Pruzanski, W.: Clinical manifestations of multiple myeloma: relation to class and type of M component. Can. Med. Assoc. J., 114:896–897, 1976.

210. Pruzanski, W., and Katz, A.: Clinical and laboratory findings in primary generalized and multiple-myeloma-related amyloidosis. Can. Med. Assoc. J., 114:906–909, 1976.

211. Pruzanski, W., and Rother, I.: IgD plasma cell neoplasia: clinical manifestations and characteristic features. Can. Med. Assoc. J., 102:1061–1065, 1970.

212. Püschel, W., and Kunath, K.: Autopsy-statistical analysis of multiple myeloma. Zentralbl. Allg. Pathol., 121:381–388, 1977.

213. Raley, L. L., and Granite, E. L.: Plasmacytoma of the maxilla: report of case. J. Oral Surg., 35:497–500, 1977.

214. Ramon, Y., Oberman, M., Horowitz, I., et al.: A large mandibular tumor with a distinct radiological "sun-ray effect" as the primary manifestation of multiple myeloma. J. Oral Surg., 36:52–54, 1978.

215. Raven, R. W., and Willis, R. A.: Solitary plasmocytoma of the spine. J. Bone Joint Surg. [Br.], 31:369–375, 1949.

216. Read, D., and Warlow, C.: Peripheral neuropathy and solitary plasmacytoma. J. Neurol. Neurosurg. Psychiatry, 41:177–184, 1978.

217. Reich, C., and Brodsky, A. E.: Coexisting multiple myeloma and Paget's disease of bone treated with Stilbamidine. J. Bone Joint Surg. [Am.], 30:642–646, 1948.

218. Renner, R. R., and Smith, J. R.: Plasma cell dyscrasias (except myeloma). Semin. Roentgenol., 9:209–218, 1974.

219. Ritz, N. D., and Meyer, L. M.: Solitary plasmacytoma of bone with subsequent multiple myeloma. Acta Haematol., 8:224–232, 1952.

220. Robbins, R.: Familial multiple myeloma: The tenth reported occurrence. Am. J. Med. Sci., 254:848–850, 1967.

221. Robins, S. M., and Chopra, D.: Multiple myeloma and multiple neoplasms. J.A.M.A., 236:1609, 1976.

222. Rodriguez, A. R., Lutcher, C. L., and Coleman, F. W.: Osteosclerotic myeloma. J.A.M.A., 236:1872–1874, 1976.

223. Rodriguez, J. M., Lam, S., and Silber, R.: Multiple myeloma with cutaneous involvement. J.A.M.A., 237:2625–2626, 1977.

224. Rondier, J., Simon, F., Cayla, J., et al.: Multiple myeloma and osteocondensation. Sem. Hop. Paris, 51:157–167, 1975.

225. Rosen, B. J.: Multiple myeloma. A clinical review. Med. Clin. North Am., 59:375–386, 1975.

226. Rosenkrantz, J. A., and Gluckman, E. C.: Coexistence of Paget's disease of bone and multiple myeloma. Case reports of 2 patients. Am. J. Roentgenol. Radium Ther. Nucl. Med., 78:30–38, 1957.

227. Roslund, J., Sundberg, K., and Tovi, D.: Plasma cell myeloma of thoracic vertebra with amyloid deposits. Acta Pathol. Microbiol. Scand., 49:273–279, 1960.

228. Rosner, F., and Grunwald, H.: Multiple myeloma terminating in acute leukemia. Am. J. Med., 57:927–939, 1974.

229. Rushton, D. I.: Peripheral sensorimotor neuropathy associated with a localized myeloma. Br. Med. J., 2:203–205, 1965.

230. Rutishauser, E.: Zur Frage der solitären Myelome. Zentralbl. Allg. Pathol., 58:355–360, 1933.

231. Ryckewaert, A., Kuntz, D., Bonhomme, J., et al.: Un cas de myélome non sécrétant avec déminéralisation vertébrale diffuse et rétention intracellulaire de la globuline myélomateuse. Rev. Rhum. Mal. Osteoartic., 36:621–627, 1969.

232. Salmon, S. E.: Expansion of the growth fraction in multiple myeloma with alkylating agents. Blood, 45:119–129, 1975.

233. Salmon, S. E.: Nitrosoureas in multiple myeloma. Cancer Treat. Rep., 60:789–794, 1976.

234. Salmon, S. E., and Durie, B. G. M.: Cellular kinetics in multiple myeloma. A new approach to staging and treatment. Arch. Intern. Med., 135:131–138, 1975.

235. Sanchez, J. A., Rahman, S., Strauss, R. A., et al.: Multiple myeloma masquerading as a pituitary tumor. Letter to the editor. Arch. Pathol. Lab. Med., 101:55–56, 1977.

236. Schmalzl, F., Keiser, G., Kresbach, E., et al.: Plasmacytoma, alkylating agents, and acute myeloid leukemia. Dtsch. Med. Wochenschr., 100:1961–1967, 1975.

237. Schmaus, K. A.: Multiples Myelom (Plasmocytom) bei einem Jugendlichen. Chirurg., 21:48–50, 1950.

238. Schoenfeld, J., Pick, A. J., Frohlichman, R., et al.: Nonsecretory plasma cell myeloma. Harefuah, 86:540–543, 1974.

239. Schwartz, C. W.: Solitary myeloma of the frontal bone. Am. J. Roentgenol. Radium Ther. Nucl. Med., 53:573–574, 1945.

240. Scurr, J. A.: Myeloma occurring in Paget's disease. Proc. R. Soc. Med., 65:725, 1972.

241. Serre, H., and Simon, L.: Maladie osseuse de Paget et myélome plasmocytaire multiple. Rev. Rhum. Mal. Osteoartic., 26:347–353, 1959.

242. Silverman, L. M., and Shklar, G.: Multiple myeloma. Report of a case. Oral Surg., 15:301–309, 1962.

243. Slavens, J. J.: Multiple myeloma in a child. Am. J. Dis. Child., 47:821–835, 1934.

244. Smêreker, J.: Inkretdrüsenveränderungen bei Plasmacytom. Virchows Arch. [Pathol. Anat.], 319:72–80, 1950.

245. Smetana, K., Gyorkey, F., Gyorkey, P., et al.: Ultrastructural studies on human myeloma plasmocytes. Cancer Res., 33:2300–2309, 1973.

246. Smith, J., and Lieberman, P. H.: An unusual case of myeloma. Clin. Bull., 4:162–163, 1974.

247. Sorenson, G. D.: Virus-like particles in myeloma cells of man. Proc. Soc. Exp. Biol. Med., 118:250–252, 1965.

248. Spitzer, R., and Price, L. W.: Solitary myeloma of the mandible. Br. Med J., 1:1027–1028, 1948.

249. Stamp, T. C. B., Child, J. A., and Walker, P. G.: Treatment of osteolytic myelomatosis with mithramycin. Lancet, 1:719–722, 1975.

250. Stewart, A., and Weber, F. P.: Myelomatosis. Q. J. Med., 26:211–227, 1938.

251. Stewart, M. J., and Taylor, A. L.: Observations on solitary plasmocytoma. J. Pathol. Bacteriol., 35:541–547, 1932.

252. Stone, R. S.: Angiosarcoma and myeloma; 2 unusual cases. Am. J. Roentgenol., 22:153–155, 1929.

253. Svien, H. J., Price, R. D., and Bayrd, E. D.: Neurosurgical treatment of compression of the spinal cord caused by myeloma. J.A.M.A., 153:784–786, 1953.

254. Tabachnick, T. T., and Levine, B.: Multiple myeloma involving the jaws and oral soft tissues. J. Oral Surg., 34:931–933, 1976.

255. Talerman, A.: Clinico-pathological study of multiple myeloma in Jamaica. Br. J. Cancer, 23:285–293, 1969.

256. Unander-Scharin, L., Waldenström, J. G., and Zettervall, O.: Surgical treatment of myelomatosis — a review of 18 cases. Acta Med. Scand., 203:265–272, 1978.

257. Valderrama, J. A. F., and Bullough, P. G.: Solitary myeloma of the spine. J. Bone Joint Surg. [Br.], 50:82–90, 1968.

258. Victor, M., Banker, B. Q., and Adams, R. D.: The neuropathy of multiple myeloma. J. Neurol. Neurosurg. Psychiatry, 21:73–88, 1958.

259. von Rustizky, J.: Multiples Myelom. Dtsch. Z. Chir., 3:162–172, 1873.

260. Waldenström, J.: Diagnosis and Treatment of Multiple Myeloma. New York, Grune & Stratton, 1970.

261. Waldenström, J.: Die Formenkreise des Plasmacytoms. Schweiz. Med. Wochenschr., 100:727–732, 1970.

262. Waldenström, J. G., Adner, A., Gyddell, K., et al.: Osteosclerotic "plasmacytoma" with polyneuropathy, hypertrichosis and diabetes. Acta Med. Scand., 203:297–303, 1978.

263. Warner, N. L., Potter, M., and Metcalf, D. (eds.): Multiple Myeloma and Related Immunoglobulin-Producing Neoplasms. UICC Technical Report Series, Vol. 13. Geneva, UICC, 1974.

264. Webb, H. E., Devine, K. D., and Harrison, E. G., Jr.: Solitary myeloma of the mandible. Oral Surg., 22:1–6, 1966.

265. Wells, H. G.: The relation of multiple vascular tumors of bone to myeloma. Arch Surg., 2:435–442, 1921.

266. Whitlock, R. I. H., and Hughes, N. C.: Solitary myeloma of mandible. Report of a case. Oral Surg., 13:23–32, 1960.

267. Wiedermann, D., Urban, P., Wiedermann, B., et al.: Multiple myeloma in two brothers. Immunoglobulin levels among their relatives. Neoplasma, 23:197–207, 1976.

268. Willis, R. A.: Solitary plasmacytoma of bone. J. Pathol., 53:77–85, 1941.

269. Wiltshaw, E.: The natural history of extramedullary plasmacytoma and its relation to solitary myeloma of bone and myelomatosis. Medicine, 55:217–238, 1976.

270. Wittig, K. H., and Motsch, H.: Solitary plasmocytoma. Zentralbl. Chir., 102:410–415, 1977.

271. Wolff, E., and Nolan, L. E.: Multiple myeloma first discovered in the mandible. Radiology, 42:76–78, 1944.

272. Wood, A. C., and Lucké, B.: Multiple myeloma of the plasma-cell type. Ann. Surg., 78:14–25, 1923.

273. Wood, G. D.: Myelomatosis. A case report. Br. Dent. J., 139:472–474, 1975.

274. Wright, C. J. E.: Long survival in solitary plasmo- cytoma of bone. J. Bone Joint Surg. [Br.], 43:767–771, 1961.

275. Wright, J. H.: A case of multiple myeloma. Trans. Assoc. Am. Physicians, 15:137–145, 1900.

276. Wright, R. S.: Acute congestive heart failure ap- parently secondary to solitary plasmocytoma and massive hemorrhage after biopsy. Case re- port. J. Bone Joint Surg. [Am.], 55:1749–1752, 1973.

27

MALIGNANT ANGIOBLASTOMA (ADAMANTINOMA) OF LONG BONES

DEFINITION

Malignant angioblastoma, often also referred to as adamantinoma, is a rare distinctive tumor of bone that usually arises in the shaft of the tibia. The light and electron microscopic features reveal both angioblastic and epithelial (adamantine) growth traits, but the exact histogenesis still remains in doubt.

SYNONYMS

Malignant angioblastoma may also be known as adamantinoma, primary epidermoid carcinoma of bone, adamantinoma-like tumor, primary epithelial bone tumor, carcinoma sarcomatodes, so-called adamantinoma, synovial sarcoma, malignant synovioma, skeletal synovioma, and dermal inclusion tumor.

SIGNS AND SYMPTOMS

Swelling, with or without pain, is the most frequent complaint. Pain associated with previous trauma, or entirely independent of it, is less commonly encountered (Fig. 27–1). The history of trauma is elicited in many patients and includes a range from simple contusions to complicated and often repeated fractures.

LOCATION

The overwhelming majority of the reported cases in appendicular sites arise in the tibia, although there are several well-documented examples in other osseous locations. At least 17 angioblastomas have been encountered in extratibial bones, including the ulna, the femur, the fibula, the humerus, the metatarsals, and the capitate

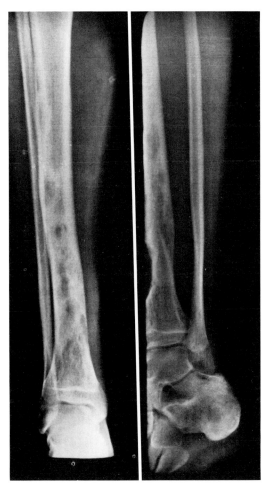

Figure 27–1. Extensive tibial malignant angioblastoma in a 16-year-old boy with a 9-month history of a slowly enlarging, painless mass. Cortical destruction and soft tissue involvement are noted. (Courtesy of Dr. J. C. Lorenzo.)

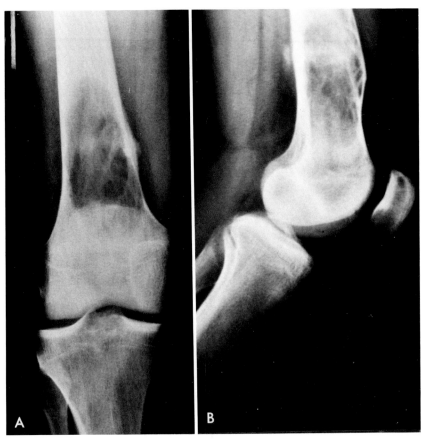

Figure 27–2. Distal femoral angioblastoma in a 20-year-old man with a preoperative clinical diagnosis of chondromyxoid fibroma.

bone (Fig. 27–2).[4, 6-8, 20, 24, 27, 39, 47, 65, 74-76, 78, 88] Synchronous polyostotic involvement may be present.[76, 83]

AGE AND SEX DISTRIBUTION

The ages of the patients studied at Memorial Hospital ranged from 13 to 67 years, with an average age of 35 years.[39] There was an equal sex distribution, although others have reported a 2:1 male to female ratio.[76]

RADIOGRAPHIC FEATURES

The characteristic radiographic findings include a sharply delineated, eccentric, lobular rarefaction in the middle or distal third of the diaphysis or in the metaphysis of a long bone associated with peripheral sclerosis (Fig. 27–3). A saw-toothed area of cortical erosion in the tibia, when present, is quite distinctive for this tumor (Fig. 27–1). Lytic and coarsely trabecular expansile lesions with honeycomb characteristics may occasionally cross the diaphysis transversely and result in extensive periosteal new bone formation. Several exceptions to these roentgenographic findings make the diagnosis of angioblastoma difficult (Fig. 27–4). Definite cortical destruction with prominent extracortical soft tissue tumor extension accompanied by marked periosteal bone formation may impart to the tibia a spindle-shaped bulge.[39] This soft tissue mass may, on occasion, be quite prominent.

The retrospective evaluation of a lesion radiographically is more often than not quite suggestive of the diagnosis, but positive identification of the tumor necessitates surgical exploration and histologic

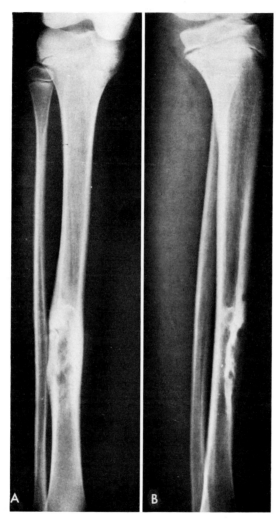

Figure 27–3.   Typical angioblastoma of the right mid-tibia in a 12-year-old girl with a 2-year history of a lump.

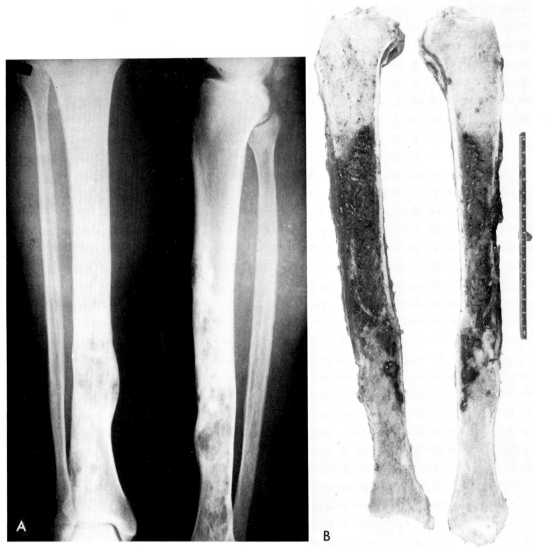

Figure 27–4.　*A*, Extensive involvement of the tibia by an ill-defined angioblastoma following several attempts at local excision. *B*, Cross-section of the specimen reveals a hemorrhagic tumor with cortical disruption.

confirmation. The most commonly entertained preoperative radiographic diagnostic alternatives include chondrosarcoma, metastatic carcinoma from an unknown primary source, eosinophilic granuloma, and hemangioendothelioma of bone.[45]

The radiographic presentation of the lesion is of paramount importance in resolving the occasional problem as to whether one deals with a metastatic carcinoma or an angioblastoma. If cortical destruction has taken place, there is no periosteal new bone formation in cases of metastatic carci-

noma; however, this is a frequent finding in a primary tumor of the tibia. The presence of a soft tissue shadow adjacent to the bone lesion is a well-known accompaniment to a tibial angioblastoma but is not seen with metastatic carcinomas.

HISTOGENESIS

Malignant angioblastoma, also known as adamantinoma of long bones, is a rare, distinctive, and controversial primary tumor of the appendicular skeleton. Unfortunately, the erroneous label "adamantinoma," meaning an ameloblastoma-like tumor, was attached to this neoplasm when, in 1913, the German pathologist Fischer first described its occurrence in the tibia.[26] In order to explain this startling happening, he incorrectly assumed that during intrauterine development the embryonal adamantine epithelium reached both the tibia and the intraoral enamel anlage in the same manner at the same time.[10, 29, 68] Actually, another case takes historical precedence; at the turn of the century, Maier described a primary epidermoid type of tumor in the ulnar diaphysis of a 20-year-old woman.[47] Since the original description, many observers have tried to portray, with variable success, how a primary, supposedly epithelial, tumor can arise in bone — a baffling occurrence that theoretically should not happen.[63] Cohnheim's theory of *Keimversprengslehre*, postulating aberrant epithelial cell nests misplaced during the course of development, had its adherents, while others preferred traumatic inclusions of skin fragments into the tibia, with subsequent tumor formation, as a more plausible source of the epithelium.[21, 67] Recently, Lichtenstein went so far as to coin the descriptive term "dermal inclusion tumor of bone" to identify this lesion.[45] The biphasic histologic growth pattern containing both epithelial and spindle cell elements gave rise to the claim that these lesions are, in fact, synovial sarcomas.[38, 43, 44, 75]

In 1957, Changus and colleagues first presented histochemical evidence to suggest that this tumor has a vascular genesis and actually represents an angioblastic neoplasm.[13] This theory was subsequently espoused by others,[23, 30, 79] and the neoplastic vascular pattern was further demonstrated.[39] Tissue culture studies also favored mesenchymal derivation.[71, 80] Several ultrastructural studies are available and, until very recently, supported an epithelial origin.[2, 41, 64, 87] These studies showed tumor cells exhibiting basement membranes, microvilli, and tonofibrils converging on the desmosomes. The tonofibrils were composed of microfilamentous fascicles with frayed ends. The desmosomes, specialized cell-to-cell attachments, accompanied by distinctive cytoplasmic

filaments, may also be demonstrated in endothelial cells, although no clumping filaments having frayed ends and attached to desmosomes have ever been demonstrated in endothelial cell junctions.[80, 82] Allegedly also supporting the epithelial genesis was the light microscopic finding of epidermoid differentiation in some portions of the lesional tissue, although such metaplastic foci are also known to occur in biphasic synovial sarcomas. The proponents of vascular histogenesis received additional ammunition from the work of Llombart-Bosch and Ortuño-Pacheco, whose ultrastructural study of a typical tibial tumor strongly supports the angioblastic nature of an "adamantinoma."[46] These investigators have identified no desmosomal tumor cell junctions. They uncovered features of mesenchymal cellular traits instead, including pinocytotic vesicles and bundles of filaments indicating endothelial derivation.

PATHOLOGIC FEATURES

On *gross examination*, the lesions are eccentrically located, even when no cortical breakthough is demonstrated. In six of the 14 cases studied at Memorial Hospital, cortical invasion with soft tissue permeation by tumor was noted.[39] The lesional tissue is characterized by a hemorrhagic cut surface with cystic areas. Aggressive lesions with adjacent soft tissue spread were often solid, fleshy, and yellow (Fig. 27–5).

Microscopically, the lesional tissue is characterized by rows of stellate cells arranged in elongated interanastomosing masses supported by a densely fibrous stroma. This pattern resembles those for tumors of skin appendages or ameloblastomas of the jaw bones (Figs. 27–6 and 27–7). Focal squamous metaplasia may be associated with such a microscopic pattern.[22] Special stains for mucin or hyaluronic acid secretion by the tumor cells are unrevealing. In addition to the so-called "ameloblastic" or "adamantine" growth traits, a wide variety of other histologic patterns may be seen (Figs. 27–8, 27–9, and 27–10).[83] Some areas may show signs of tubular, alveolar, or vessel formation, while others are entirely devoid of such features (Figs. 27–11, 27–12, and 27–13). Here and

Text continued on page 442

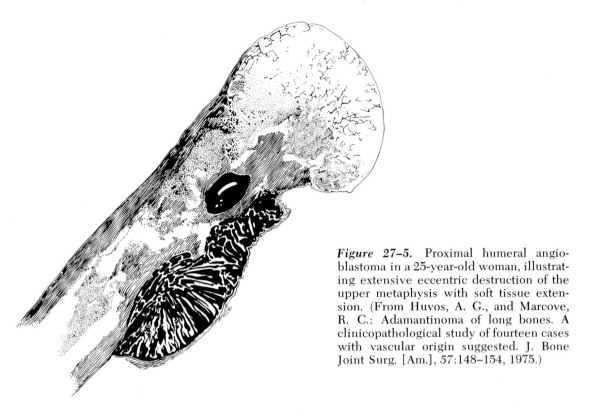

Figure 27–5. Proximal humeral angio-blastoma in a 25-year-old woman, illustrating extensive eccentric destruction of the upper metaphysis with soft tissue extension. (From Huvos, A. G., and Marcove, R. C.: Adamantinoma of long bones. A clinicopathological study of fourteen cases with vascular origin suggested. J. Bone Joint Surg. [Am.], 57:148–154, 1975.)

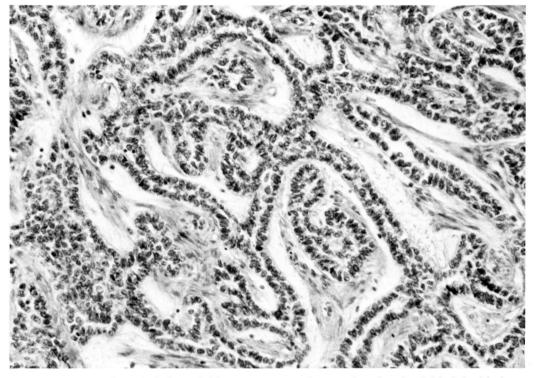

Figure 27–6. Typical epithelial ameloblastic pattern with convoluted and infolded double-layered structures and scanty intervening stroma. (Hematoxylin-eosin stain. Magnification ×50.) (From Huvos, A. G., and Marcove, R. C.: Adamantinoma of long bones. A clinicopathological study of fourteen cases with vascular origin suggested. J. Bone Joint Surg. [Am.], 57:148–154, 1975.)

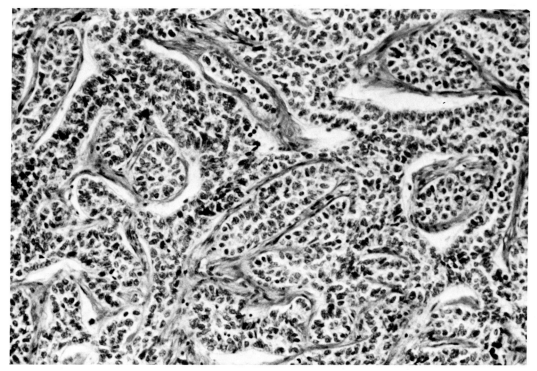

Figure 27–7. Follicular ameloblastic growth traits with discrete islands of tumor cells forming a distinct pattern. (Hematoxylin-eosin stain. Magnification ×50.) (From Huvos, A. G., and Marcove, R. C.: Adamantinoma of long bones. A clinicopathological study of fourteen cases with vascular origin suggested. J. Bone Joint Surg. [Am.], 57:148–154, 1975.)

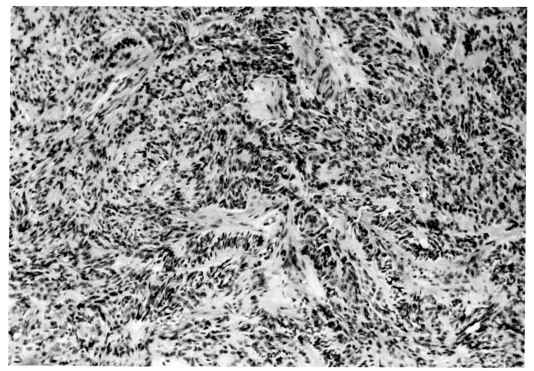

Figure 27–8. Fibrous spindle cell pattern in an angioblastoma with palisading columns of cells. (Hematoxylin-eosin stain. Magnification ×50.)

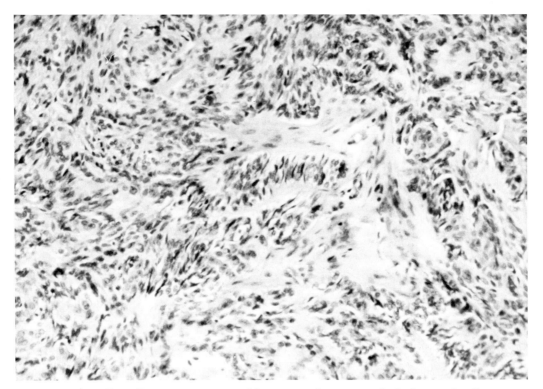

Figure 27–9. Spindle cell pattern in an angioblastoma with occasional whirling and collagenization. (Hematoxylin-eosin stain. Magnification × 80.)

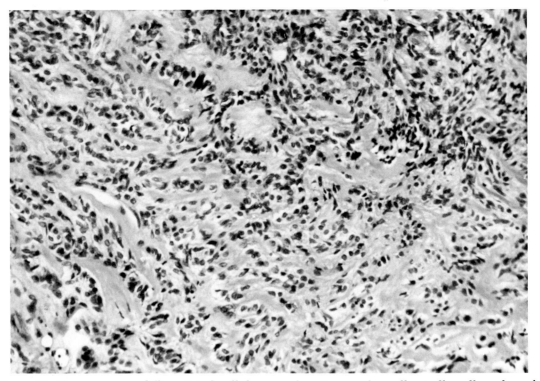

Figure 27–10. A more undifferentiated cellular growth pattern with small spindle cells and ample intercellular matrix. (Hematoxylin-eosin stain. Magnification × 80.)

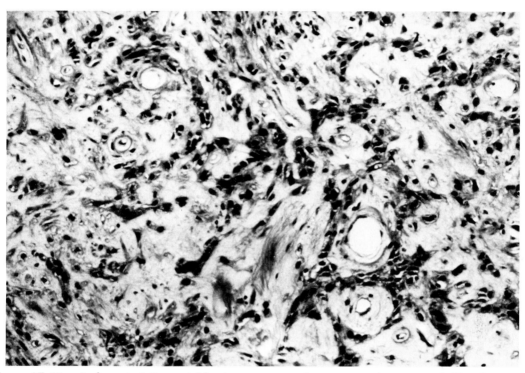

Figure 27-11. A characteristic angioblastic tumor growth pattern with merging fields of more undifferentiated tumor cells. (Hematoxylin-eosin stain. Magnification × 80.)

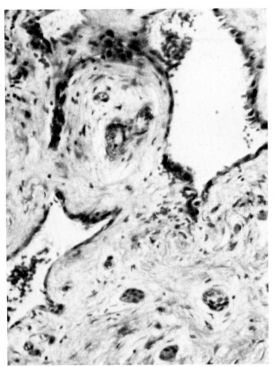

Figure 27–12. Telangiectatic vascular pattern in an angioblastoma with small islands of more typical tumor cell clusters. (Hematoxylin-eosin stain. Magnification × 80.)

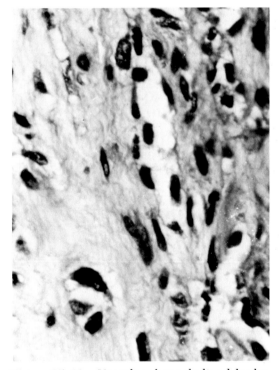

Figure 27–13. Vascular channels lined by hyperplastic endothelial cells in an angioblastoma which otherwise exhibited a typical pattern. (Hematoxylin-eosin stain. Magnification × 200.)

there, neoplastic vessel formation may be demonstrated with hyperplastic endothelial lining cells. These channels are seen to merge with areas of solidly growing tumor cells. These transitional and imperceptibly merging microscopic fields between a typical adamantine and a vascular pattern suggest that an angioblastic origin for these tumors is more than likely. Foci of osteoid production may be seen in some of the lesions, the significance of which has not been established.[13]

Several groups of investigators, particularly from the Mayo Clinic, have described osteolytic areas associated with, but independent of, "adamantinomas" of long bones.[6, 14, 21] This component was initially identified as osteitis fibrosa[21] and later as fibrous dysplasia.[6, 14] Others followed suit and have described similar features.[18] Recent critical re-evaluation of the same data at the Mayo Clinic has prompted the conclusion that these areas neither radiographically nor microscopically represent classic fibrous dysplasia and are only vaguely reminiscent of it.[76] An interesting combination of angioblastoma with intracortical fibrous dysplasia and congenital pseudoarthrosis has been reported, an association that has been interpreted as favoring a vascular origin for this tumor.[40] Markel observed two cases of ossifying fibroma in combination with angioblastoma of long bones.[50] The histologic interpretation of the lesion as being an ossifying fibroma has been questioned.[51, 62] Of the more than 30 cases of angioblastomas studied by this author, not one showed an association with fibrous dysplasia or ossifying fibroma.

TREATMENT AND PROGNOSIS

Most of the lesions are treated primarily by curettage, although such attempts only rarely result in long-term cure, except in small circumscribed lesions.[39] Analysis of follow-up data underlines the unreliability of curettage as a definitive treatment modality. *En bloc* resections also seem to yield less than dependable results, since in three such attempts recurrence was noted in each, probably due to an unexpected soft tissue component of the lesion.[39] The slow progression of angioblas-

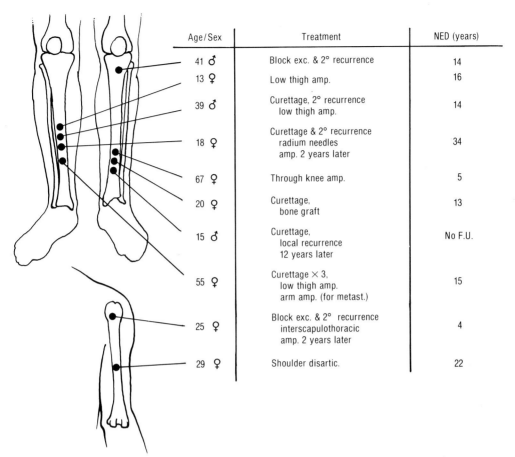

Figure 27–14. Follow-up information on 10 surviving patients treated at Memorial Hospital. (From Huvos, A. G., and Marcove, R. C.: Adamantinoma of long bones. A clinicopathological study of fourteen cases with vascular origin suggested. J. Bone Joint Surg. [Am.], 57:148–154, 1975.)

Age/Sex	Treatment	NED (years)
41 ♂	Block exc. & 2° recurrence	14
13 ♀	Low thigh amp.	16
39 ♂	Curettage, 2° recurrence low thigh amp.	14
18 ♀	Curettage & 2° recurrence radium needles amp. 2 years later	34
67 ♀	Through knee amp.	5
20 ♀	Curettage, bone graft	13
15 ♂	Curettage, local recurrence 12 years later	No F.U.
55 ♀	Curettage × 3, low thigh amp. arm amp. (for metast.)	15
25 ♀	Block exc. & 2° recurrence interscapulothoracic amp. 2 years later	4
29 ♀	Shoulder disartic.	22

Age/Sex	Treatment	Died
47 ♂	RT, amputation	5 years pulmonary metastases
38 ♂	Curettage, curettage 4 years later, block exc. 2 years later block exc. 10 years later	Unrelated cause 3 years later No clinical metastases
45 ♂	Curettage, bone chips, amp. 1 year later	2 years pulmonary metastases
33 ♂	Curettage, amputation 3 mos. later	Postop death (M.I.) autopsy: no metastases

Figure 27–15. Follow-up information on four nonsurviving patients treated at Memorial Hospital. (From Huvos, A. G., and Marcove, R. C.: Adamantinoma of long bones. A clinicopathological study of fourteen cases with vascular origin suggested. J. Bone Joint Surg. [Am.], 57:148–154, 1975.)

tomas may permit successful attempts at eradication by *en bloc* excision in spite of the high recurrence rate, especially if the tumor is relatively well-circumscribed. Suspicious regional lymph nodes should also be excised if an *en bloc* excision is undertaken. The likely explanation for the relatively high rate of local recurrence of angioblastomas may be the fact that some of the tumors are genuinely multicentric or are more extensive at the time of initial presentation than would be surmised from the radiographic examination alone.[11]

The analysis of the clinical data of patients treated at Memorial Hospital clearly demonstrates that ablation of the limb is the preferred and ultimately most successful method of treatment (Figs. 27–14 and 27–15). The prolonged natural history of tibial angioblastomas, their propensity to remain localized for protracted periods, and the surgeon's ability to control the tumor, even in the face of local recurrence, will encourage many to attempt to curet or excise an apparently limited lesion. If this conservative surgical approach is chosen, one must be on close guard for eventual local recurrence, which, in turn, will probably necessitate amputation. More advanced surgical techniques utilizing radical *en bloc* excision and appropriate endoprosthesis may be reasonable alternatives to consider in the future.

Various treatments are employed in the cases that originate in bones other than the tibia.[39] Local resection and *en bloc* excision were most commonly employed, but amputation yielded the most consistent long-term curative results.

All malignant angioblastomas of the appendicular skeleton are highly aggressive tumors with proved potential for regional and distant metastasis. It remains to be determined which neoplasm will actually do so, and no dependable histologic features have been found to herald such behavior.

Approximately 15 per cent of malignant angioblastomas have been reported to metastasize preferentially to other bones, lymph nodes, and lungs.[39, 49, 55, 56, 57, 76] Metastases developing within two years following diagnosis usually involve regional lymph nodes, in contrast to those manifesting after several years that habitually appear in the lungs or in other bones.[83]

REFERENCES

1. Agarwal, S., Manjrekar, P. S., Koshal, K. D., et al.: Adamantinoma of the tibia. Indian J. Cancer, 4:257–262, 1967.
2. Albores Saavedra, J., Diaz Gutierrez, D., and Altamirano Dimas, M.: Adamantinoma de la tibia. Observaciones ultrastructurales. Rev. Med. Hosp. Gen. Mexico, 31:241–252, 1968.
3. Allegreni, R., and Dell'Orto, R.: Adamantinoma of the long bones. Case report. Arch. Ortop., 80:465–471, 1967.
4. Anderson, C. E., and Saunders, J. B.: Primary adamantinoma of the ulna. Surg. Gynecol. Obstet., 75:351–356, 1942.
5. Baker, A. H., and Hawksley, L. M.: A case of primary adamantinoma of the tibia. Br. J. Surg., 18:415–421, 1930.
6. Baker, P. L., Dockerty, M. B., and Coventry, M. B.: Adamantinoma (so-called) of the long bones. Review of the literature and a report of 3 new cases. J. Bone Joint Surg. [Am.], 36:704–720, 1954.
7. Bell, A. L.: A case of adamantinoma of the femur. Br. J. Surg., 30:81–82, 1942.
8. Besemann, E. F., and Perez, M. A.: Malignant angioblastoma, so-called adamantinoma, involving the humerus. A case report. Am. J. Roentgenol. Radium Ther. Nucl. Med., 100:538–541, 1967.
9. Braidwood, A. S., and McDougall, A.: Adamantinoma of the tibia. Report of two cases. J. Bone Joint Surg. [Br.], 56:735–738, 1974.
10. Brocheriou, C., Hauw, J. J., Auriol, M., et al.: Ultrastructural study of 6 cases of ameloblastoma. Ann. Anat. Pathol., 20:231–244, 1975.
11. Bullough, P. G., and Goldberg, V. M.: Multicentric origin of adamantinoma of the tibia. A case report. Rev. Hosp. Spec. Surg., 1:71–74, 1971.
12. Campanacci, M., Giunti, A., and Leonessa, C.: Adamantinoma delle ossa lunghe. Chir. Organi Mov., 58:385–394, 1970.
13. Changus, G. W., Speed, J. S., and Stewart, F. W.: Malignant angioblastoma of bone. A reappraisal of adamantinoma of long bone. Cancer, 10:540–559, 1957.
14. Cohen, D. M., Dahlin, D. C., and Pugh, D. G.: Fibrous dysplasia associated with adamantinoma of the long bones. Cancer, 15:515–521, 1962.
15. Crehalet, Y. L., and Puccinelli, A. D.: Un adamantinome solitaire du tibia. J. Radiol. Electrol. Med. Nucl., 50:517–518, 1969.
16. De Santis, E., and Porfiri, B.: L'adamantinoma delle ossa lunghe: aspetti ultrastrutturali du un adamantinoma della tibia. Arch. Putti Chir. Organi Mov., 28:129–135, 1977.
17. Delarue, J., Chomette, G., and Bousquet, M.: Les "adamantinomes" du tibia. A propos de deux observations. Ann. Anat. Pathol., 5:336–351, 1960.
18. Delarue, J., Chomette, G., and Brocheriou, C.: Adamantinome du tibia et "dysplasie fibreuse." Ann. Anat. Pathol., 9:373–378, 1964.
19. Desaive, P.: Les épithéliomes des os long. Bull. Acad. R. Med. Belg., 20:105–124, 1955.

eosinophilic granuloma, which is often asymptomatic, has been noted. Pulmonary symptoms, when present, resolve spontaneously or progress to a bilateral interstitial infiltrate and fibrosis. This event is manifested by a honeycomb-type of lung, culminating in cor pulmonale and right-sided heart failure. Spontaneous pneumothorax may complicate the clinical course in some cases.

Laboratory investigations are uniformly noncontributory, and their results are nonspecific. A slight to moderate leukocytosis in the differential blood count may be noted, with a relative increase in the eosinophilic leukocytes. Even if the peripheral blood smear fails to reveal a markedly elevated eosinophil count in a solitary eosinophilic granuloma, it is quite possible that the bone marrow aspiration from an uninvolved portion of bone will yield such increased values.[82]

LOCATION

Almost any bone may be the site of origin. The skeletal distribution varies in the series of cases reported, but, in general, the skull (particularly the calvarium), the mandible, the ribs, the vertebrae, and the long tubular bones of the extremities (specifically the femur and the humerus) are most frequently involved. Most of the rib lesions are found in adults while the long bones are predilected in children.[79] Lesions involving the pelvic bones are quite common and are most frequently located in the ilium, especially directly above the acetabulum. Hands or feet are practically never affected. In the long tubular bones, eosinophilic granuloma appears in the shaft, with an equal distribution in the diaphysis and metaphysis. Epiphyseal location is exceptional.[99, 128]

Additional bone lesions developing subsequent to an apparently solitary lesion are usually noted within six months of the original.

AGE AND SEX DISTRIBUTION

Solitary eosinophilic granuloma is a disease of childhood and young adults, although a few cases may be encountered in patients over the age of 30. About half of the cases with solitary lesions occur in the first decade of life, with the ages ranging from 16 months to 61 years.[79] An overall average age of 13.5 years has been noted.[83] Most patients with mandibular presentation are older and in their third decade of life. The average age of patients with lesions in the jaw is 26 years.[91] Its occurrence in older persons should be viewed with scepticism, raising the suspicion of Hodgkin's disease instead of eosinophilic granuloma. A moderately increased male to female ratio that may reach 2:1 has been noted among the multifocal cases.

RADIOGRAPHIC FEATURES

The osseous lesions that occur in either the solitary or the multifocal forms of eosinophilic granuloma are radiographically indistinguishable. Eosinophilic granulomas most commonly arise in the medulla; however, on occasion, some may originate in the cortex. Erosion of the cortex elicits a periosteal reaction.

In multifocal eosinophilic granuloma, extraskeletal manifestations may be featured without skeletal involvement. Close follow-up of the patients, however, will reveal bony defects in many of the cases. The osseous lesions represent the classic presentation, usually demonstrable early in the course of the disease. As emphasized by Moseley, the skeletal lesions are no longer considered abolutely indispensable for the diagnosis of eosinophilic granuloma.[88, 89] They may be entirely absent, or they may not become clinically apparent until extraosseous lesions are well established. The lesions, as already stated, may involve any bone but have a predilection primarily for the skull and pelvic bones, the femur, and the ribs. The bones of the hands and feet are affected only very rarely.

The typical radiographic features of early lesions are those of a destructive radiolucent oval area of rarefaction with varying sizes in the spongiosa. These are usually well-demarcated, "punched out," without peripheral sclerosis.[88, 89]

The lesional area may show a solitary bone defect, or, occasionally, a tight cluster of partially overlapping lesions may be

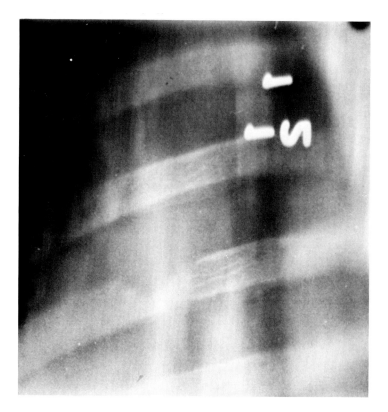

Figure 28–1. Tomogram of an eosinophilic granuloma of the rib in an adult male presenting with a pathologic fracture. (Courtesy of Dr. D. R. Dahlenburg.)

encountered. In such instances, the superimposed areas of rarefaction present with a "hole within a hole" appearance.[88, 89] A distinct and characteristic feature of many lesions is the slanting or beveling of the edges, which provides the lesion with a visual illusion of depth.[88, 89] In the experience of many, this three-dimensional aspect has been found to be a time-honored feature of the diagnosis. On occasion, the lesions may be poorly demarcated, and the periphery gradually merges with the adjacent normal bone. The bone destruction by the lesion may be quite uneven and patchy, manifested by coarse intralesional trabeculations by columns of retained bone.

Thinning of the adjacent cortex by compression may be noted with scalloping of the endosteal surface. Cortical destruction or fractures may be present directly due to the lesion (Fig. 28–1). Periosteal bone formation, especially in long bones, may occur, giving a typical onionskin lamellated appearance. This feature closely imitates the periosteal changes seen in osteomyelitis, Ewing's sarcoma, or

non-Hodgkin's lymphoma[84] (Fig. 28–2). Calvarial lesions are entirely devoid of periosteal reaction. Involvement of the ribs may exhibit expansion of the bony contours, a feature that is quite rare in lesions arising in the long bones.[111] This apparent expansion is usually due to periosteal bone formation and not actual bone distention.

Despite the fact that the skull is one of the most frequently involved bones, in some cases it is spared entirely. The radiolucent skull lesions vary markedly in size from small defects to large, irregularly outlined, geographic areas of bone destruction. During the process of healing, the sharp lesional borders become smudged and hazy. The "button sequestrum," a calvarial doughnut-shaped lesion originally described by Wells, has been thought to be almost diagnostic of eosinophilic granuloma of the skull.[144] However, this calvarial radiolucent defect with a central bony density has been seen in tuberculosis, staphylococcal osteomyelitis, and metastatic carcinoma, in addition to a great many other benign or malignant lesions,

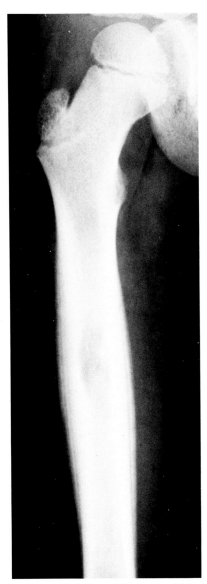

Figure 28–2. Mid-femoral eosinophilic granuloma in a 5-year-old girl with multifocal affection. The lytic, medullary, poorly delineated lesion is accompanied with periosteal onionskin-type lamellations.

including those of Paget's disease and multiple myeloma.[125] It seems that, in cases in which a typical "button sequestrum" of the skull is seen, a prompt biopsy examination is clearly indicated to establish the correct diagnosis.

The rapidly progressing skull lesions erode the diploë and extend through the inner and outer tables. Typically, no periosteal bone production is present, in contrast to the periosteal changes accompanying cortical perforation in long tubular bones. Temporal bone involvement usually goes hand in hand with base of skull disease and otitis media. A base of skull lesion may be present in the absence of calvarial or temporal bone involvement. The signs of otitis media are reliable indicators of temporal bone involvement.[4] Multifocal lesions may affect the sella turcica and the sphenoid, which may account for some of the patients having diabetes insipidus. Orbital bone destruction results in unilateral exophthalmos.

Mandibular lesions may be present and are usually located around the apices of the teeth (Fig. 28–3). By active growth, the lamina dura of neighboring teeth, in addition to surrounding bone is eroded. The characteristic complaint of loose teeth and the radiographic features of "floating teeth" describe the finding of teeth being enveloped by radiolucent lesional tissue.

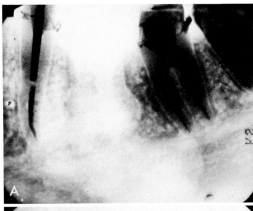
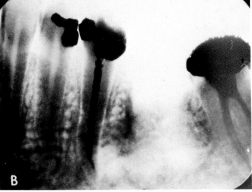

Figure 28–3. Both radiographs reveal a 2 cm area of rarefaction in the molar region of the mandible of a 21-year-old woman with a solitary eosinophilic granuloma.

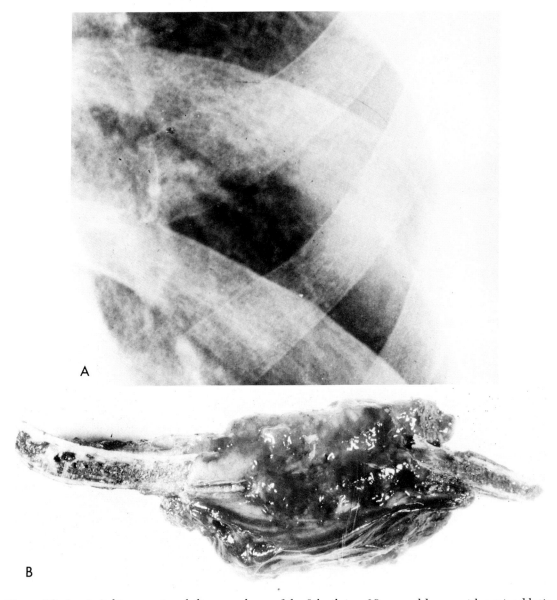

Figure 28–4. *A,* Solitary eosinophilic granuloma of the 9th rib in a 28-year-old man with a mixed lytic and sclerotic bone destruction. *B,* The resected rib specimen reveals tumor replacing bone with soft tissue extension. The patient is disease-free 14 years later.

Rib lesions may expand the bony contours dissimilarly to the affection in the long tubular bones. The lack of expansion, however, is not synonymous with limited involvement. Pathologic fractures may occur (Fig. 28–4). Involvement of the pelvic bones produces well-defined osteolytic defects with peripheral sclerosis.

It has become increasingly evident that Calvé's disease, the so-called vertebra plana in children and adolescents, which was previously considered to be due to aseptic necrosis of the vertebral body, is in fact the direct result of eosinophilic granuloma.[13, 23, 44, 65, 92, 146] This is characterized by a wedge-shaped collapse of the affected vertebral body, which sometimes becomes flat and thereby resembles a silver dollar.[27, 61] Rarely, if only the posterior aspect of the vertebral body, the neural arches, or

s are eroded, vertebral body in-
· eosinophilic granuloma does
⌐dging collapse.[64] The ver-
˙e either unilaterally or
' but characteristically
ι is involved. Finding
ⁿollapse in a child or
⸗ a skeletal radiogra-
·r the presence of
'nophilic granulo-
ι unusually slow-
· granuloma may
ᴏn of multiple
.es with adjacent

of eosinophilic
⸗ diaphysis of a
ιl considerations
· bone cyst. In
⸗ to recall that eo-
⸗ is more frequently
ꞃaft, and a simple bone
y to be at, or close to,
the ℮ⱽⱽ   ⸗aft. Bone cysts are usually
larger on ⱼ ꞓsentation and are definitely
less painful than eosinophilic granulomas.

The peculiar feature of eosinophilic granuloma is the *"tempo phenomenon."* In this
disease, the pace of the development, progression, and disappearance of the bone
lesions is quite brisk. Lesions may come
and go entirely within a few months; new
lesions may develop in the same bone just
adjacent to, or far removed from, the previous site of involvement. Although the
tempo of the cycle is rapid in most instances, occasionally the development of
the lesions is slow and they linger for a
considerable period of time. After a one
year disease-free period, it is unlikely that
a reasonably well-documented solitary eosinophilic granuloma will undergo multifocal dissemination. Patients with a solitary
focus of disease involving the craniofacial
bones or the ilium are more likely to progress to multifocal eosinophilic granuloma.[78]

Therapy-induced, or even spontaneous,
healing results in the rarefied osseous
areas acquiring sclerotic confines. Progressive healing is manifested by diminishing
intralesional opacifications, and the mar-
gination gradually becomes ill defined.
The lesion finally blends imperceptibly
into the surrounding bone. The gradual
lessening of the density may make the le-

sion hard to visualize, and, in such cases,
only the adjacent cortical scalloping can
be appreciated. Radiotherapy is usually
followed by increasingly sclerotic lesions
manifesting endosteal bone deposition.
Even these sclerotic lesions may eventually
resolve, leaving no telltale signs of their
previous existence behind.

When multifocal disease is suspected,
skeletal survey must precede biopsy so
that the most accessible, rather than the
presenting, lesion may be selected.

PATHOLOGIC FEATURES

In the earliest phases of inception, the
lesions are hemorrhagic and cystic, with
soft brownish-yellow streaked lesional tissue (Fig. 28–4B).

On histologic examination, conspicuous
sheets and clusters of mononuclear histiocytes, some with striking phagocytic activity, admixed with collections of eosinophilic leukocytes are present (Figs. 28–5 and
28–6). In some foci, hemorrhage and necrosis are featured, with multinucleated
phagocytic giant cells in adjacent fields
(Fig. 28–7). The phagocytic capacity of
both mononuclear and multinucleated histiocytic cells is demonstrated by ingestion
of erythrocytes, eosinophils, and hemosiderin granules. Some of these features are
displayed to a better advantage with meth-
ylene blue and Giemsa preparations. The
cytoplasm of the phagocytic cells often exhibits double refractile neutral fat deposition (Fig. 28–8).

The presence of mature eosinophilic
leukocytes is characteristic of this lesion,
although the basic proliferating cell is tra-
ditionally considered to be a histocyte, despite the fact that proof of this is still lacking. The eosinophils have irregularly
outlined bilobed and indented nuclei (Fig.
28–9). If the lesional tissue has been overly decalcified, the eosinophilic cells become less readily identifiable. In areas
where the eosinophilic leukocytes are
undergoing fragmentation, proteinace-
ous crystalline structures, the so-called
Charcot-Leyden crystals, are demonstrable, a feature already noted to be associated with eosinophilic granuloma by Taratynov as early as 1913 and 1914.[130, 131]

Fracture through a lesion results in ex-

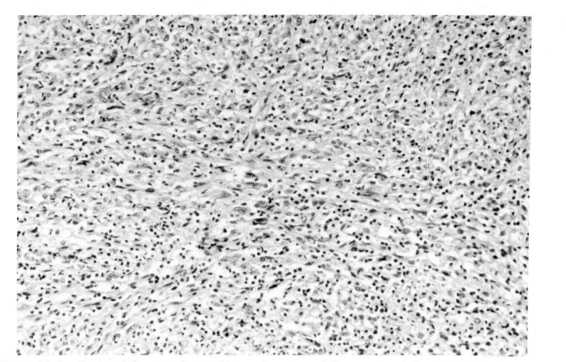

Figure 28–5. Eosinophilic granuloma of bone showing a diffuse eosinophilic infiltrate with an admixture of scattered histiocytes. (Hematoxylin-eosin stain. Magnification ×50.)

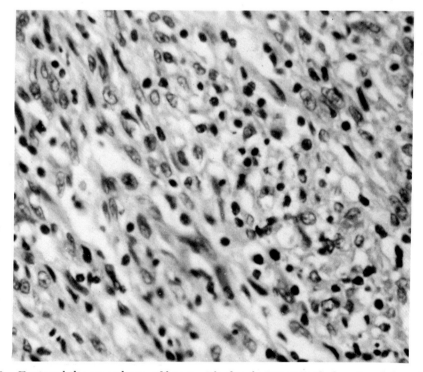

Figure 28–6. Eosinophilic granuloma of bone with closely intermingled eosinophils and histiocytic cells. (Hematoxylin-eosin stain. Magnification ×80.)

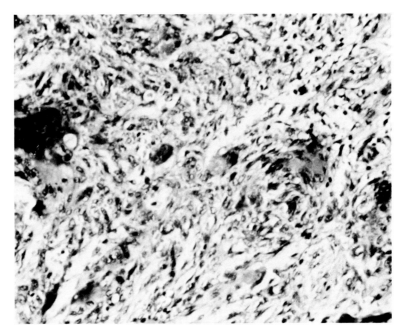

Figure 28–7. Eosinophilic granuloma of bone featuring multinucleated phagocytic giant cells and fibrosis. (Hematoxylin-eosin stain. Magnification × 80.)

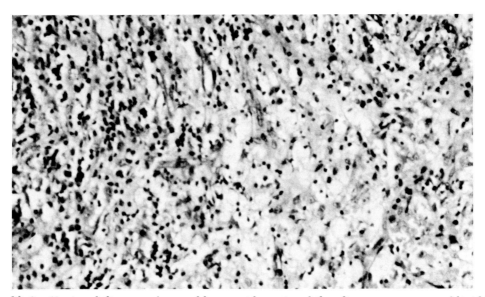

Figure 28–8. Eosinophilic granuloma of bone with eosinophils adjacent to an area of lipid-laden "foam cells." (Hematoxylin-eosin stain. Magnification × 80.)

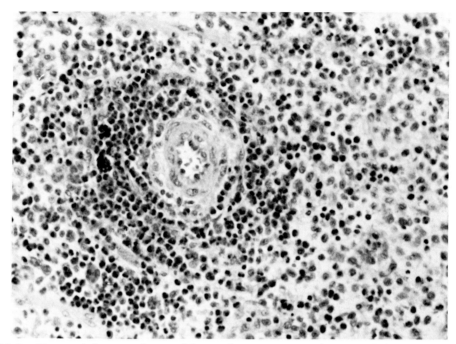

Figure 28–9. Eosinophilic granuloma of bone showing a typical eosinophilic cell infiltrate in a largely perivascular arrangement resembling an allergic reaction. Hematoxylin-eosin stain. Magnification × 200.)

aggerated fibrous tissue proliferation, which may obscure the typical histologic features of an eosinophilic granuloma. Closer examination, however, will still reveal clusters of histiocytes intermixed with eosinophils separated by irregular fibrous septa. In these areas, periosteal connective tissue scarring and reactive new bone and callus formation are demonstrable.[60] This fibrosis is the inevitable consequence of a previous fracture and, therefore, should not be construed as evidence of healing.

In 1942, Green and Farber delineated the progressive, histologically identifiable, phases of eosinophilic granuloma during its evolutionary cycle.[49] They found that the eosinophils markedly diminish in number and finally disappear as the lesion matures. Instead, the large mononucleated histiocytes become the predominant cell type with some fibrous tissue elements. In their view, which is not uniformly shared, an intermediate stage of obligatory lipidization is seen, characterized by lipid-laden mononuclear histiocytic cells (foam cells) that are eventually transformed into bone through fibrosis. Careful histologic study of untreated healing lesions, however,

demonstrates that resorption of the lesional tissue proceeds via gradual resolution and fibrosis and not by lipidization or lipogranuloma formation. In our experience, foci of xanthomatous foam cells are only occasional concomitants of eosinophilic granuloma, appearing in close association exclusively with chronic suppuration, and are neither requisite nor dominant components. In histologically ambiguous cases in which the lipid-laden histiocytic foam cells dominate the picture, serious consideration should be given to another disease process described in 1930 by Chester as "skeletal lipid (cholesterol) granulomatosis," sometimes also referred to as "Chester-Erdheim disease."[20]

Eosinophilic granuloma may involve extraskeletal sites in addition to bones. These sites include the skin, vulva, gingiva, salivary glands, lungs, and lymph nodes.

During the process of spontaneous healing, a solitary focus of eosinophilic granuloma histologically may resemble a fibrous cortical defect or a nonossifying fibroma with a prominent xanthomatous component. The matted, pinwheel growth pattern of the fibroblastic cells clearly separates these lesions from an eosinophilic granuloma. Foam cells also are only occasional and minor components of eosinophilic granuloma.

In many instances of eosinophilic granuloma, *ultrastructural studies* revealed rodlike or tennis racket–shaped cytoplasmic inclusions in the histiocytic cells identical to those seen in the normal Langerhans' cells of the epidermis. These so-called Langerhans' or Birbeck granules are absent in normal histiocytes. Characteristically, they are lined by a trilaminar membrane and contain a central lamella showing a periodicity of approximately 6 nm. It is assumed that they develop by infolding of the plasmalemma and probably represent secondary cell membrane alterations directly resulting from antigenic challenge.

TREATMENT

Depending on the location, solitary eosinophilic granuloma should be treated by curettage with or without placing of bone chips. Inaccessible skeletal lesions, such as in the spine, or those involving the long bones of the lower limb require supervoltage fractionated irradiation with a total dose in the 300 to 600r range. This low-dose schedule results in good control of the disease process and stimulates lesional resorption.

Chemotherapy has been employed in the treatment of multifocal eosinophilic granuloma. Methotrexate, prednisone, and vinblastine in small doses have been used successfully to abort the progressive stages of the disease and to decrease its morbidity.[78] Supervoltage fractionated radiation therapy with a total dose of about 300 to 600r delivered to vertebral or other lesions should yield an immediate healing response.

REFERENCES

1. Abt, A. F., and Denenholz, E. J.: Letterer-Siwe's disease: splenohepatomegaly associated with widespread hyperplasia of nonlipoid-storing macrophages: discussion of the so-called reticulo-endothelioses. Am. J. Dis. Child., 51:499–522, 1936.

2. Arcomano, J. P., Barnett, J. C., and Wunderlich, H. O.: Histiocytosis X. Am. J. Roentgenol. Radium Ther. Nucl. Med., 85:663–679, 1961.

3. Augereau, B., Thuilleux, G., and Moinet, Ph.: Eosinophil granuloma of bones. Report of 15 cases including 10 survivals with an average follow up of 4 years. J. Chir., 113:159–170, 1977.

4. Avery, M. E., McAfee, J. G., and Guild, H. G.: The course and prognosis of reticuloendotheliosis (eosinophilic granuloma, Schüller-Christian disease and Letterer-Siwe disease): a study of 40 cases. Am. J. Med., 22:636–652, 1957.

5. Avioli, L. V., Lasersohn, J. T., and Lopresti, J. M.: Histiocytosis X (Schüller-Christian disease): a clinicopathological survey, review of ten patients and the results of prednisone therapy. Medicine, 42:119–147, 1963.

6. Barth, R. F., Vergara, G. G., Khurana, S. K., et al.: Rapidly fatal familial histiocytosis associated with eosinophilia and primary immunological deficiency. Lancet, 2:503–506, 1972.

7. Batson, R., Shapiro, J., Christie, A., et al.: Acute nonlipid disseminated reticuloendotheliosis. Am. J. Dis. Child., 90:323–343, 1955.

8. Beck, W.: Über das gutartige Knochenmarkretikulom mit Eosinophilie. Virchows Arch. [Pathol. Anat.], 311:569–592, 1944.

9. Beeson, P. B., and Bass, D. A.: The Eosinophil. Philadelphia, W.B. Saunders Co., 1977.

10. Berk, O., and Atasagun, H.: Eosinophilic granuloma: A case report. Kanser, 5:30–35, 1975.

11. Bopp, J. H., and Günther, D.: Die Strahlenbehandlung des eosinophilen Granuloms. Strahlentherapie, 140:143–147, 1970.

12. Buchman, J.: Osteochondritis of the vertebral body. J. Bone Joint Surg., 9:55–66, 1927.

13. Calvé, J. A.: Localized affection of the spine suggesting osteochondritis of vertebral body, with clinical aspects of Pott's disease. J. Bone Joint Surg., 7:41–46, 1925.

14. Campbell, J. B., and Alexander, E., Jr.: Eosinophilic granuloma of skull — report of case. J. Neurosurg., 1:365–370, 1944.

15. Cardozo, L. J., Bailey, I. C., Billinghurst, J. R., et al.: Non-osseous eosinophilic granuloma presenting as acute transverse myelitis. Br. J. Surg., 61:747–749, 1974.

16. Case records of the Massachusetts General Hospital. Case 9-1973. N. Engl. J. Med., 188:459–463, 1973.

17. Castrup, W., and von Koppenfels, R.: Contribution to the so-called eosinophilic soft-tissue granuloma. Strahlentherapie, 148:139–145, 1974.

18. Cederbaum, S. D., Niwayama, G., Stiehm, E. R., et al.: Combined immunodeficiency manifested by Letterer-Siwe syndrome. Letter to the editor. Lancet, 1:958, 1972.

19. Chacha, P. B., and Khong, B. T.: Eosinophilic granuloma of bone. A diagnostic problem. Clin. Orthop., 80:79–88, 1971.

20. Chester, W.: Über Lipoidgranulomatose. Virchows Arch. [Pathol. Anat.], 279:561–602, 1930–1931.

21. Cheyne, C.: Histiocytosis X. J. Bone Joint Surg. [Br.], 53:366–382, 1971.

22. Christian, H. A.: Defects in membranous bone, exophthalmos and diabetes insipidus. An unusual syndrome of dyspituitarism: a clinical study. Med. Clin. North Am., 3:849–871, 1920.

23. Compere, E. L., Johnson, W. E., and Coventry, M. B.: Vertebra plana (Calvé's disease) due to eosinophilic granuloma. J. Bone Joint Surg. [Am.], 36:969–980, 1954.

24. Cruthirds, T. P., and Johnson, H. R.: Solitary primary eosinophilic granuloma of bone. J.A.M.A., 196:295–296, 1966.

25. Curtis, A. C., and Cawley, E. P.: Eosinophilic granuloma of bone with cutaneous manifestations. Arch. Dermatol., 55:810–818, 1947.

26. Daneshbod, K., and Kissane, J. M.: Histiocytosis. The prognosis of polyostotic eosinophilic granuloma. Am. J. Clin. Pathol., 65:601–611, 1976.

27. Davies, P. M.: Xanthomatosis associated with vertebra plana. Br. J. Radiol., 22:725–728, 1949.

28. de Man, J. C. H.: Rod-like tubular structures in the cytoplasm of histiocytes in "Histiocytosis X." J. Pathol. Bacteriol., 95:123–126, 1968.

29. Dingley, A. R.: Eosinophil granuloma of the temporal bone. J. Laryngol. Otol., 66:285–287, 1952.

30. Doede, K. G., and Rappaport, H.: Long-term survival of patients with acute differentiated histiocytosis (Letterer-Siwe disease). Cancer, 20:1782–1795, 1967.

31. Dundon, C. C., Williams, H. A., and Laipply, T. C.: Eosinophilic granuloma of bone. Radiology, 47:433–444, 1946.

32. Engelbreth-Holm, J., Teilum, G., and Christensen, E.: Eosinophil granuloma of bone — Schüller-Christian's disease. Acta Med. Scand., 118:292–312, 1944.

33. Ennis, J. T., Whitehouse, G., Ross, F. G. M., et al.: The radiology of bone changes in histiocytosis X. Clin. Radiol., 24:212–220, 1973.

34. Enriquez, P., Dahlin, D. C., Hayles, A. B., et al.: Histiocytosis X: A clinical study. Mayo Clin. Proc., 42:88–99, 1967.

35. Farber, S.: The nature of "solitary or eosinophilic granuloma" of bone. Am. J. Pathol., 17:625–626, 1941.

36. Ferris, R. A., Pettrone, F. A., McKelvie, A. M., et al.: Eosinophilic granuloma of the spine: an unusual radiographic presentation. Clin. Orthop., 99:57–63, 1974.

37. Fèvre, M.: Eléments du diagnostic positif du granulome éosinophile des os. Toulouse Med., 9:705–711, 1954.

38. Fèvre, M.: Aspects radiologiques du granulome éosinophile des os, en particulier au fémur et à la clavicule. Rev. Chir. Orthop., 41:3–31, 1955.

39. Fèvre, M., and Bertrand, P.: Existence du granulomes éosinophiles épiphysaires. Rev. Chir. Orthop., 56:345–353, 1970.

40. Finzi, O.: Mieloma con prevalenza delle cellule eosinofile circoscritto all'osso frontale in un giovine di 15 anni. Minerva Med., 9:239–241, 1929.

41. Fowles, J. V., and Bobechko, W. P.: Eosinophilic granuloma in bone. J. Bone Joint Surg. [Br.], 52:238–243, 1970.

42. Fraser, J.: Skeletal lipoid granulomatosis (Hand-Schüller-Christian's disease). Br. J. Surg., 22:800–824, 1934–1935.

43. Friedman, B., and Hanaoka, H.: Langerhans cell granules in eosinophilic granuloma of bone. J. Bone Joint Surg. [Am.], 51:367–374, 1969.

44. Fripp, A. T.: Vertebra plana. J. Bone Joint Surg. [Br.], 40:378–384, 1958.

45. Galeotti-Flori, A., and Parenti, G. C.: Reticuloendoteliosi iperplasica infettiva ad evoluzione, granuloxantomatosa (tipo Hand-Schüller-Christian). Riv. Clin. Pediatr., 35:193–263, 1937.

46. Glanzmann, E.: Infektiöse Retikuloendotheliose (Abt-Letterer-Siwe'sche Krankheit) und ihre Beziehungen zum Morbus Schüller-Christian. Ann. Paediatr., 155:1–8, 1940.

47. Goldner, M. G., and Volk, B. W.: Fulminant normocholesteremic xanthomatosis (histiocytosis X). Report of incidence in an aged woman. Arch. Intern. Med., 95:689–698, 1955.

48. Gray, J. D., and Taylor, S.: Acute systemic reticuloendotheliosis terminating as a monocytic leukaemia. Cancer, 6:333–337, 1953.

49. Green, W. T., and Farber, S.: "Eosinophilic or solitary granuloma" of bone. J. Bone Joint Surg., 24:499–526, 1942.

50. Güthert, H.: Zur Morphologie des eosinophilen Granuloms des Knochens. Zentralbl. Allg. Pathol., 89:388–392, 1952–1953.

51. Hamilton, J. B., Barner, J. L., Kennedy, P. C., et al.: The osseous manifestations of eosinophilic granuloma. Report of nine cases. Radiology, 47:445–456, 1946.

52. Hand, A., Jr.: Polyuria and tuberculosis. Arch. Pediatr., 10:673–675, 1893.

53. Hansen, P. B.: The relationship of Hand-Schüller-Christian's disease, Letterer-Siwe's disease and eosinophilic granulomas of bone (with report of 5 cases). Acta Radiol. (Stockh.), 32:89–112, 1949.

54. Hatcher, C. H.: Eosinophilic granuloma of bone. Arch. Pathol., 30:828, 1940.

55. Held, A. J., and Rutishauser, E.: L'histiocytoréticulose dite granulomatose éosinophile des maxillaires. Bull. Acad. Suisse Sci. Med., 4:415–432, 1948.

56. Hill, R. M.: Non-specific (eosinophilic) granuloma of bone. Br. J. Surg., 37:69–76, 1949.

57. Hodgson, J. R., Kennedy, R. L., and Camp, J. D.: Reticuloendotheliosis. Radiology, 57:642–652, 1951.

58. Holst, G., Husted, E., and Pindborg, J. J.: On the eosinophilic bone granuloma with regard to localization in jaws and relation to general histiocytosis. Acta Odontol. Scand., 10:148–179, 1953.

59. Hunter, T.: Solitary eosinophilic granuloma of bone. J. Bone Joint Surg. [Br.], 38:545–557, 1956.

60. Jaffe, H. L., and Lichtenstein, L.: Eosinophilic granuloma of bone: a condition affecting one, several or many bones, but apparently limited to the skeleton, and representing the mildest clinical expression of the peculiar inflammatory histiocytosis also underlying Letterer-Siwe disease and Schüller-Christian disease. Arch. Pathol., 37:99–118, 1944.

61. Jansson, G.: Zur Kenntnis der Skelettveränderungen bei der Schüller-Christian'schen Krankheit (Xanthomatöse Spondylose mit paravertebraler Schattenbildung). Acta Radiol., 16:59–73, 1935.

62. Kaplan, C., Shamoto, M., and Katoh, A.: An appraisal of histiocytosis X. J. Surg. Oncol., 4:180–189, 1972.

63. Kaufman, A., Bukberg, P. R., Werlin, S., et al.: Multifocal eosinophilic granuloma ("Hand-Schüller-Christian disease"). Report illustrating H-S-C chronicity and diagnostic challenge. Am. J. Med., 60:541–548, 1976.

64. Kaye, J. J., and Freiberger, R. H.: Eosinophilic granuloma of the spine without vertebra plana. A report of two unusual cases. Radiology, 92:1188–1191, 1969.

65. Kieffer, S. A., Nesbit, M. E., and D'Angio, G. J.: Vertebra plana due to histiocytosis X: serial studies. Acta Radiol. [Diagn.] (Stockh.), 8:241–250, 1969.

66. Kierland, R. B., Epstein, J. G., and Weber, W. E.: Eosinophilic granuloma of skin and mucous membrane. Association with diabetes insipidus. Arch. Dermatol., 75:45–54, 1957.

67. Kothe, W.: Das eosinophile Granulom des Knochens. Fortschr. Geb. Roentgenstr. Nuklearmed., 79:453–461, 1953.

68. Lahey, M. E.: Histiocytosis X — comparison of three treatment regimens. J. Pediatr., 87:179–183, 1975.

69. Lahey, M. E.: Histiocytosis X — an analysis of prognostic factors. J. Pediatr., 87:184–189, 1975.

70. Laurent, R., Oppermann, A., Agache, P., et al.: Histiocytose X chronique disséminée (Maladie de Hand Schuller Christian). Etude au microscope électronique. J. Med. Besançon, 7:365–384, 1971.

71. Lefebvre, J., and Chaumont, P.: Le devenir du granulome éosinophile chez l'enfant. J. Radiol. Electrol., 39:705–712, 1958.

72. Letterer, E.: Aleukämische Retikulose (ein Beitrag zu den proliferativen Erkrankungen des Retikuloendothelialapparates). Frankf. Z. Pathol., 30:377–394, 1924.

73. Lewes, D., and Valentine, J. C.: Alcohol-induced pain due to eosinophil granuloma of bone. Lancet, 1:461–462, 1962.

74. Lichtenstein, L.: Histiocytosis X. Integration of eosinophilic granuloma of bone, "Letterer-Siwe disease" and "Schüller-Christian disease" as related manifestations of a single nosologic entity. Arch. Pathol., 56:84–102, 1953.

75. Lichtenstein, L.: Pathology: diseases of bone. N. Engl. J. Med., 255:427–433, 1956.

76. Lichtenstein, L.: Histiocytosis X (Eosinophilic granuloma of bone, Letterer-Siwe disease, and Schüller-Christian disease): further observations of pathological and clinical importance. J. Bone Joint Surg. [Am.], 46:76–90, 1964.

77. Lichtenstein, L., and Jaffe, H. L.: Eosinophilic granuloma of bone — with report of a case. Am. J. Pathol., 16:595–604, 1940.

78. Lieberman, P. H.: Eosinophilic granuloma and related syndromes. In Beeson, P. B., and McDermott, W. (eds.): Textbook of Medicine, Vol. II. 14th ed. Philadelphia, W. B. Saunders Co., 1975, pp. 1529–1531.

79. Lieberman, P. H., Jones, C. R., Dargeon, H. W. K., et al.: A reappraisal of eosinophilic granuloma of bone, Hand-Schüller-Christian syndrome and Letterer-Siwe syndrome. Medicine, 48:375–400, 1969.

80. Lindenbaum, B., and Gettes, N. I.: Solitary eosinophilic granuloma of the cervical region. A case report. Clin. Orthop., 68:112–114, 1970.

81. Mallet, R., Ribierre, M., Labrune, B., et al.: Deux observations d'histiocytose X du jeune enfant. Présence dans les lésions osseuses de filaments intracytoplasmiques d'apparence virale. Bull. Soc. Med. Hop. Paris, 117:385–391, 1966.

82. Marcove, R. C.: Bone-marrow eosinophilia with solitary eosinophilic granuloma of bone: a report of two cases. J. Bone Joint Surg. [Am.], 41:1521–1525, 1959.

83. McGavran, M. H., and Spady, H. A.: Eosinophilic granuloma of bone. A study of twenty-eight cases. J. Bone Joint Surg. [Am.], 42:979–992, 1960.

84. McKenzie, A. H., and Day, F. G.: Eosinophilic granuloma of the femoral shaft simulating Ewing's sarcoma. J. Bone Joint Surg. [Am.], 39:408–413, 1957.

85. Meyer, E.: Hand-Schüller-Christian disease or eosinophilic xanthomatous granuloma. Am. J. Med., 15:130–133, 1953.

86. Mickelson, M. R., and Bonfiglio, M.: Eosinophilic granuloma and its variations. Orthop. Clin. North Am., 8:933–945, 1977.

87. Morales, A. R., Fine, G., Horn, R. C., Jr., et al.: Langerhans cells in a localized lesion of the eosinophilic granuloma type. Lab. Invest., 20:412–423, 1969.

88. Moseley, J. E.: Patterns of bone change in the reticuloendothelioses. J. Mt. Sinai Hosp., 29:282–321, 1962.

89. Moseley, J. E.: Bone Changes in Hematologic Disorders (Roentgen Aspects). New York Grune & Stratton, 1963, pp. 161–179.

90. Mukadum, F. K., and Pinto, J. M.: Eosinophilic granuloma. Indian J. Cancer, 14:92–96, 1977.

91. Mutschelknauss, R., Becker, R., and Machtens, E.: Klinik und Therapie des eosinophilen Granuloms der Kiefer. Fortschr. Kiefer. Gesichtschir., 14:90–97, 1970.

92. Nesbit, M. E., Kieffer, S., and D'Angio, G. J.: Reconstitution of vertebral height in histiocytosis X: a long-term follow up. J. Bone Joint Surg. [Am.], 51:1360–1368, 1969.

93. Nesbit, M. E., Wolfson, J. J., Kieffer, S. A., et al.: Orbital sclerosis in histiocytosis X. Am. J. Roentgenol. Radium Ther. Nucl. Med., 110:123–128, 1970.

94. Newton, W. A., Jr., and Hamoudi, A. B.: Histiocytosis: A histologic classification with clinical correlation. In Rosenberg, H. S., and Bolande, R. P. (eds.): Perspectives in Pediatric Pathology. Vol. 1. Chicago, Year Book Medical Publishers, 1973, pp. 251–283.

95. Nezelof, C.: L'histiocytose X. Rev. Fr. Etud. Clin. Biol., 11:22–39, 1966.

96. Nezelof, C., Despres, S., Barbey, S., et al.: Histiocytose X. Eléments histochimiques et autoradiographiques en faveur d'une synthèse lipidique en culture in vitro. Biomedicine, 20:414–424, 1974.

97. Nyholm, K.: Eosinophilic xanthomatous granulomatosis and Letterer-Siwe disease. Acta Pathol. Microbiol. Scand. [A], *216* (Supplement):1–79, 1971.

98. Oberman, H. A.: Idiopathic histiocytosis: A clinicopathologic study of 40 cases and review of the literature on eosinophilic granuloma of bone, Hand-Schüller-Christian disease and Letterer-Siwe disease. Pediatrics, 28:307–327, 1961.

99. Ochsner, S. F.: Eosinophilic granuloma of bone. Experience with 20 cases. Am. J. Roentgenol. Radium Ther. Nucl. Med., 97:719–726, 1966.

100. Otani, S.: A discussion on eosinophilic granuloma of bone, Letterer-Siwe disease and Schüller-Christian disease. J. Mt. Sinai Hosp., 24:1079–1092, 1957.

101. Otani, S., and Ehrlich, J. C.: Solitary granuloma of bone simulating primary neoplasm. Am. J. Pathol., 16:479–490, 1940.

102. Panner, B., and Carter, A. C.: Histiocytosis X. Chronic disseminated form (Schüller-Christian disease) with marked arteriosclerosis in a young woman. Am. J. Med., 26:974–978, 1959.

103. Peeters, F. I.: Die Differentialdiagnosis benigner solitärer Defekte im Schädeldach. Fortschr. Geb. Roentgenstr. Nuklearmed., 117:625–629, 1972.

104. Prager, P. J., Menges, V., DiBiase, M., et al.: Eosinophilic granuloma of the bone in adults. Radiologe, 16:21–28, 1976.

105. Prete, K.: Über das sogenannte Eosinophile Granulom des Knochens und seine Beziehungen zur Hand-Schüller-Christianschen Krankheit. Wien. Klin. Wochenschr., 62:841–845, 1950.

106. Rashkovskaya, M. I.: Bone xanthomatosis in a child four-and-a-half years old. Pediatriia, 2:82–83, 1956.

107. Ratomski, R., Król, J., Bruszewski, J., et al.: Granuloma eosinophylicum. Beitr. Orthop. Traumatol., 17:12–16, 1970.

108. Ritter, R. A., Jr.: Histiocytosis-X. A case report with electron microscopic observations. Cancer, 19:1155–1164, 1966.

109. Rodrigues, R. J., and Lewis, H. H.: Eosinophilic granuloma of bone. Review of literature and case presentation. Clin. Orthop., 77:183–192, 1971.

110. Rubbiani, U., and Russo, S.: Su una rara osservazione di granuloma eosinofilo a sede tibiale. Arch. Ital. Patol. Clin. Tumori, 2:1225–1237, 1958.

111. Saenger, E. L., and Johansmann, R. J.: Letterer-Siwe's disease. Problems in diagnosis and treatment. Am. J. Roentgenol. Radium Ther. Nucl. Med., 71:472–483, 1954.

112. Sbarbaro, J. L., and Francis, K. C.: Eosinophilic granuloma of bone. J.A.M.A., 178:706–710, 1961.

113. Schairer, E.: Über eine eigenartige Erkrankung des kindlichen Schädels (Osteomyelitis mit eosinophiler Reaktion). Zentralbl. Allg. Pathol., 71:113–117, 1938.

114. Schajowicz, F., and Slullitel, J.: Eosinophilic granuloma of bone and its relationship to Hand-Schüller-Christian and Letterer-Siwe syndromes. J. Bone Joint Surg. [Br.], 55:545–565, 1973.

115. Schneider, K., Erd, W., Lobenwein, E., et al.: Eosinophiles Granulom (Histiozytosis X) mit pulmonaler und ossärer Manifestation. Wien. Klin. Wochenschr., 87:486–488, 1975.

116. Schüller, A.: Über eigenartige Schädeldefekte im Jugendalter. Fortschr. Geb. Roentgenstr. Nuklearmed., 23:12–18, 1915.

117. Schüller, A.: Dysostosis hypophysaria. Br. J. Radiol., 31:156–158, 1928.

118. Schulze, E., and Schnepper, E.: Erfahrungen bei der Diagnose und Behandlung des eosinophilen Knochengranuloms mit besonderer Berücksichtigung der Telekobalt-Strahlentherapie. Strahlentherapie, 132:173–183, 1967.

119. Sholkoff, S. D., and Mainzer, F.: Button sequestrum revisited. Radiology, 100:649–652, 1971.

120. Sigala, J. L., Silverman, S., Jr., Brody, H. A., et al.: Dental involvement in histiocytosis. Oral Surg., 33:42–48, 1972.

121. Siwe, S.: Die Reticuloendotheliose — ein neues Krankheitsbild unter den Hepatosplenomegalien. Z. Kinderheilkd., 55:212–247, 1933.

122. Siwe, S.: The reticulo-endothelioses in children. *In* Levine, S. Z., Butter, A. M., Holt, L. E., Jr., et al. (eds.): Advances in Pediatrics. Vol. 4 New York, Interscience Publishers, 1949, pp. 117–143.

123. Smith, D. G., Nesbit, M. E., Jr., D'Angio, G. J., et al.: Histiocytosis X: Role of radiation therapy in management with special reference to dose levels employed. Radiology, 106:419–422, 1973.

124. Soboleva, N. I., and Ryabinkina, A. I.: On the etiology and pathogenesis of Taratynov's disease (eosinophilic granuloma of bones or benign bone-marrow reticuloma with eosinophilia). Arkh. Patol., 15(4):37–46, 1959.

125. Som, P. M., Anderson, P. J., and Wolf, B. S.: A malignant calvarial doughnut lesion ("button sequestrum?"). Mt. Sinai J. Med. N.Y., 45:390–393, 1978.

126. Sonnenburg, I.: The eosinophilic granuloma of the jaws. Stomatol. DDR, 27:614–618, 1977.

127. Stelzner, F.: Über das eosinophile Granulom des Knochens. Zentralbl. Chir., 75:846–849, 1950.

128. Stern, M. B., Cassidy, R., and Mirra, J.: Eosinophilic granuloma of the proximal tibial epiphysis. Clin. Orthop., 118:153–156, 1976.

129. Takahashi, M., Martel, W., and Oberman, H. A.: The variable roentgenographic appearance of idiopathic histiocytosis. Clin. Radiol., 17:48–53, 1966.

130. Taratynov, N. I.: Connection between local eosinophilia and the formation of crystals (Charcot-Leyden's?) in tissues. Kazan. Med. J., 13:39–54, 1913.

131. Taratynov, N. I.: Zur Frage über Beziehungen zwischen lokaler Eosinophilie und Charcot-Leydenschen Kristallen. Frankf. Z. Pathol., 15:284–296, 1914.

132. Thompson, J., Buechner, H. A., and Fishman, R.: Eosinophilic granuloma of the lung. Ann. Intern. Med., 48:1134–1145, 1958.

133. Tos, M.: E.N.T. manifestations of Letterer-Siwe disease. Acta Otolaryngol., 56:84–92, 1963.

134. Tos, M.: A survey of Hand-Schüller-Christian's disease in otolaryngology. Acta Otolaryngol., 62:217–228, 1966.

135. Tusques, J., and Pradal, G.: Analyse tridimensionnelle des inclusions rencontrées dans les histiocytes de l'histiocytose "X", en microscopie électronique. Comparaison avec les inclusions des cellules de Langerhans. J. Microscopie, 8:113–122, 1969.

136. van Creveld, S.: Xanthomatosis generalisata osseum chez les enfants. La maladie de Schüller-Christian. Réticulo-endothélioses infectieuses avec localisation particulière dans le squelette. Rev. Fr. Pediatr., 13:314–335, 1937.

137. Vazquez, J. J., and Ayestaran, J. R.: Eosinophilic granuloma of the stomach similar to that of bone. Light and electron microscopic study. Virchows Arch., 366:107–111, 1975.

138. Virenque, J., Pasquié, M., and Glaubert, J.: Notes sur le granulome éosinophile des os. Presse Méd., 68:2304–2307, 1960.

139. Vogel, J. M., and Vogel, P.: Idiopathic histiocytosis: a discussion of eosinophilic granuloma, the Hand-Schüller-Christian syndrome, and the Letterer-Siwe syndrome. Semin. Hematol., 9:349–369, 1972.

140. von Albertini, A.: Histologische Geschwulstdiagnostik. Stuttgart, Georg Thieme Verlag, 1974, pp. 484–487.

141. Waldman, R. S., and Powell, T.: Eosinophilic granuloma of the clavicle simulating primary bone neoplasm. Clin. Orthop., 64:150–152, 1969.

142. Wallgren, A.: Systemic reticuloendothelial granuloma. Nonlipoid reticuloendotheliosis and Schüller-Christian disease. Am. J. Dis. Child., 60:471–500, 1940.

143. Walthard, B., and Zippinger: Das eosinophile Granulom des Knochens. Schweiz. Med., Wochenschr., 79:618–623, 1949.

144. Wells, P. O.: The button sequestrum of eosinophilic granuloma of the skull. Radiology, 67:746–747, 1956.

145. West, W. O.: Velban as treatment for diffuse eosinophilic granuloma of bone. Report of a case. J. Bone Joint Surg. [Am.], 55:1755–1759, 1973.

146. Yabsley, R. H., and Harris, W. R.: Solitary eosinophilic granuloma of a vertebral body causing paraplegia. Report of a case. J. Bone Joint Surg. [Am.], 48:1570–1574, 1966.

147. Zinkham, W. H.: Multifocal eosinophilic granuloma. Natural history, etiology and management. Am. J. Med., 60:457–463, 1976.

INDEX

Page numbers in *italics* indicate illustrations.
Page numbers followed by (t) indicate tables.

A

Abscess, Brodie's. See *Brodie's abscess.*
  of bone, similarity to osteoid osteoma, 23
Absorption of bone, spontaneous, 356
Aclasis, diaphysial. See *Osteochondroma, multiple.*
Adamantinoma, 432
  and ossifying fibroma, 10
Adrenogenital syndrome, giant cell tumor associated
  with, 268
Alkaline phosphatase, in osteogenic sarcoma, 53–55,
  54, 109
  in Paget's disease, 120
  normal values of, 53, 53(t)
Ameloblastoma. See also *Adamantinoma.*
  similarity to myxoma of facial bones, 199
Amputation, Berger, for chondrosarcoma, 225
  for chondromyxoid fibroma, 198
  for fibrosarcoma, 260
  for malignant angioblastoma, 444
  for malignant fibrous histiocytoma, 318
  for malignant hemangioendothelioma, 367
  for non-Hodgkin's lymphoma of bone, 398
  for osteogenic sarcoma, 74–76
Amyloidosis, with multiple myeloma, 422
Anaplasia. See *Dedifferentiation.*
Anemia, in multiple myeloma, 414
Aneurysmal bone cyst, differential diagnosis of, 274(t)
  radiographic characteristics of, 37(t)
  recurrence rate of chondroblastoma associated
    with, 185, *186*
  secondary to chondroblastoma, *180,* 181
  secondary to giant cell tumor, 273
  secondary to osteoblastoma of sacrum, 38
  similarity to osteogenic sarcoma, 72
  vs. malignant hemangioendothelioma, 367
Angioblastic sarcoma, 358
Angioblastoma, malignant, 432–446
  age and sex distribution of, 434

Angioblastoma (*Continued*)
  malignant, bones involved in, 432, 434
    definition of, 432
    gross appearance of, *436,* 437, *438*
    histogenesis of, 436, 437
    metastasis of, 444
    microscopic appearance of, 437, 442, *438–442*
    mistaken for chondromyxoid fibroma, *434*
    prognosis of, 442, *443,* 444
    radiographic appearance of, 434, 436, *433–436*
    signs and symptoms of, 432
    synonyms for, 432
    treatment of, 442, *443,* 444
    vs. metastatic carcinoma, 436
Angioendothelioma, 358, 359
Angiofibrosarcoma, 358
Angioglomoid tumor, 352
Angiography, diagnostic, for chondrosarcoma of
    craniofacial bones, 239
    for chordoma, 377
    for Ewing's sarcoma, 328, 329
    for hemangioma of bone, 351
    for juxtacortical osteogenic sarcoma, 103
    for malignant fibrous histiocytoma, 312
    for malignant hemangioendothelioma, 361
    for myeloma of calvarium, 418
    for osteoblastoma, 37, *38*
    for osteogenic sarcoma, 73
    for osteoid osteoma, 23
Angioma, malignant, 358, 359
Angiosarcoma of bone, 358–368. See also
  Hemangioendothelioma, malignant.
Annular sequestrum, in osteoid osteoma, 23
  of tissue, from osteoblastoma, 35
Arthritis, chronic, post-irradiation sarcoma in, 129
  degenerative, hypertrophic, as symptom of osteoid
    osteoma, 20
Arthrodesis, for giant cell tumor, 285
Atrophy, of bone, progressive, 356

463